Pediatric
Clinical Skills

Pediatric Clinical Skills

THIRD EDITION

Richard B. Goldbloom, OC, MD, FRCPC

Chancellor and Professor of Pediatrics,
Dalhousie University,
IWK Health Centre
Halifax, Nova Scotia, Canada

SAUNDERS

An Imprint of Elsevier

SAUNDERS
An Imprint of Elsevier

The Curtis Center
Independence Square West
Philadelphia, PA 19106

PEDIATRIC CLINICAL SKILLS, Third Edition

Notice

Pediatrics is an ever-changing field. Standard safety precautions must be followed, but as new
research and clinical experience broaden our knowledge, changes in treatment and drug therapy
may become necessary or appropriate. Readers are advised to check the most current product
information provided by the manufacturer of each drug to be administered to verify the
recommended dose, the method and duration of administration, and contraindications. It is the
responsibility of the treating physician, relying on experience and knowledge of the patient, to
determine dosages and the best treatment for each individual patient. Neither the Publisher nor the
editor assume any liability for any injury and/or damage to persons or property arising from this
publication.

The Publisher

Library of Congress Cataloging-in-Publication Data

Pediatric clinical skills / [edited by] Richard B. Goldbloom.—3rd ed.
    p. ; cm.
    Includes bibliographical references and index.
    ISBN-13: 978-0-7216-9475-7   ISBN-10: 0-7216-9475-6
    1. Children—Medical examinations. 2. Children—Diseases—Diagnosis. 3. Medical
history taking. 4. Physical diagnosis. 5. Pediatrics. I. Goldbloom, Richard B.
    [DNLM: 1. Pediatrics. WS 200 P37045 2003]
RJ50.P4 2003
618.92'0075—dc21   2002017676

Acquisitions Editor: Judith Fletcher
Project Manager: Jodi Kaye

ISBN-13: 978-0-7216-9475-7
ISBN-10: 0-7216-9475-6

EH/MVY

Printed in the United States of America

Last digit is the print number: 9 8 7 6

To the world's seven best grandchildren—
Michael, Ellen, Katie, Amy, Stephen, Daniel, and William
—with love.

Foreword

The popularity of *Pediatric Clinical Skills* is underlined by the fact that this represents the third edition of the book within a decade. Richard Goldbloom and his collaborators have again provided us with a delightful, effective addition to the teaching of pediatrics. The book is written clearly, in a style that is informal, personalized, and often humorous. Most important of all, every page yields abundant practical, useful information. Dr. Goldbloom's gentle, but critical, hand is detectable throughout the text.

The third edition includes three new chapters that address issues of increasing importance to clinicians. The chapter on cross-cultural pediatric care by Richard Goldbloom is particularly welcome, since today each of us is called on regularly to do our best for children and families from increasingly diverse cultural, ethnic, and linguistic backgrounds. Knowledge of, and sensitivity to, such differences are vitally important clinical skills. Another new chapter by Richard Goldbloom addresses the special competences required for effective care of children with chronic conditions and for providing effective support for their families. Finally, Paul Dyment has contributed a new chapter on the skills required for physical evaluation of children prior to athletic participation. He offers valuable, practical guidance on performing such assessments quickly and effectively.

As with its predecessors, the third edition of *Pediatric Clinical Skills* will be valuable to every one of us ... from medical students at the very beginning of their pediatric clinical experience to the most senior of pediatricians. Students will find a wealth of practical guidance in conducting family interviews that are both informative and empathetic. They will learn how to elicit every possible clue to understanding the child, the family, and their environment. They will also acquire the knowledge and skills required for carrying out a thorough and informative physical examination. Even the most experienced pediatricians will find in these pages the means to enhance their clinical skills. One of the great benefits of such skills is the ability to avoid costly, anxiety-producing, and unnecessary investigations in many cases.

Had this book been available when I began my career in pediatrics, my knowledge and skills would have received an immeasurable boost. Standard, comprehensive textbooks of pediatrics cannot devote the space required for the kind of attention and care this book devotes to issues such as family interviewing and history-taking, or to its wealth of information about astutely observing and examining infants, children, and adolescents.

I recommend this book unequivocally, and I wish the Editor and his collaborators continued success and many future editions.

Sydney S. Gellis
Professor and Chairman Emeritus,
Department of Pediatrics,
Tufts University School of Medicine
Boston, Massachusetts

Preface to the Third Edition

The first edition of *Pediatric Clinical Skills* was published in 1992, the second in 1997. All of us who participated in the authorship of the first two editions have been deeply gratified by the book's popularity with undergraduate and postgraduate students of pediatrics, and even with some of the "old dogs" who have acquired a few "new tricks" from these pages.

Each of our contributors sets great value on the amount of diagnostic gold that can be mined through the application of well-trained listening skills, acute powers of observation, and sensitive antennae for non-verbal cues. Notwithstanding all the technological and scientific marvels of the age, the family interview remains unchallenged as our most sophisticated and productive diagnostic instrument, and often our most powerful form of therapy as well. We are keenly aware that in the diagnosis and treatment of illness, understanding how the child and family feel is often as important as diagnosing and treating disease. The talents required are learned rather than innate, and none of us is too old to perfect them. They are the hallmarks of the skilled clinician, and we hope this book helps its readers further along the path to such expense.

Today, clinical rounds are too often conducted in hospital corridors with more time devoted to flipping through charts and reviewing laboratory results than to visiting the patient and family, which we believe should be our first priority. The old facetious statement "If the x-ray warrants it, we'll do a physical examination" sometimes seems closer to truth than to satire.

Since most clinical skills have changed little, if at all, since the previous edition appeared, readers may wonder why we decided to produce a new edition rather than simply reprinting the previous one. Updating our contributors' hairstyles in the illustrations hardly seemed sufficient to justify the effort and expenses. The fact is that, on reflection, we recognized several important omissions in the early editions. For example, we realized that because the ethnocultural kaleidoscope of most communities has been expanding steadily, clinicians must acquire new knowledge and special sensitivity to provide effective cross-cultural care. We all carry an obligation to ensure that the families of every cultural, ethnic, and linguistic tradition have equal access to quality care and are treated with equal respect and understanding. We have therefore added a new chapter dealing with this issue.

A second deficiency of the earlier editions was the absence of guidance concerning the special skills required for evaluating children and adolescents prior to participation in sports. Paul Dyment, an acknowledged expert in the field, has provided an excellent new chapter on this topic.

Finally, research advances in diagnosis and treatment have changed the spectrum of pediatrics, such that many children now require skilled long-term care for a variety of chronic, disabling conditions. Compared with acutely ill children and those requiring preventive health care, these children, adolescents, and their families need caregivers who are team players and possess the special clinical skills required from the moment the child's diagnosis is first disclosed to the parents. In exploring this issue in a new chapter, I felt it would be useful to draw directly on the comments of three families who have had years of first hand experience with a large number of caregivers. They have been remarkably frank. Their comments are the most effective type of illustration, and I have quoted them with their generous permission.

All chapters have been revised to varying degrees, and several new and improved illustrations have been added. We hope readers agree that these changes have significantly enhanced the scope and value of the book.

Richard B. Goldbloom, OC, MD, FRCPC

Acknowledgments

Thanks to the outstanding expertise and collaboration of three individuals, compiling the third edition of this book was an especially easy task and a thoroughly pleasant experience: working with Judith Fletcher, Executive Editor at Saunders was, as always, a pleasure. Jodi Kaye provided meticulous and efficient overall management of the project, and Bernice MacLellan, my good friend and assistant for the past 14 years, dealt with masses of manuscript, illegible editorial scribblings, and recalcitrant contributors with extraordinary equanimity and good grace. Finally, a special word of gratitude to the three families who, by sharing their personal experiences and lessons learned, made invaluable contributions to our new chapter on "Caring for Children with Chronic Conditions and Their Families." These wise and sensitive coauthors include Carol and John Young, Jane, Donna, and Ian Thompson, and Andrea and Anne Crowe.

Contributors

Philip C. Bagnell, MD
Professor, Department of Pediatrics. Executive Associate Dean for Academic and Faculty Affairs, James H. Quillan College of Medicine, East Tennessee State University, Johnson City, Tennessee
Clinical Evaluation of Gastrointestinal Symptoms in Children

Elizabeth A. Cummings, MD
Assistant Professor, Dalhousie University, Halifax, Nova Scotia, Canada
Clinical Endocrine Evaluation of the Child

Joseph M. Dooley, MB, BCh, FRCPC
Professor of Pediatrics, Dalhousie University, Head, Division of Pediatric Neurology, IWK Health Centre, Halifax, Nova Scotia, Canada
Pediatric Neurologic Examination

Paul G. Dyment, MD
Former Professor of Pediatrics and Vice Chancellor for Academic Affairs, Tulane University, New Orleans, Louisiana; Clinical Professor of Pediatrics, University of Vermont, Portland, Maine
The Sports Preparticipation Physical Examination

Laura A. Finlayson, MD, FRCPC
Assistant Professor, Dalhousie University, Chief of Dermatology, IWK Health Centre, Halifax, Nova Scotia, Canada
Clinical Assessment of the Skin in Children

Jan E. Fleming, MD, FRCPC
Psychiatric Assessment of Children and Adolescents

D. A. Gillis, CM, MD, FRCSC
Professor and Former Head, Department of Surgery, Dalhousie University, Former Chief of Surgery, IWK Health Centre, Halifax, Nova Scotia, Canada; Former Chief Medical Officer, National Guard Health Affairs, Riyadh, Saudi Arabia; Currently Vice President, Professional and Academic Affairs, IWK Health Centre, Halifax, Nova Scotia, Canada
Surgical Assessment of the Child's Abdomen

Alan L. Goldbloom, MD, FRCPC
Associate Professor, Department of Paediatrics, University of Toronto; Executive Vice President and Chief Operating Officer, The Hospital for Sick Children, Toronto, Ontario, Canada
Examination of the Head and Neck

Richard B. Goldbloom, OC, MD, FRCPC
Chancellor and Professor of Pediatrics, Dalhousie University, IWK Health Centre, Halifax, Nova Scotia, Canada
Family Interviewing and History-Taking; Skills for Culturally Sensitive Pediatric Care; Assessment of Physical Growth and Nutrition; Caring for Children with Chronic Conditions and Their Families

Alexandra A. Howlett, MD
Assistant Professor of Pediatrics and Obstetrics and Gynecology, Dalhousie University; Neonatologist, IWK Health Centre, Halifax, Nova Scotia, Canada
Evaluating the Newborn Infant: Diagnostic Approach

Daniel M. Hughes, MD, FRCPC
Assistant Professor of Pediatrics, Division of Respirology, Dalhousie University, Pediatric Respirologist, IWK Health Centre, Halifax, Nova Scotia, Canada
Evaluating the Child's Respiratory System

Ellen Jamieson, MEd
Research Associate, Department of Psychiatry and Behavioural Neurosciences, Canadian Centre for Studies of Children at Risk, McMaster University, Hamilton, Ontario, Canada
Psychiatric Assessment of Children and Adolescents

Krista A. Jangaard, MD, FRCPC
Assistant Professor of Pediatrics and Obstetrics and Gynecology, Dalhousie University; Neonatologist, IWK Health Centre, Halifax, Nova Scotia, Canada
Evaluating the Newborn Infant: Diagnostic Approach

Nuala P. Kenny, OC, MD, FRCPC
Professor and Chair, Department of Bioethics, Dalhousie University, Halifax, Nova Scotia, Canada
Skills for Assessing the Appropriate Role for Children in Health Decisions

Bianca A. Lang, MD, FRCPC
*Associate Professor of Pediatrics, Dalhousie University;
Active Staff and Head, Division of Rheumatology, IWK
Health Centre, Halifax, Nova Scotia, Canada*
Pediatric Musculoskeletal Examination

G. Robert LaRoche, MD, FRCSC
*Associate Professor, Ophthalmology, Dalhousie
University, Head, Ophthalmology, IWK Health Centre,
Halifax, Nova Scotia, Canada*
Examining the Visual System in Children

Mark D. Ludman, MD, FRCPC
*Adjunct Professor of Pediatrics, Dalhousie University,
Halifax, Nova Scotia, Canada; Medical Geneticist,
Department of Medical Genetics, Rabin Medical Center,
Beilinson Campus, Petach Tikva, Israel*
Assessing the Child with Congenital Anomalies

Harriet L. MacMillan, MD, MBCh, FRCPC
*Associate Professor, Departments of Psychiatry and
Behavioural Neurosciences and Pediatrics, Canadian
Centre for Studies of Children at Risk, McMaster
University; Director, Child Advocacy and Assessment
Program, McMaster Children's Hospital, Hamilton
Health Sciences, Hamilton, Ontario, Canada*
Psychiatric Assessment of Children and Adolescents

Elihu P. Rees, BSc, MDCM, FRCPC
*Associate Professor, Pediatrics (Retired), Dalhousie
University, Medical Staff (Life), IWK Hospital for
Children, Halifax, Nova Scotia, Canada*
Evaluating the Newborn Infant: Diagnostic Approach

Douglas L. Roy, MDCM, FRCPC
*Professor of Pediatrics (Retired), Former Head,
Division of Pediatric Cardiology, Dalhousie University,
School of Medicine; Former Head, Division of Pediatric
Cardiology, IWK Health Centre, Halifax, Nova Scotia,
Canada.*
Cardiovascular Assessment of Infants and Children

Sonia R. Salisbury, MD
*Professor of Pediatrics, Dalhousie University, Halifax,
Nova Scotia, Canada*
Clinical Endocrine Evaluation of the Child

Sarah Shea, AB, MD, FRCPC
*Associate Professor, Department of Pediatrics,
Dalhousie University, Director, Child Development
Clinic, Izaak Walton Killam Health Centre, Halifax,
Nova Scotia, Canada*
Developmental Assessment

Linda E. Skinner, BA, BEd
*Part-time Faculty, Child and Youth Studies, Mount
Saint Vincent University; Chief, Child Life and School
Services, IWK Health Centre, Halifax, Nova Scotia,
Canada*
Skills for Assessing the Appropriate Role for Children
in Health Decisions

Joan B. Wenning, BSc, MD, FRCSC
*Associate Professor, Department of Obstetrics and
Gynecology, Dalhousie University; Active Staff,
Department of Obstetrics and Gynecology, IWK Health
Centre, Halifax, Nova Scotia, Canada*
Pediatric Gynecologic Assessment

Contents

1 FAMILY INTERVIEWING AND HISTORY-TAKING 1
Richard B. Goldbloom

2 SKILLS FOR CULTURALLY SENSITIVE PEDIATRIC CARE 19
Richard B. Goldbloom

3 ASSESSMENT OF PHYSICAL GROWTH AND NUTRITION 27
Richard B. Goldbloom

4 EVALUATING THE NEWBORN INFANT: DIAGNOSTIC APPROACH 55
Alexandra A. Howlett
Krista A. Jangaard
Elihu P. Rees

5 ASSESSING THE CHILD WITH CONGENITAL ANOMALIES 75
Mark D. Ludman

6 DEVELOPMENTAL ASSESSMENT 91
Sarah Shea

7 EXAMINATION OF THE HEAD AND NECK 111
Alan L. Goldbloom

8 EXAMINING THE VISUAL SYSTEM IN CHILDREN 127
G. Robert LaRoche

9 EVALUATING THE CHILD'S RESPIRATORY SYSTEM 151
Daniel M. Hughes

10 CARDIOVASCULAR ASSESSMENT OF INFANTS AND CHILDREN 169
Douglas L. Roy

11 CLINICAL EVALUATION OF GASTROINTESTINAL SYMPTOMS IN CHILDREN 191
Philip C. Bagnell

12 SURGICAL ASSESSMENT OF THE CHILD'S ABDOMEN 207
D. A. Gillis

13 PEDIATRIC NEUROLOGIC EXAMINATION 223
Joseph M. Dooley

14 PSYCHIATRIC ASSESSMENT OF CHILDREN AND ADOLESCENTS 249
Harriet L. MacMillan
Jan E. Fleming
Ellen Jamieson

15 PEDIATRIC MUSCULOSKELETAL EXAMINATION 261
Bianca A. Lang

16 CLINICAL ENDOCRINE EVALUATION OF THE CHILD 287
Sonia R. Salisbury
Elizabeth A. Cummings

17 THE SPORTS PREPARTICIPATION PHYSICAL EXAMINATION 311
Paul G. Dyment

18 PEDIATRIC GYNECOLOGIC ASSESSMENT 317
Joan B. Wenning

19 CLINICAL ASSESSMENT OF THE SKIN IN CHILDREN 331
Laura A. Finlayson

20 CARING FOR CHILDREN WITH CHRONIC CONDITIONS AND THEIR FAMILIES 343
Richard B. Goldbloom

21 SKILLS FOR ASSESSING THE APPROPRIATE ROLE FOR CHILDREN IN HEALTH DECISIONS 349
Nuala P. Kenny
Linda E. Skinner

chapter 1

Family Interviewing and History-Taking

RICHARD B. GOLDBLOOM

Most textbooks deal with the history-taking interview as a diagnostic procedure—a systematic data-gathering process designed to identify problems and to arrive at a diagnostic formulation, leading ultimately to a treatment plan. To achieve its maximum value, however, the family interview should be as therapeutic as it is diagnostic. Treatment begins as the family walks in the door.

Whenever I have asked parents to tell me what qualities in a physician are most important to them, their answers have been remarkably consistent. You might imagine that their first priority would be professional competence, but this is rarely, if ever, mentioned. Their first concern is usually "a doctor who gives us enough time." Some physicians are able to leave families satisfied that they have given them enough time even in a relatively short visit. Others, despite taking more time, may leave families dissatisfied by permitting frequent interruptions or distractions, by interrupting the parents, or simply by not being attentive listeners. Such transgressions can markedly impair family satisfaction.

A familiar sight around hospitals is the presence of a physician standing and conversing with patients or family members, the latter often visibly anxious. If it were possible to legislate changes in body language, the first law to be passed should be that everyone involved in such conversations be required to sit down. Being seated does not need to prolong conversations. But the mere act of sitting down, even for a few moments, conveys a powerful message to the patient or family. It says unmistakably, "I *have time* to listen to you and to talk to you."

The second priority mentioned by most parents is to have a physician who explains things to them in language that they understand. Communication skills— good listening and clear talking; mostly the listening— count for more than anything else with parents. In your conversations with parents, use lay terms whenever possible, avoiding jargon and unintelligible alphabetical abbreviations, such as ECG, EEG, BUN, ICU, CT, and MRI. Also, try to avoid using words such as pulmonary, renal, cardiac, allergy, and a hundred others that may mean little or nothing to many parents and can strike terror into the hearts of some.

The lexicon of fear-inducing terms contains words such as *pneumonia, meningitis, epilepsy, asthma,* and *mental retardation,* each of which can have very different meanings for parents than they do for you. Use such words sparingly—and only after finding out exactly what they mean to the parents.

The qualities that most parents seek in their physicians tell us a lot about our job definition. The late Dr. Harry Gordon, a distinguished pediatrician, put it neatly: "The physician's mission is to relieve anxiety— and all our knowledge, research, diagnosis, and treatments are only means to that end." This concept underlines the importance of differentiating between disease (the pathologic condition) and illness or "dis-ease" (how the patient feels). Diagnosis and treatment of the two are not identical, and treatment of both is essential to successful management.

Key Point

It has been documented that, as students advance through undergraduate and postgraduate years, two unfortunate changes tend to develop in the content of their patient interviews: They tend to focus progressively more on disease and less on illness.

Finding out how the child and family feel and expressing your appreciation of those feelings can be highly therapeutic. Do not hesitate to season your comments with regular expressions of empathy and support (e.g., "This must have been a difficult time for you"; "You must be pretty worried about this problem"; and "I think you've done a great job with this youngster— and I know it hasn't been easy.") Such expressions also help lay the foundation for successful management plans in dealing with a child's problems.

Empathy alone is certainly no substitute for scientific knowledge, nor for first-class clinical skills of diagnosis and treatment. However, empathy also should not be regarded as some form of "warm and fuzzy" bedside manner that features a gentle touch and a velvet voice. Empathy is the expression of true insight into how patients and families feel and an appreciation of the difficulties they face.

INTERVIEWING AND HISTORY-TAKING SKILLS

Two clinical skills—interviewing and history-taking—deserve practice and polish more than others, because the more highly developed the interviewer's skills, the more benefit accrues to patients and their families. Like any good productive conversation, a successful medical interview incorporates the following basic actions:

1. Establish a warm, friendly atmosphere.
2. Maintain privacy and eliminate distractions.
3. Sustain eye contact.
4. Continue a steady logical flow of content and conversation to nudge the most and the best out of the interviewees.
5. Listen carefully.
6. Observe carefully.
7. Season your conversation with regular expressions of empathy and support.

Note-Taking

During family interviews and pediatric physical examinations, it is easy to become distracted by personal concerns—trying to remember questions that you should ask or fearing that you will forget some critical element of the physical examination. Such preoccupations make it difficult to give your undivided attention to the family's needs. Nothing destroys the flow of an interview more than frequent pauses to take notes. Two useful tips are (1) maintain eye contact with the person you are interviewing and (2) take as few written notes as possible, jotting down only important details. Following these tips will help you avoid writing pauses, recognize important nonverbal communications from and between parents and child, and contribute verbal and nonverbal feedback.

Different Styles of Questions

Become familiar with the appropriate use of different techniques for asking questions, which can help elicit a good history.

DIRECT VERSUS OPEN QUESTIONS

To determine whether there is a family history of migraine in a child who complains of headaches, you can ask the key question in several possible ways. The reliability of the answer may depend heavily on *how* the question is framed.

The Direct Question

The "Does anyone in your family have migraine?" question is based on the following assumptions:

1. Parents understand what the word *migraine* means, which they often do not.
2. If someone in the family does have migraine, it has been diagnosed correctly, which often is not so.
3. The opening words "Does anyone" will prompt the parents to perform a thorough mental review of all family members, which they frequently do not.

Many lay individuals do not have a clue what the word *migraine* really means. Many adults have headaches that have been diagnosed previously as "sinus headaches," "tension headaches," or "temporomandibular joint (TMJ)" syndrome. Review of the symptoms of such patients may reveal that they actually have characteristic migraine.

Key Point

Because parents often are reluctant to admit they do not understand the question, they may answer in the negative, thereby omitting important information.

An alternative would be a directive, almost confrontational type of question given in the form of an instruction. "Tell me who has headaches in your family" puts the question in a totally different form that is likely to elicit a more reliable and useful response. This question differs from the earlier one in that:

1. It uses words everyone understands.
2. It does not prediagnose anyone's headache or accept previous headache diagnoses.
3. The directive phrasing ("Tell me who ...") is more likely to induce a thorough mental review of individual family members.

The Open Permissive Question

Consider the depersonalized question, "I don't know about you, but many people who have a child with this problem ...." This approach is excellent for bringing up sensitive issues such as guilt, sex, and fear of serious illness. As a nonaccusatory introduction to a question, it is less likely to elicit anxiety and inhibit parents from discussing the subject. The mere acknowledgment that it is usual for other people in their situation to have similar feelings or fears often greatly helps parents or children to acknowledge similar concerns. Suppose, for example, that a child has been brought to you because of pallor and cervical adenopathy. Parents rarely verbalize an overwhelming fear that the youngster may have leukemia. That frightening idea may have arisen from knowing of another child who had similar symptoms and turned out to have leukemia, or the parents may simply have read about the disease or have seen a television program about it.

Parents of children who have "minor" signs or symptoms—that is, minor from the physician's perspective—frequently have secret fears about serious or potentially fatal disease. Such fears are often too upsetting to verbalize without some form of facilitation. Interviewers who fail to recognize the widespread existence of such fears and to alleviate them often overlook what is, in fact, the primary issue on the parents' agenda. One investigation of more than 800 doctor-patient pediatric clinical studies found that 24% of the parents had never revealed to the physician their single greatest concern! If ever there was a lesson in the importance of actively ferreting out hidden agendas, this was it.

An effective way to raise such covert issues is to say, "I don't know about you, but many parents whose child has these symptoms worry that it might turn out to be something really bad." Then, pause, look for nonverbal acknowledgment, and listen. Add "Like leukemia, for instance." Then ask, "Have you worried about that sort of thing, too?" Because this question format often identifies the parent's chief anxiety, it sets the stage for you to assure them that other parents worry about the same point and to alleviate their fears.

Parents acknowledge their concerns verbally or nonverbally, with an instant smile of relief or a nod of agreement. No matter how they admit their concerns, do not postpone resolving the issue. Use the interview as therapy. Whenever possible, state or prove unequivocally and without delay that the child does *not* have leukemia. Also, try to identify the real source of their particular fears—often an affected relative or friend whose diagnosis may have been missed at first assessment. Ask, "Who do you know who has had a child with leukemia?"

Key Point

If it is humanly possible, do not equivocate or qualify your reassurances when you are trying to ease parent's anxiety.

The Offhand, Screening Question

Some innocent-sounding questions, tossed casually into the conversation, can be incredibly valuable in screening for problems of parent-child interaction. Checking for maternal depression is one example. An offhand question such as "Are you having fun with the baby?" is useful, because the repertoire of potential responses is limited. The most positive, reassuring answer is an instantaneous, emphatic "Yes!" or "Sure!" delivered with a smile or chuckle and with an immediate positive nonverbal response. The latter response may include, affectionate interaction between parent and baby, such as eye contact, smiling, patting, or tickling. Any of these responses provides powerful prima facie evidence for a healthy parent-infant relationship.

However, the parent may hesitate and respond with a puzzled look or a grudging affirmative, suggesting that the interaction may be less than ideal. The time lapse between the end of the question and a parent's response can sometimes be a measure of the anxiety generated by the question.

Genuinely worrisome replies include the inability to respond, an unhappy downward gaze, a shaky voice, and tears—sure signs of difficulties that should lead to a quest for details. Resist any temptation to switch the conversation to another topic, as some interviewers do when they feel uncomfortable about having touched on a sensitive or painful area. Instead, immediately verbalize your recognition that there is a problem. Statements such as "You don't look very happy. Would you like to tell me about it?" may open the door for the parent to reveal the central concern, allowing you to begin dealing constructively with the distress.

Dressing for the Interview

How should you dress for clinical encounters with children and their families? Does it really matter? Do white coats frighten children? Support for every viewpoint on this long-standing debate is largely anecdotal, although several studies have shown that adults tend to associate more conservative, traditional dress with their expectation of competence. Given that ours is a serving profession with the mission of relieving anxiety, how we look, what we say, and what we do should always support that mission to the greatest extent possible. The whiteness of the coat has a long-standing cultural association with cleanliness and purity. By tradition, it may also serve to legitimize procedures, such as pelvic or rectal examinations, that would otherwise be considered socially taboo. We do not fool children by dressing in nontraditional attire or by donning coats of many colors. When families from cultures other than our own are concerned, nontraditional attire may even be disconcerting. The most important question is not whether you opt for the white coat but whether you have considered all sides of the issue and made your final decision in the best interests of the majority of your patients and their families.

Establishing the Tone

Establishing the most favorable atmosphere for a family interview can be helped in several ways that may seem trivial at first. For example, some busy physicians in private offices or clinics simply ask an assistant to "send in the next patient"—an impersonal approach that can begin the encounter on a note of intimidation. It takes only seconds to go to the waiting area, greet the child and family by name, and escort them back to the office. This simple gesture can set the right tone of concern and respect. It also provides a great opportunity to observe how the child and parents interrelate and to observe the child's gait if he or she is at walking age. I always take advantage of this moment to compliment youngsters on any handy subject—an article of clothing, a haircut, or a favorite toy. I also offer my hand to a younger child for the walk back to the office. These little gestures go a long way toward starting the clinical encounter on friendly terms and keeping it that way.

In many cultures, it is considered thoroughly rude to "get down to business" right away, whether the business is commerce or health care. Common courtesy demands pleasant preliminary banter about the weather, the crops, or the family. We can learn a lot from such traditions, which help put people at their ease.

Key Point

In health care interviews, the introductory conversation helps establish the caregiver as friendly, unhurried, and supportive, qualities of major importance to all patients and families.

Shake hands with the parents and greet each family member by name. Be sensitive about the best way to address parents. Some physicians call just about everyone by the first name, a habit that sounds a bit phony and that some parents simply do not like. It is also rather impersonal to address parents simply as "Mom" or "Dad." Initially, it is always better to err on the side of formality and call parents "Mr. and Mrs. Jones," unless and until they specifically request you to do otherwise. Do not patronize parents or use meaningless terms of endearment.

If you are a student or a resident, give parents both your first and last names and explain your status and role. Do not allude to yourself simply by your first name, and always wear a legible name tag. In their anxiety, it is easy for parents to forget a name, especially if they have to deal with several health care personnel in the same office.

Key Point

During discussions with parents or in written communications, refer to the child by name whenever possible, rather than using the impersonal "he" or "she." This communicates your appreciation of the child's individuality and focuses your concern.

In hospital conversations, case presentations, or written communications, do not refer to a child impersonally as "a 3-year-old white female." A phrase such as "Mary Ann is a healthy-looking, 3-year-old, red-headed girl" conveys a totally different feeling about a child and is a mark of your respect for the youngster's individuality.

THE SETTING

Whenever possible, conduct the interview in a physical setting that offers comfort, privacy, and a minimum of interruption. Try to avoid interposing physical barriers, such as a desk, between yourself and the parents. Although these details of the process may seem trivial, each contributes in its own way to the ultimate diagnostic and therapeutic value of the interview.

RESPECT FOR OTHER PEOPLE'S TIME

In the hospital setting, after exchanging initial greetings with the parents, always ask whether they are under particular time constraints that may limit their ability to give a relaxed, nondistracted interview. Ask questions such as the following:

- "Have you missed a meal?"
- "Do you have other children who are expected home from school soon or who have to be met?"
- "Do you have household (or farm) chores to do?"
- "Are you late for work?"

Key Point

Always demonstrate by word and deed that the patient's time is every bit as valuable as yours.

Individual physicians or outpatient clinics that assign the same appointment time to more than one patient send a loud, clear message that they consider the patient's time less valuable than theirs.

Occupying the Child

Always have age-appropriate play materials on hand to entertain and relax the child and any siblings who are along for the visit. Toys, puzzles, and coloring books provide more than mere diversion. Watching children use play materials gives you valuable insight into their development. Also, gaining the child's interest, confidence, and friendship early in the encounter can make all the difference between an easy physical examination and a difficult one.

The Problem Seen from Different Perspectives

In the classic Japanese film *Rashomon*, three witnesses to a murder give strikingly different individual accounts of the same dramatic event. Similarly, each of us may interpret the same situation in highly subjective ways. It is important to learn how each parent interprets a child's problem. Having both parents present for the initial interview has many valuable payoffs. For one thing, it furnishes immediate insight into how the family works and an understanding about family dynamics that can help in your work with the individual members. Observe whether one parent is domineering or is a supportive leader of the family group. How does each parent relate to the child? How do they relate to each other?

In certain circumstances, it is essential to have both parents on hand. These situations include examination of the child with behavioral or learning problems, developmental delays, or serious or chronic illness. Successful management often depends on negotiating an agreement with both parents that calls for them to share the day-to-day responsibilities for treatment (see the later discussion of the therapeutic contract).

The Parent's Opening Statement

A good interviewer usually begins by asking the parents to describe their main concern and their expectations of the visit. "Tell me why you've come to see me and how you think I may be able to help" is a useful opener. The most important sequel to this invitation is letting the parent or patient *complete* their opening statement without interrupting them.

When patients' opening statements have been analyzed, they have been rarely found to exceed 1.5 minutes. However, it has also been found that the majority of patients are never allowed to complete that statement, because doctors often interrupt with distracting questions from their own agenda. Here is an example:

Patient: "Two weeks ago, Jack started to cough, and—"
Doctor: "Was it a wet cough or a dry cough?"

Establishing the Ground Rules

After exchanging the opening pleasantries, making everyone comfortable, and listening *without interruption* to the parents' or patient's opening statement, you should describe the ground rules of the interview and its objectives. Explain that some questions may seem to have nothing to do with the child's presenting problem but are nevertheless essential to a comprehensive medical evaluation. If the child is old enough to answer questions, involve him or her in the interview. Finally, always urge parents to interrupt you if there is something they do not understand or if they have any questions or important issues they wish to raise.

Uncovering Hidden Agendas

> **Key Point**
>
> The child's presenting complaint may or may not be the biggest problem, and sometimes the child is not the real patient.

For some families, the child serves as the "key in the door" in their search for help. Certain hidden agendas recur with remarkable frequency in pediatric clinical encounters. If you unearth such family secrets, you can offer enormous help and relief. If you miss these issues, you may fail to relieve the family's anxiety, although you may have diagnosed and treated the presenting complaint or disease appropriately.

The presenting complaint may be excessive crying, abdominal pain, sleep disturbances, poor school performance, or headaches—all common pediatric problems. Yet a sensitive interview may disclose that the family's biggest problem is a depressed mother, a father who drinks excessively or is having an extramarital relationship, or serious financial difficulties. If the child's symptoms are to be relieved, the physician must recognize and, when possible, remedy the root problem.

PARENTAL GUILT FEELINGS

Most parents who bring a child to medical attention experience some degree of self-blame for their youngster's difficulties, perceiving themselves as guilty of perceived sins of omission or commission. Their child's clinical problem may be as "routine" as an earache, but a parent speculates silently, "If I hadn't let him out without his sweater," or "If only I had brought her to the doctor last week instead of waiting until now, maybe she wouldn't be so sick." Recognizing how frequently self-blame occurs should help you uncover the issue during the initial interview and deal with it on the spot—another example of the interview as therapy. Reassurance that self-blame is universal and normal, that hindsight alone confers 20/20 vision, and that the child's current condition could not have been predicted truly relieves most parents. To reveal this issue, use a variation on the depersonalized question, such as "I don't know about you, but many parents I see wonder whether this problem was caused by something they had done or not done." A pause is then appropriate. If there is no response, ask, "Have you worried about that sort of thing?"

Key Point

Generally, the more serious a child's problem, the more likely parents are to indulge in feelings of self-blame.

Guilt feelings are often so deeply felt and so disturbing that parents cannot bring themselves to verbalize them spontaneously, although the associated tension may be sensed by all concerned. This is an example of a typical "secret in the family": feelings or situations, real or imagined, that family members know about but that no one dares mention, as if there were an unspoken pact of silence.

Feelings of self-blame for causing an illness often occur in families of children with developmental delays, multiple congenital anomalies, or serious chronic disease. It is vital to ask the right questions to elicit the parents' individual perceptions of what caused the problem, with a question such as "What are your thoughts about what might have caused her problem?"

Some time ago, I interviewed the father of a teenaged girl with a severe developmental delay. She had been seen by several physicians and had undergone various psychological assessments over the years, but the father was clearly still searching for something. During our conversation, I said, "I don't know about you, but most parents of children with this condition have their own ideas about what may have caused it. What are your thoughts about what might have caused her problem?"

He immediately exclaimed, "I know what caused this, Dr. Goldbloom!" He then described walking beside a swimming pool with his daughter when she was 2 years old. He let go of her hand, and she fell into the pool. Although she was immersed for less than 30 seconds and had never lost consciousness, he was convinced that he was personally responsible for her condition. For all those subsequent years, he had remained silent, but he had always blamed himself for her mis-

fortune. If no one had asked him that fundamental question, the issue would have remained unresolved for him, perhaps permanently. Because his daughter's antecedent history made it clear that her development had never been normal, I was able to persuade the father he was not culpable.

Sometimes one parent blames the other, either openly or secretly. If the marriage is unstable, this can be a serious problem calling for expert help.

UNARTICULATED FEARS OF DEATH

Many parents harbor unexpressed fears that their child may die, another common "secret in the family." Becoming aware of how frequently parents fear serious illness and possible death in their children helps you ask the key questions that allow them to acknowledge the fear and enable you to defuse the concern quickly and unequivocally.

Key Point

One of the most common clinical situations eliciting a fear of death occurs when a child has a generalized convulsion, usually a "benign" febrile seizure.

Although it is well documented that most parents who witness their child having a first febrile seizure believe that their child is actually dying or has already died,[1] general pediatrics and pediatric neurology textbooks often fail to mention this issue, a clear example of how medical teaching focuses on disease (the physician's problem) rather than illness (the patient's problem). Parents rarely express such fears spontaneously, presumably because the mere thought is simply too frightening to verbalize. Even if the child never has another seizure, unless the issue has been confronted openly, parents may live in fear of a repetition of the seizure and of death resulting from it.

Many physicians are reluctant to raise the issue of death if the parents have not done so, either because the topic makes them uncomfortable as well or because they believe they will upset the parents by the mere mention of such an issue. Unless you help parents admit this fear and then deal with it unequivocally, any advice and reassurance you offer on other seizure-related issues will do little to relieve their anxiety. Your words may not even be heard because the parents are so preoccupied by the awful fear that they cannot bring themselves to verbalize.

As for other "hidden" issues, you should ask a depersonalized question, such as "I don't know about you, but many parents who have seen their baby have a convulsion tell me they were afraid the child was dying. Were you afraid of that?" If the parents acknowledge the fear, either verbally or nonverbally, make the following points immediately:

1. Most parents feel the same way.
2. There is absolutely no risk of death in febrile convulsions, although the child may look awful—blue, unconscious, not breathing—for a few moments.
3. About 5% of "normal" children younger than 5 years have convulsions with fever at some time.
4. The child may have another such convulsion and may look just as bad, but the child will not die.

OBTAINING THE INITIAL HISTORY

Format

It is traditional and appropriate to begin a written history by identifying the informant and indicating whether he or she appears to be reliable. When the document is to become part of a child's hospital record, remember that you are writing it for the information and guidance of future readers. Keep it legible, and maintain a logical sequence of information.

LISTING THE CHIEF COMPLAINTS

List the chief complaints in temporal sequence, noting the duration of each. Wherever possible, quote the parents verbatim rather than translating their statements into medical jargon. If they say their child has trouble breathing, do not write "dyspnea" as the complaint.

HISTORY OF THE PRESENT ILLNESS

A precise sequential description of the evolution of a child's illness is the most valuable diagnostic aid, usually even more helpful than the physical examination, which, like imaging procedures and laboratory tests, usually confirms suspicions raised by the history.

Dating the onset of complaints is important. "When was he or she last perfectly well?" Quote liberally from the informants, putting their statements in quotation marks. The evolution of the child's problems should then flow in a clear, concise temporal sequence, leading up to the present moment. Always seek a history of similar problems in contacts or relatives.

PRIOR HISTORY

Prenatal History

Document the mother's age, previous pregnancies, miscarriages, and abortions. Indicate whether this pregnancy was planned or unplanned; if the pregnancy was unplanned, ask the parents how they felt upon learning of it. Record the pregnancy duration—term, preterm (by how many weeks), or post-term. Note the mother's (and father's) smoking, drinking, and drug exposure history and details about the mother's health during pregnancy (hyperemesis, bleeding, illnesses, or accidents).

Birth

Was the onset of labor spontaneous or induced? If induced, why? Note the duration of labor and whether any unusual problems occurred during its course. Record the birth weight. Finally, note whether the baby breathed and cried spontaneously or required resuscitation, oxygen, or other special care. Today, parents often know the baby's Apgar scores.

Neonatal Period

List any health problems during the newborn period—jaundice, breathing problems, feeding problems, seizures, or other difficulties. Ask whether the baby went home with the mother or was kept in hospital for any reason.

The "Vulnerable Child" Syndrome. When you talk to parents about the history of the pregnancy and neonatal period, remember that in some families, health problems during those periods may induce parental anxiety that can persist through the child's infancy and childhood even though the original condition is long past. For example, an infant may have had transient respiratory difficulty or jaundice in the newborn period followed by complete recovery. Despite the completeness of that recovery, some parents may continue to show what appears to be excessive anxiety when the youngster experiences minor illnesses, because the earlier experience has led them to perceive their child as vulnerable (hence the "vulnerable child" syndrome). We should therefore be careful not to label parents as "overanxious"—a pejorative label that can affect the doctor-family relationship adversely. When parents seem "overanxious" there is usually a valid reason. Uncovering the origin of the anxiety can benefit all concerned.

Feeding History

The amount of detail required is highly problem- and age-dependent. For an infant, first establish the feeding method—breast or formula. For a breast-fed infant, record the duration and any associated problems. For formula-fed, younger infants, note the type of formula, its dilution, any formula changes that have been made, the feeding frequency, and the amount taken at each feeding.

For older infants, record the age at introduction of solid foods, the current diet composition, and any problems, such as difficulty feeding, regurgitation, or vomiting. Note whether vitamin and fluoride supplements are taken; if so, record the dose.

Bowel Movements. Many parents volunteer vivid descriptions of their infant's bowel movements. Unless an infant has significant constipation or true diarrhea, neither parents nor the physician should fall victim to the syndrome of "fecal fascination." This caution is especially important for a breast-fed infant. Breast-fed infants may produce many stools over a 24-hour period with a wide spectrum of color and consistency. They may also go for days (a week or more) without producing any stools whatsoever—all these phenomena representing variations of normal. Generally speaking, the less inspection and discussion of stools, the better for all concerned.

Growth and Development

The baby's birth weight has already been registered, but it can be helpful, depending on the nature of the problem, to chart any subsequently recorded weights or heights.

Tailor the developmental history to the child's age. It is pointless to ask the parent of a 10-year-old girl how old she was when she first smiled. Unless there is an obvious developmental delay, begin by asking for her current school grade to determine whether it is age-appropriate; then ask whether she has repeated any grades and whether she receives resource help or tutoring. Find out her best and worst school subjects, because this information may help identify learning problems. If the patient is experiencing academic difficulties, find out whether she has been tested by a school (or other) psychologist.

Remember that as children grow older, the normal age range for attainment of specific developmental milestones usually widens. For example, a normal infant begins to smile in response to stimulation between 5 and 7 weeks of age. Compare this narrow 2-week range of normality with the fact that a normal child may begin to sit unsupported at any time between 5 and 8 months of age.

Immunizations

Key Point

Avoid vague statements such as "immunizations are up to date." Instead, become familiar with the normal immunization schedule, and keep the child's record as specific and accurate as possible.

Many parents have difficulty remembering the number and types of immunizations their children have received. It helps greatly to provide them with a written record of their child's immunizations.

Previous Illnesses

Previous illnesses include hospital admissions, emergency room visits, operations, and accidents. Record these in chronologic order, by age or dates.

Functional Inquiry (Review of Systems)

Items to include in a systems' review are listed in Table 1–1.

Family and Psychosocial History

The family history and psychosocial history are frequently poorly detailed in a patient's medical record. This fact is amazing and disconcerting, because often this history yields information crucial to understanding the child's problems and planning effective management.

The frequent omission of systematic psychosocial inquiry from pediatric interviews has been documented. In one study, involving interviews of the mothers of 234 children aged 6 months to 14 years, visits were audiotaped, and the dialogue was coded for the interviewers' (1) questions about psychosocial issues, (2) statements of support and reassurance, and (3) statements indicating sympathetic, attentive listening. It was noteworthy that *none* of the parents had given a psychosocial concern as the reason for the visit. Nevertheless, many parents disclosed psychosocial concerns, at an average time of 10 to 15 minutes into the interview. Not surprisingly, psychosocially oriented interviewing techniques were associated with greater disclosure of problems in the following four topic areas:

- Parental medical or emotional impairment
- Family disruption
- Use of physical punishment
- Aggressive or overactive child behavior

Key Point

Although the traditional "organic" history may become so systematized and routine that practitioners can reiterate its format easily by rote, recording a thorough family and psychosocial history has not been traditionally systematized the same way.

A useful approach is described in the following sections. First, describe the family structure, preferably in a typical genetic format that may include parental occupations.

Table 1–1 REVIEW OF SYSTEMS IN HISTORY-TAKING

Ear, nose, throat, and respiratory	Infections: How many? Febrile or afebrile? Duration? Respiratory difficulty: Croup, wheezing? Cough: Under what circumstances? Earache: Discharge? Hearing loss? Do older children turn up the TV unusually loud? Sore throats: Swallowing difficulty? Swollen glands?
Cardiovascular	For infants: Fatigue or sweating during feedings? Respiratory difficulty? For older children: Syncopal episodes? Murmurs detected previously?
Gastrointestinal	Appetite, weight gain, height growth? Bowel movements: Frequency, consistency? Blood, mucus, pain before or during defecation? Abdominal pain: Site, duration, radiation? Effect on normal activity? Associated symptoms and signs?
Central nervous system	Headaches? Seizures? Weakness?
Rashes	Any?
Genitourinary	Urinary: Frequency? Dysuria? Enuresis (daytime, nocturnal, primary, or secondary)? Adolescents: Sexually active? (Question best asked without parental presence and comfortably introduced; e.g., "Some boys of your age are sexually active—how about you?") Menstruation: Age at menarche? Regularity? Dysmenorrhea? Menorrhagia? Discharge, pruritus, rashes? Sexually transmitted diseases?

CONSANGUINITY

Although many pediatric hospital admissions are for genetically determined conditions, every admission history should include a statement about the presence or absence of consanguinity. Do not be shy about asking the question directly, because parents are not offended. Begin by asking "Are you and your husband (wife) related in any way?" or "Is there anyone in your family who is related to both of you?" In smaller communities, especially those with fairly stable populations, consanguinity is not uncommon, because the original community may have been settled by only three or four families. In such circumstances, parents may be unaware of consanguineous relationships; for clues, ask whether any family names appear on both paternal and maternal sides.

FAMILY HISTORY OF DISEASE

When taking the family history of a child with a serious disease, adapt it, when possible, to the child's particular complaint or condition.

For a child who is complaining of chronic abdominal pain or has rectal bleeding, it is essential to ask whether any family member has had chronic inflammatory bowel disease, such as Crohn disease or ulcerative colitis. Roughly 15% of children with Crohn disease have a positive family history of inflammatory bowel disease, so a positive family history can help in establishing the diagnosis.

Here are some important—but frequently overlooked—questions to ask about family history of disease:

1. Is there a family history of problems similar to those of the patient?
2. Is there a family history of myocardial infarction in family members younger than 50 years? This fact can be a clue to the possibility of hyperlipidemia in children.
3. Is there a family history of headaches?

In relation to the third question, remember that migraine is a common cause of headache in children. Although many people have at least one relative with migraine, affected children often have a strong family history, with two or more affected members on one side of the family. When there is a history of headache in other family members, follow up this issue by requesting a description of their symptoms, including duration and severity, aura, lateralization, photophobia, sensitivity to noise (phonophobia), visual disturbances, paresthesias, and nausea or vomiting. Choose your words carefully to avoid medical terms with which parents may be unfamiliar.

FAMILY DYNAMICS

At the initial interview, begin thinking about how this family seems to work. Certain attributes help families work well, be reasonably happy, and function effectively as a group with minimum risk of serious emotional dysfunction in the children. A family is a unit of individuals who cohabit in a psychodynamic equilibrium. To develop successfully as a unit and maintain their particular homeostasis, a family requires three principal components: (1) leadership, (2) shared labor, and (3) good, warm, and supportive communication.

Every group that works effectively, including families, needs leadership, a quality that should be carefully distinguished from domination. Domineering rule weakens the members of any group, but leadership strengthens them by bringing out the best in each member. Observe both parents together as the dynamics are played out verbally and nonverbally. Use both your eyes and your ears well. During each family interview, ask yourself three basic questions: (1) How do they look? (2) What do they say to you and to each other? and (3) What do they do?

PSYCHOSOCIAL HISTORY

Asking questions about the nine specific issues listed here screens effectively for most psychosocial problems, a process that takes only a couple of minutes.

Important Screening Issues

- Occupations and employment history (including frequent or prolonged parental absences).
- Household—space, number, and identity of occupants, frequency of domiciliary moves.
- Support systems—relatives and friends on whom they can depend, especially at difficult times.
- Financial problems, including any social assistance.
- Recreational history—What do they do as a family for fun?
- Major life events (e.g., serious illness, death, separation, divorce).
- Psychiatric illness, especially depression.
- Substance abuse (alcohol, drugs).
- Marital stability.

OCCUPATIONAL HISTORY OF EACH PARENT

Key Point

Obtaining an occupational history may be important for various reasons: Parents may be exposed to particular infections or toxins in their occupations. Some jobs, such as those in the armed services, merchant marine, or sales, require a parent to be absent frequently or for long periods.

Prolonged, frequent parental absences can sometimes destabilize family life profoundly. Such absences place a disproportionate burden of responsibility on the homebound parent, often leading to exhaustion, resentment, and marital dysfunction. Recurrent or prolonged absence of one parent eliminates many of the normal opportunities for shared labor, a key element in determining a family's emotional health. To complicate matters further, the absentee parent (most often the father) may continue to play the uninvolved role during visits home. Alternatively, he may try to establish his parental authority by assuming a domineering posture or a downright punitive role, a phenomenon rarely appreciated by other family members.

DESCRIBING THE HOUSEHOLD

A brief physical description of the home can be extremely useful. How many rooms? How many occupants? Crowding can put enormous strains on family relationships.

Household Moves

The impact of a household move is a frequently underestimated major life event. Next to divorce, serious illness, and death, moving can be one of life's greatest traumas. Too often, its impact on family homeostasis is underestimated. The powerful negative effects of moving from one community to another include detachment of family members from critical support systems, such as relatives and close friends. Most people form no more than two or three truly deep friendships in an entire lifetime—the kind of friends to whom parents would turn unhesitatingly for help and support in times of major personal trouble. Generally, those two or three special friendships date either from childhood or from the early adult years. Household moves, many of which occur in the middle adult years, often separate families from their vital anchors and support systems. For the mother who works at home raising a family, the impact of a household move can be especially traumatic and isolating. For children, it may mean separation from close friends (their support systems) and adaptation to a new school.

Special Considerations

Take special note of the family that lacks a telephone. The lack of a telephone may not be simply a sign of poverty, although the family in question may be poor.

Key Point

Usually, families without phones lack them for a reason far more compelling than poverty alone: They may simply have no one to talk to.

Such families badly need extra support to overcome their isolation. Although they have no phone, they may have a television set, which may be their sole source of a social life, albeit a fantasy one, serving as a temporary distraction from isolation and other disadvantages.

SUPPORT SYSTEMS

Briefly define the family's support system. Are there grandparents, other relatives, or neighbors who help regularly with baby-sitting or in other supportive ways?

RECREATIONAL ACTIVITIES

What does the family do for recreation as a group, and how often? How often do the parents go out together as a couple—for a meal, a movie, sports, with friends, or just for a walk? Recreational activities tell you a lot about family relationships. It can be surprising to learn how many couples have had no conjoint activities outside the home for weeks or months—sometimes for years! When discussing these issues, pay attention to the nonverbal messages as well as the spoken answers.

MAJOR LIFE EVENTS

Note any major illnesses, deaths, accidents, separations, divorces, or other major life events in the family, and record the dates. Such events can play a major direct or indirect role in a child's health problems.

PSYCHIATRIC ILLNESS

After the common cold, depression is the most prevalent of human afflictions. Major depression is reported to occur in 3% of adult men and 4% to 9% of adult women. It can affect both the victim and the family in many adverse ways, but its existence is often not revealed unless the question is specifically asked: "Has anyone in your family ever suffered from serious depression?" Also ask about other significant emotional or psychiatric conditions requiring treatment or hospitalization.

SUBSTANCE ABUSE

Ask "Has anyone on either side of the family ever had a problem with alcohol? Or with drugs?" Only when you ask this question of all families does it become obvious that alcohol abuse is a far more widespread family problem than is commonly recognized. One of

every six children in the United States is reported to have an alcoholic parent.

Eliciting an accurate history of adult drinking habits can be tricky. Asking people directly how much they drink commonly produces significant underreporting, especially in alcohol abusers. You can obtain a more accurate record by first asking what individuals drink when they do take a drink—beer, wine, or liquor. Then ask for the estimated daily intake by suggesting a relatively large amount. "How many beers do you usually drink a day—six or eight?" The question style hints that such an intake is not unusual and seems to reduce the tendency of problem drinkers to understate their actual intake. The drinking problem in many families may go unnoted if you do not question the parents specifically on this issue.

MARITAL STABILITY

The recreational history may give useful clues to marital stability. Also, open-ended questions such as "How would you describe your marriage in a single word?" and "What do you do as a family for fun?" elicit valuable insights into the partner and parent-child relationships, especially if you watch the parent's expressions and body language during the responses.

DEVELOPING A PROBLEM LIST AND TREATMENT PLAN

Once you have completed and recorded the family interview, history-taking, and physical examination, tabulate a list of the problems identified and connect each problem with a specific management plan or solution. A problem-based strategic management plan focuses on the entire patient—the child and the family—not just on a disease, a symptom, or an organ system.

Key Point

The problem-oriented approach to medical record-keeping goes beyond focusing on a single underlying disease, because it produces a comprehensive list of all the significant problems that affect the child and the family.

The following case history shows how multiple problems require individual attention to provide comprehensive care for a child who might otherwise be treated simply as a "case of asthma." Ultimately, dealing with issues that might be rated as subsidiary may improve the child's health and welfare more than a management plan that is limited to medicating the focal disease.

Mary J., aged 6 years, presents with recurrent wheezing episodes over the preceding 2 years. She currently is treated with a bronchodilator (salbutamol), given with a "puffer" three times daily. Mary's father is unemployed; her mother works as a grocery cashier. The family has moved twice in the past 5 years, and they have no other relatives in their present community. Mother describes her husband as a "weekend alcoholic." She states that Mary seems rather agitated and emotionally labile at home, and her teacher confirms this observation. Mary coughs when excited, when tickled, or after running and tires easily.

There is a significant family history of atopy. Both parents smoke. There is a cat at home. On questioning, mother confirms that Mary frequently exhibits the "allergic salute" (see Fig. 9–2). On examination, Mary is well nourished, with height and weight in the 25th percentile. She has "allergic shiners" and coughs occasionally. Her nasal turbinates are swollen and pale, obstructing the nasal airways. Pneumatic otoscopy suggests fluid in the middle ears. Her chest is slightly hyperresonant to percussion. On auscultation, expiration is slightly prolonged, with occasional musical expiratory rhonchi at both bases posteriorly.

The problem list and management plan are shown in the following table:

Problem	Management Plan
Allergic rhinitis	Trial of steroid nasal spray
Tobacco smoke exposure	Parents counseled regarding smoking cessation and referred to Lung Association to enroll in smoking cessation program
Possible allergy to cat hair	Mary to be skin tested for cat hair sensitivity. If test positive, parents agree to remove cat for 1 month, followed by extensive housecleaning
Asthma inadequately controlled, partly exercise-induced	Trial of inhaled steroid therapy
Agitation and emotional lability	Reaction to salbutamol? In consideration of other interventions, discontinue salbutamol therapy and see whether symptoms improve; report in 1 week
Paternal alcohol abuse	Mother to contact Alcoholics Anonymous for assistance with intervention
Lack of family support systems	Parents to join local branch of Asthma Association. Community health nurse called; she will visit home to follow up recommendations and report progress

THE FINE ART OF DIFFERENTIAL DIAGNOSIS

Key Point

If the cause of the child's complaints is not immediately obvious, making a differential diagnosis and establishing a plan of investigation may be necessary.

Include a differential diagnosis in the child's medical record only when there is genuine doubt about the clinical diagnosis. To be useful, it must be a differential diagnosis for the particular child, never of the symptom or sign; thus, it should not attempt to list most known causes of a presenting clinical problem, such as cough, jaundice, or splenomegaly. The differential diagnosis list should be short and realistic, showing only conditions that could plausibly explain most or all of this child's symptoms and signs.

Because clinical phenomena almost never exist in total isolation, each must be interpreted in its unique context. In descending order of probability, list the conditions that might offer a rational explanation for the manifestations of the youngster's illness. Focus the plan of investigation on the most likely diagnosis first. Always begin with the fewest, least expensive, least painful, and least invasive procedures that offer the greatest likelihood of confirming clinical suspicions.

THE THERAPEUTIC CONTRACT

The final moments of the interview call for good listening. It is extremely valuable to ask parents to reiterate their understanding of the child's problem and what should be done about it. Their response will tell you whether you and the parents are on the same wavelength. Once that is determined, establish the therapeutic contract with the family.

Therapeutic Contract

The three basic operating principles of a therapeutic contract remain constant, whether the child's problem is a recurrent sore throat, chronic renal disease, or a behavior problem. They are as follows:

1. Agree about the tasks to be performed.
2. Agree on who is responsible for each task, preferably sharing the work among different family members.
3. Agree on the time and means of reporting back in the short term (e.g., 1 to 2 weeks) to assess progress and decide further management. Reporting back in the near future is one of the best guarantees of compliance with a treatment plan.

INTERVIEWING AND EXAMINING ADOLESCENTS

The form and content of your first clinical encounter with any adolescent patient should be well planned in advance. The entire ambiance, conversation, and examination procedure should reflect your sensitivity to each teenager's particular level in the transition between childhood and adulthood.

It has been said, in reference to visits to hospital facilities, that the most important person in the institution is the first person you meet. This concept is especially true for teenagers, whether the setting for the clinical encounter is a hospital, clinic, private office, school, or other site. The initial greeting, whether by you or someone else, sets the tone for what follows.

Depending on the adolescent's age and the nature of the problem, it is often best to have one or both parents present during the first part of your meeting. At that time, assure the teenager and the parents that you will make time available for separate private discussions. Many adolescents are far more communicative when interviewed alone. Before taking the history, establish a mutual understanding of the ground rules and the objectives of the visit. The essential elements of this contractual agreement are as follows:

- Assurance of privacy and confidentiality: Parents need to understand that there may be issues you would like to discuss privately with the teenager. Assure the teenager that any such conversation will be strictly confidential unless otherwise agreed. This assurance carries a powerful message of respect for the teenager.
- Informed consent.
- Mutual agreement about who will be in the room during the interview.

Explaining the Purpose of the Interview

You owe the teenager an explanation of why you are asking a wide range of questions, some of which many seem unrelated to the presenting complaint. Explain that this step is essential to obtaining a thorough assessment and to pointing the way to better overall health. Advise the patient that a few questions will be of an awkward personal nature so that there are as few surprises as possible. The emphasis should always be on the ultimate objective, which is helping the youngster (or family) feel better.

Picking Up Nonverbal Cues

Nonverbal cues are particularly important in the evaluation of adolescents. Looks, gestures, and signs such as personal grooming and facial expressions often speak louder than words in expressing a teenager's mood and feelings. Recognize the significance of apathy, fatigue, and depression. Polishing your observational and intuitive skills can be the most valuable aid to understanding and helping teenagers.

Many teenagers who are brought to physicians show degrees of reluctance that can vary from shyness or embarrassment to outright hostility and mutinous muteness. An inexperienced interviewer can easily become frustrated (even angry) when a teenager's responses to questions consist chiefly of shrugs, monosyllables, or "I don't know." Such responses are more likely to occur when parents are in the room. Often, teenagers have been brought to physicians because they have problems that their parents view negatively. You must carefully avoid becoming a partner to the negative or deprecating comments or attitudes of parents. Similarly, do not overidentify with the attitude of the teenager.

As an effective interviewer who wants to help teenagers, you must constantly be aware of the need to recognize the patient's positive attributes as a therapeutic key to improving the negative ones. Accentuating the positives begins with the very first greeting—"I like your outfit," "I'm glad to meet you."

By the same token, it often helps to start the interview with a topic unrelated to the presenting complaint, especially if the latter is a "hot" topic. This approach also helps establish better rapport. You can always find something (no matter how trivial) that deserves positive recognition. Take the first part of the history directly from the adolescent. This approach expresses unequivocally your respect for the youngster's individuality.

Do not start with the sensitive issues, and when parents are present, try not to let a diffident teenager defer to the parents when you ask about his or her main health concerns. When you ask a question, some reluctant teens immediately appeal to the parent, either verbally or by an appealing look, to provide the reply. You can always put the ball right back in the youngster's court by saying, "I really want to hear what *you* think—then we'll talk to your Mom [Dad] in a few minutes." Many teens respond positively to such expressions of personal interest and respect.

Avoid a heavy-handed approach. Judicious use of humor (of the nondeprecating variety) can help relax a tense or anxious adolescent and make it a lot easier to deal with sensitive issues later.

There is no magic formula for a successful interview with all adolescent patients. Each conversation must be custom tailored to the unique characteristics of the patient and family and to the nature of the individual problem. However, if you apply the principles described here, you are more likely to obtain a diagnostically and therapeutically effective interview.

Incidentally, you do not facilitate the process by trying to dress or talk like an adolescent or using a lot of current teenage jargon. Most teenagers sense the phoniness of such an approach and may be made uncomfortable as a result.

You may want to ask a teenager to describe the family—their ages and occupations and some details of family life. He or she can also be questioned directly about issues such as school performance, sports participation, social activities with family and peers, and daily habits—rest (bedtime, how he or she feels on awakening), nutrition (does he/she eat breakfast?), daily health habits, and safety. This conversation should be punctuated by expressions of approval for positive attributes and empathy for any difficulties the teenager is experiencing. Starting with such topics will make the teenager feel a lot more comfortable when you come to discuss more sensitive issues. For some issues, it will be more appropriate for the parent to respond to questions; examples are history of birth, immunization, early development, and past illnesses.

As suggested earlier, the framing of each question needs to be selected carefully. It often helps to start with an open-ended, general question, such as "How are things at home?" "Do you have fun as a family?" "How are you doing at school?" or "Do you have lots of friends?"

In increasingly cosmopolitan communities, you should be well informed about cultural and ethnic customs and differences that affect behavior (your own and the family's) in clinical settings. In some cultures, adolescent girls carefully avoid eye contact with the physician, particularly one of the opposite sex. In such circumstances, it may be preferable for a teenager to be seen by a physician of the same sex, if it can be arranged (see Chapter 2).

Talking About the "Hot" Topics

When the time comes to explore more sensitive issues, it is important to set the stage, by saying something like "Now I need to ask you some questions that a lot of people your age worry about." Substance abuse, sexuality, anxiety, depression, eating disorders, and family dysfunction head the list of "hot" topics that must be handled with particular sensitivity and tact. The best prelude to such questions is to give the reason for asking them and to "permit" the adolescent to be concerned about such issues. For example, "I know that many kids of your age are sexually active—how about you?" Always make sure your question has been well understood. A story, possibly apocryphal, is told about a teenage girl who was asked by her physician whether she was sexually active. "No," she replied, "I just lie there." Neither a nod nor a "yes" or "no" guarantees comprehension of the question.

Finally, remember that as with playing a musical instrument well, skilled interviewing requires constant

practice and that there is always room for improvement in your performance. Videotaping or audiotaping a few of your interviews with adolescents and their families and reviewing the tapes critically is one of the best ways of identifying and correcting weaknesses.

The Physical Examination

Most technical details of the physical examination are explained in other chapters throughout this book, but certain skills apply particularly to adolescents. Explain the various examinations and the reasons for each as you proceed. At the beginning, ask teenagers whether they would like a chaperone to be present. A chaperone is always advisable when examining an adolescent of the opposite sex. Be especially sensitive to the adolescent's modesty, especially when it comes to undressing. Suitable gowns of the nongaping variety should be provided, and the patient should be given enough time and privacy to change. Only the body part being examined must be exposed at any time, and it can be covered when you are done.

Explain each part of the examination as you go along, and tell the patient when your findings are normal. Maintaining a good flow of light conversation and asking questions during the examination relieves much of the anxiety that teenagers feel under these circumstances. Blood pressure is particularly sensitive to anxiety levels in some adolescents. Sphygmomanometry should therefore be deferred until the patient is as relaxed as possible. If blood pressure is elevated on the first reading, repeat the measurement at least twice at intervals and with the youngster standing and lying down, using distraction and reassurance to achieve as much relaxation as possible; document any postural effects on blood pressure.

Finding certain normal variants should remind you to mention them specifically and reassure the teenager that such findings are entirely normal. Like other patients with hidden agendas, teenagers rarely verbalize their concern about such problems. This does not mean they are not worried. Common examples are as follows:

Asymmetric breast development: In some girls, one breast develops more rapidly than the other. Such asymmetry almost always corrects itself as puberty progresses.
Asymmetric scrotum: One testicle may be situated lower in the scrotum than the other—another normal finding that can worry some teenage boys.

Concluding the Visit

This is the time to review the problems identified. Finding out what the adolescent has learned from the visit is more important than your delivering a verbal summary as a monologue. The final portion of the visit should include the following ingredients:

Concluding Questions. Ask questions such as "Are there any other questions you would like to ask me?" or "Do you feel this visit has helped you?" If the answer is "Yes," ask "In what way?" .

Note whether the teenager looks and acts differently at the end of the visit compared with your initial impression. If you believe that the visit has been less than satisfactory from the adolescent's, parents', or your own perspective, a further appointment should be made to continue the discussion. For some adolescents, as with some adults, several visits may be required to deal effectively with certain problems, especially ones that have been years in the making. Remember that the interview should be as therapeutic as it is diagnostic; an effective therapeutic contract often requires selection, by mutual agreement, of a single problem (rather than an array of issues) to deal with initially. Successful management of a single problem often has a valuable spin-off in correcting other difficulties. When the problem is of a psychosocial nature, it may be best to have the adolescent and parents select the issue they wish to deal with as their first priority.

Parental Involvement. With the teenager's agreement, invite the parent or parents to join you for a final review of the problems, the management plan, and follow-up arrangements.

Summary. Summarize the problems you have identified, and negotiate a plan for management and follow-up. The latter should often include a telephone contact within 1 week or so, preferably initiated by the teenager and scheduled for a specific date and time. Tell the teenager to feel free to contact you, and give him or her the necessary information for doing so (telephone number and the best time to reach you).

More Hidden Agendas

Hidden agendas may be even more common in clinical encounters with adolescents than in those with families of younger children. The one feature common to such issues is that teenagers rarely volunteer the relevant information unless specifically asked.

It helps to have a "shopping list" of topics you wish to explore. The most common hidden agenda topics for adolescents are follows:

- Substance abuse (by the teenager, friends, or family members)
- Depression
- Suicidal thinking (an estimated 30% of teenagers have suicidal ideation at some time)
- Fears of serious illness or somatization related to a recent serious illness or death in a relative or close friend

- Concerns about sexuality—sexual identity, birth control, sexually transmitted diseases, pregnancy
- School problems
- Sexual or physical abuse
- Family turmoil
- Problems with peers (e.g., gang involvement)

Clinical skills for eliciting emotional and behavioral problems in adolescents are discussed in more detail in Chapter 14.

CLINICAL SKILLS FOR SPECIAL SITUATIONS

Hospital Rounds

Whether your first attention on rounds is given to the patient or to the chart says something about whether your first concern is for the child or the disease. Even from the viewpoint of efficiency, if you see and speak to the child and family first, you need to spend remarkably little time with the paperwork.

Consultations

In the early part of the 20th century, the attending physician always spoke directly to the consultant when requesting a consultation. The protocol and courtesies were rigorously observed, whether the consultation took place in the hospital or in the patient's home. The family was informed of the consultation in advance, and both physicians arrived dressed in their best finery. As a courtesy, the attending physician would arrive 5 or 10 minutes ahead of the consultant, to introduce the patient and family properly. The consultant would examine the patient and discuss the problem privately with the attending physician, and then both would meet with the family to offer their opinion and respond to the family's concerns.

Compare that scenario to a typical contemporary hospital consultation: The attending physician or a delegate places a consultation request form with two or three lines of telegraphic information in the "Out" basket or types it into a computer. The impersonal request ultimately reaches the consultant, who arrives at a time of his or her choosing. The family often lacks advance knowledge that the consultation has been requested. If they are present when the consultant arrives, it may be more by luck than by design. Too often, the attending physician or resident, who knows the child best, is not present when the consultant arrives. Faced with such handicaps, the consultant is expected to provide expert evaluation and wise counsel in a kind of diagnostic and therapeutic vacuum. The final event in this unfortunate saga is the reappearance of the completed, sometimes illegible, consultation sheet, possibly several days later or even after the patient's discharge, in the physician's "In" basket.

Meanwhile, the family may never have heard the assessment or recommendations from the consultant's lips and may never have had a chance to ask the consultant any questions. Often, the child's regular caregivers (staff physicians) have missed a golden opportunity to acquire new knowledge and skills directly from the consultant (in either the child's interest or their own)—and so the sad chronology ends.

Key Point

Enormous dividends can be reaped through selectively retaining the best elements of a more traditional consultation protocol.

Here are some specific recommendations for making a consultation valuable for the physician, the consultant, the child, and the family:

1. Complete the consultation request, but always telephone the consultant. A 2-minute chat can transmit much more useful information than two written lines.
2. Try to negotiate a mutually satisfactory time to meet for the consultation. Watching a good cardiologist for 5 minutes is more productive than reading a two-page consultation report.
3. Let the child and family know when and where the consultation will occur. The parents and the consultant can be invaluable to each other in serving the child's best interests.
4. Arrive ahead of the consultant to make the necessary introductions. Remain behind for a few minutes to see whether the child and family have other questions—some consultants have a bad habit of leaving in a hurry.

Helping the Irate Parent

Sooner or later, often without warning, every physician faces an angry or hostile parent. It may happen in a busy emergency department, on a ward, or in an office. Physicians who have never calmly analyzed the causes of parental anger are unlikely to handle the situation effectively and constructively.

A previously planned, step-by-step strategy can help you manage this clinical situation in such a way as to defuse parental anger and be genuinely helpful to the family.

Most parents who express anger do so toward physicians, nurses, receptionists, or others whom they have never met before. If you realize that the parents usually are not angry with you personally, you will not take their anger personally. As a well-known saying puts it, "Don't get the idea that everybody hates you—everybody hasn't met you!"

Parental anger is usually an expression of anxiety, frustration, or of loss of control over the parent's own, or the child's, destiny. It needs to be understood as such.

Having recognized that the parent's hostility is not personal, first acknowledge the anger with words such as "I can see that you are upset." Either begin to move everyone to a quiet room with privacy and comfort or suggest "Why don't you come over here with me and sit down, and I'll see how we can help." Most of us react reflexively to anger with anger. The natural response to a raised voice is to compete by raising your own vocal volume. With an irate parent, however, it is essential to *lower*, rather than raise, your voice in volume and pitch. Try that maneuver in an ordinary friendly conversation with two or three other people; note how, as your voice descends toward a whisper, your listeners quiet, and their attention becomes progressively more rapt.

Once the parent is settled in a quiet comfortable environment, let him or her ventilate feelings without interruption. Often within minutes, the anger will cool sufficiently that the parent becomes receptive to help.

It is not unusual to discover that the triggering event seems inconsequential. As more information about the family comes out, however, it often becomes apparent that this triggering event was simply "the last straw" in a succession of stresses, some of which may have little direct connection to the child's current illness. Any of the common psychosocial stresses mentioned earlier in this chapter (financial problems, feelings of isolation due to a lack of support systems, marital discord, substance abuse, psychiatric difficulties) or sometimes even a mundane stress, such as not having eaten for several hours, can precipitate an outburst. If you understand a family's problems as well as the child's presenting complaint, you can be truly helpful to the family in distress.

The Child With Chronic or Recurrent Illness

Interviewers should be especially sensitive to the needs of parents whose child has a chronic or recurrent health problem requiring frequent visits or hospital admissions. The special clinical skills required for dealing with children with chronic conditions are discussed in detail in Chapter 20.

Breaking News of a Child's Death

Few tasks test your clinical counseling skills more than having to tell parents their child has just died. No matter how often you have done it before, or for how long the child's death had been expected, there is no easy way of breaking such awful news. Nevertheless, there are good, bad, and indifferent ways of helping parents deal with this terrible tragedy. Here are a few general guidelines:

1. Be prepared to spend as much time as required with the parents after telling them the news.
2. Be sure to break the news in a private, quiet setting—never in a waiting room or corridor.
3. Always sit with the parents before telling them—never give them bad news while you are standing.
4. Always refer to the child by name.
5. Avoid euphemisms. The child has died, not "passed away," "left us," or "gone to heaven."
6. When a particular nurse has been involved in the child's care, the nurse should share in the task of informing the parents.
7. Parents should be offered the opportunity to see their child after death, hold the youngster if they wish, and say goodbye in their own way—either in privacy or with your supportive presence, whichever seems more appropriate.
8. The support of those who cared for the child during life should never end with the child's death. They can express their sympathy and concern verbally or in writing and by attending the funeral, if possible.
9. Make arrangements to meet the parents again soon afterward and as often as required. This provides an opportunity to answer their questions, enables parents to ventilate their feelings, and allows for interpretation of the findings when an autopsy has been performed.

When a child's death is sudden and unexpected, as in sudden infant death syndrome or after a motor vehicle accident, parents' reactions may follow a pattern different from that observed when a youngster has died after a prolonged illness. Their initial grief reactions may include shock, numbness, disbelief, and anger, in any sequence or combination.

Whatever the events leading to a child's death, a skilled, understanding clinician can play a critical role in helping parents achieve as accepting an adjustment as possible in this great tragedy.

Breaking Other Difficult News

The late Dr. Bronson Crothers was one of the great pediatric neurologists of the first half of the 20th century. Parents came from all over the world to the Children's Hospital in Boston to have him assess their developmentally delayed or neurologically disordered children. He was a master in helping parents come to

terms with such agonizing problems. A pediatric resident once asked him, "How do you tell parents for the very first time that their child is retarded?" Crothers replied, "I never tell them. I always let them tell me."

Underlying his response was a concept that is truly fundamental. The transmission of difficult information to families is not a transfer of information. It is a subtle process of inducing understanding. There is a world of difference between imparting information and inducing understanding. Transmitting information involves much talking and little listening. By contrast, inducing understanding calls for much listening and relatively little talking. It requires supersensitive "antennae" to detect what parents can understand and to recognize when to conclude an interview and return later, at an agreed-on time and place, because the parents have had all they can handle for the moment. Inducing understanding and enhancing the family's ability to adapt to a difficult or chronic problem are almost never achieved in a single conversation. Repeated discussions may be needed over days, weeks, or months, each one building on the understandings generated by its predecessors.

The style of questions that help parents understand is rather special. For example, in the case of a developmentally delayed child, it may be appropriate to ask, "At what age level would you say [child's name] is functioning right now?"

Key Point

Parents' estimate of their child's level of functioning is often remarkably accurate.

The parents' appreciation of the future educational and occupational significance of that delay may be less precise or realistic, and it may require several years of guidance and support to help them come to terms with it. Do not destroy parents' natural defenses by insisting on immediate concordance with your own long-range prognosis. It may be appropriate to pose questions such as "Do you think he/she will be able to go to school at the usual age?" or "What do you see [child's name] being able to do 2 (or 5) years from now (or when he/she is an adult)?"

If the parents' future vision seems overly optimistic, do not feel obliged to disagree or contradict them. Given the chance, parents often ask, "What do you think?" A physician can gently plant a tiny seed of doubt with an answer such as, "Well, I hope so—I'm not really too sure." The issue can be raised again at a subsequent session, and you often find, after the passage of time, that parents' expectations have become more tempered and more realistic.

Skills for effective initial disclosure of the diagnosis of a chronic or disabling condition are discussed in detail in Chapter 20.

Encouraging Second Opinions

When parents first hear bad news about their child, one early reaction, spoken or unspoken, is often one of denial. Reactions such as "Maybe he's wrong" and, a little later, "Perhaps someone else knows a treatment or cure that our doctor doesn't know about" are understandable, wishful thoughts to which any of us would be susceptible in similar circumstances. Parents often do not verbalize such thoughts because they may be afraid of upsetting the physician with any expression of lack of confidence. Therefore, you should always anticipate this question and raise the issue.

Physicians should be comfortable with their limitations and ready to admit them openly. You might raise the issue by saying, "None of us has a monopoly on knowledge about Jane's condition. If you'd like to have an expert in these conditions look at her and advise you, I approve of that, and I will be happy to help you arrange it." This suggestion usually elicits a strong mixture of relief and gratitude in parents, whether or not they decide to take advantage of the offer.

Key Point

No matter how trivial the problem seems to the physician, every patient has the right to a second opinion, and the family physician should never interfere with that right or disapprove of it by word, silence, or facial expression.

That wish for a second opinion is not an expression of lack of confidence in the physician's ability, but an admirable expression of the parents' concern for their child's welfare, and it should be supported. Generally, a physician's readiness to solicit additional opinions strengthens the family's trust and confidence in the physician's judgment on most issues.

SUMMARY

Of all the diagnostic aids available, a well-conducted family interview and a thorough history are the best "imaging procedures" available. Although the quality of the picture depends on the interviewer's skills, no other technology can provide as clear an appreciation of the child and family, their problems, and the psychosocial backdrop against which the problems have developed. Recognition of both the therapeutic and the diagnostic value of the interview brings the discovery that, as with musical performance, technique is perfected only through regular, conscientious practice.

REFERENCE

1. Baumer JH, David TJ, Valentine SJ, et al: Many parents think their child is dying when having a first febrile convulsion. Dev Med Child Neurol 23:462, 1981.

chapter 2

Skills for Culturally Sensitive Pediatric Care

RICHARD B. GOLDBLOOM

Many years ago, a resident was presenting the case history of a sick Latino child to a distinguished American professor of pediatrics. Describing the information he had obtained from the child's mother, he reported, "I wasn't able to obtain a complete history because of the mother's language difficulty."

"Just a moment!" the professor interjected. "*Whose* language difficulty?"

This vignette says it all about a fundamental aspect of effective communication: We have a responsibility to provide sensitive care for families whose ethnic or religious background, color, language, or culture differs from our own. As a caregiver, you owe it to your patients to familiarize yourself with the customs and beliefs of as many groups as possible in your own community. It is simply an issue of respect.

Each distinct ethnic, religious, and cultural group has its particular values and beliefs; traditions of acceptable and unacceptable behaviors; special patterns of speech and gestures; gender roles; health practices; customs; beliefs about the causes and cures of illness; birth and death rites; attitudes about transfusion, autopsy, organ donation, and organ transplants; food practices and intolerances; attitudes toward authority; and child-rearing practices. Each group also has its own way of displaying emotions such as fear, pain, grief, concern, pleasure, and disagreement.[1] Skilled clinical assessment requires both a knowledge of and a respect for those differences. It also requires preparatory work. Faced with a family from a culture different from your own, you have no time to excuse yourself so you can brush up on their beliefs and customs. So come prepared, as often as possible.

GROWING SCOPE OF MULTICULTURALISM

The racial and cultural kaleidoscope of most developed countries is diversifying rapidly. In 1990, about 75% of the U.S. population was of white European descent. It is estimated that by 2020, this proportion will have decreased to 53%. Currently, 25% of all children younger than 5 years in the United States come from minority backgrounds, and this percentage is predicted to rise to 48% by 2025. In Canada's 1996 census, more than 10% of the population consisted of visible minorities, with a high proportion of immigrants coming from a wide variety of ethnic and cultural backgrounds, and about 25% of these being in the pediatric age group. These trends emphasize the growing importance of culturally sensitive health care. Concurrent with these striking demographic changes, marriages between people of different races and cultural backgrounds are increasing steadily.

Key Point

Do not assume, on the basis of language, dress, or ethnicity, what the ideas and beliefs of an individual or family may be. Characteristics common to a group do not necessarily predict those of the individual or family.

DANGERS OF STEREOTYPING

We are all at risk of stereotyping linguistic, cultural, or religious groups, usually on the basis of limited exposure. The populations of most countries are heterogeneous with respect to language, traditions, and customs, and beliefs and practices vary as much within as between groups.[2] Thus, characteristics that may be common within a cultural group do *not* necessarily predict those of a particular individual or family. Therefore, do not assume, from language, dress, or culture, what an individual's ideas or beliefs may be.[1]

CULTURAL DISADVANTAGE IN HEALTH CARE

Several studies have demonstrated that children whose racial or ethnic backgrounds differ from those of the mainstream population suffer disadvantage in the health care they receive.[3] Many complex factors undoubtedly contribute to this discrepancy, including economic disadvantage, an undersupply of culturally competent caregivers, transportation difficulties, and unmet needs for child care. Some families may also have difficulty following instructions for medications or other treatments. In the United States, even after adjustments are made for socioeconomic factors, health conditions, and number of physician visits, black and Hispanic children have been found (1) to be less likely to receive prescription medications and (2) to receive fewer services when hospitalized.[3, 4]

FAMILY HIERARCHIES—WHO ARE THE AUTHORITIES AND DECISION-MAKERS?

Although many western cultures have evolved over recent decades from a patriarchal to a more egalitarian model of family authority, others have very different traditional hierarchies. These structures must be understood and respected by anyone caring for children. Among Vietnamese, for example, the father is traditionally the decision-maker, and the mother defers to him. The same is true in Saudi Arabian families, and during family interviews, the father may answer questions directed at the mother. Physicians who address questions or comments to a parent who is *not* the traditional family leader may inadvertently upset *both* parents. Among traditional Chinese, the loyalty and deference of younger to older family members is strictly observed by people of all ages, and preservation of family honor ("saving face") is very important. In Japanese families, children's unacceptable behavior may be regarded as reflecting unfavorably on their parents. In some Southeast Asian cultures, parents may be reluctant to make decisions about their children without consulting their traditional community leaders, whom they may regard as part of the extended family.

GET THE NAMES RIGHT

Many cultures do not follow the traditional western naming system, in which everyone's personal name is followed by a surname. Among traditional Chinese, for example, the family name comes first, followed by a personal name that is often in two parts, sometimes hyphenated. The Vietnamese use a similar system.

South Asian Muslims have no tradition of a family name. Traditional Sikhs do not use a family name, only a first name plus a male or female title—*Kaur* for women, *Singh* for men. Make every effort to use, pronounce, and record names correctly. This is another important expression of respect.

A Word or Two Can Make all the Difference

Language can be the greatest single barrier to quality care, and speaking at least one other language with reasonable fluency is a major asset for any caregiver. However, no matter how linguistically challenged you may be, make it a point to acquire at least a handful of words and phrases of greeting in each of the languages spoken by significant numbers of families in your community. There is no faster way to bring a smile to the face of a parent or child or to ease the anxiety of a family who are already intimidated by a strange environment and a foreign culture. There is no better way to signify your appreciation of the family's cultural individuality. A simple "Buon giorno" (Italian), "Buenos dias" or "Buenos tardes" (Spanish), "Salaam aleikum" (Arabic), "Ohayo gozaimasu" (Japanese), "Shalom" (Hebrew), "Bonjour" (French), "Gin Dobre" (Polish), or "Guten tag" (German) is a good start. If, however, your community contains significant numbers of families of a particular linguistic tradition, improving your relevant language skills can do a world of good.

Some people are under the mistaken impression that speaking (English) louder helps people of other languages understand. This is never true and, worse still, is often upsetting to the family. Culturally insensitive care amounts to involuntary racism. The inverse, *cultural competency*, has been defined as "acting with grace across lines of difference."[5] You can learn much from discussing these cross-cultural issues with colleagues and friends from different cultural backgrounds and by keeping one or two reliable reference sources handy.

The Variable Meanings of Looks and Gestures

Some of the involuntary physical gestures that accompany or amplify our side of conversations can have very different meanings for other cultural groups. In North America and Western Europe, for example, we shake hands with great regularity on meeting with or saying goodbye to others; however, in some cultures, shaking hands with people of the opposite gender is strictly taboo. In Thailand, shaking hands is often avoided entirely. Among Finns, conversing with the hands in the pockets is considered impolite. Similarly, in the western world, we encourage eye contact with both adults and children, whereas North American aboriginals and people from India and Asia may specifically avoid direct eye contact, as a sign of respect. In western cultures, we often nod our heads to signify understanding or agreement, but in some cultures, a nod implies neither and may simply mean "I hear you speaking" or "If you say so."

Some cultures are highly tactile (e.g., French, Italian, Russian, Jewish, and Greek), others much less so. Physical touch between genders may be distinctly uncomfortable for conservative Arab Muslims. Observant Muslims never use the left hand to eat in the presence of others. Doctors and physiotherapists may be puzzled if they find the parents of a child with a right hemiplegia to be "uncooperative" when they try to encourage the child to use the left hand instead; if the family observes the Muslim faith, this "solution" is unacceptable.

To reduce the risk of sudden infant death syndrome (SIDS), we currently discourage parents from sleeping with their infants. However, in some cultures, such as that of the Maoris of New Zealand or the Hmong of Laos, such sleeping situations are the norm and should be respected and accepted. Korean children may sleep with their parents until they are 4 years old. Similarly, although we discourage consanguinity for genetic reasons, it is the norm for some groups, and our traditional approach to genetic counseling may be both impractical and offensive to them.

Key Point

When a parent nods his or her head in apparent assent while you are talking, don't assume that this means "I understand" or "I agree." The best way to find out what parents have understood is to ask them to reiterate their understanding of the situation toward the end of the interview.

DISCIPLINARY PRACTICES

In some cultures, physical punishment has been a traditional form of parental discipline, and it should not be equated automatically with child abuse. Likewise, what is considered a problem behavior by one culture may be seen in a very different light by another.

ATTITUDES TOWARD CHRONIC CONDITIONS

Clinicians need to know and understand the variation in attitudes that prevails in different cultures toward a family member with a chronic condition. In North America and Europe, typical attitudes emphasize both survival and functional capacity. As a result, every effort is directed to cure or toward minimizing disability. By contrast, in some Asian cultures, the emphasis is on living in harmony with nature, and a chronic condition may be accepted as part of that harmony.

LIFE AND DEATH ISSUES

It is important to be aware of a patient's traditional or religious views on issues such as abortion, organ transplantation, cremation, and burial. Detailed discussion of these issues is available in references on cross-cultural care, but the following example illustrates how vital it is to know and respect such differences: In most Muslim countries, organ transplantation is practiced, including some cadaveric transplants. Muslim tradition, however, requires same-day burial. Autopsies are permitted under certain circumstances, such as suspected foul play. Cremation is strictly prohibited. When an infant dies, ritual washing is required, and the baby is draped in a white shroud made of two pieces of cloth. Islam permits in vitro fertilization. Abortion may occasionally be allowed prior to "ensoulment" of the fetus (generally considered to occur at about 120 days), although many Shiah and some Sunni Muslims do not permit abortion at any stage of pregnancy.

RECENT IMMIGRANT FAMILIES

It is valuable to keep handy a pocket reference that provides basic health-relevant information about people from a wide range of specific countries and cultures. Several available guides offer summaries of basic issues such as languages spoken, race-specific or endemic diseases, health care beliefs, authority patterns in families, customs of eye contact and touch, child-rearing practices, birth and death rites, national childhood immunization practices, perceptions of time, and the family's traditional role in the care of children in the hospital. Several valuable guides are listed in the "Suggested Readings" at the end of this chapter.

EFFECTIVE CONVERSATION

Conversing effectively with families from different cultures requires even greater emphasis on the elements that should characterize all clinical interviews with families from our own cultural background. These elements are as follows:

Bidirectional conversation: Give as much time to listening as to talking.
Respect: Treat all views as legitimate.
Responsiveness: Do not predetermine outcomes. As in all patient-doctor encounters, family members should be treated as partners—therapeutic allies—in the development of a management plan for the child.

Empathy: Include expressions of your understanding that the child's problem is causing the parents concern in every conversation you have with them.

CONSENT FOR TREATMENT

Anxious parents are often willing to sign a consent form placed before them, whether or not they understand its contents. Such signatures, however, confer no legal validity whatsoever on the document. It is therefore our individual and institutional duty to ascertain that any written or verbal consent is truly informed, that is, it is clearly understood by the parents in their own language. Translations of such documents into other languages should be readily available. If necessary, make use of an interpreter to ensure the parents' full comprehension.

Using Interpreters Effectively

Interpreters can be valuable, especially if they have professional training in medical assessment methods and are experienced cultural as well as linguistic interpreters. Such individuals should be sensitive to nonverbal as well as verbal messages, because effective interpretation involves far more than the mere translation of words. Many larger hospitals maintain lists of skilled, culturally competent health interpreters.

Use of an interpreter is bound to prolong any clinical encounter, so be sure to allow for the extra time required. Sometimes, giving adequate care to a child from another culture requires scheduling of additional visits. Before meeting with the family, discuss the goals of the interview with the interpreter. At the beginning of the interview, ask the family whether they feel comfortable speaking through an interpreter, and ask the interpreter to translate as literally as possible. Then introduce the interpreter and explain his or her role. Always look at the parent (*not* the interpreter), and speak slowly, clearly (*not* loudly), and in short sentences, using simple words and allowing enough time for the interpreter to translate. Encourage the family to ask questions. Stay alert for any hint that a family member may not understand something. After the interview, ask the interpreter whether he or she has additional relevant observations to contribute.

Key Point

There is a world of difference between a translator and an interpreter. A *translator* deals only in words. An *interpreter* understands and communicates the meaning of looks, gestures, customs, traditions, and health practices in both directions between families and caregivers.

False Fluency

Even the use of interpreters does not eliminate the possibility of miscommunication, which may occasionally have serious consequences. Overestimation of your own or an interpreter's fluency in the patient's language can lead you to overlook or misinterpret important information. This situation has been termed *false fluency.*

Interpreters may not be available on the short notice necessitated by emergency situations. In such cases, health care providers can contact the AT&T Language Line Services in the United States or Canada at 1-800-752-6096. A fee for this translation service is charged to the health care provider.

SPECIAL FEATURES OF CROSS-CULTURAL HISTORY-TAKING

In addition to the usual historical information outlined in Chapter 1, the following issues require special attention for patients from other cultures, especially for recent immigrants:

1. Linkage of immunization history with information about current immunization policy and practice in the country of origin.
2. History of tropical diseases if the family has come from a tropical country.
3. Inquiry concerning hereditary conditions, infections, nutritional deficiencies, and other disorders known to occur with increased frequency in the family's ethnic group or country of origin. This issue is especially important in evaluation of recent immigrants, because significant or transmissible conditions may be asymptomatic. For example, tuberculosis is still endemic in many countries. Children from Central America, the Caribbean, South America, and Africa may carry intestinal parasites. Other commonly silent infections are human immunodeficiency virus and hepatitis B.

When you obtain the psychosocial history in families of different cultural backgrounds, it is useful to determine which family members are responsible for child-rearing and to ask about sleeping arrangements. It may be important to know whether a preschool-aged child is participating in a school readiness program.

Developmental Assessment of the Preschool-Aged Child

Before applying developmental screening tests to preschoolers from diverse backgrounds, you must know whether any test you propose to use has been validated in diverse populations or translated into the family's language. For detailed information on these issues, consult the review by Li and colleagues.[6]

Family Perceptions of the Child with Chronic Illness

In many cultures, chronic illness or disability in a child may be viewed as a form of punishment, a sign of divine displeasure, a loss of spirit, or a curse. In societies that believe in reincarnation, a disability may be seen as evidence of transgression in a previous life. Although a family may listen to and accept your "rational" scientific explanation for an illness, their doing so does not necessarily eradicate their traditional beliefs.

In some societies, a child's gender can play a role in determining the extent to which parents seek medical help. In traditional East Indian and Chinese families, for example, less attention may be paid to illness in girls than in boys.

Another factor that may affect family attitudes and behavior is the parent's expectation for the child's survival. In some cultures, views about inevitability may be different from our own, and these views may influence the amount of energy the family devotes to the child's care as well as the extent to which they cooperate with caregivers.

Asking a few open-ended questions, such as those listed here, can give you valuable insights into how a patient or family from another culture perceives an illness:

- What do you think caused this problem?
- Why do you think it started when it did?
- How bad is it?
- How long do you think it will last?
- What are you most afraid of about [child's name]'s illness?
- What are the main problems this illness has caused you?
- What kind of treatment do you think he/she should receive?
- What do you hope the treatment we decide on will do for you?

In her book *The Spirit Catches You and You Fall Down*, Anne Fadiman[7] captures with extraordinary insight and eloquence the collision of cultures surrounding the health care of a young Hmong* child with epilepsy. Consider the following excerpt:

---

* A tribal group originating in Laos, Hmong refugees came to the U.S. after the Vietnam War. They have deep-rooted belief in spirits and shamanism. They practice animal sacrifice and believe deeply in the inviolability of the body—hence can be deeply offended by procedures such as blood sampling and lumbar puncture.

"All of [the American physicians] had spent hundreds of hours dissecting cadavers and could distinguish at a glance between the ligament of Hesselbach and the ligament of Treitz, but none of them had had a single hour of instruction in cross-cultural medicine. To most of them, the Hmong taboos against blood tests, spinal taps, surgery, anesthesia and autopsies—the basic tools of modern medicine—seemed like self-defeating ignorance. They had no way of knowing that a Hmong might regard these taboos as the sacred guardians of his identity, indeed, quite literally, of his very soul."

This book should be required reading for anyone seeking a better understanding of cross-cultural health issues. It emphasizes the need for respect and compromise that are essential to the effective care of a child from another culture.

Alternative Therapies and Folk Medicine

Every society, *including our own*, uses a wide variety of "folk medicines," unproven remedies, and alternative therapies. In North America, physicians prescribe vast quantities of cough syrups, oral decongestants, teething remedies, and other over-the-counter products whose efficacy is unproved or, more often, nonexistent. Today, many families also use herbal and "natural" remedies or consult nontraditional therapists.

We therefore have no justification for any feelings of superiority or skepticism about folk remedies used in other cultures. It is important to identify *all* the treatments a child has received. Gathering information about such treatments is best achieved through a step-wise approach to questioning, as follows:

1. People have told me that there are ways of treating children with this kind of illness that doctors don't know about. Have you heard of any of these remedies or treatments?
2. (If yes) Are they effective?
3. Have you tried (such a remedy) for this child's illness?
4. Was it helpful?

In areas with a large Puerto Rican population, it is common for people to patronize local *botanicas* to purchase traditional herbal remedies. For many parents, however, using traditional remedies does not exclude the use of others. Generally speaking, it is best not to discourage ethnomedicine if there is no evidence that it is harmful.

In caring for Hispanic or Latino families, caregivers should be familiar with the following common beliefs and customs:

Mal de ojo: The evil eye. Typical childhood symptoms attributed to mal de ojo include loss of appetite, crying, weight loss, and listlessness. Among Mexicans, mal de ojo is often believed to be caused by excessive admiration of the child.

Empacho: An illness thought to occur when a substance gets "stuck" to the wall of the stomach, usually attributed to dietary indiscretion and treated by diet change, laxatives, massage and, possibly, a visit to a folk healer, known as a *sobadora* or *curandero* in Mexican American communities and as a *santiguadore* among Puerto Ricans.

You can bring out the parents' views of the cause and management of their child's illness by asking the following series of open-ended, general questions:

1. What do you think is wrong with [child's name]?
2. Some parents have told me about an illness called [folk-name]. Have you heard of it?
3. (If yes) Have you ever seen someone with it?
4. Has [child's name] ever had it?
5. Do you think he/she has it now?
6. Why do you think your child developed it?
7. What do you think caused it?
8. Why do you think it started when it did?
9. What do you think is happening inside [child's name]'s body?
10. What are the symptoms that make you know your child has this illness?
11. What are you most worried about with this illness?
12. How do you treat it?
13. Is the treatment helpful?
14. What will happen if the problem is not treated?
15. What do you expect from the treatment?

Breaking Bad News Across Cultures

The specific clinical skills for breaking bad news described in Chapter 1 are even more important when the family comes from a different cultural background. The following additional issues must be considered.

- Whenever possible, the family should be encouraged to bring close relatives with them, to provide support and understanding. Remember that in most (more than 90%) cultures of the world, what we regard as the "nuclear" family is a rarity, and much more extended families are the norm. This essential difference must be respected.[1]
- If possible, address the family in their own language, and use a culturally sensitive health interpreter, if required, to facilitate two-way interpretation and understanding.
- Make sure everyone is comfortably seated and that you are prepared to commit as much time as necessary for a mutually satisfactory interview.
- Speak directly to the family, *not* to the interpreter.
- Do not leap directly into a discussion of the diagnosis. Some introductory "small talk" is expected in many cultures. It helps relax anxious parents, so they are better prepared to receive any bad news.
- Always begin by saying something positive and complimentary about the child before discussing the specifics of diagnosis, management or prognosis.
- Avoid all medical jargon, and offer information in a nonpatronizing manner.
- Be completely honest but, if possible, finish on a note of hope.
- Give the family ample opportunity to ask questions. You can often discover their main concerns by asking "What is it you are most worried about?" Two-way communication throughout the interview is critical.
- Make the diagnosis clear and unambiguous. Give the parents a brief, jargon-free, *written* report. Parents of any culture can be so anxious that they may have difficulty remembering the diagnostic term for the child's condition later, hence the value of a written report, preferably in the family's first language.
- Toward the end of the interview, always ask the parents to reiterate their understanding of the child's condition, the name of the condition, and what can or should be done to help.
- Finally, give the family the names and phone numbers of key contacts in writing, and set a specific date and time for the next follow-up appointment. A second meeting within 1 to 2 weeks (sooner, if necessary) is highly recommended, because most parents (of any culture) think of additional questions within hours or days of receiving bad news.

Cross-Cultural Skills for Physical Examination

Conditions such as rashes, petechiae, and jaundice may differ markedly in people of different skin color. In dark-skinned individuals, an alteration in skin consistency can indicate a rash as much as or more than a change in color (see Chapter 19 for further details). Petechiae may be easier to detect in the nail beds, palms, soles, and oral mucosa than elsewhere. Cyanosis may also be more apparent in the nail beds, palms, soles, and conjunctivae than in other sites. In dark-skinned individuals, the peripheral part of the sclerae may normally be yellowish, so jaundice may be best appreciated close to the iris or on the palate. Pallor is more likely to be detected through examination of the conjunctivae, nail beds, palms, and soles.

Children from some cultures may show physical evidence of having received certain folk medicine treatments. Among the most striking examples are patterned petechial eruptions, seen most often in children from Southeast Asia, caused by the treatment known as coin rubbing. In this common traditional treatment, the patient's skin is rubbed with heated coins or spoons (which may have been dipped in oil) to treat a condition such as sore throat or bronchitis. Typically, this treatment leaves linear, dark, petechial eruptions on the skin. Clinicians unfamiliar with this practice and its characteristic physical signs have been known to mistake its skin manifestations for signs of child abuse. Similar false accusations of child abuse have been made by health professionals unfamiliar with the blue birthmarks known as mongolian spots, which occur in a high percentage of dark-skinned individuals of all racial backgrounds and which can be mistaken for bruises.

Culturally Sensitive Prescribing

Race and ethnic background can affect patient responses to prescribed medications. Significant ethnic differences in the distribution of genetic variants of enzymes involved in metabolizing many drugs can result in important variations in drug response and toxicity. For example, glucose-6-phosphate dehydrogenase (G6PD) deficiency is found in some African Americans, Southeast Asians, and people from the Mediterranean region, in whom it may cause hemolysis in response to medications such as sulfonamides and antimalarial agents. Asians and African Americans may be more sensitive than whites to some psychotropic drugs. Variations in the way drugs are metabolized can alter their therapeutic effects. Hypertensive black patients tend to respond better to calcium channel blockers and diuretics than to beta-blockers or angiotensin-converting enzyme inhibitors. Such examples underline the importance of "pharmaco-cultural" awareness in prescribing medications for patients of various racial and cultural backgrounds.

Gaining Wisdom by Hindsight

After you have had a clinical encounter with a family whose cultural background differs from your own, review the experience and ask yourself, "How could I have done better for this child and family?" Such reflection helps refine your cross-cultural sensitivity and makes your subsequent experiences with families from different cultures more satisfying for all concerned.

SUMMARY

We live in an era of increasing multiculturalism and racial diversity. To deliver a comparable quality of care to *all* children and their families, each of us must acquire a solid working knowledge of the customs and beliefs of other population groups, including their traditional family relationships, authority structures, and perceptions of illness and disability. Effective communication, with the use of experienced health interpreters whenever necessary, is the single most important skill required to ensure understanding and effective therapeutic collaboration among the physician, child, and family.

REFERENCES

1. Groce NE, Zola IK: Multiculturalism, chronic illness and disability. Pediatrics 91:1048–1055, 1993.
2. Flores G: Culture and the patient-physician relationship: Achieving cultural competency in health care. J Pediatr 136:14–23, 2000.
3. Wilson PA, Griffith JR, Tedeschi PF: Does race affect hospital use? Am J Public Health 75:263–269, 1985.
4. Hahn B: Children's health: Racial and ethnic differences in the use of prescription medications. Pediatrics 95:727–732, 1995.
5. Bettez S: Personal Communication quoted by Brown W, Barrera I: Enduring problems in assessment: The persistent challenges of cultural dynamics and family issues. Inf Young Children 12:34–42, 1999.
6. Li C, Walton JR, Nuttall EV: Preschool evaluation of culturally and linguistically diverse children. In Nuttall EV, Romero I, Kalesnik J (eds): Assessing and Screening Preschoolers: Psychological and Educational Dimensions, 2nd ed. Needham Heights, MA, Allyn & Bacon, 1998.
7. Fadiman A: The Spirit Catches You and You Fall Down: A Hmong Child, Her American Doctors and the Collision of Two Cultures. New York, Farrar, Straus & Giroux, 1997.

SUGGESTED READINGS

American Medical Association: Culturally Competent Health Care for Adolescents. Chicago IL, American Medical Association, 1994.
Canadian Pediatric Society: Children and Youth New to Canada: A Health Care Guide. Ottawa, Canadian Pediatric Society, 1999.
Geissler EM: Pocket Guide to Cultural Assessment. St. Louis, Mosby–Year Book, 1995.
Kinsman SB, Sally M, Fox K: Multicultural issues in pediatric practice. Pediatr Rev 17:349–355, 1996.
Kleinman A, Eisenberg L, Good B: Culture, illness and care: Clinical lessons from anthropologic and cross-cultural research. Ann Intern Med 88:251–258, 1978.
MacKune-Karrer B, Taylor EH: Toward multiculturality: Implications for the pediatrician. Pediatr Clin North Am 42:21–30, 1995.
Pachter LM: Practicing culturally sensitive pediatrics. Contemp Pediatr 14:1–12, 1997.
Waxler-Morrison N, Anderson J, Richardson E: Cross-Cultural Caring: A Handbook for Professionals in Western Canada. Vancouver, University of British Columbia Press, 1990.

chapter 3

Assessment of Physical Growth and Nutrition

RICHARD B. GOLDBLOOM

How short is too short? How fat too fat? When is a child really too thin or too tall? Pathologic disturbances of growth are easy enough to recognize when they are extreme. However, most children who are brought to physicians because their parents are concerned about abnormalities of growth or nutrition turn out to be in the "gray areas" of physical growth—at the extremes of the normal distribution curves where normality and abnormality overlap. Thus, in many clinical situations, the first problem is to decide whether the child is expressing an extreme of normality or true abnormality. Three procedures are required for making good clinical decisions: (1) accurate measurements, (2) comparison with appropriate normal standards, and (3) (too often neglected) careful assessment of the child's genetic endowment, both of somatotype and of growth pattern or trajectory.

Key Point

It is often forgotten that children resemble their parents, not only in their ultimate body configuration but also with respect to the route (trajectory) they travel to attain that final appearance.

Therefore, in children with growth deviations that are possibly "constitutional," it is essential to find out what father and mother looked like around the same age. Looking at old family photos often helps. These may show that the heavy-set, 190-cm (6-ft, 3-in.) father of an abbreviated, needle-shaped 10-year-old boy was, like his son, the shortest and thinnest in his class until he was 15, when he underwent a major adolescent growth spurt and bypassed his classmates. Or asking the skinny girl's plump, anxious mother how much she herself weighed on her wedding day may surprisingly divulge that this woman, 152 cm (60 in.) tall, who now weighs 66 kilos (145 lb), weighed only 43 kilos (95 lb) "soaking wet" at the time of her marriage.

MEASUREMENTS AND GROWTH CHARTS

Recumbent Length versus Height

Because most babies younger than 10 to 12 months cannot stand alone and most toddlers refuse to stand still, any child younger than 2 years should be measured for length in the recumbent position. In children of this age group, recumbent length and standing height are not the same, the former being significantly greater. Standard growth charts for younger children are based on measurements of recumbent length. Various accurate measuring devices, some cheap and others expensive, are available for determining recumbent length and height. The essential point is to use a stable, accurate, fixed device if both individual and serial measurements are to mean anything (Figs. 3–1 and 3–2). Accuracy is a

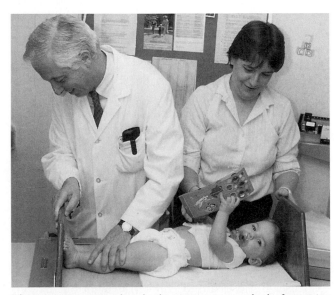

Figure 3–1 Measuring length: the appropriate method of assessing linear growth in children younger than 2 years. Keeping the youngster entertained improves accuracy.

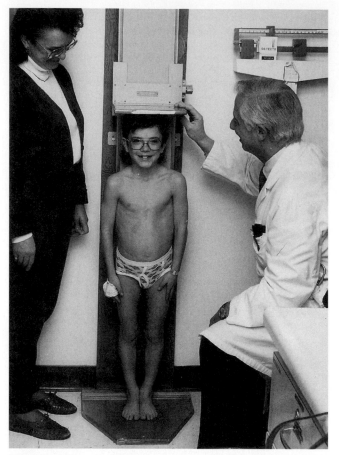

Figure 3–2 Measuring height: The apparatus should be fixed and accurate. The child should be positioned with the head and heels touching the back board.

must but never more than when there is the slightest concern about the child's growth. To be absolutely sure, check all measurements at least twice, and never accept anyone else's measurements as reliable.

Finally, never commit the unpardonable sin of eyeball approximation—as, unfortunately, many still do. Notoriously unreliable methods include putting pen or pencil marks on a piece of paper on which the baby is lying, to approximate crown and heel, then removing the baby and measuring the distance between marks, or laying a tape measure beside or under the baby. These disreputable practices are highly inaccurate and can lead to unreliable charting of growth and misdiagnoses of disproportion between linear and ponderal growth.

Weight

Infants and young children should be weighed naked or with a diaper at most, with the weight of the diaper subtracted afterward. The scales should be reliable and should be checked for accuracy and balance before each use. In hospitalized children, weight fluctuations often influence management. Therefore, infants should be weighed at the same time each day, ideally in the morning before being fed and by the same caregiver.

Any unusual or unexpected fluctuation calls for reweighing. If a sudden gain or loss of weight is validated, a reasonable explanation (e.g., edema causing a sudden gain, or inadequate intake, diuresis, or diarrhea causing a sudden loss) should be sought.

Occasionally, young children resist sitting or standing alone on a scale to be weighed. In such cases, rather than struggling for success, have a parent stand on the scale holding the child in the arms. Then weigh the parent alone, and determine the child's weight by subtraction.

Head Circumference

The technique for measuring head circumference is described in Chapter 7. Remember to check the measurement at least once to be certain it is accurate.

LARGE AND SMALL HEADS

> **Key Point**
>
> By far the most common cause of an unusually large head in an apparently normal infant or child is having a parent with a large head—often the father, who may or may not be present at the visit.

For some reason, it is more often the father who has the oversized cranial vault. Therefore, if a child's head circumference is two standard deviations or more above the mean, simply apply a tape measure to each of the parents' heads to see where *their* measurements fit on the chart before creating anxiety or considering further investigation. Once it has been established that this is a familial characteristic and that the affected parent and child are both otherwise normal, no further investigation is necessary. This normal variant is known as *benign familial megalencephaly.*

Below-normal head circumference can occasionally also be familial and benign (i.e., without associated developmental problems). More often, it is associated with developmental delay, even when familial. The usual cause of poor cranial growth is poor brain growth. Much less commonly, it can result from premature fusion of several cranial sutures (*premature synostosis*). If all cranial sutures fuse prematurely, the head circumference will be small and the child eventually may show evidence of increased intracranial pressure, such as papilledema and radiographic evidence of increased pressure by the cerebral gyri on the inner table of the skull—exaggeration of the so-called digital impressions. This condition is quite rare.

More often, premature synostosis involves a single suture or pair of sutures. It may be recognized clinically in two ways. First, an elevated bony ridge is often palpable along the length of the fused suture. Second, the

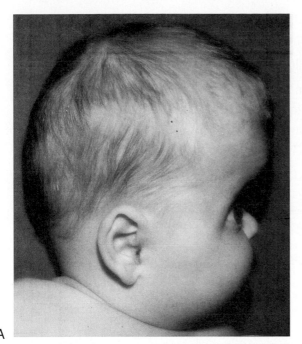
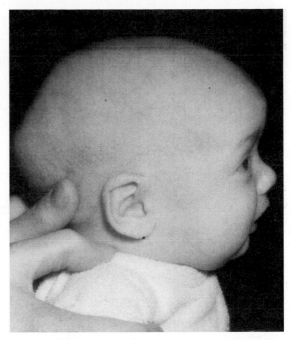

A   B

Figure 3–3 *A*, Distortion of skull growth caused by premature synostosis (fusion) of coronal sutures. *B*, Distortion of skull growth caused by premature synostosis of sagittal suture (dolichocephaly).

cranial shape is distorted in a predictable, recognizable way, depending on which sutures have closed prematurely. Remember that the direction in which the skull bones grow is perpendicular to the suture lines; the directions in which the skull can and cannot grow after synostosis of a suture are therefore predictable, as is the shape of the resulting cranial distortion. For example, if the sagittal suture fuses prematurely, further lateral growth of the skull is prevented. Anteroposterior growth will continue (perpendicular to the coronal sutures), and the skull will become long and narrow (*dolichocephaly*) (Fig. 3–3).

Graphic Recording of Measurements

The child's recumbent length or standing height, body weight, and head circumference should be recorded and plotted on appropriate age- and sex-specific growth charts. In North America, the 1977 National Center for Health Statistics (NCHS) growth charts have been replaced by the Centers for Disease Control and Prevention (CDC) Growth Charts for the United States (Fig. 3–4).[1] Unlike the 1977 charts, the 2000 CDC growth charts represent the current mix of breast-fed and formula-fed infants in the United States. In addition, CDC charts are now available for plotting body mass index (BMI) in percentiles for age and sex.*

Special growth charts have been developed for children with certain dysmorphic conditions, including Down syndrome, Turner syndrome, and achondroplasia (see Suggested Reading).

Proportion and Disproportion

When a child seems unusually short, first determine whether the growth retardation is proportional or disproportional; that is, whether there is significant disproportion between the growth of the head, trunk, and extremities. The chondrodysplasias, of which the best recognized is achondroplasia, are characterized by shortening of the limbs with normal linear growth of the trunk. Thus, the achondroplastic child (terms such as *dwarf* and *midget* should never be used, because they have very disturbing connotations for parents) has a normal sitting height but a markedly reduced standing height.

ARM SPAN AND ITS RELATIONSHIPS

If a child is old enough to cooperate, you can measure the arm span by having the youngster stand with the back and heels touching the wall and the arms fully extended parallel to the floor, palms facing forward. With parental assistance and using a *steel* tape measure, measure the distance between the third fingers of each hand. The span-height difference and span-to-height ratio then can be determined (Fig. 3–5).

---

*The 2000 CDC Growth Charts are available on the Internet (at: www.cdc.gov/growthcharts) and the CDC's Epi Info software, in which both exact percentiles and z scores can be calculated (software available from the CDC, Atlanta, GA).

Text continued on page 40.

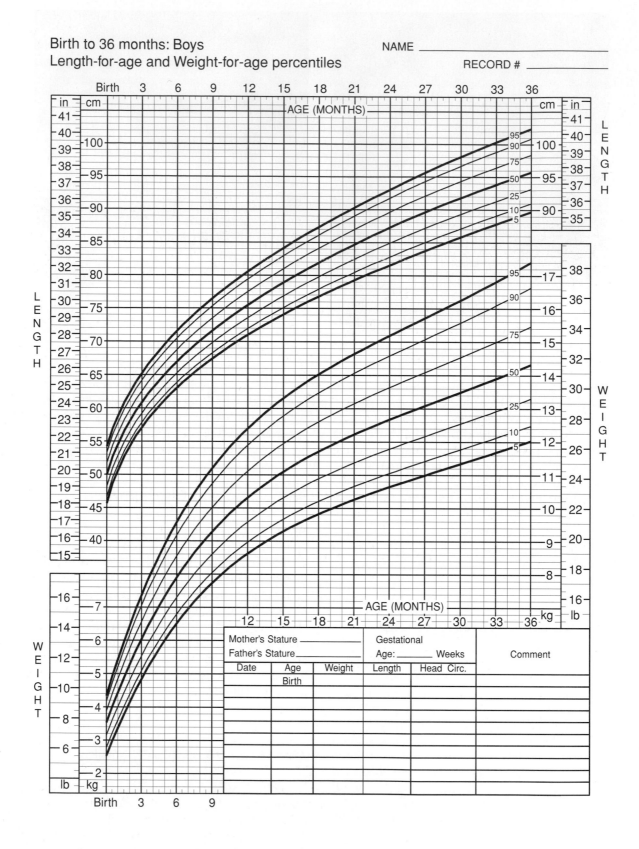

Birth to 36 months: Boys
Length-for-age and Weight-for-age percentiles

NAME _____

RECORD # _____

A

Figure 3–4 Growth charts for children from birth to 20 years. *A* through *D*, Sex-specific growth charts for infants (birth to 36 months): length-for-age and weight-for age percentiles (*A* and *B*), and head circumference–for-age and weight-for-age percentiles (*C* and *D*). *E–H*, Sex-specific growth charts for older children (2 to 20 years): stature-for-age and weight-for-age percentiles (*E* and *F*), and body mass index–for-age percentiles (*G* and *H*). *I* and *J*, weight-for-stature percentiles. (Redrawn from Ogden CL, Kuczmarski RJ, Flegal KM, et al: Centers for Disease Control and Prevention 2000 growth charts for the United States: Improvements to the 1977 National Center for Health Statistics version. Pediatrics 109:45–60, 2002.)

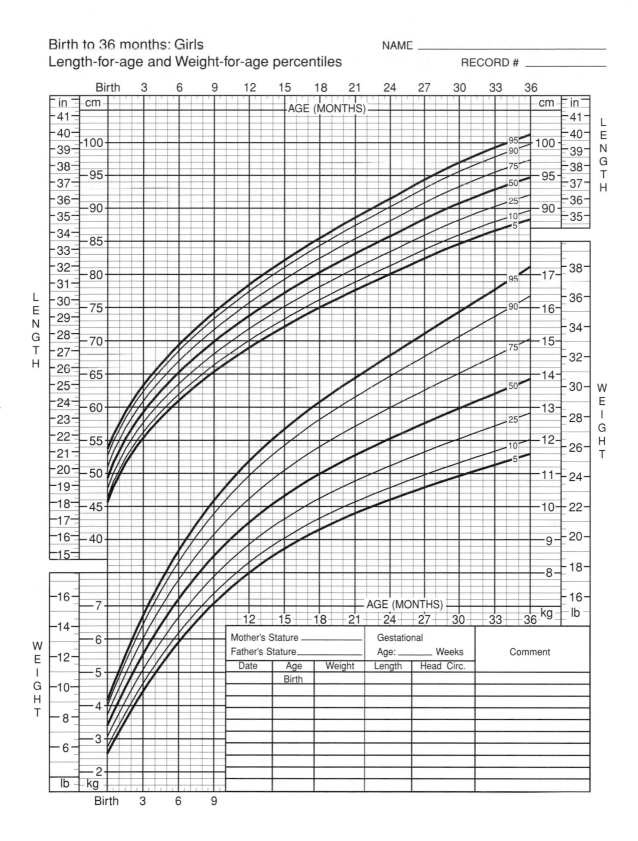

Birth to 36 months: Girls
Length-for-age and Weight-for-age percentiles

B

Figure 3–4 *Continued*

Birth to 36 months: Boys
Head circumference-for-age and
Weight-for-length percentiles

NAME _____

RECORD # _____

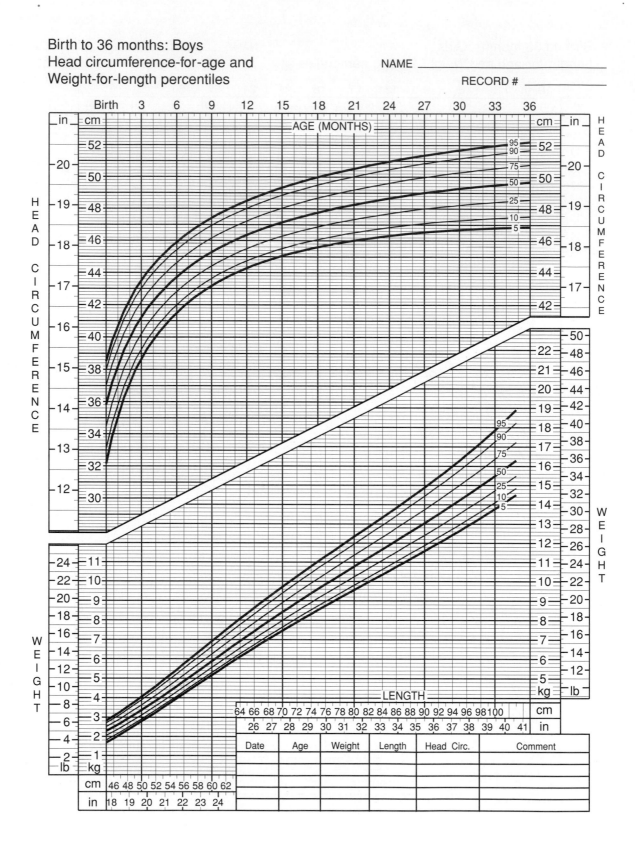

C

Figure 3–4 *Continued*

Birth to 36 months: Girls
Head circumference-for-age and
Weight-for-length percentiles

NAME _____

RECORD # _____

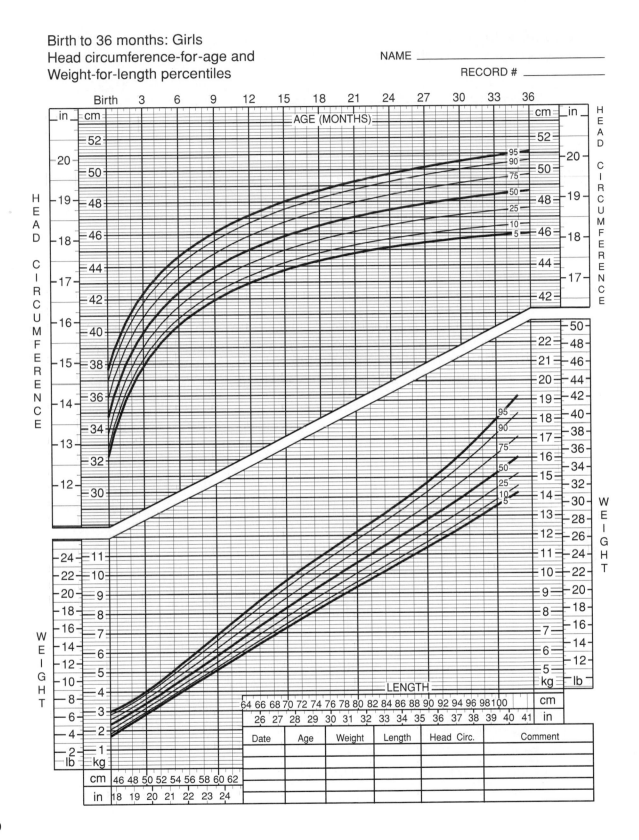

D

Figure 3–4 Continued

2 to 20 years: Boys
Stature -for-age and Weight-for-age percentiles

NAME _____

RECORD # _____

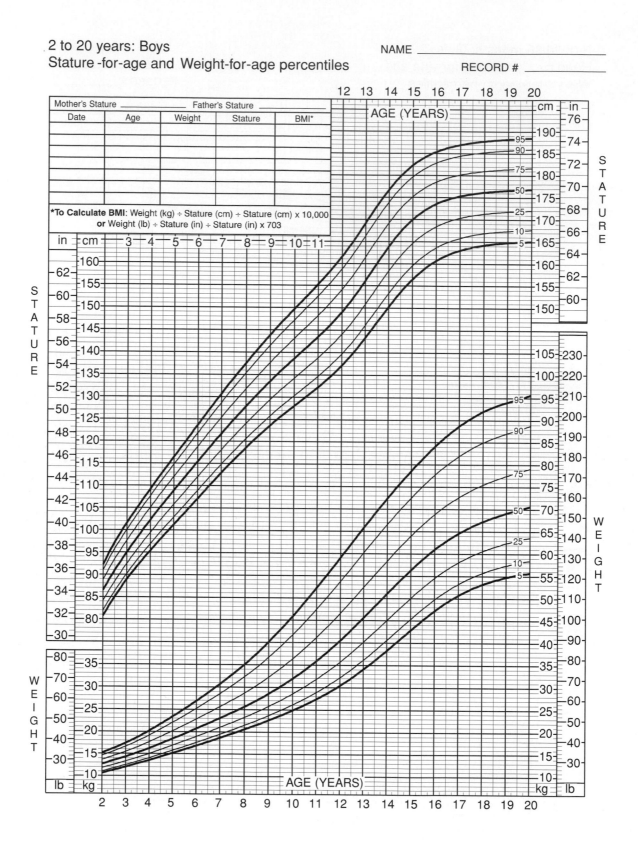

E

Figure 3–4 *Continued*

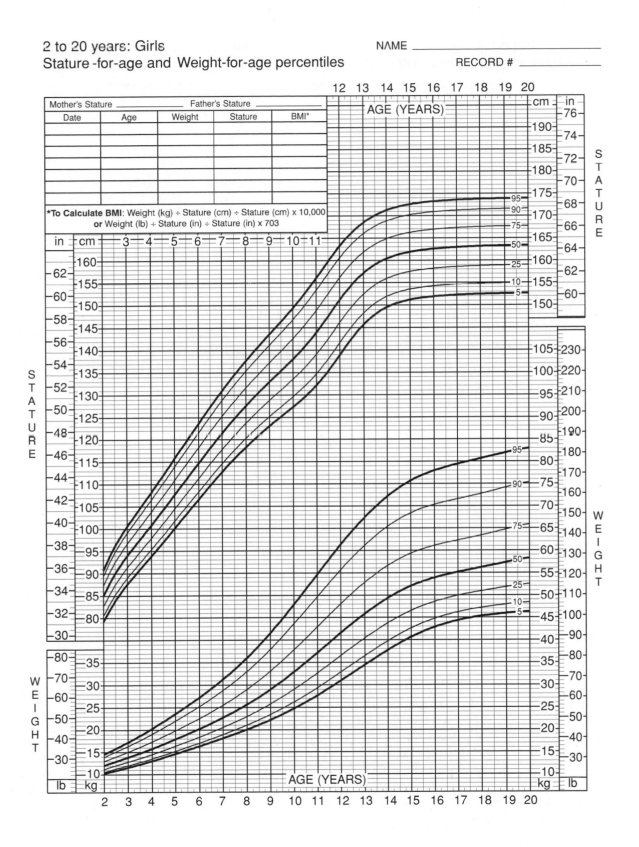

2 to 20 years: Girls
Stature-for-age and Weight-for-age percentiles

F

Figure 3–4 *Continued*

2 to 20 years: Boys
Body mass index-for-age percentiles

NAME _____

RECORD # _____

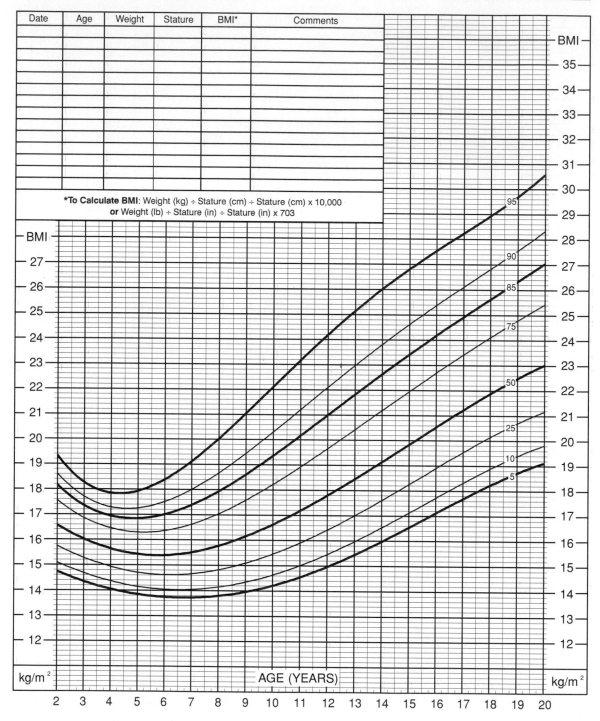

*To Calculate BMI: Weight (kg) ÷ Stature (cm) ÷ Stature (cm) x 10,000
or Weight (lb) ÷ Stature (in) ÷ Stature (in) x 703

G

Figure 3–4 *Continued*

2 to 20 years: Girls
Body mass index-for-age percentiles

NAME _____

RECORD # _____

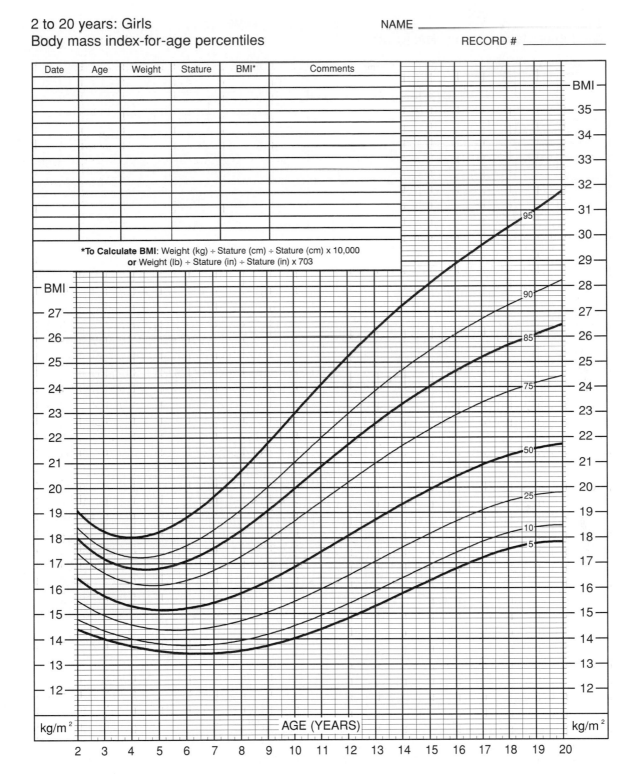

Date	Age	Weight	Stature	BMI*	Comments

*To Calculate BMI: Weight (kg) ÷ Stature (cm) ÷ Stature (cm) x 10,000
or Weight (lb) ÷ Stature (in) ÷ Stature (in) x 703

H

Figure 3–4 *Continued*

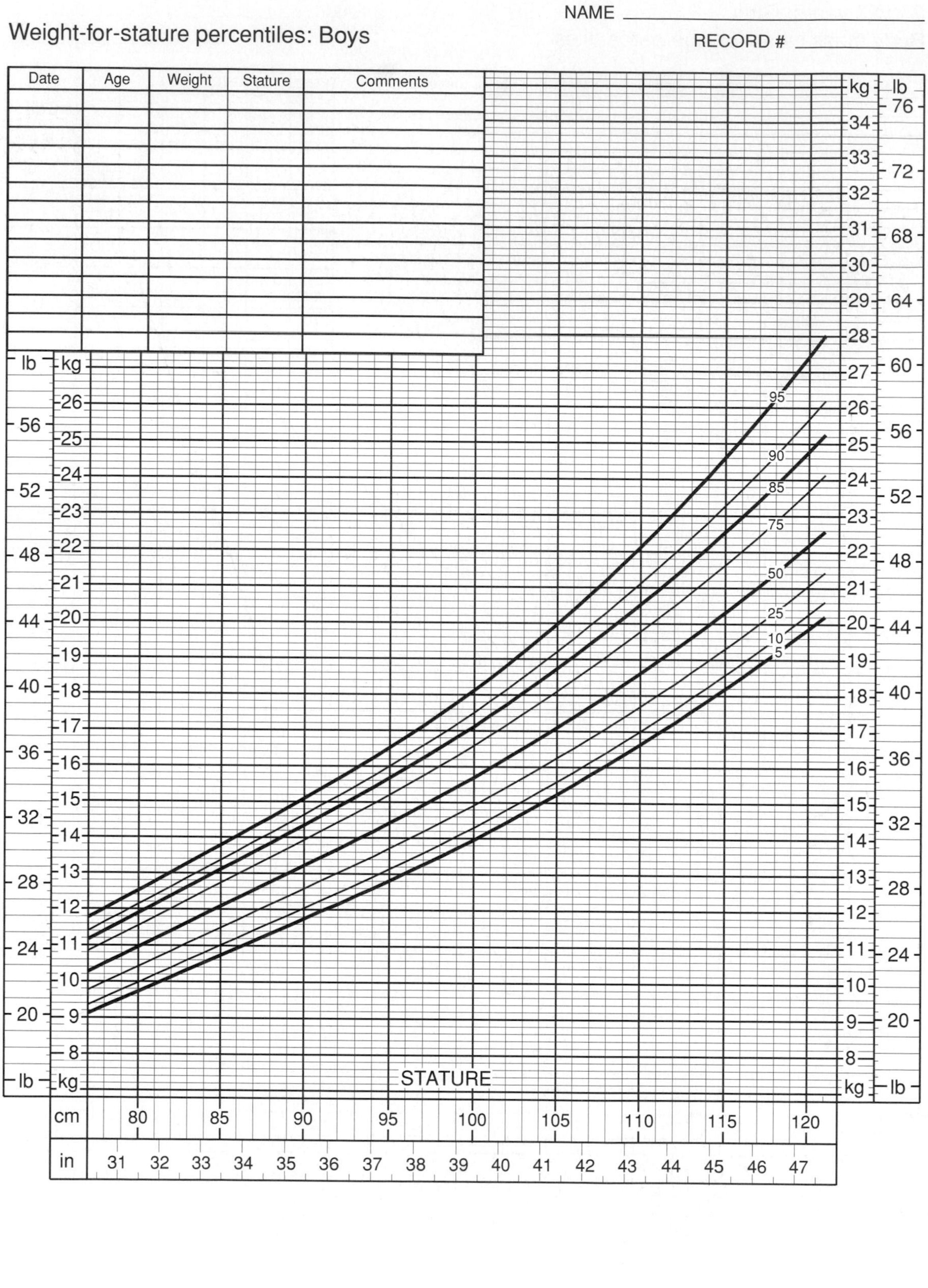

NAME
RECORD #
Weight-for-stature percentiles: Boys
Date
Age
Weight
Stature
Comments
kg
lb
95
90
85
75
50
25
10
5
STATURE
cm
in

Figure 3–4 *Continued*

Weight-for-stature percentiles: Girls

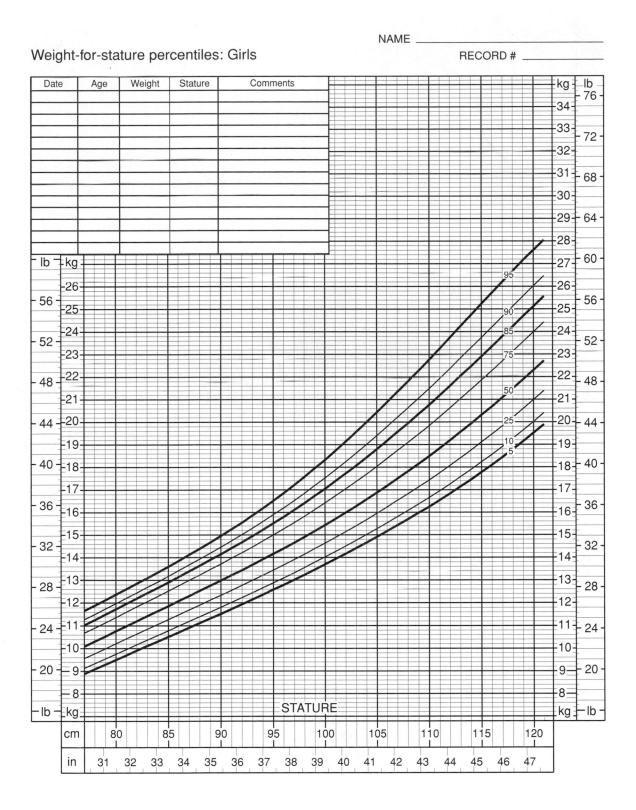

J

Figure 3–4 *Continued*

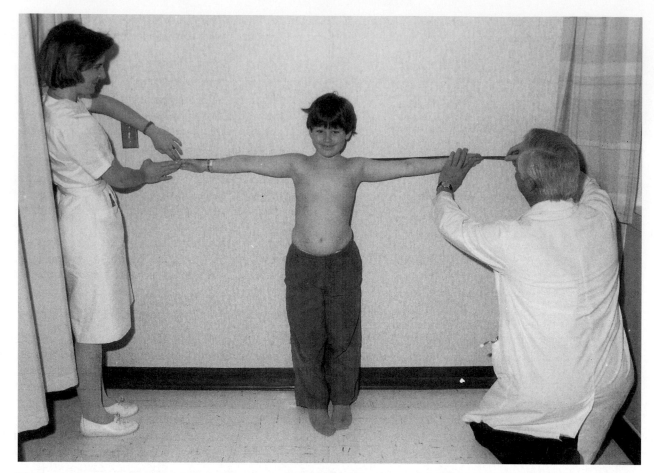

Figure 3–5 Measuring arm span. It is preferable to use a steel tape measure. Measure the distance between the tips of the third fingers.

MEASURING THE UPPER AND LOWER SEGMENTS

Measuring the upper and lower segments is tricky and not always supremely accurate. It requires identifying the top of the pubic ramus and marking it on the skin with a pen or wax pencil. This sounds easier than it is, especially in a chubby youngster in whom you must indent the adipose lower abdominal-suprapubic area to locate the top of the pubic bone. After you make the mark and release the pressure, the abdominal wall springs back, and the mark does not always stay where you thought it was relative to the pubis. Make sure the youngster does not bend forward to look; this movement can distort the measurement. Measure the lower segment by dropping a steel tape perpendicularly from the mark to the floor (Fig. 3–6*A*). Then determine the length of the upper segment by subtracting the lower segment length from the height. Figure 3–6*B* shows the average upper-to-lower segment ratio at different ages. Remember that there are ethnic and familial differences in these ratios, so it is sometimes necessary to measure the parents as well.

IMPORTANCE OF SEQUENTIAL MEASUREMENTS

Key Point

A single measurement can establish whether the growth attained is in the normal range but does not reveal the past or predict the future.

When growth deviates from normal, sequential measurements over significant periods are needed to evaluate the underlying problem adequately and, when necessary, monitor the response to treatment. The older the child, the longer the measurement interval required to assess the significance of an apparent deviation in growth. Measurement of growth velocity, as described later in this chapter, can be more informative than "snapshot" anthropometric measurements taken at a particular moment in time.

Regular charting of height and weight should be part of every child's routine health care. Parents should be encouraged to keep their own records of these measure-

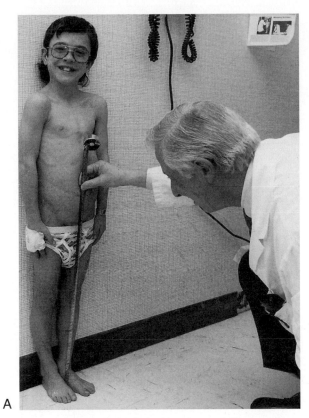

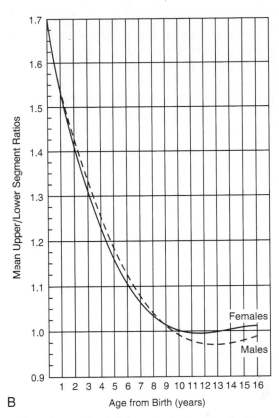

A   B

Figure 3–6 *A*, Measuring the lower body segment. Subtract this measurement from the standing height to obtain the upper body segment measurement. *B*, Upper-to-lower body segment ratio for males and females, birth to 16 years. (*B* from Greene MG [ed]: The Harriet Lane Handbook, 12th ed. St. Louis, Mosby–Year Book, 1991.)

ments. During the first year of life, it is not unusual for a child's height and weight measurements to cross at least one percentile line. After 18 months to 2 years of age, however, measurements in most healthy children tend to stay within the same percentile channel (or an adjacent channel) until the onset of puberty, unless obesity develops or some form of significant growth delay occurs.

Once normal head circumference has been established in infancy, usually it is not necessary to continue measuring the head circumference regularly unless specifically indicated (e.g., by the presence of a neurologic or developmental problem).

Useful as they are, growth charts are no substitute for good judgment. Children march to individual drummers and often follow the growth timetables of their antecedents. Remember that the curves on published growth charts are smoothed-out representations of observations on many healthy youngsters. Individual children, not having read this textbook, may not follow such idealized curves precisely, because their growth may occur in rather irregular spurts.

When you find any deviation from these "normal" curves, ask yourself what a deviation means in terms of the child's genetic, medical, and psychosocial history. Whenever possible, use growth charts derived from the same geographic area or ethnic population as that of the child under consideration. For example, many

Southeast Asian children have heights and weights below the third percentiles of North American growth charts. These differences may reflect a mixture of ethnic (genetic) and nutritional (environmental) factors. When the economy of a region improves dramatically over a few years, average heights and weights of children can increase remarkably. In fact, average height for age in a particular population over time is a telling measure of the health of a nation's economy.

A Language for Communicating Information About Children's Growth

From time to time, a child is described as being "below the third percentile for height and weight." That popular style of description is an abomination and a curse. In the first place, by definition, 3% of the normal population rightfully belongs below the third percentile of any growth parameter. This placement does not automatically categorize them as abnormal. Also, such phrasing tells absolutely nothing about (1) how far below the third percentile the measurements fall or (2) whether the child's linear and ponderal growth are impaired proportionally or disproportionally.

Several ways of expressing growth measurements are more meaningful and useful. One is to determine the child's "height-age" or "weight-age" (i.e., the age for which a particular measurement represents the 50th percentile on a standard growth chart) (Fig. 3–7). Figure 3–7 shows that the boy in question, whose chronologic age is 10 years 4 months, has a height-age of 7 years and a weight-age of 5 years 2 months. Stating each measurement in these terms immediately communicates the image of a child who is a little shorter than average but is also underweight or undernourished, even in relation to his reduced height.

Weight as a Percentage of Ideal

A useful way to express the ponderal aspect of a child's nutritional status is weight as a percentage of ideal.

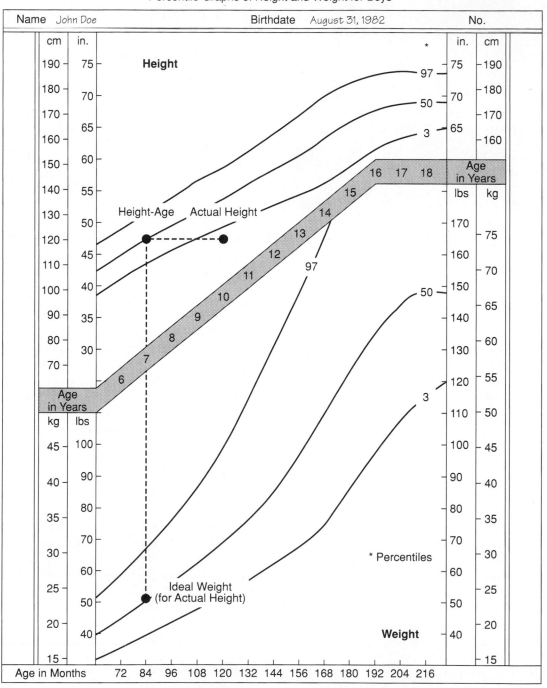

Percentile Graphs of Height and Weight for Boys

Name   John Doe   Birthdate   August 31, 1982   No.

Figure 3–7 Determination of height-age, weight-age, and ideal weight for (actual) height.

Ideal, in this case, means the ideal (average) weight for the child's actual recumbent length or standing height. This value is simple to determine, as illustrated in Figure 3–7. The boy's height is 120 cm. Extrapolating horizontally to the 50th percentile shows that he has a height-age of 7 years. If you drop a perpendicular line to the weight graph from his height-age until it meets the 50th percentile weight line, you see that the ideal weight for his actual height is approximately 23.5 kg.

Express his actual weight as a percent of ideal as shown in the following equation:

$$\frac{\text{Actual weight (kg)}}{\text{Ideal weight for actual height (kg)}} \times 100 = \text{Weight as \% ideal}$$

Table 3–1 shows the classification of protein-energy malnutrition according to McLaren and Read's[2] arbitrary system. This system of expression conveys an immediate and vivid image of the severity of a child's undernutrition, irrespective of the underlying cause.

Children with Delayed Growth

There are many causes of growth delay; those due to growth hormone or thyroxine deficiency are discussed in Chapter 16.

Key Point

By far the most common growth problem seen in clinical practice is constitutional growth delay, a normal variant seen predominantly in boys, in whom the onset of puberty may be delayed in tandem with slow linear growth.

In children with constitutional growth delay, bone maturation is typically delayed (i.e., bone age is significantly less than chronologic age), and there is frequently a history of similar linear growth and pubertal delay in one of the parents.

Table 3–1   CLASSIFICATION OF PROTEIN-ENERGY MALNUTRITION

Classification	Weight as Percentage of Ideal (for Actual Height)
Normal	90–110
Mild protein-calorie malnutrition	85–90
Moderate protein-calorie malnutrition	75–85
Severe protein-calorie malnutrition	<75

From McLaren DS, Read WC: Classification of nutritional status in early childhood. Reprinted with permission of Elsevier Science, The Lancet, 1972, Volume 2, p 146.

Anxieties of the Short Child

The boy with constitutional growth and pubertal delay, whose classmates seem to tower over him, often fantasizes that he is destined to remain forever frozen in stature at his current height and in his hairless, undersized, microgenital state. For such a youngster, vague reassurance that he will "probably" attain normal height offers cold comfort at best. By contrast, giving him and his parents a reliable prediction of his adult height will immediately improve his self-image and his vision of the future. Furthermore, if you use either an orchidometer or a centimeter rule and determine that the testes have begun to enlarge beyond the usual prepubertal volume of approximately 1 mL, you can state *unequivocally*, despite the absence of adult sweat odor or of pubic or axillary hair, that the miracle of puberty is already under way and that further exciting developments are imminent.

Predicting Ultimate Adult Height

Several methods are available for predicting adult height in children who have no underlying skeletal abnormality, endocrinopathy, or other disease. The technique developed by Roche and colleagues[1] (named the *RWT method,* after its authors) is one of the most accurate, simple, and practical.

The original RWT method required only a knowledge of the child's age, weight, height, bone age (as determined from a radiograph of one wrist and comparison with normal standards), and the midparent stature (the sum of mother's and father's heights divided by 2). Each measure was then multiplied by a positive or negative weighting factor derived from the calculated mathematical contribution of each to the determination of final adult height. The sum of values of the positive products minus the sum of the values of the negative products yields the predicted adult height in centimeters. The original article on this method provides the necessary tables and instructions to do this simple calculation,[1] which takes only a few moments, especially if you use a pocket calculator.

The most recent modification of the RWT method, known as the Khamis-Roche method,[3] does not require the determination of skeletal age and has only marginally less accuracy and reliability than the original method.

GROWTH (HEIGHT) VELOCITY

For children who have significant disturbances of growth, for those receiving treatments that may impair growth, and for those being treated for growth disturbances, measurement of growth velocity can provide far more meaningful information than static measurements of height and weight. Tanner and Davies[4] have pointed out that once puberty has begun, the use of cross-section population curves to plot the growth of children is misleading, because, for example, the course of the 50th percentile line is not always followed by individual children. If a child happens to be an early or late maturer, the deviation is particularly marked. The growth velocity charts devised by Tanner and Davies[4] include standard curves for early and late maturers (Fig. 3–8). When you are using this system to record height velocity, remember that the height incre-

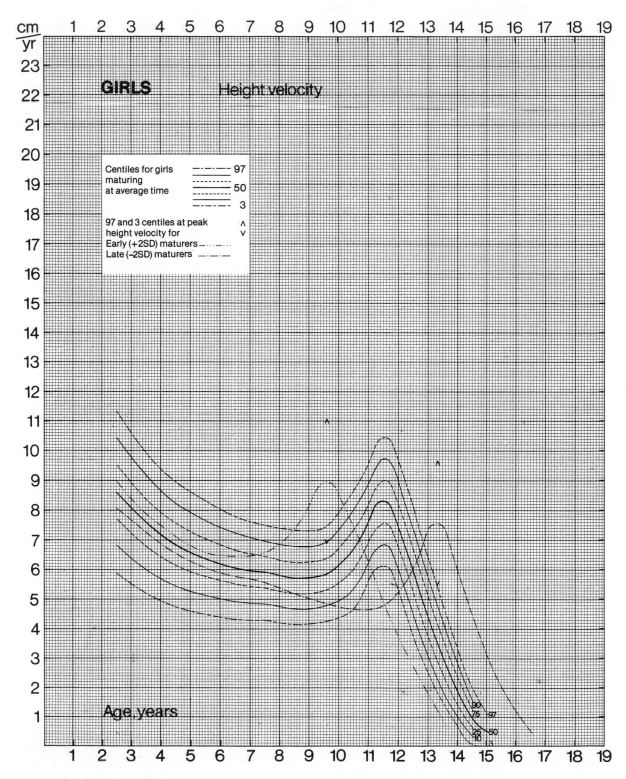

Figure 3–8 Growth velocity charts for North American girls (*A*) and boys (*B*). (From Tanner JM, Davies PSW: Clinical longitudinal standards for height velocity for North American children. J Pediatr 107:317, 1985.)

ments on which the charts are based are whole-year increments.

Like trees, children grow faster in the spring and summer and slower in the fall and winter. Therefore, height measurements used to determine growth velocity should be made at no less than approximately 1-year intervals.

Staging Pubertal Development

In normal children and in children with any disorder of secondary sexual development, the stage of puberty must be defined as precisely as possible whenever a physical examination is performed. Generalizations such as "early breast development," "scant pubic hair,"

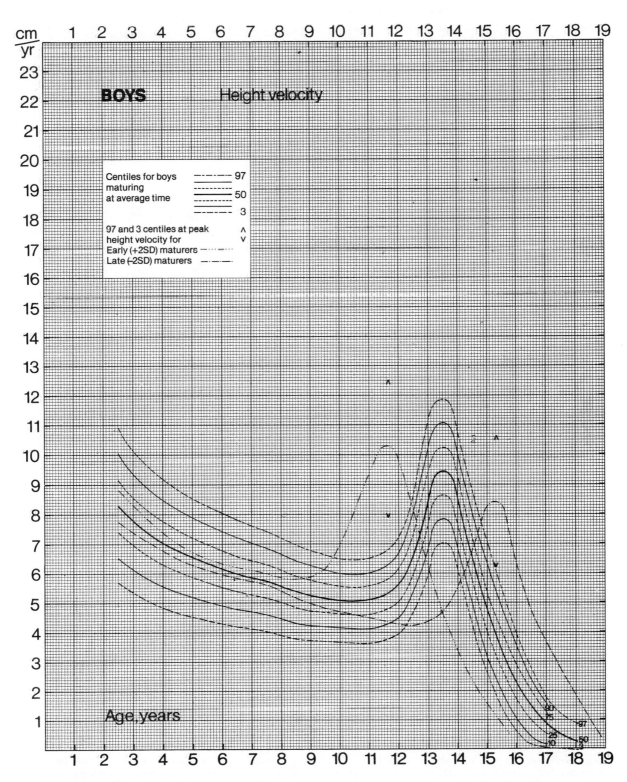

B

Figure 3–8 *Continued*

and "prepubertal testes" are too vague and imprecise for documenting the progression of normal or abnormal secondary sexual development with the required accuracy, especially when the interval between consecutive examinations may be months or years, and memory for such details cannot be trusted.

Tanner and Davies[4] divided the process of breast and pubic hair development into stages, as outlined in Figure 3–9. Their system of staging these elements of pubertal development is now used worldwide. In most girls, breast budding is the earliest physical manifestation of puberty, although in some perfectly normal girls,

Pubertal development in size of male genitalia.

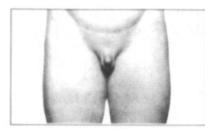

Stage 1. The penis, testes, and scrotum are of childhood size.

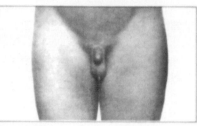

Stage 2. There is enlargement of the scrotum and testes, but the penis usually does not enlarge. The scrotal skin reddens.

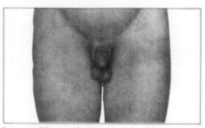

Stage 3. There is further growth of the testes and scotum and enlargement of the penis, mainly in length.

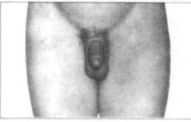

Stage 4. There is still further growth of the testes and scrotum and increased size of the penis, especially in breadth.

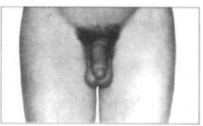

Stage 5. The genitalia are adult in size and shape.

Pubertal development of male pubic hair.

Stage 1. There is no pubic hair.

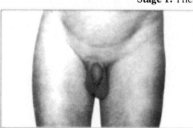

Stage 2. There is sparse growth of long, slightly pigmented, downy hair, straight or only slightly curled, primarily at the base of the penis.

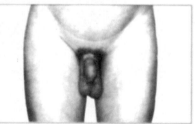

Stage 3. The hair is considerably darker, coarser, and more curled. The hair spreads sparsely over the junction of the pubes.

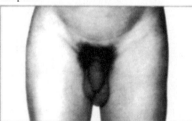

Stage 4. The hair, now adult in type, covers a smaller area than in the adult and does not extend onto the thighs.

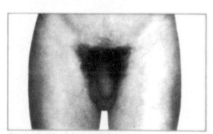

Stage 5. The hair is adult in quantity and type, with extension onto the thighs.

A

Figure 3–9 Tanner stages of breast and pubic hair development in boys (*A*) and girls (*B*). (Used with permission of Ross Products Division, Abbott Laboratories Inc., Columbus, OH 43215. From Johnson TR, Moore WM, Jeffries JE: *Children Are Different: Physiology,* 2nd ed. Columbus, OH, Ross Products Division, Abbott Laboratories Inc, 1978.)

adrenarche (pubic and axillary hair development) may precede *thelarche* (breast development). The idea that girls enter puberty much earlier than boys has been somewhat overstated, simply because the physical manifestations of the onset of puberty are more obvious in girls. On average, girls show their earliest secondary sexual changes only about 6 months ahead of the earliest manifestations in boys. The first pubertal change in most girls takes the form of breast budding. In boys, however, the typical earliest evidence of secondary sexual development is testicular enlargement. Thus, unless you make it a regular practice to use an orchidometer or other means to measure testicular size, you can easily miss a 1- or 2-mL increase in testicular volume between visits, whereas you would rarely miss a newly evident breast nodule.

Pubertal development in size of female breasts.

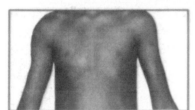 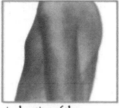 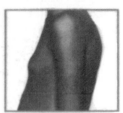

Stage 1. The breasts are preadolescent. There is elevation of the papilla only.

Stage 2. Breast bud stage. A small mound is formed by the elevation of the breast and papilla. The areolar diameter enlarges.

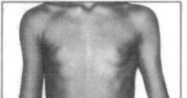 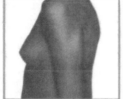 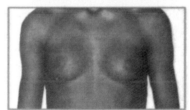 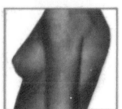

Stage 3. There is further enlargement of breasts and areola with no separation of their contours.

Stage 4. There is a projection of the areola and papilla to form a secondary mound above the level of the breast.

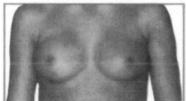 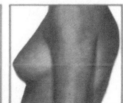

Stage 5. The breasts resemble those of a mature female as the areola has recessed to the general contour of the breast.

Pubertal development of female pubic hair.
Stage 1. There is no pubic hair.

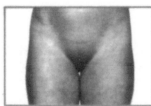 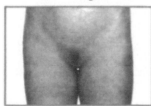 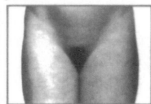 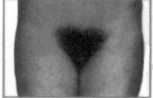

Stage 2. There is sparse growth of long, slightly pigmented, downy hair, straight or only slightly curled, primarily along the labia.

Stage 3. The hair is considerably darker, coarser, and more curled. The hair spreads sparsely over the junction of the pubes.

Stage 4. The hair, now adult in type, covers a smaller area than in the adult and does not extend onto the thighs.

Stage 5. The hair is adult in quantity and type, with extension onto the thighs.

B

Figure 3–9 Continued

> ### Key Point
>
> Two phenomena of early breast development in girls deserve special attention. First, in many perfectly normal girls, breast development is asymmetric. A breast nodule may appear on one side months before the other. Second, it is not unusual for an early breast nodule to be a little tender or sensitive to the friction of overlying clothing.

Parents who discover a unilateral "breast lump," a firm tender nodule under the areola in their 8-year-old daughter, sometimes begin to worry that the child may have cancer. Let no physician ever fall in with such a suspicion or think of performing a biopsy of such a nodule, which represents the child's entire endowment of breast tissue. Breast malignancy is, for practical purposes, unknown in children.

DENTAL DEVELOPMENT

Children vary considerably in the ages at which their teeth erupt, depending partly on genetic factors. Table 3–2 summarizes the average ages for calcification and eruption of primary and secondary dentition and, for primary dentition, the usual ages of tooth shedding.

Teething—Myths and Realities

For centuries, the normal process of tooth eruption in infants and toddlers has been blamed for an endless variety of symptoms and illnesses. To this day, many people (including a good many clinicians) are convinced that, at the very least, complaints of drooling and irritability can be attributed to the teething process. Others add to this list of purported clinical associations fever, loose stools, rashes, colds, and even convulsions. Such convictions have resulted in various over-the-counter remedies being marketed for application to the gums, ostensibly to relieve discomfort. The problem is that people (parents or physicians) who believe in a causal association between teething and symptoms tend to examine the baby's gums only when the child is symptomatic. Because children are teething nonstop from a few months of age onward, such assumptions of guilt by association become self-fulfilling prophecies. In the few, well-designed prospective studies of the clinical correlates of tooth eruption that have been conducted—including a Finnish investigation that consisted of regular daily recording of symptoms and signs and careful examination for gum tenderness—no clinically significant associations between tooth eruption and the traditionally assumed clinical manifestations have been found. Old ideas die hard, however, and centuries-old beliefs in a causal linkage between teething and symptoms in infants are no exception.

> ### Key Point
>
> The evidence clearly indicates that physicians who attribute a baby's unexplained symptoms to teething are seeking the last haven of refuge for the diagnostically destitute.

Table 3–2 CHRONOLOGY OF HUMAN DENTITION

	Calcification		Eruption		Shedding	
	Begins at	Complete at	Maxillary	Mandibular	Maxillary	Mandibular
Primary or deciduous teeth						
Central incisors	5th fetal mo	18–24 mo	6–8 mo	5–7 mo	7–8 yr	6–7 yr
Lateral incisors	5th fetal mo	18–24 mo	8–11 mo	7–10 mo	8–9 yr	7–8 yr
Cuspids (canines)	6th fetal mo	30–36 mo	16–20 mo	16–20 mo	11–12 yr	9–11 yr
First molars	5th fetal mo	24–30 mo	10–16 mo	10–16 mo	11–11 yr	10–12 yr
Second molars	6th fetal mo	36 mo	20–30 mo	20–30 mo	10–12 yr	11–13 yr
Secondary or permanent teeth						
Central incisors	3–4 mo	9–10 yr	7–8 yr	6–7 yr		
Lateral incisors	Max: 10–12 mo Mand: 3–4 mo	10–11 yr	8–9 yr	7–8 yr		
Cuspids (canines)	4–5 mo	12–15 yr	11–12 yr	9–11 yr		
First premolars (bicuspids)	18–21 mo	12–13 yr	10–11 yr	10–12 yr		
Second premolars (bicuspids)	24–30 mo	12–14 yr	10–12 yr	11–13 yr		
First molars	Birth	9–10 yr	6–7 yr	6–7 yr		
Second molars	30–36 mo	14–16 yr	12–13 yr	12–13 yr		
Third molars	Max: 7–9 yr Mand: 8–10 yr	18–25 yr	17–22 yr	17–22 yr		

Mand, mandibular; Max, maxillary.
From Behrman RE, Vaughan VC: Nelson Textbook of Pediatrics, 13th ed. Philadelphia, WB Saunders, 1987.

Nutritional Assessment

A child's height and weight and the weight-to-height relationship remain the best general guides to overall nutritional status with respect to protein-calorie sufficiency.

Today, with the exception of iron deficiency (with or without associated anemia), deficiencies of specific nutrients due to inadequate intake are relatively rare in developed countries. Nutritional rickets (vitamin D deficiency) virtually disappeared after the introduction of legal requirements to supplement cow's milk with vitamin D. Similarly, universal supplementation of infant formula products with vitamin C eliminated scurvy from the clinical scene. By far the most common clinical nutritional disorders are protein-calorie malnutrition, secondary either to disease or to psychosocial deprivation, and nutritional iron deficiency. Other specific nutrient deficiencies are more likely to be associated with particular diseases; examples are deficiencies of fat-soluble vitamins in steatorrheic states and of vitamin B_{12} in chronic ileal disease.

Clinical Assessment of the Child with Possible Iron Deficiency

HISTORY

Several questions have special importance when an infant is suspected of iron deficiency, but the two most useful are "How much milk does the baby drink?" and "Is he or she still on the bottle?" These questions are more informative than trying to quantify dietary iron intake from various solid food sources. If, for example, a 1-year-old boy with iron deficiency is consuming 1350 mL (45 oz) of whole cow's milk every 24 hours, it is possible to calculate instantly what this intake represents in terms of the child's daily energy requirement, because whole milk provides approximately 20 kcal/oz, or 66.6 kcal/100 mL: 45 oz × 20 kcal/oz = 900 kcal. If the youngster weighs 11 kg and you remember that an average 1-year-old's total daily energy requirement is roughly 80 to 90 kcal/kg body weight, it is obvious that this boy's daily intake of 900 kcal in the form of milk is providing nearly 100% of his total daily energy requirement. The implications for treatment, aside from the need for iron supplementation, are obvious.

Parents of an iron-deficient infant often report that the baby refuses all solids. In such infants, severe reduction or temporary elimination of milk intake, coupled with discontinuation of bottle feeding, invariably results in rapid acceptance of solid foods. Severe restriction of milk intake not only increases the child's appetite for solid foods but removes the dietary cause of gastrointestinal mucosal alterations that may result in erythrocyte and protein losses into the gut—which further aggravate the iron deficiency state and may cause hypoalbuminemia and edema.

It is also important to ask whether the child has a history of pica (ingestion of foreign materials such as dirt and starch). For reasons that are poorly understood, iron deficiency states are sometimes associated with pica, which usually disappears when the iron deficiency is corrected.

> **Key Point**
>
> Nutritional iron deficiency in North America is frequently a marker for psychosocial deprivation. Thus, a detailed evaluation of family circumstances, relationships, and problems is essential for comprehensive management and support.

EXAMINING THE PALE CHILD

When a child appears pale, the first issue to be settled is whether the pallor is synonymous with anemia. Pseudoanemia is one of the most common nondiseases of early childhood. Some children are congenitally pale or white-skinned because their skin is less pigmented than average, a phenomenon that is usually hereditary. This hypopigmentation (usually associated with blond or blondish hair color) increases the transparency of the skin. Usually one or both parents are white-skinned as well. The greater transparency of the skin causes the bluish veins to be unusually visible (e.g., on the face or upper anterior chest wall). In clinical assessment, the key point is to examine areas such as the conjunctivae, nail beds, and oral mucosa. In the child with pseudoanemia, the color is normally red, the dietary history usually reveals an adequate intake of iron-containing foods (e.g., infant cereals, egg yolk, meat), and there is no apparent loss of energy. Always ask whether the child is happy and normally active.

If the history does suggest the possibility of iron deficiency and the child is anemic, the mucous membranes may appear pale. The iron-deficient, milk-fed infant often appears large and doughy. Other particular physical findings to be noted are (1) hepatosplenomegaly and (2) peripheral edema—because severe iron deficiency is sometimes associated with hypoproteinemia.

Evaluating the Obese Child

> **Key Point**
>
> Obese youngsters rarely visit physicians' offices willingly or on their own initiative. Their unhappiness about their obesity is often magnified by the prospect of exposure to medical scrutiny.

The fact that our society is so biased against the obese and so worshipful of pathologic thinness as the ideal human form undoubtedly magnifies the discomfiture and low self-esteem of obese youngsters. The first step in preparing to be genuinely helpful to an obese child is to search your own soul and ask yourself how you really feel about obese people in general. When I put this question to groups of physicians, the initial response is usually an embarrassed silence. After a few moments, the hesitant confessions begin, often as single adjectives—"frustrated," "depressed," "angry," or even "disgusted." A medical degree confers no immunity against societal bias. Feelings of frustration among health professionals are also understandable, because with only a few exceptions, most long-term results of attempts to treat obesity and achieve sustained weight loss, especially in children, have been disappointing. To some extent, such frustration results from trying to treat the obesity rather than attempting to help the child who happens to be obese. How you begin the interview and the tenor and content of the conversation are therefore critical.

It is a good idea for your first words to the youngster to consist of a compliment (on any handy topic—clothing, good looks, etc.). They should be followed by a statement that you are glad to see the child. It also helps to verbalize your recognition that the child may be unhappy about coming to see you but that you would like to try to help him or her anyway.

You must take great care not to reinforce, by verbal or nonverbal slips, the poor self-image that is almost universal among obese youngsters. Even parents of an obese youngster, who often are obese themselves, may inadvertently contribute to this negativism, perhaps because they recall the unhappiness they experienced growing up obese. They may see themselves reflected in the child and do not like what they see.

SPECIAL FEATURES OF THE OBESE CHILD'S HISTORY

When parents of an obese youngster are asked to tell you their concerns, they often describe a succession of problems, worries, and disappointments related to issues such as the child's eating habits, lack of physical activity, and problems with peer relationships. Understandably, listening to such a recital is not calculated to strengthen the child's self-image, even though the parents' concerns are based in reality. When this happens, I usually try to turn the conversation in a more positive direction, by saying something like "Now that you've told me your concerns about Jenny, I'd like you to tell me all the things that are really good about her—her special talents and what you think are her best qualities as a person." I often record the positives and negatives in two-column fashion—both sides of the youngster's personal ledger. If weight loss is allowed to become the sole criterion of successful management of the obese child, all concerned

are often doomed to further disappointment and frustration. More important, such a narrow approach does a major disservice to the child and family.

Details of the family history are of major importance. I always obtain as much accurate information as possible about the heights and weights of parents, grandparents, aunts, and uncles. When possible, I weigh and measure both parents myself.

Key Point

In the overwhelming majority of patients with childhood-onset obesity, the principal determinants are genetic, and this fact is often confirmed by a detailed family history.

When a parent is also obese, I usually ask for memories about his or her own childhood. The answers are often deeply moving and revealing. Such parents may remember being called names and having difficulties with peer relationships, and they often say things like "I don't want her to go through what I went through."

Recent evidence suggests that some obese individuals may have inherited disorders in the regulation of energy balance, which may partly explain why, for many obese children, dietary energy intake is not greater than average. In others, the genetic regulation of satiety may be at fault. Obesity is not the result of a character defect or a lack of willpower! Therefore, you must carefully avoid approaches that, inadvertently or otherwise, blame the victim.

The next important item in history-taking is a rough estimate of the child's energy output. An excellent indirect indicator is an estimate of the total number of hours of television-watching, computer activity, and video game play per day. I review the youngster's average day, hour by hour and program by program, with the child and family. This usually provides a good estimate of the youngster's kinetic output and the level of immobility. The inactive child is often a reflection of inactive parents.

I usually avoid questioning the child about food intake at the first interview, for the following three reasons:

- The child has already been imbued with the belief that he or she eats too much.
- Dietary restriction alone is a notoriously unsuccessful mode of treatment.
- Adiposity is not the youngster's sole problem, and among the various difficulties identified, it may be the one least amenable to modification.

Of greater importance to management is a full description of the family's usual mealtime scene. Do they eat together as a family? Do the parents make disapproving remarks about or focus accusatory looks on each mouthful of food consumed or request for a second helping? Having the child and parents describe a typical mealtime scenario often reveals that what should be a happy, mutually supportive family gathering is, in fact, a dreaded, miserable experience for the youngster. This fact has important implications for management.

In the same vein, the history of the family's group recreational activities may help identify interventions that may be useful in increasing the youngster's energy output. If family meals represent unhappy times for obese children, their school day may be even worse, as a result of name-calling and other forms of harassment by their peers. A telephone call to the child's teacher may help, both to assess the child's academic performance and to sense the teachers' attitudes toward the youngster. This discussion may offer an opportunity to develop a therapeutic alliance designed to make the child's day happier by raising the youngster's self-esteem through interventions such as assignment of new responsibilities in the classroom coupled with extra praise and recognition.

When the time does come to evaluate the child's energy intake, do not overlook the liquid calories—soft drinks, juices, and milk. It may be possible to reduce the youngster's daily energy intake significantly by substituting diet soft drinks, low-fat milk, and water. These simple changes may be readily acceptable to youngsters and parents alike.

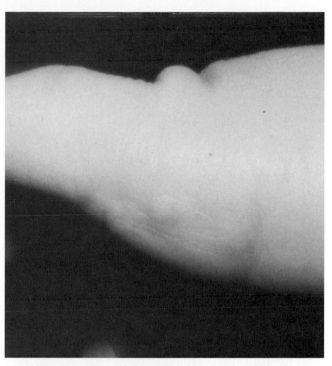

Figure 3–10 A barely visible stellate scar at the base of the fifth finger is the sole evidence of a "skin tag" (actually a rudimentary supernumerary digit) that was tied off in the newborn period. This finding is an important clue to the cause of this child's obesity, which is Laurence-Moon-Biedl syndrome.

PHYSICAL EXAMINATION OF THE OBESE CHILD

Key Point

Do not begin the physical examination of an obese youngster by putting the child on the scale!

Most prepubertal children with obesity that cannot be ascribed to a specific syndrome or endocrine disturbance, in other words, the majority of obese children, tend to be taller than average for their genetic endowment. The obese child who is short for age deserves a closer look for a specific cause.

A useful way to begin is by examining the hands and feet. In obese youngsters, always check the area of skin over the base of the fifth finger and fifth toe. The presence of a small stellate scar is a telltale sign that a "skin tag" was removed soon after birth with a suture tied tightly around it (Fig. 3–10). In fact, such a skin tag was almost certainly a rudimentary supernumerary digit; this finding, coupled with obesity, raises the likelihood that the child has Laurence-Moon-Biedl syndrome, in which obesity is often associated with polydactyly, retinitis pigmentosa, progressive loss of vision, some developmental delay, and, often, a progressive nephropathy.

Another uncommon but important sign to look for in the hands of obese children is the "metacarpal sign." Children with pseudohypoparathyroidism (a syndrome associated with obesity) often have strikingly short fourth and fifth metacarpals and metatarsals. Elicit the metacarpal sign by having the youngster make a fist. When the fourth and fifth metacarpals are hypoplastic, the relevant knuckles are absent, often replaced by dimples (Fig. 3–11). Incidentally, this sign is also seen in females with Turner syndrome (XO anomaly).

"Stretch marks" are often observed in the skin of the abdomen and thighs of obese children. (See Chapter 16 for the distinction between Cushing syndrome and obesity of other causes.)

Another obesity syndrome that can usually be suspected simply from the history and physical findings is the *Prader-Willi syndrome.* In affected children, obesity typically develops between 6 months and 6 years of age and is usually associated with mild to moderate developmental delay, hypotonia, and feeding problems in infancy. The facies is characteristic, with prominent forehead and rather almond-shaped eyes. The hands and feet are small. Compulsive overeating usually appears by 3 years of age. In boys, the penis and scrotum are often small, and in girls, the labia poorly formed. The syndrome is usually caused by a defect in the paternal chromosome 15.

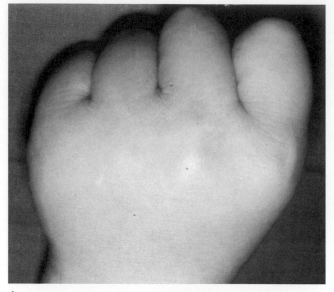

A

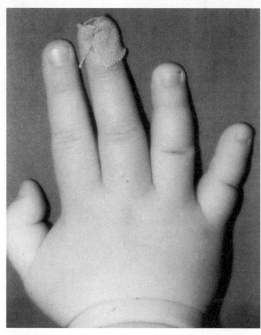

B

Figure 3–11 The "metacarpal sign" (unusually short fourth and fifth metacarpals) seen in pseudohypoparathyroidism and in Turner syndrome. *A*, No fourth and fifth knuckles are seen when the child makes a fist. *B*, Extension of the fingers shows unusually short fourth and fifth fingers due to hypoplasia of the metacarpals.

Evaluating the Child with Failure to Thrive

The central issue in a child with failure to thrive is usually whether the child's nutritional or growth deficiency is due to underlying (unrecognized) organic disease or to some form of psychosocial deprivation. As with other growth disturbances, the history, physical examination, and observation of the child's behavior and the family interaction are by far the most powerful tools in the diagnostic armamentarium.

Key Point

It is well established that when the history and physical findings in infants or children with failure to thrive do not suggest a specific underlying organic disease, unfocused protocols of laboratory investigations and imaging studies almost never provide the answers.

Besides, when there are no clear-cut signs suggesting organic disease, a complete psychosocial history and direct observation of the child and family (as described in Chapter 1) usually allow a diagnosis of deprivational growth failure and malnutrition to be made on distinct positive grounds rather than by exclusion.

ENERGY INTAKE AND REQUIREMENTS

Once the history, family observation, and physical examination are complete, the most useful subsequent clinical observation is quantitation of the youngster's daily energy intake—a process that is often best accomplished with the help of a therapeutic nutritionist. Quantitation is the key. A casual qualitative observation that an undergrown or undernourished child is "eating well" can be extremely misleading and may prejudice the child's recovery. The daily energy intake required for normal growth and that required for growth recovery are two vastly different quantities.

Two bits of knowledge are essential for proper clinical evaluation and for a successful plan of management:

- Knowledge of the normal (average) intake for a child of this age (or of this height-age)
- Appreciation of the fact that the achievement of growth recovery ("catch-up" growth) requires a daily energy intake that averages 50% more than the normal daily intake of a well-nourished child of the same height.

Average daily energy intakes at different ages are listed in Table 3–3. Whether a child's growth and nutritional deficits are rooted in organic or psychosocial disease, the final common pathway of pathogenesis is usually that insufficient kilocalories are reaching the circulation. As Keys and colleagues[5] showed in their classic studies of experimental human starvation, the problem is complicated by the fact that one of the prime clinical manifestations of prolonged undernutrition is anorexia. The combination of anorexia and a greatly increased energy requirement for recovery makes for a major challenge, which explains why hyperalimentation methods (enteral or parenteral) are so often required at the outset to induce nutritional and growth recovery in these youngsters.

To understand why such supernormal energy intakes are required for catch-up growth, consider the case of a

Table 3–3 DAILY ENERGY REQUIREMENTS AT DIFFERENT AGES

Age	Sex	Units (kcal/kg/day)
0–2 mo	Both sexes	100–120
3–5 mo	Both sexes	95–100
6–8 mo	Both sexes	95–97
9–11 mo	Both sexes	97–99
1 yr	Both sexes	101
2–3 yr	Both sexes	94
4–6 yr	Both sexes	100
7–9 yr	M	88
	F	76
10–12 yr	M	73
	F	61
13–15 yr	M	57
	F	46
16–18 yr	M	51
	F	40

Modified from Canada Bureau of Nutritional Sciences: Recommended Nutrient Intaktes for Canadians. Ottawa, Health and Welfare Canada, Canadian Government Publication Centre, 1983.

child whose weight is well below the 3rd percentile line and whose weight is low for height. If such a child is fed (and assimilates) a normal daily intake, the youngster will grow at a normal incremental rate. The weight curve, therefore, will rise at a slope parallel to the 3rd percentile, but the gap will not be narrowed. Nutritional recovery, or catch-up growth, calls for a daily rate of weight gain that is well above normal (often as much as 50% above normal). A supernormal growth rate clearly requires an above-normal energy intake.

SUMMARY

Accurate measurements over time and comparisons with established standards are essential for the early recognition, diagnostic evaluation, and successful management of growth and nutritional problems in infants and children. In evaluating children with suspected growth problems, you should always first ask, "Is the child normal?" The concepts of height-age, weight-age, and weight as a percentage of ideal provide useful, meaningful, and accurate expressions for communicating information about children's growth. The trajectory and outcome of every child's growth must always be considered in relation to those of the parents.

The mythology that continues to be associated with teething as an explanation for symptoms and signs in infants should be put to rest permanently.

Understanding the special anxieties of the short child, the fat child, and the child with delayed puberty should dictate the style and content of the history interview and of the physical examination. For children with constitutional delay of growth and puberty, calculation of the predicted adult height is as valuable therapeutically as it is diagnostically.

For the obese child, understanding the central role of heredity and appreciating how obesity colors and complicates the child's life allows you and the family to focus on the potentially remediable associated problems rather than reinforcing everyone's belief in the impossible dream of thinness as the sole path to health and happiness.

At the other nutritional extreme, when a child fails to thrive, a truly thorough history and physical examination, coupled with observation of family interaction, rarely leave much doubt as to whether the child's problem is rooted in organic disease or in psychosocial deprivation. In either instance, the distinction is based on positive findings, not on exclusion.

Protein-calorie malnutrition and iron deficiency are by far the most common nutritional abnormalities encountered in North American children. In the latter condition, the history of prolonged bottle-feeding and the child's consumption of most of his or her energy requirement in the form of milk are key to understanding the pathogenesis and designing a successful program of management.

REFERENCES

1. Roche AF, Wainer H, Thiessen D: The RWT method of height prediction. Pediatrics 56:1026, 1975.
2. McLaren DS, Read WC: Classification of nutritional status in early childhood. Lancet 2:146, 1972.
3. Khamis HJ, Roche AF: Predicting adult stature without skeletal age: The Khamis-Roche method. Pediatrics 94:504, 1994 [published erratum appears in Pediatrics 95:457, 1995].
4. Tanner JM, Davies PSW: Clinical longitudinal standards for height velocity for North American children. J Pediatr 107:317, 1985.
5. Keys A, Brozek J, Henschel A, et al: The Biology of Human Starvation. Minneapolis, University of Minnesota Press, 1950.

SUGGESTED READING

Hall JG, Froster-Iskenius, Allanson JE: Handbook of Normal Physical Measurements. New York, Oxford University Press, 1989. (An invaluable, comprehensive, pocket-sized [large pocket] desk reference on all variety of physical measurements, both in normal infants and children and in those with various congenital anomalies and dysmorphic syndromes.)

chapter 4

Evaluating the Newborn Infant: Diagnostic Approach

ALEXANDRA A. HOWLETT, KRISTA A. JANGAARD, AND ELIHU P. REES

Ideally, if you are going to care for a newborn, you should get to know the family before the child's birth. This step is often taken by physicians in private practice but should be encouraged more widely. It makes antenatal care more comprehensive and helps the family care for the baby with as little anxiety as possible. Meeting the parents well before the delivery helps you become familiar with the prenatal history and makes you aware of important family issues.

Your main sources of information should be the following:

1. Talking with the parents.
2. Talking with the obstetrician or family physician.
3. Reviewing the mother's antenatal health record.
4. Reviewing the mother's hospital chart.

OBTAINING THE HISTORY

Table 4–1 lists the important questions that should be asked for any antenatal history.

APPROACH TO PHYSICAL EXAMINATIONS OF THE NEWBORN: WHEN, WHY, AND HOW

The First Examination

Examine every newborn infant at least twice (preferably three times) during the first few days of life. If possible, perform the first assessment in the hospital's delivery area to (1) identify any obvious major and minor congenital malformations, (2) assess gestational age, nutritional status, and vigor; and (3) determine how well the baby handles the transition from intrauterine to extrauterine life. Most babies make the major physiologic adaptations of this transition smoothly. The few who do not adapt

normally—those born prematurely or after perinatal stress or asphyxia—will need help to adapt successfully.

The method used almost universally in delivery rooms to evaluate the central nervous system (CNS) status and general adaptation of the neonate to extrauterine life is the Apgar score. This scoring system, summarized in Table 4–2, evaluates the baby in five different respects: heart rate, respiration, color, muscle tone, and reflex irritability (response to stimulation). These signs are usually evaluated at 1 minute and 5 minutes after birth. The Apgar score is the total of the baby's scores for each of the five signs. To be consistent, have the Apgar score recorded by an experienced observer (nurse or physician) whose principal responsibility is caring for and evaluating the baby. Interobserver variation in scoring may be considerable, and therefore, experience is essential. Evaluate the signs at exactly 1 minute and 5 minutes to establish the score, especially in relation to muscle tone and reflex irritability. The latter is usually elicited by flicking the sole of the foot; the appropriate response to this stimulation is a vigorous cry.

Recording the Apgar score serves two purposes. First, it ensures a careful evaluation of the baby during the immediate newborn period. Second, it helps to determine the presence and level of CNS depression and whether there is a need to continue resuscitation. In babies who need resuscitation, serial scores measured at 1, 2, 5, and even 10 minutes furnish a semi-quantitative method of recording recovery. The relationship of low Apgar scores and neurologic abnormality later in infancy is not reliable.

> **Key Point**
>
> Do not use the Apgar score as a means of defining asphyxia. A low score does not necessarily mean that the infant is suffering from asphyxia, as was previously believed.

Table 4–1   SIGNIFICANT ISSUES TO ASK ABOUT WHEN TAKING THE HISTORY FOR A NEWBORN

Mother's past pregnancies and their outcome	Number of pregnancies
	Stillbirths
	Abortions
	Neonatal deaths
	Cesarean section
	Health of surviving children (in neonatal period and to present)
	Specific concerns that parents may have about current pregnancy because of past experiences
Preexisting systemic illness in mother and maternal medications	Hypertension
	Depression
	Diabetes
	Seizure disorder
	Thyroid disease
	Cardiac disease
	Metabolic disorder (phenylketonuria)
Genetic history	History of inherited disorders
	Consanguinity
	Unexplained neonatal deaths in the family
History of current pregnancy	Date of last menstrual period
	Estimated date of conception by dates (and by ultrasonography if early ultrasonogram [9–13 weeks] available)
	Results of ultrasonography, amniocentesis, cordocentesis, chorionic villus sampling
	Pregnancy-induced hypertension, gestational diabetes
	Note maternal weight gain and blood pressure, fetal growth, blood type
	History of alcohol use, drug use (prescribed or illicit), cigarette use
	Group B *Streptococcus* status (if known)
	History of maternal surgery during pregnancy
	Concerns about placenta (placenta previa, thickening, etc.)
	Use of magnesium sulfate, betamethasone
Current labor and delivery	Induced or spontaneous labor (if induced, why?)
	Time of rupture of membranes and quality of amniotic fluid (bloody, meconium-stained)
	Length of second stage
	Use of medications (analgesics and time prior to delivery)
	Intrapartum fever and antibiotics
	History of fetal distress
	Presentation (vertex, breech, transverse)
	Vaginal or cesarean delivery (if cesarean, why?)
	Use of forceps or vacuum extraction
Adaptation to extrauterine life	Apgar scores
	Resuscitation needed? If so, what and for how long?
	Need for naloxone

Table 4–2   PARAMETERS OF EVALUATION USING THE APGAR SCORE

Sign	0 Points	1 Point	2 Points
Heart rate (beats/min)	Absent	Slow (<100)	>100
Respiratory effort (breaths/min)	Absent	Slow and irregular	Good, crying
Muscle tone	Flaccid	Some flexion of extremities	Active motion
Reflex irritability	No response	Grimace	Vigorous cry
Color	Pale	Cyanotic	Completely pink

The Apgar scoring system produces more than just a number. The presence or absence of individual signs should tell you not just that an infant had "an Apgar 6" but that this score was assigned because certain func-tions were absent or suboptimal. For example, a baby with congenital neuromuscular disease may score well for heart rate, respiratory effort, and color but poorly for muscle tone and reflex irritability. A preterm infant scores lower than a full-term baby because an immature baby's muscle tone is always less than that of a normal-term infant.

The accurate diagnosis of perinatal asphyxia is not easy and requires not only evaluation of the clinical condition at birth but also evaluation of umbilical cord arterial blood gases and subsequent clinical neurologic sequelae in the newborn period (hypoxic-ischemic encephalopathy). Low Apgar scores may be caused by many conditions affecting the baby, such as sepsis, neuromuscular disorders, and perinatal asphyxia.

The Second Examination

The best place to carry out the second physical examination is in the mother's room, preferably with both parents present. Having the parents there makes it possible to obtain further history details, complete the initial physical examination, answer questions on the spot, demonstrate and discuss normal variations or abnormalities discovered during the physical examination, and offer some valuable anticipatory guidance. This second, more thorough examination should be conducted within the first 12 hours of life. It is designed to identify congenital malformations, ascertain that adaptation to extrauterine life is proceeding normally, and detect any prenatally or perinatally acquired illnesses. The sooner it is performed, the happier the parents will be.

The Third Examination

The main purposes of the third examination are to discover postnatally acquired problems, such as infection and excessive jaundice, and to detect any malformations that were not apparent at the first or second examination, such as some forms of congenital heart disease whose murmurs are not audible on the first day of life. In past years, the third examination was often performed at 3 or 4 days of age. The current trend toward early discharge of mothers and infants from the hospital means discharge may occur as early as 24 hours after birth, and discharge is common by 48 hours after a normal vaginal delivery. Thus, the third examination often takes place after the mother has been discharged from the hospital. Early hospital discharge guidelines now recommend assessment of a newborn by a health care provider within 72 hours of discharge. It is, however, important that this third examination and assessment of the baby's condition be carried out within the first week of life. The third examination may be performed by a physician or by an experienced nurse or midwife and may take place in the hospital, in the home, or at a clinic or office.

Many of us learned physical examination initially with cooperative adult patients, in whom it was easy to start at the top of the head and work downward in a systematic cephalocaudal manner. Because infants are not always cooperative, you must be prepared to examine a newborn infant thoroughly but to keep the sequence of procedures flexible. For example, if the baby is resting quietly, first listen to the heart and chest, then palpate the abdomen. Carry out other parts of the examinations when the baby is active, moving, or even crying, but be sure to examine all systems and record the findings systematically.

CLINICAL OBSERVATIONS AND WHAT THEY MEAN

Encourage the parents to participate as much as possible in the examination—undressing the baby, holding the baby on the lap or the bed, and providing a stabilizing finger for the baby to grasp (Fig. 4–1). The first part of the examination is the most important. Do not touch the baby except to remove all clothing gently. The baby should be naked, warm, and well illuminated and should be helped to feel stable and secure on the examining surface. Improving the baby's stability and relaxation by letting him or her grasp the parent's or your finger allows an immediate appreciation of the strength of the baby's reflex grasp and reduces the tendency for instinctive startle reflexes that occur when the baby feels unstable and rolls on the examining surface.

The ideal time to examine a newborn is a couple of hours after a feeding, when the baby may not be too deeply asleep, as babies often are just after a feeding, nor awake and screaming, as they often are just before a feeding. Stand back and take a long hard look.

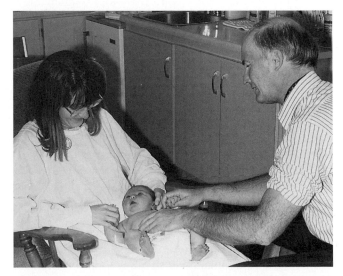

Figure 4–1 The newborn feels more stable and tends to relax if you allow the infant to hold your hand during the examination.

Educated observation often reveals far more than touching, poking, and kneading; while observing, answer the following questions:

1. Does the baby look normal or abnormal?
2. Do the body proportions, face, head, and neck appear grossly normal?
3. Are there any obvious deformities, malformations, or unusual appearances? If you have any doubts about the normality of the baby's facial appearance, look at the mother and father's features before jumping to conclusions.
4. Is the baby distressed or resting comfortably? Distress may be respiratory (or cardiopulmonary), with intercostal, subcostal, or suprasternal retractions (indrawing), tachypnea, and expiratory grunting. Other signs of neonatal distress are unusual irritability, and excessive crying, or the reverse—apathy, lethargy, and hypotonia.
5. What color is the baby's skin? A normal baby's skin is well oxygenated or pink; in babies of more pigmented races, the pinkness is best seen on the palms, lips, buccal mucosa, and conjunctivae. It is normal for babies to exhibit *acrocyanosis* (bluish or purplish color of the hands and feet). Parents may need reassurance that this is entirely normal. The extremities may be somewhat mottled with a netlike pattern if they are cool (*cutis marmorata*, literally, "marble skin") (Fig. 4–2). Generalized mottling may signify acidosis or vascular instability. Another variation of skin color is the so-called harlequin color change, seen mostly in low-birth-weight infants, in which the skin is dark pink or reddish on the dependent half of the baby but the upper half appears comparatively pale, with the two colors sharply demarcated along the midline. This is a striking phenomenon but has no pathologic significance.

Look for hematomas, hemangiomas, ecchymoses, and petechiae. The last can be associated with increased intravascular pressure during delivery, thrombocytopenia from the presence of platelet antibodies, or congenital infections. Cutaneous hemangiomas are often absent or minimally apparent at birth but develop and grow over the first weeks or months of life, only to regress spontaneously later. Ecchymoses may indicate more than usual trauma or an underlying coagulation disorder.

You can perform much of the newborn's neurologic examination without touching the baby. Do all four extremities move equally and maintain a general posture of flexion, with alternating flexion and extension movements? The eyes should move if they are open, and there may be sucking and tongue movements, yawning, facial grimacing, and spontaneous startle responses. The four most important parts of the neurologic assessment are (1) judging the baby's level of alertness, (2) observing

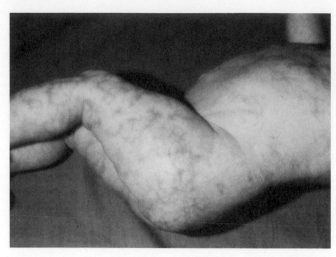

Figure 4–2 Cutis marmorata ("marble skin") can occur as a normal phenomenon when the baby is exposed.

spontaneous movement, (3) listening to the baby's cry, and (4) observing facial movements.

A baby's level of alertness varies with the time of day and the time of last feeding; normal newborns spend about 20 of the 24 hours asleep. Visual alertness is temporarily limited if erythromycin ointment or silver nitrate drops have been instilled in the eyes as prophylaxis for gonococcal ophthalmia.

LISTENING TO THE CRY

Babies normally cry when they are uncomfortable, disturbed, or hungry. Train yourself to listen carefully to infant cries because there is much to be learned from them. The normal cry should be strong; hoarseness, weakness, or an unusually high-pitched or low-pitched cry may indicate laryngeal or neurologic abnormalities. Repetitive inconsolable crying is also abnormal. An experienced nurse or mother can quickly tell you whether a particular baby's cry is normal and is sometimes the first to suspect a disorder simply on the basis of an unusual cry: the high-pitched "cerebral" cry; the low throaty cry of congenital hypothyroidism; the characteristic catlike cry of the cri du chat syndrome, or the weak, poorly sustained cry of the infant who is sick or cerebrally damaged or has Down syndrome.

MUSCLE TONE

By carefully examining many babies, you will become familiar with the differences among normal, increased, and diminished muscle tone of newborns. The differences cannot be described in words. Only by making it a regular practice to flex and extend babies' arms and legs repeatedly during every examination of newborns can you develop an instinctive "feel" for normal, increased, and decreased muscle tone. When a newborn baby is pulled to the sitting position from the supine, the head lags behind the trunk; a healthy full-term baby makes some effort to bring the head in line with chest. Once lifted to a sitting position, a full-term infant can keep the head upright for several seconds.

PRIMITIVE REFLEXES

Many so-called primitive reflexes can be elicited that may already have been observed during the earlier part of the examination.

Key Point

Reflexes should be symmetric, and the tone and strength of infant's limbs and truncal reflexes should be normal.

Asymmetric Tonic Neck Response

Assess for the asymmetric tonic neck response by turning the baby's head from midline to one side and noting the arm's gradual extension on the side to which the head is turned along with flexion of the other arm. The position resembles the classic fencing or boxing posture. Because of this reflex, it is important to ensure

that the baby's head is midline before you elicit any of the other responses.

Moro Reflex

Newborns often demonstrate the Moro, startle, or embrace reflex spontaneously when they are suddenly moved, exposed to a sudden loud noise, given the feeling of falling, or feel unstable on a flat surface. You can most reliably elicit this reflex by allowing the infant's head to drop (while supporting it gently) below the level of the rest of the body while the baby is in a reclining position. The baby extends the arms suddenly and rapidly with the hands open, then brings them back together more slowly in an embrace type of movement. The initial rapid movement may be accompanied by a grimace or cry (Fig. 4–3). Symmetry of movement is important. Weakness of one arm (e.g., in brachial plexus injury) results in an asymmetric Moro reflex.

Palmar Grasp

Find the palmar grasp by placing your index fingers in each of the baby's open hands; the baby's fingers should close around your fingers with strength enough to lift the baby's body part of the way off the bed or table (Fig. 4–4).

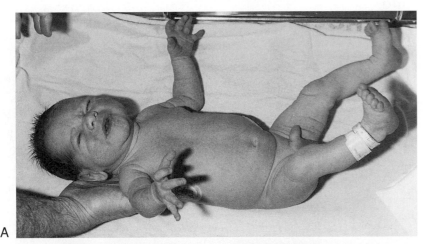

A

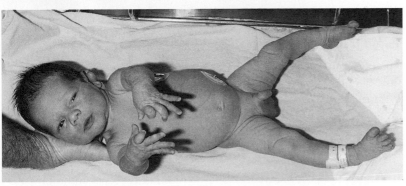

B

Figure 4–3 Induce the Moro or "embrace" reflex by giving the infant the feeling of falling. The response begins with a sudden extension of the arms and legs (*A*), which is followed by a slower embracing movement bringing the arms together (*B*). The Moro reflex is sometimes accompanied by a cry.

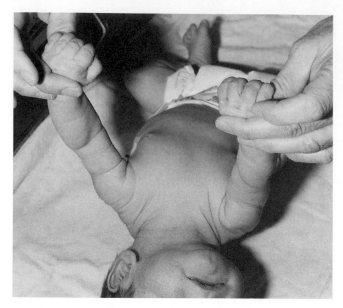

Figure 4–4 In the newborn, the prehensile grasp of the fingers is often strong enough to support the baby's weight.

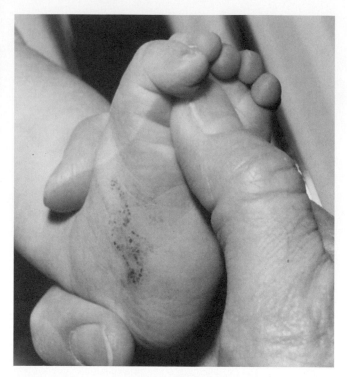

Figure 4–5 The plantar grasp typically is strongest in the newborn period.

Plantar Grasp

A strong plantar grasp usually can be demonstrated if you place your thumb on the sole of the baby's foot in the space under the toes (Fig. 4–5).

Placing and Propulsive (Stepping and Walking) Reflexes

Holding the baby upright, touch the dorsum of the feet to the bed or a table, and it will seem as if the baby is trying to walk. Parents are invariably fascinated and delighted by the demonstration that their newborn baby "can walk."

If there is any doubt about the integrity of the baby's CNS, either because of the history (difficult labor, delivery, traumatic procedures, or birth asphyxia) or because of associated physical findings, such as an abnormal cry, major deformities, or malformations, a more complete neurologic examination should be conducted (see Chapter 13).

WEIGHING AND MEASURING

For the physician's and the parents' records, it is important to measure the baby's head circumference, length, and weight accurately and to assess the nutritional status. Measure the head circumference, preferably with a disposable tape measure, around the largest occipital-frontal diameter across the forehead, just above the eyes and over the most prominent part of the occiput (Fig. 4–6). Head circumference normally measures 33

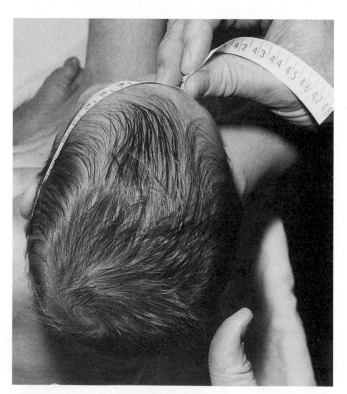

Figure 4–6 Measuring the head circumference.

to 37 cm in a full-term infant. If a baby's head circumference measures slightly above or below the normal for age, check the parents' head circumferences before "pushing the panic button." Benign familial megalencephaly, a normal variant, is the most common cause of a larger than average head. The condition can be verified by checking the head circumference of both parents. Megalencephaly is usually handed down by the father.

Although chest circumference is not measured routinely in a newborn, it is a good indicator of body proportion if there is doubt. Chest circumference normally measures 30 to 37 cm and is usually 1 to 2 cm smaller than the head circumference during the first 6 months of life. It is measured around the nipple line with the baby lying supine.

Measuring length is important, but it *must* be done accurately. Measuring with a tape measure or by making pencil marks on a piece of paper underneath the baby are notoriously inaccurate. Accurate length measurement is best accomplished by using one of the commercially available fixed measuring devices, with the baby lying supine and the head touching a fixed object (Fig. 4–7). Extend the baby's body and legs and hold them flat; record resulting length, which is normally 47 to 55 cm. Plot the weight, length, and head circumference on a sex-appropriate fetal growth chart (Fig. 4–8) to see whether the baby is (1) within the normal range for gestational age and (2) proportional in terms of head circumference, length, and weight. If there is doubt about a baby's upper and lower segment proportions, remember that the newborn's midpoint is normally at about the umbilicus. The ratio of crown-to-pubis length to pubis-to-heel length in the newborn is normally1.7:1. Making these measurements may help if a short-limbed growth disorder, such as a chondrodystrophy, is suspected.

The average healthy full-term North American baby weighs approximately 3500 g. The range of normal variation is defined in either percentiles or standard deviations from the mean on the growth charts. Assess the baby's nutrition from its growth in relation to gestational age (which may be deficient in weight alone or in all three measurements), and determine whether there is wasting of tissues. Wasting may be most

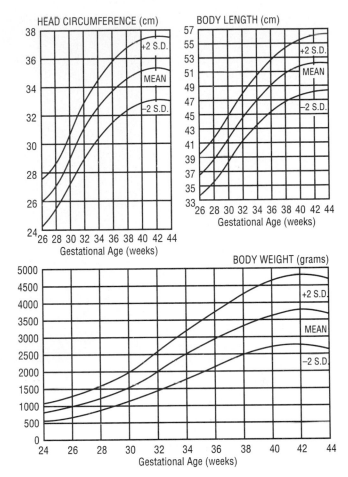

Figure 4–8 Growth charts for the newborn male (in Nova Scotia). Measurements are related to gestational age. (From Lubchenco LO, Hansman M, Dressler M, Boyd E: Intrauterine growth as estimated from liveborn birth weight data at 24 to 42 weeks of gestation. Reproduced with permission from Pediatrics, Vol. 32, Page 794, Figure 1, Copyright 1963.)

obvious over the anterior thighs, where the quadriceps bulk and subcutaneous fat are most easily assessed. Babies with moderate to severe wasting of the subcutaneous and muscular tissues or those whose body weight is more than two standard deviations below the mean for gestational age may have significant problems that should be evaluated during the newborn period. Such problems are congenital malformations and metabolic disturbances such as hypoglycemia and hypocalcemia. You should follow the future growth and development of such infants closely.

ASSESSING GESTATIONAL AGE

The physical examination can help you determine whether a baby is truly full term (37 weeks' gestation or more) or preterm (premature) (less than 37 weeks' gestation).

The full-term baby has deep creases crisscrossing the sole of the foot from the ball to the heel (Fig. 4–9). The preterm baby does not.

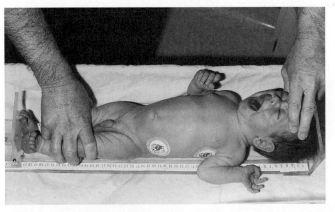

Figure 4–7 Measuring the length. A stable accurate measuring device and proper positioning are essential. Note that many infants do not relish this procedure. Leave it to the last.

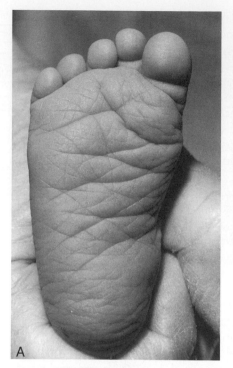
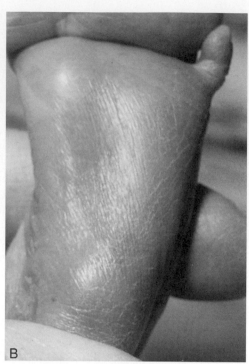

Figure 4–9 *A*, Typical sole creases of a full-term infant. *B*, Comparatively smooth sole of a premature infant.

The preterm baby's ear has fewer folds and is more pliable than the springy, cartilaginous, well-formed ear of the full-term infant (Fig. 4–10).

In the full-term male, the scrotum is full, rugated, and pendulous with the testes fully descended; in the preterm baby, the scrotum is smaller and smoother, and the testes are either high in the scrotum or in the inguinal canal (Fig. 4–11). The testes are usually palpable in the upper scrotum by 36 weeks' gestation and are fully descended by 40 weeks'.

The preterm female has relatively prominent labia minora and small labia majora, whereas in a full-term girl, the labia majora fully cover the vaginal opening and obscure the labia minora (Fig. 4–12).

The preterm infant's scalp hair is fine and woolly, like fluffed-up cotton wool; the full-term baby has straight silky hair, and each strand is separate.

In the well-nourished full-term baby, the breast nodule under the areola is approximately half a centimeter in diameter, whereas in the preterm infant, it measures 3 mm or less. This is an unreliable sign for gestational age, however, because undernourished babies may have little or no breast tissue even at full term.

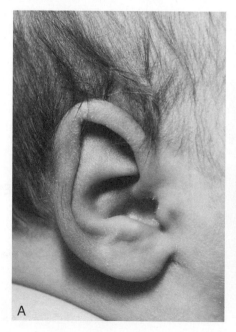
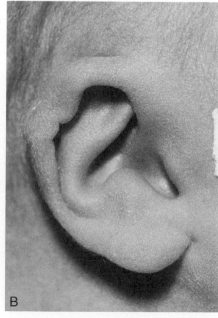

Figure 4–10 *A*, The springy cartilaginous ear of the full-term baby. *B*, The softer, less well formed ear of the premature infant.

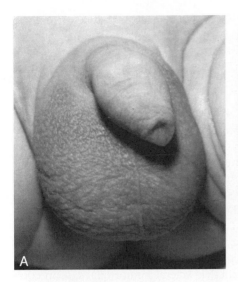
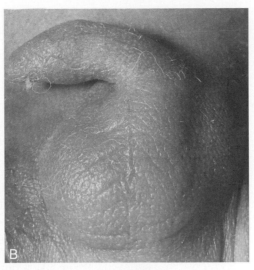

Figure 4–11 *A*, The well-formed rugated scrotum of the full-term male infant. *B*, The smoother immature scrotal surface in the premature infant. In the preterm infant, the testes are often highly placed or located in the inguinal canal.

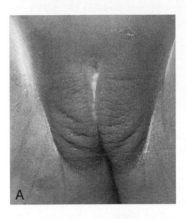
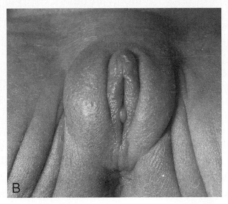

Figure 4–12 *A*, The typical prominent labia majora of the full-term female infant. *B*, The premature female genitalia. The labia majora are less prominent and the labia minora more prominent, than in the full-term infant.

More detailed systems exist for evaluating and scoring the gestational age of infants, the most popular of which was described by Dubowitz in 1970 and refined by Ballard and associates[1] in 1991. The Dubowitz assessment is a useful tool for which considerable practice and experience are required to achieve accuracy. The scale involves assessing 10 neurologic and 11 physical criteria on a numerical scale and calculating a total score. That score is then matched to a table giving approximate gestational age. The physical criteria, including those already described, are more accurate than the neurologic criteria, because the neurologic score is falsely low in a sick or neurologically compromised infant, as well as in many preterm infants. Detailed assessment tools, such as the Brazelton Neonatal Behavioral Assessment Scale, are available to study neurologic behaviors.[2]

THE HEAD

Newborns' heads vary considerably in shape and symmetry, depending on intrauterine position and pressures, presentation at delivery, and the amount of molding that has taken place during labor and delivery. A baby born by breech delivery or cesarean section characteristically has a fairly round, symmetric head, whereas the head of a baby born by vaginal vertex delivery is usually elongated occipitally, with some overriding (overlapping) of the sutures and possibly a caput succedaneum (Fig. 4–13) or a cephalhematoma. A *caput succedaneum* is a collection of subcutaneous edema fluid caused by constricting pressure during passage through the birth canal; it normally resolves within the first few days of life. A *cephalhematoma* is a subperiosteal collection of blood limited by the periosteal attachments to the area over a single bone of the skull. Soft and fluctuating, it feels like a fluid-filled cyst, and it may last for several weeks, gradually getting smaller. During its resolution, a cephalhematoma usually calcifies initially at the edges, giving the impression on palpation of depression of the skull in the center with an eggshell-like bony margin, raising fears of skull fracture. In general, the baby's skull is smooth without any obvious depressed areas. Depressed fractures are rare but can occur.

Key Point

You should be able to feel all the sutures in a baby's head, which may override one another for the first day or so after vaginal delivery or may be slightly separated, but normally not by more than 0.5 cm.

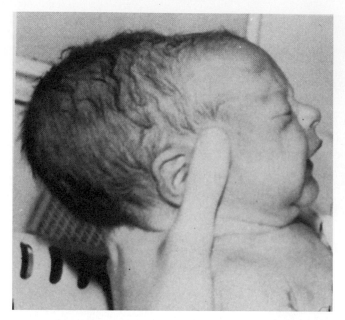

Figure 4–13 Caput succedaneum. The subcutaneous edema was caused by the pressure of the passage through the birth canal. (From Cunningham FG, MacDonald PC, Grant FG: Williams Obstetrics, 18th ed. East Norwalk, CT, Appleton & Lange, 1989. Reproduced with permission from Pediatrics, Vol. 32, Page 794, Figure 1, Copyright 1963.)

The normal size of the diamond-shaped anterior fontanel varies considerably; it usually admits at least one fingertip, but often admits two fingers or more. The anterior fontanel should be flat or slightly sunken when the baby is held in the upright position and is quiet. The posterior fontanel often barely admits one fingertip and may be difficult to appreciate in the first few days because of the overlapping sutures.

Transillumination

Transillumination of the head is not performed as part of the routine physical examination. This maneuver can, however, be a useful screening test in any baby with an unusually large, asymmetric head or with wide sutures, before you resort to more accurate forms of intracranial diagnosis, such as ultrasonography and computerized tomography (CT) scan. Use a full-sized flashlight (not a penlight) with a soft rubber rim at the light end so that a tight seal against the scalp can be achieved. Take the baby into a completely darkened room. Apply the light closely to the scalp, and move it over the entire head. Normally, a rim of light—approximately 1 to 2 cm wide—is visible around the margins of the flashlight lens, but it may be reduced in infants who have pigmented skin, prematurity, or scalp edema (*caput succedaneum*) and over the frontal areas. The rim of light is often strikingly larger in a baby with increased amounts of fluid in the subarachnoid, subdural, or ventricular space; therefore, in conditions such as severe hydrocephalus, chronic subdural hematoma,

or effusion and hydranencephaly, there is usually a significant increase in transillumination.

The Eyes

Examination of a newborn baby's eyes may seem difficult at first, but as with other aspects of the examination, it is surprising how much you can learn without touching the infant. First, establish that both eyes are of normal size with normal-appearing corneas, pupils, and sclera, and make sure that red reflexes are present bilaterally and that there are no anterior chamber hemorrhages or visible cataracts or other malformations of the lens or iris. The main ingredient of success in this examination is patience. See Chapter 8 for details.

Small subconjunctival scleral hemorrhages, seen commonly in newborns (Fig. 4–14), are caused by increased intravascular pressure during delivery. They are unsightly but harmless and usually disappear in a few days. If you do find some, reassure the parents immediately.

Getting a good look at a newborn's eyes is not always easy, but a several useful tricks make doing so less frustrating for all concerned. First, babies open their eyes in a darkened or dimly lit room more readily than in brightly lit surroundings. If babies are in the quiet alert state, they often open their eyes spontaneously. Truly quiet and alert babies may fix their gaze on you, looking at you rather than through you (see Chapter 8). You can establish that the baby will follow your face through an arc of at least 90 degrees. This finding, coupled with the presence of bilateral red reflexes, gives good first-line reassurance about the baby's vision.

Although it is sometimes possible to separate the baby's eyelids with your fingers, with or without pieces of gauze wrapped around them, this practice is not recommended. In the first place, during the first few hours of life, the eyelids are often covered with slippery

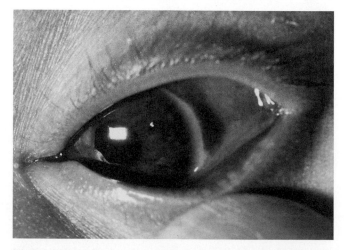

Figure 4–14 Scleral subconjunctival hemorrhage, which is a common, transient, and harmless phenomenon in newborns.

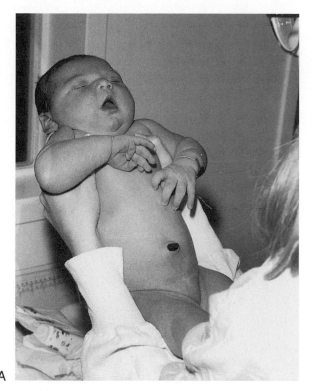
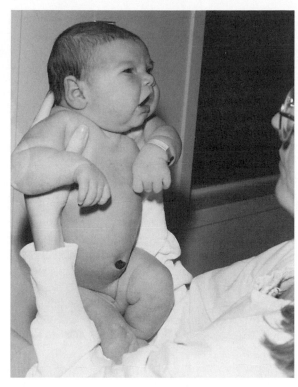

A   B

Figure 4–15 *A,* Using the vestibular reflex to induce a newborn to open the eyes. *B,* Gentle rocking back and forth often produces the desired result.

vernix, making it no easy task to get a grip. Second, this approach often makes babies cry and try to close their eyes even more tightly. If it is impossible to catch the baby in the quiet alert state, try taking advantage of the vestibular reflex as a means of getting an infant to open the eyes. Pick the baby up, supporting the head with a hand, and hold the baby upright with the face at your eye level; then slowly rock the baby back and forth, toward and away from you (Fig. 4–15). If the baby is quiet and not crying, the eyes usually open for a few moments at least, letting you check the red reflexes and pupillary responses. Do not be surprised if the baby appears to have a strabismus (to be "cross-eyed"), because conjugate movement of the eyes in young infants is only intermittent.

Ophthalmoscopy is not performed routinely in newborns. It is usually limited to infants in whom there are specific concerns about the eyes, such as those who may be subject to retinopathy of prematurity, and infants with congenital infections, such as toxoplasmosis, rubella, and cytomegalovirus. This examination is generally performed by ophthalmologists after dilation of the baby's pupils.

The Ears

Ear examination in the newborn is generally limited to the external ear and outer ear canal. Observe the formation of the external ear—its folds, stiffness, symme-

try, and placement on the head—and the patency of the ear canal. It is possible to examine the ear canal and tympanic structures with an otoscope, but this is not usually part of the routine physical examination of newborns. You should, however, examine the ear canals carefully in any infant who has any malformation of the external ear. The newborn's eardrum is placed more horizontally than in older children and requires careful orientation to see it; moreover, the ear canals are often blocked with vernix and amniotic debris during the first couple of days of life, making it difficult to visualize the eardrums. External ear malformations, such as low-set ears, abnormalities in shape or formation, skin tags, and pits, are important both cosmetically and as indicators of possible associated congenital malformations that may be part of specific syndromes (see also Chapter 5).

The Nose

The main purpose of examining a newborn's nose is to assess the patency of both nares. You can establish patency by blocking first one nostril and then the other with a finger while the baby's mouth is closed, and listening to each unblocked nostril in turn (with or without a stethoscope) for air movement. If you suspect an obstruction such as choanal atresia or stenosis, try to pass a small, soft catheter through the nasal passage. Because babies at rest breathe primarily through the nose, patency of the nasal airway is essential. A baby with bilateral choanal atresia usually presents with respiratory distress and cyanosis. If the baby's mouth is opened or if the baby opens it to cry and the distress and cyanosis are relieved, consider this diagnosis. Use an oral airway, and confirm the diagnosis as described.

The Mouth

If the baby happens to cry during the examination, seize the opportunity to examine the mouth. Check whether the palate is intact. Although many babies appear to have the tongue tethered to the bottom of the mouth by a frenulum that sometimes reaches the tip of the tongue ("tongue tie"), it is always mobile enough allow the baby to suck and to establish breast-feeding, which are all that is necessary at this age (Fig. 4–16). Cutting the tongue frenulum used to be widely practiced but is no longer considered a useful or acceptable procedure. True tongue tie is exceptionally rare if it exists at all.

Note the uvula's configuration. A bifid uvula may be the only sign of a submucous (invisible) cleft of the palate.

Check for the presence of prematurely erupted teeth. Whitish epidermal inclusion cysts are occasionally seen along the gums or the palate. They are harmless and disappear after awhile.

Stroke the face beside the baby's mouth with a finger to elicit the rooting reflex, in which the baby turns the head toward the finger and opens the mouth as if to grasp a nipple (Fig. 4–17). By putting a finger in the baby's mouth, you can elicit the suck reflex and check

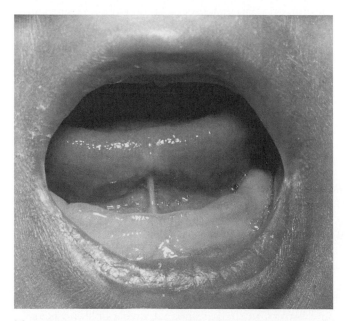

Figure 4–16 A prominent tight frenulum of the tongue, mistakenly referred to as "tongue tie." These normal variants cause no problem and should be left alone.

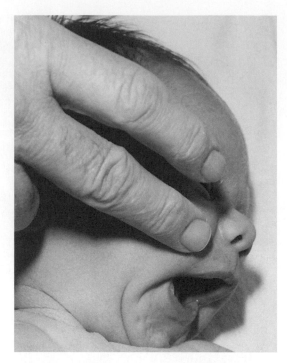

Figure 4–17 Eliciting the rooting reflex. Stroking the infant's face near the mouth causes the baby to open the mouth and turn toward the stimulus. Breast-feeding mothers often use this reflex to advantage in initiating nursing.

the palate. It is unnecessary to test for the gag reflex unless there are specific concerns about neurologic function. When the baby cries, note whether the mouth and face are symmetric. Asymmetric crying may be the one and only tipoff to a unilateral facial palsy that is not apparent when the baby is quiet. In a baby with unilateral facial palsy, the affected side does not move as well as the other side, the nasolabial fold remains flat, and the corner of the mouth droops (Fig. 4–18). Facial palsy is often associated with compression of the facial nerve during delivery (i.e., by forceps). The majority of facial palsies resolve without permanent damage.

Some babies have some mucus or saliva drooling from the mouth, with the bedding under the head being frequently wet. In the first few hours of life, this may be a normal phenomenon if the baby has swallowed much amniotic fluid and is regurgitating stomach contents. Yet it also may reflect an inability to swallow properly, from either neuromuscular problems or esophageal obstruction, as with esophageal atresia. Isolated neuromuscular swallowing difficulties are uncommon and would become evident as abnormal neurologic findings in other tests of the cranial nerves. Suspect an esophageal obstruction if (1) there is excessive mucus and drooling and (2) a soft plastic nasogastric tube inserted into the mouth and throat fails to reach the stomach. Learn the procedure for the tube insertion from an experienced nurse. In infants with esophageal obstruction or atresia, a nasogastric tube may *appear* to have gone in far enough to have

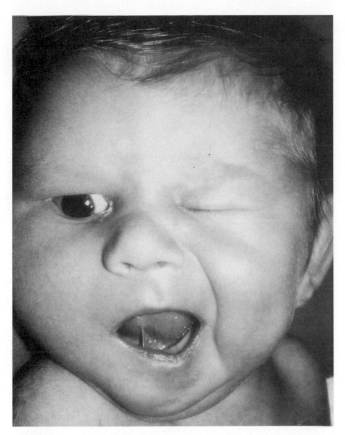

Figure 4–18 Asymmetric crying is caused by a right-sided facial paralysis. Milder degrees of unilateral facial paralysis may be demonstrable only when the baby is made to cry.

reached the stomach, but in fact, it may be curled up on itself in the blind-ended pouch. To ensure that the tube is in the stomach, aspirate from the tube and test the secretions for pH. If they are from the stomach, the pH should be acid. You can also inject air into the tube and listen for bubbling sounds over the stomach with a stethoscope. This second method is less reliable, because sound can be transmitted well within the chest and abdomen. If there is still any doubt that the tube has reached the stomach, a radiograph of the chest and abdomen will decide the issue. The association of esophageal atresia with tracheoesophageal fistula is extremely high; therefore, if atresia is found, assume there is a fistula. At this stage, consult with a pediatric surgeon and radiologist.

THE NECK

Examine the baby's neck for fibroma of the sternomastoid muscle (fibrous sternomastoid tumor). This tumor is often misdiagnosed as a hematoma and may be associated with facial asymmetry and a head tilt due to an associated shortened hypotrophic sternomastoid muscle. More rarely, there may be a fistula representing a remnant of the branchial arch system, opening anywhere from the ear down along the anterior border of the sternomastoid. Inspect and feel the thyroid area to make sure that there is no thyroid enlargement, especially if the mother has taken iodides during pregnancy or there is a family history of thyroid disease.

> **Key Point**
>
> Remember that the newborn's neck muscles are not strong; therefore, whenever lifting a baby, you should always support the head separately with one hand (Fig. 4–19).

Routinely palpate the clavicles, which are the most common sites of fracture during delivery. Unusually large or macrosomic infants are at increased risk for

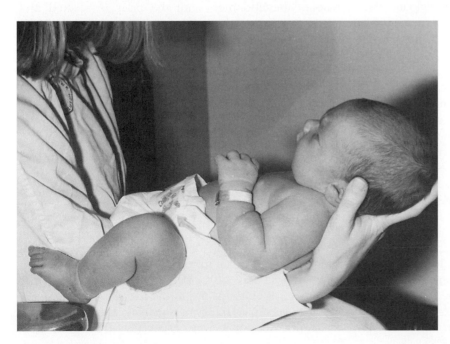

Figure 4–19 Proper way to pick the baby up, always supporting the head.

clavicular fractures, which may manifest as pseudo-paralysis of one arm. The baby can move the arm but does not because movement causes pain. Palpation over the clavicle may reveal crepitus in the first few days. Soon after, a sizable lump of callus forms at the fracture site; it will gradually disappear over many months. No treatment is necessary.

THE CHEST

The newborn's respirations are normally irregular in both amplitude and frequency, with pauses that should last less than 10 seconds. This irregular breathing pattern is even more marked in preterm infants. The respiratory rate averages 30 to 40 breaths/min in a resting, full-term baby. Breath sounds should be heard well in the front and the back, and although a few crackles may be heard immediately after birth, no significant crackles or wheezes should be heard within a few hours. Signs of respiratory distress, such as subcostal, intercostal, or suprasternal retractions, should not be evident.

While the baby is quiet, listen to the heart. The heart rate is usually 120 to 130 beats/min, with a normal range of 100 to 160 beats/min. Occasional extrasystoles are common. The two heart sounds are usually equal in intensity, and the normal variation in the width of the split in the second sound with respiration may be difficult to appreciate because the respiratory and heart rates are so rapid. During the first few days, it is common to hear a soft precordial systolic murmur. If this murmur is not associated with other signs of congenital heart disease and disappears in a day or two, it was probably due to flow through the ductus arteriosus, which remains patent immediately after birth, closing gradually over subsequent hours or days.

Feel the peripheral pulses. Always palpate the femoral region to be certain that femoral pulses are present, are equal bilaterally, are equal in strength to the brachial pulses, and are of normal volume. If the pulses are present at the initial examination, do not assume that they are still there at the next examination; recheck the femoral pulses at each examination of the baby for the first year. Failure to check and recheck the femoral pulses in the newborn is a "capital crime." The arteries are found at the lateral side of the femoral triangle just below the inguinal ligament (Fig. 4–20). Make sure that you have *really* felt the femoral pulsations—if you only think you have felt them, you have not. Absence or weakness of femoral pulsations indicates possible aortic coarctation and *warrants an urgent cardiology consultation.* Provide a record of four-limb blood pressures to the cardiologist for the examination. Adequate peripheral perfusion manifests as warm pink extremities with good capillary refill.

Some newborns have hypertrophy of glandular breast tissue. This condition is caused by maternal hormonal

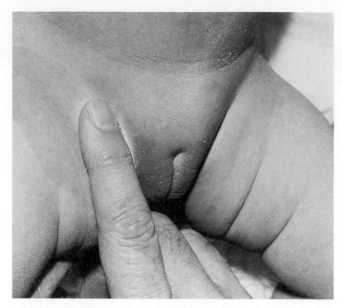

Figure 4–20 Palpating for a femoral pulse. Lay your examining finger flat along the course of the inguinal ligament and just below it. Gentle pressure with the fingertip should elicit the pulsation. (If you are not sure, you have not felt it.)

stimulation in utero, and the breast may continue to enlarge during the first few days of life. Newborns may even secrete milk from the nipples ("witches' milk"). Never treat or manipulate engorged breasts. Spontaneous regression of breast engorgement is the rule.

THE ABDOMEN

The normal newborn's abdomen looks slightly protuberant, and a separation is frequently felt between the two rectus muscles (*diastasis recti*). Do not try to palpate the abdomen until the baby is relaxed and quiet. Gentle, steady pressure with warm hands is the most effective means of getting the baby to relax the abdominal muscles.

Key Point

Trying to palpate the liver, spleen, or kidneys against resistance is unrewarding and potentially harmful.

In most babies, the soft, poorly defined liver edge is palpable in the right upper quadrant. Applying your thumb or fingers gently to the skin surface, you should feel a resistance that falls away as your fingers move downward. The liver edge is normally felt 1 to 2 cm below the right costal margin in the right nipple line. In newborns, it may be palpable right across the upper abdomen, sloping upward to the mid-left costal margin. Inability to palpate the liver edge may suggest diaphragmatic paralysis or hernia, especially if the finding is associated with respiratory distress. The spleen may or may not be palpable in the newborn. When palpable, it should be felt just below the left costal margin. The spleen, too, is soft and may be difficult to feel.

Abdominal palpation should include a search for unusual masses and for renal size. The firm, rounded left kidney can usually be felt fairly easily. The lower pole of the right kidney should also be relatively easy to palpate below the liver. No other masses are normally felt in the abdomen at this age except for a full bladder.

The umbilical cord may be in varying states of dryness, depending on the baby's nutritional state and age at the time of examination. The cord contains a jelly (Wharton jelly) in which three vessels are normally embedded—two umbilical arteries and one umbilical vein—which spiral down the umbilical cord to the placenta. If there is only 3 or 4 cm of cord below a clamp, it can be difficult to determine how many vessels are present from looking at the crushed end of the cord. Approximately 1% of babies have only a single umbilical artery; 10% of these infants have other congenital malformations. As a solitary finding, a single umbilical artery does not call for extensive investigation beyond a thorough physical examination and a notation on the chart and office record to maintain awareness of the possibility of internal malformations if problems arise. In a baby with intrauterine growth restriction, the cord is often thin and stringy with little Wharton jelly. In a baby who has been bathed in meconium in utero for more than a few hours, the cord may be stained green.

Always inspect the anus to be sure that it is patent. Obviously, its patency is ensured if the baby has already passed meconium and the anus looks normal. If a rectal temperature can be taken, the anus is patent. Digital rectal examination normally is not performed unless there is good reason to suspect an internal anomaly. On the rare occasion that it is required, use your fifth finger, well lubricated, and proceed as slowly and gently as possible. Gentle pressure against the anal orifice usually induces relaxation within a minute or so, allowing the finger to be inserted with less trauma.

THE GENITALIA

Examine the genitalia carefully to help estimate gestational age and to ascertain normal anatomy. The female newborn has relatively large labia majora that cover and occlude the labia minora and vaginal introitus. The vaginal opening usually is largely occluded by the hymenal membrane. Vaginal discharge is often present, especially on the second and third days of life, when there also may be some minor bleeding, resulting from withdrawal of maternal progesterone stimulation. The clitoris is easily seen, but it should not be so large as to appear phallic. There are frequently small tags of tissue near the introitus. Palpate the labia majora carefully to exclude the presence of gonads that, if located there, may indicate sexual ambiguity or, more rarely, herniation of the ovaries into the labia.

In males, the glans penis is normally covered completely by foreskin that cannot and should not be fully retracted. Retracting it slightly allows you to easily see whether the opening in the prepuce is adequate for urination. It may or may not be possible to see the urethral meatus, which should be slitlike and located at the tip of the glans. If the baby voids during the examination, you can note the quality and strength of the stream. The scrotum of the full-term boy is pendulous and well rugated, and it may be more pigmented than the rest of the skin in dark-skinned babies. The testes should be completely descended. The normal testis is 1 to 2 cm long, the size and consistency of a small seedless grape, and about 1 mL in volume. Remember that if your hand is cold or the baby is unusually irritable, the cremasteric reflexes may quickly retract the testes to the top of the scrotum or even into the inguinal canals. The scrotum is best examined in a quiet baby and with a warm hand. Sliding one hand medially along the inguinal ligament toward the top of the scrotum before touching the scrotum blocks the escape route of the testis in an infant who has a very active cremasteric reflex.

Many developmental variations and anomalies can involve the external genitalia, the only parts of the reproductive system available for immediate examination. These variations and anomalies may also involve the internal sexual organs, having serious implications for the health of the child and future reproductive capability. In addition, abnormalities of the external genitalia may be linked with anomalies of the renal system. One of the most common anomalies of the male genital system is *hypospadias*, a ventral displacement of the urethra on the meatus or shaft of the penis. It can be of varying severity: in primary hypospadias, the urethra is still on the glans; in secondary hypospadias, the urethra is at the junction of the glans and the shaft of the penis; in tertiary hypospadias the urethra is somewhere on the shaft of the penis. Primary hypospadias is generally isolated, but more severe manifestations may be associated with renal anomalies, requiring renal ultrasonography and consultation with a pediatric urologist. Babies with hypospadias should not be circumcised because the foreskin may be needed for later surgical repair.

Key Point

If the genitalia do not appear normal, it is important to find out whether there has been a family history of unexplained infant deaths. Salt-losing congenital adrenal hyperplasia, often manifesting as apparent virilization in a female, can be a life-threatening condition.

Immediately after birth, evaluate any infant with apparently ambiguous or abnormal genitalia. Potentially life-threatening adrenal insufficiency is associated with some forms of ambiguous genitalia. One abnormality that is frequently found in an apparent female is a large phallus with hypospadias. The labia may or may not be fused, and it may be possible to feel gonads in what appear to be labial folds. Conversely, the infant may seem to be a male with an unusually small phallus, undescended or nonpalpable testes, and a small scrotum. Many variations are possible, including hypospadias with or without *cryptorchidism* (undescended testes). It is important to find out whether similar problems exist within the family, because some of these problems are hormonally determined or chromosomally inherited.

Early definitive assignment of the infant's sex is important for both medical and psychological reasons. It is important to identify infants with potentially life-threatening adrenal insufficiency so they can be treated promptly and to diagnose other potentially treatable conditions, such as Smith-Lemli-Optiz syndrome. Also, for family reasons, the child must be assigned a sex. This sex assignment will not necessarily reflect chromosomal sex, but after due consultation and appropriate investigations, the assignment should reflect the more appropriate sex for potential sexual functioning in later life. Tell the parents initially that their infant's genitalia are not completely developed and that special tests, performed as quickly as possible, will determine the sex that is the most appropriate for rearing. Advise the parents not to give the baby a name immediately, and tell hospital staff not to assign a sex to the baby for paperwork purposes—refraining from using "Baby Boy Jones" or "Baby Girl Jones," and using merely "Baby Jones." Complete the sex assignment within 2 or 3 days.

Investigations for ambiguous genitalia may include chromosome analysis, urine and blood hormone analyses, and internal examination by ultrasonography or radiography with contrast enhancement. Often, consultations with an experienced pediatrician or neonatologist, endocrinologist, geneticist, and pediatric urologist are needed to help make a quick and accurate diagnosis. (See Chapters 5 and 16 for detailed discussions of this issue.)

HERNIAS AND HYDROCELES

Hydroceles are common in newborn boys (see Chapter 12). An isolated hydrocele without hernia usually disappears within weeks or months, rarely requiring repair. If you find a hernia, make sure that it is easily reducible. If it is not, consult a surgeon immediately, because early repair may be required. Hernias in girls are rare and always call for careful palpation for aberrant gonads as well as exclusion of sexual ambiguity before and during surgical exploration.

THE HIPS

Do not assume that the hips are not dislocated or subluxable in a baby who kicks the legs vigorously. Congenital dislocation of the hip occurs in approximately 1 in 500 to 1 in 1000 babies. If diagnosed early, the condition is treatable with good results. The most common screening maneuver combines those described by Barlow[3] and Ortolani[4] (Fig. 4–21).

Key Point

Failure to diagnose hip dislocation in the newborn can cause major problems requiring long treatment, with results that may range from less than ideal to downright disabling.

With the baby relaxed and supine on a firm surface, flex the thighs to a right angle to the abdomen and the knees to a right angle with the thighs. Then, grasp each thigh with your forefinger along the outside of the shaft of the femur, your middle fingertip on the greater trochanter and your thumb medially. With the baby at rest, first adduct the femora fully and push down toward the bed. If either femoral head is felt to leave the acetabulum posteriorly, it has dislocated (Barlow maneuver).

Then gently abduct each leg from the position of full adduction so that the knees come to lie laterally on the mattress. During abduction, push the greater trochanters medially and forward with your fingers. If you feel (or hear) a click during either adduction or abduction, if there is resistance as the knee approaches full abduction, or if there is a spasm or discomfort of the adductor muscles of the femur, the baby probably has a congenitally dislocated or subluxable hip (Ortolani test) and needs orthopedic assessment.

THE EXTREMITIES

Now move your hands down over the baby's legs to judge symmetry and equality of length, quickly checking the number of toes and for the presence or absence of syndactyly on each foot. Slight syndactyly of the second and third toes is a common minor congenital anomaly without special significance (Fig. 4–22). If you have not already looked at the creases of the soles of the feet to assess gestational age, now is a good time to do so. Most normal newborns have slight bowing of the legs, reflecting intrauterine position. This disappears gradually as the infant gets older. Often, if the baby 's legs are "folded up" accordion style, gentle pressure on the soles of the feet induces the baby to resume the intrauterine posture, allowing a greater appreciation of how the legs became bowed.

Differentiate true clubfoot, a fixed deformity, from apparent but pliable and transient foot deformations

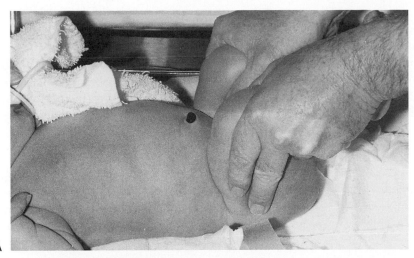

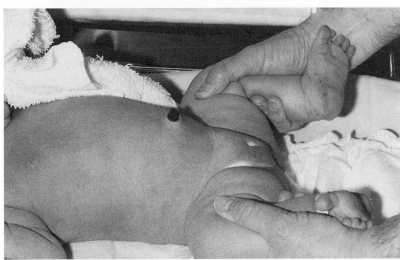

Figure 4–21 *A* and *B*, Proper technique for examining the newborn for congenital subluxation or dislocation of the hip.

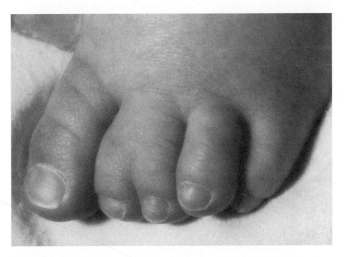

Figure 4–22 Partial syndactyly of the second and third toes is a common minor anomaly in otherwise healthy infants.

caused by in utero positioning. The latter can be straightened out easily with gentle pressure from the fingers to bring the feet into normal position and alignment. These transient abnormalities become less obvious over the first weeks and months of life. The deformities of clubfoot, however, are not completely correctable by hand pressure and require orthopedic management as early as possible. They may or may not be associated with neurologic problems.

Rudimentary skin tags at the lateral border of either the fifth finger or the fifth toe usually represent rudimentary supernumerary digits (*polydactyly*), which may be a signpost for associated malformations or syndromes. Many well-intentioned physicians tie these tags off with a bit of silk suture for cosmetic reasons, but the evidence should not be destroyed until its significance has been determined. Check the nails on the fingers and toes; extra-long nails are common in post-term infants, and hypoplastic nails are part of many dysmorphic syndromes, such as Williams syndrome and fetal alcohol syndrome (FAS).

THE BACK

Now, turn the baby over and examine the back. Check the creases at the thigh-buttock area for symmetry. Asymmetry may reveal early signs of leg shortening associated with congenital dislocation of the hip. Examine the midline of the back particularly carefully, because midline congenital defects on the dorsal surface may signal important internal anomalies. Starting at the lower end, look at the top of the cleft between the buttocks at the base of the spine. Many babies have a pilonidal dimple in this area (Fig. 4–23) that will disappear and has no special significance. In the rare circumstance that there seems to be no bottom to the dimple or that it is a sinus tract, further investigation (with ultrasonography) should be initiated, because the tract may communicate with the spinal canal and may be associated with other malformations. Any hemangioma, lipoma, or tuft of hair that crosses the midline of the lower back carries a high probability of being associated with an internal structural spinal abnormality, such as spina bifida occulta or tethering of the spinal cord by a bony spicule or fibrous band (*diastematomyelia*). Run a finger up and down the spine, noting lumps or gaps between the spines, or gaps where there should be spines, which could indicate spina bifida or lipomeningocele. Continue the examination right up to the base of the neck and the occiput, looking for defects. Neural tube defects may be small, but they are always in the midline. There is frequently a small flat area hemangioma at the nape of the neck, popularly known as "stork bite," which is insignificant; it will become less obvious as the infant gets older, either by disappearing or by being covered by hair.

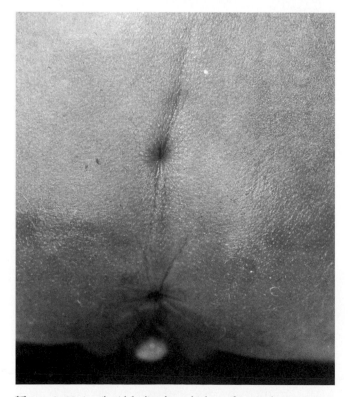

Figure 4–23 A pilonidal dimple, which is frequently present in normal newborns. Most are shallow blind tracts that disappear in a few months.

SKIN OF THE NEWBORN

Vernix Caseosa

The skin of the head and face of a newborn may exhibit a variety of changes. Most of them have little significance, but it is important to reassure the parents that they are normal and do not require treatment. At birth, the normal full-term infant is covered to varying degrees with *vernix caseosa*. The literal translation of this term from Latin is "cheesy varnish"; it is a greasy substance that protects the skin during the lengthy immersion in amniotic fluid, much as the skin of a long-distance swimmer is protected by heavy grease applied to it. This is the normal sebaceous secretion of the skin.

Skin Changes in Postmaturity

Unusual dryness, flakiness, or cracking of the skin may be associated with postmaturity or sometimes, if severe, with a true dermatologic disorder, *congenital ichthyosis* (literally, "fish skin").

Angiomatous Lesions

There are frequently small, flame-shaped, flat hemangiomas over the eyelids, the roof of the nose, and, as previously noted, the back of the neck and occiput. They go by colorful popular names, such as "angel's kisses" on the upper lids, "stork bites" at the base of the occiput, and nevus flammeus or flame-shaped nevus on the forehead in the midline. These lesions are insignificant and usually disappear over the first few months. Differentiate these lesions from significant flat hemangiomas, such as port-wine stains, which are generally larger and permanent and may involve areas of the face or head in a particular nerve distribution. Port-wine stains in the distribution of any branch of the trigeminal nerve may be associated with intracranial vascular malformations.

Milia

Milia, small white spots on the skin, particularly over the nose and cheeks, represent hyperactive sebaceous glands with visible retained secretions. They do not require treatment.

Key Point

The skin lesions that should cause concern and warrant close observation, investigation, and treatment include vesicles, pustules, areas lacking skin (either congenital or acquired), and large, bulky subcutaneous hemangiomas.

Petechiae

Petechiae on the face are quite common. Pinpoint in size, they do not blanch with pressure; they usually result from increased pressure in the venous system during a vertex vaginal delivery. They may therefore be especially numerous and associated with some edema after a face presentation or may appear over the buttocks after breech delivery. These petechiae resolve in a few days.

Generalized petechiae suggest either a vascular or platelet disorder or a congenital infection. Bruising (*ecchymoses*) also may be related to delivery trauma or, rarely, to a coagulopathy, most likely a thrombocytopenia. The extent and resolution of these lesions should help to differentiate them.

Erythema Toxicum

The most common skin lesion in newborns and the one that often causes anxiety to parents is *erythema toxicum,* or newborn rash, which is extremely common in full-term infants. The lesions usually appear as yellowish white "pustules" on an erythematous base, 1 to 3 mm in diameter, that occur singly or in groups anywhere on the baby's body. There may be a few or hundreds that frequently come and go in a matter of hours. Their significance is unknown, but they are harmless and require no treatment. Differentiate these lesions from true infectious pustules that contain pus. If the identity of such lesions is in doubt, quickly smear the contents of a lesion on a slide and perform a Gram stain. Erythema toxicum lesions contain many eosinophils, whereas pustule contents are characterized by neutrophils and gram-positive cocci.

Pigmented and Depigmented Lesions

Patches of unusual pigmentation may be normal or abnormal. More than five or six patches of brownish pigmentation (café au lait spots) suggest the possibility of congenital neurofibromatosis; check both parents for the presence of similar lesions.

It is common to find one or more large deep bluish lesions over the buttocks or lower spine in nonwhite infants or dark-skinned, dark-haired white infants. These are called mongolian spots. They occur in most Asian infants, in more than 90% of black infants, in most East Indian infants, and in many dark-skinned white infants. Do not confuse this pigmentation with bruising. Occasionally, when such confusion has occurred, parents have been wrongly suspected of child abuse.

Areas of depigmentation may be significant, because they may be the earliest, and for a time the only, manifestations of tuberous sclerosis, a progressive degenerative neurologic disease. The typical lesions often occur in the shape of an ash leaf (Fig. 4–24) and may occur singly or in multiples. Their appearance is intensified by examination under ultraviolet illumination (a Wood lamp).

Small, slightly elevated hemangiomas, called *strawberry hemangiomas,* typically enlarge as the infant grows but are not associated with deeper problems. They may be unsightly because they tend to grow considerably over the first few months of life, and they may be a nuisance, but most are insignificant, and they will resolve over a few years. Strawberry hemangiomas require treatment only occasionally—when they overlie cartilage, which they can erode, or when they obstruct vision or the airway. Not commonly present at birth, these lesions develop over the first few weeks of life.

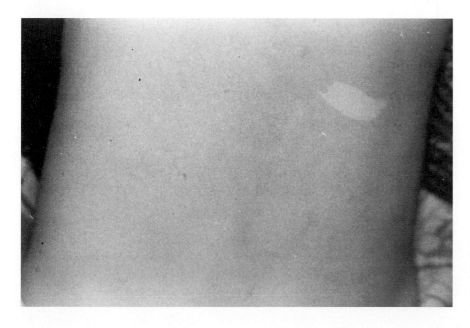

Figure 4–24 Typical "ash leaf" depigmented lesion. Often the first and, for some time, the only sign of tuberous sclerosis in a newborn infant. (From Solomon LM, Esterlee NB: Major Problems in Clinical Pediatrics: Neonatal Dermatology. Philadelphia, WB Saunders, 1973.)

Occasionally, a small area of the scalp appears to have a well-circumscribed defect that is hairless. The patch is shiny, a deeper pink than surrounding scalp, and slightly indented. This is a congenital epidermal defect called *cutis aplasia*, which is most often harmless. However, defects more than 1 cm in diameter can be associated with other anomalies in the infant, such as trisomy 13. If such a scalp lesion is found, careful examination of the infant is crucial. Infants with large defects should be seen by a pediatrician.

SUMMARY

Remember that normality is far more common and far more variable than abnormality. Approximately 95% of babies are normal. Five percent of newborns have abnormal features of greater or lesser significance. There is no substitute for examining as many babies as thoroughly as possible to acquire the warm secure feeling that comes with an appreciation of the immense breadth of normal variation. If you are in doubt about a particular finding in a specific baby, always ask someone with more experience for advice. A good videotape demonstrating physical examination of the newborn is also available.[5]

REFERENCES

1. Ballard JL, Khoury JC, Wedig K, et al: New Ballard score, expanded to include extremely premature infants. J Pediatr 119:417–423, 1991.
2. Brazelton TB: Neonatal Behavioral Assessment Scale, 2nd ed. (Spastics International Medical Publications Clinics in Developmental Medicine, Monograph 88.) London, Blackwell Scientific Publications, 1984.
3. Barlow TG: Early diagnosis and treatment of congenital dislocation of the hip. J Bone Joint Surg Br 44:292, 1962.
4. Ortolani M: La lussazione congenital dell'onca. Bologna, Capelli, 1948.
5. Association of Women's Health, Obstetric and Neonatal Nurses (AWHONN): Newborn Assessment (videotape). Baltimore, Williams & Wilkins, 1986.

SUGGESTED READING

Wimmer JE: Neonatal resusitation. Pediatr Rev 15:255–265, 1994.

chapter 5

Assessing the Child with Congenital Anomalies

MARK D. LUDMAN

Parents who seek help because their child has a congenital anomaly deserve a high level of competence and sensitive understanding from their physician. They want reliable, well-informed answers and an appropriate management plan. First and foremost, an accurate diagnosis is needed. Parents ask many questions, such as the following:

"Why did this happen?"
"What is going to become of my child?"
"What problems will she have in the future?"
"Will she go to school?"
"Will he be 'normal'?"
"What are the chances that something like this will happen again?"

The importance of recognizing parents' needs throughout the interview cannot be overemphasized. This issue is especially vital when you are dealing with the parents of a child who has a birth defect, as underlined in Chapter 1. Remember the spectrum of emotions they may feel at the child's birth and long afterward: shock, guilt, shame, anger, denial.

Key Point

It is imperative that you be sensitive to the parents' concerns and feelings as you interview them and examine their child.

Such parents have just given birth to a child who is less than perfect, who has a "defect." Yet over the past 9 months, they had developed all sorts of fantasies about this child: "Will it be a boy or girl?" "Who will it look like?" "Will he have my nose?" Never did it occur to them that something like this could happen to them. When parents look over their new baby for the first time in the delivery room, they often begin by counting the baby's fingers and toes, never imagining that they would find anything other than ten of each. When

asking questions about topics such as drug and chemical exposures during the pregnancy, maternal employment conditions, or family history, remember that these particular parents are likely to feel guilt. Try not to add to their guilt feelings inadvertently, and do not allow yourself to be misled by such feelings either.

Comfort and counsel the parents throughout the interview; try to set them at ease, reassure them, and give them feedback and encouragement while eliciting information. Point out that we all vary in our appearance, otherwise we could not recognize one another. Emphasize that many features of a baby that an experienced clinician detects as unusual would never be noticed by the average person on casual observation.

One important point deserves emphasis: NEVER use demeaning, insensitive, or inappropriate terms, such as "funny-looking kid" or "FLK," to describe the child either to the parents or to colleagues. If you use such terms when talking to a colleague, you can be sure some child's parents will overhear and resent it.

THE LOGIC BEHIND THE DIAGNOSTIC APPROACH

Thousands of congenital anomalies have been identified, ranging from mild conditions with only minor cosmetic concerns to more serious, possibly lethal conditions. Congenital anomalies are *the* leading cause of death in infancy.

Major anomalies that affect the child's function or social acceptability adversely are found in 2% to 3% of newborns. Many anomalies, although present at birth, are not detectable until later. Thus, 8% to 9% of 7-year-olds have a major anomaly. Examples include certain congenital heart defects, some types of craniosynostosis, and dental abnormalities. Minor abnormalities of no medical or cosmetic consequences may be seen in as many as 15% of births.

These statistics highlight the importance of an organized approach to detecting these problems. Only a careful methodical approach to diagnosing structural defects enables you to provide optimal care to the family. Furthermore, you will need great sensitivity in conducting the procedure; diagnostic labels may produce untoward results, such as stigmatization, as well as beneficial ones, for the child and family.

The "Four Cs"

I use a sequential "four C" approach to the diagnosis of a child with congenital anomalies:

1. *Collect* the data.
2. *Catalog* and organize the data.
3. *Categorize* the defect or defects.
4. *Compare* with references and make the diagnosis.

The bulk of this chapter deals with step 1, collecting the data, which is primarily the process of history-taking and physical examination, often aided by laboratory investigations. Step 2 involves listing the pertinent positive features that have been found. If the diagnosis is not instantly obvious, move to the subsequent steps.

DEFINITION OF TERMS

> **Key Point**
>
> Before you can collect data, you must become familiar with the precise meaning of the terms used to describe anomalies: *major* or *minor anomaly, malformation* and *deformation, sequence* and *syndrome*.

The words *malformation* and *deformation* have specific meanings to dysmorphologists. This chapter deals with the child who has congenital anomalies rather than the child who has congenital malformations. *Congenital anomaly* is a more inclusive term covering all problems commonly referred to as "birth defects," whereas *congenital malformation* is a defect specifically caused by an intrinsic developmental abnormality. A major external anomaly, such as a cleft lip and palate, may be apparent on superficial examination, but the specific nature of that defect, and its association with more subtle features, may be meaningful because anomalies like cleft lips and palates occur not only as isolated defects but also as individual features of more than 250 different syndromes. Your approach to problems such as cleft lip, then, requires that the range of the genetic/dysmorphologic history and physical examination be comprehensive, as it will be if you use the information from each chapter of this book.

Congenital Anomalies

Congenital anomalies have been noted throughout recorded history. Sculptures showing anomalies have been found dating back to 6500 BC, and records dating back to ancient Babylon indicate a keen awareness of congenital anomalies. However, it was only after 1966 that classification of an organized approach to these problems received serious attention. In that year, Dr. David W. Smith coined the term *dysmorphology* to refer to the clinical identification and assessment of structural anomalies, or "birth defects." Over the decades since then, much dysmorphology work was devoted to developing anomaly classification schemes. Such schemes help us understand at what point in development, and often how, the anomaly or constellation of anomalies occurred.

> **Key Point**
>
> After cataloging the child's anomalies, the next task is to decide (1) whether they represent a single isolated defect or multiple defects and (2) which are major anomalies and which are minor.

Isolated versus Multiple Defects

Begin to classify and categorize structural abnormalities by deciding whether the observed defect is isolated or one of multiple defects. If the anomaly is an isolated one, few additional investigations will be necessary, and generally, the prognosis will be clear, and management less complex. However, a child with multiple congenital anomalies represents a diagnostic challenge that may entail considerable investigation. The prognosis may be more grave, especially if the central nervous system (CNS) is involved. If a chromosomal or mendelian disorder is present, the family may face a significant risk of recurrence in a subsequent pregnancy. Further, management of the child is likely to be much more complicated, requiring coordination of care by multiple specialists. Thus the approach to the child with a cleft palate, a ventricular septal defect, or polydactyly is quite different from that for the child with all three anomalies.

Major Anomalies

Next, differentiate between major and minor anomalies. *Major malformations* have serious cosmetic, surgical, or functional consequences. Examples are cleft lip, congenital heart defects, spina bifida, anencephaly, and gastrointestinal obstructions such as duodenal atresia and imperforate anus. Major anomalies involve structures such as the CNS, heart, lungs, kidneys, gastrointestinal tract, and genitalia and are detected readily when organ dysfunction develops. Assessment for internal anomalies may be triggered by signs found on physical examination, such as a heart murmur or a scaphoid abdomen accompanied by bowel sounds in the chest. The diagnosis, however, generally requires further investigations such as imaging studies. Cardiac evaluation may require a chest radiograph, electrocardiogram, and echocardiogram; computed tomography or magnetic resonance imaging may be indicated to assess the central nervous system. Assessment of the limbs and spine often involves reviewing skeletal radiographs.

Minor Anomalies

Although individual minor anomalies may not be surgically or medically significant, their existence is clinically important to dysmorphologists. The presence of several minor anomalies alerts the astute clinician to the possibility that more serious major defects may also be present. Although single minor anomalies are common in the general population, the occurrence of two is less common, and the occurrence of three or more is cause for concern.

Key Point

Ninety percent of newborns who have three or more minor anomalies also have a major malformation. Often, it is the minor anomalies that allow establishment of a specific diagnosis.

Constellations of Minor Anomalies

Most minor anomalies are detected simply by careful observation—the key element of the dysmorphologic examination. When examining individual characteristics, each of which is a minor abnormality, remember that it is not so important that a particular feature is "abnormal."

Key Point

Few, if any, minor anomalies are pathognomonic for a specific syndrome. Although such features are individually nonspecific, it is the constellation of variations that constitutes an identifiable pattern of maldevelopment or syndrome, just as a particular constellation of features lets you instantly recognize your uncle in a crowd.

The constellation of minor anomalies gives the facies typical of certain so-called syndromes their characteristic appearance. In Down syndrome, for example, 79%

of the malformations detectable by clinical examination are minor anomalies. When diagnosis of Down syndrome is made, the "whole" (i.e., the constellation of minor anomalies) is more important than the sum of the individual parts. Many of these individual minor anomalies can also be found as isolated anomalies in perfectly "normal" people in the general population. This is where clinical experience plays an important role, because it is often easier to recognize individual anomalies than to spot the composite pattern that signals a particular syndrome.

Key Point

There is generally wide variation in the expression of any syndrome, and the severity and frequency of the individual minor anomalies may vary.

Minor anomalies include upward- or downward-slanting palpebral fissures, small or low-set ears, ear tags or pits, *clinodactyly* (incurving of the finger, generally the fifth, often associated with a dysplastic middle phalanx), or widely spaced nipples. Variations in features found frequently in the population; (in more than 4% of individuals) are considered normal variants, not minor anomalies. They include mild webbing (*syndactyly*) between the second and third toes (see Fig. 4–22) and *hydroceles* (fluid accumulation surrounding the testes). Because of the large numbers of minor anomalies and potential variations, it would be impractical to list them all here.

Key Point

More than 70% of minor anomalies involve the hand or the face, including the eyes, ears, and mouth. Minor anomalies are therefore valuable clues in syndrome diagnosis.

Nearly 50% of minor anomalies affect the head and face, reflecting both the complexity and variability of the structures involved. Remember the saying "The face reflects the brain"; craniofacial anomalies may be significant predictors of CNS abnormalities.

Anomalies are subdivided according to the mechanism of their abnormal morphogenesis, being classified as *malformations, deformations,* or *disruptions.* This classification poses the question of what happened in utero.

Malformations

A *malformation* is a structural defect caused by an intrinsic abnormality in the developmental process; that part of the body never developed normally. Malformations generally occur during the embryonic period and rarely correct spontaneously. Examples are anencephaly, spina bifida, cleft lip and palate, polydactyly, duodenal atresia, and congenital heart defects.

Deformations

A *deformation*, by contrast, is an abnormal shape, form, or position of a previously normally formed body part because of a mechanical force. Such forces generally result from uterine constraint because of insufficient amniotic fluid, malpresentation or uterine abnormalities, or lack of fetal movement. Sometimes the fetus is restrained; other times, severe neurologic problems cause the fetus to move less. Deformations generally arise later in the fetal period than malformations and often are corrected either spontaneously or through splinting. Examples are clubfoot, congenital hip dislocation, and some congenital contractures.

Disruptions

A *disruption* is a structural defect resulting from destruction of, or interference with, an originally normally formed body part. Typical examples are the anomalies produced by aberrant amniotic tissue bands that may cause amputation of digits, limb constrictions, or bizarre facial clefts. Vascular compromise can also lead to deprivation of blood supply to specific regions of the developing fetus, interfering with continued development. This process is thought to be the underlying cause of some unilateral limb reduction defects and of *gastroschisis*, an abdominal wall defect.

Sequences and Syndromes

After categorizing a child's defects as malformations, deformations, or disruptions, determining the developmental point at which they probably occurred, and arriving at a specific diagnosis, you turn to the next key question: Do the multiple anomalies seem to have occurred as a sequence or do they likely represent a syndrome?

Dysmorphologists distinguish among different patterns of multiple anomalies as *syndromes* and *sequences*.

SEQUENCE

A *sequence* is a pattern of multiple anomalies, a cascade of malformations or deformations, all developing as the result of a single initiating abnormality. An excellent example is the so-called Potter sequence. The initiating event is oligohydramnios, which leads to pulmonary hypoplasia and respiratory insufficiency.

Oligohydramnios may have arisen for different reasons, such as an amniotic fluid leak or a lack of kidney development with no fetal urine production. The fetal compression in utero caused by the lack of fluid leads to (1) a characteristic facial deformation that has been described as looking as if a silk (or nylon) stocking had been pulled down over it, (2) abnormal positioning of the hands and feet, (3) joint contractures, (4) growth deficiency, and (5) often, a breech presentation. Whatever the cause, the obvious detectable features— the multiple minor facial anomalies, the joint contractures, and the pulmonary abnormalities—are all secondary to a lack of amniotic fluid.

SYNDROME

A *syndrome* is a pattern of multiple anomalies all thought to be pathogenetically related but not known to represent a single sequence. Thus, all the congenital anomalies seen in the child with Down syndrome result from the presence of extra chromosome 21 material, but they do not all result as a cascade of events from a single initiating defect. In other syndromes, a single mutant gene, rather than a chromosomal defect, causes an intrinsic disturbance in multiple groups of embryonic tissues, resulting in a recognizable pattern of abnormality.

If the pattern of anomalies detected in a particular child is a syndrome, you must determine whether the constellation of defects is unique to this child or constitutes a recognizable pattern that has been identified previously in many other patients.

This consideration brings up the last stage of the "four C" diagnostic dysmorphologic approach: comparison with references.

Comparing Patterns

The number of recognizable patterns of structural abnormalities and syndromes is enormous, and more are being recognized all the time. The pattern, such as Down syndrome, may be familiar, but if it is not, take heart.

Key Point

There are about 1700 identified syndromes, most of them rare. The average general practitioner may have seen 12 syndromes throughout his or her career, and a typical pediatrician, 50. Even the dedicated geneticist may have a working knowledge of only about 200.

Even experienced dysmorphologists generally cannot remember all the anomalies that constitute any specific syndrome. The amount of information concerning the individual features of specific syndromes is simply too vast to memorize. Luckily, there are many useful reference books for comparing the patient's characteristics with descriptions and photographs of identified syndromes. Perhaps the most widely used is *Smith's Recognizable Patterns of Human Malformation*,[1] which has invaluable tables listing the differential diagnosis of specific individual anomalies. These tables allow you to create a short list of syndromes that manifest as the particular anomalies you have identified in a given patient.

When using these tables to generate a list of diagnostic possibilities, start with the rarest and most distinctive feature you have noticed. Starting with features such as low-set ears or epicanthic folds would result in an unwieldy list, whereas starting with a white forelock or a dislocated lens would be much more manageable. Likewise, if all you identify are several very common features, such as short stature, broad nasal bridge, and clinodactyly, you are very unlikely to attain a specific diagnosis.

Also, several computer programs are now available that can generate such lists, after a constellation of identified anomalies has been entered.[2, 3] These programs provide descriptions and often photographs of patients with different syndromes. The major advantage of such programs is their encyclopedic quality, but their usefulness is always limited by the accuracy of the history and physical findings that the physician "feeds" them. Computer programs cannot take the history or perform the physical examination; only a clinician can.

As a result of the many advances in our understanding of the molecular basis of development and the progress of the Human Genome Project, we are learning the genetic basis for many syndromes. Nevertheless, although we may know the molecular basis for a syndrome, we still may not have any diagnostic laboratory test for it. For some syndromes, a test may be available to confirm a diagnosis made on clinical grounds. Despite your best efforts, and the use of all diagnostic modalities, you may never reach a diagnosis. In fact, in more than half of children with multiple anomalies, no diagnosis can be established. Do not be afraid to admit that you cannot reach a diagnosis when that situation arises: Remember that assigning an incorrect diagnosis can be worse than not coming up with one.

OBTAINING THE HISTORY

To make the proper diagnosis required to manage the patient and counsel the family, the clinician must elicit accurate and complete information.

History of Pregnancy, Labor, and Delivery

Elements of this complete history that require special attention are the pregnancy, labor, and delivery.

PREGNANCY HISTORY

The pregnancy history is outlined in Chapters 1 and 4. Be sure to relate calendar dates to gestation time. For example, note that the mother had a viral illness at 7 gestational weeks, not "on January 16." Specifically inquire about the course of the pregnancy.

Ask about fetal growth. Were any size-date discrepancies noted? Did fetal growth rate seem to diminish? Uterine size may provide clues to both fetal growth and fetal physiology. Polyhydramnios (increased amniotic fluid volume) indicates either increased fetal urine excretion or, more typically, difficulties with fetal swallowing that may be seen with fetal neuromuscular disease, gastrointestinal tract obstruction, or heart failure. Lack of fundal growth may indicate intrauterine growth retardation or oligohydramnios. As mentioned earlier, one cause of the latter is poor fetal renal function. The deformations associated with the oligohydramnios sequence could be expected. Information from prenatal ultrasound examinations may help assess these situations, because other fetal anomalies, fetal position, and activity or uterine abnormalities may have been recognized at the time of the ultrasonography.

Significant Questions

1. Were any prenatal studies, such as amniocentesis, chorionic villus sampling, detailed ultrasonography, maternal serum screening, or cordocentesis, performed?
2. Did the mother or father experience any chronic medical problems, such as diabetes, seizures, phenylketonuria, or idiopathic thrombocytopenic purpura?
3. Did any accidents, illnesses (such as fever or infections), or unusual events, such as medical or dental procedures, occur during the pregnancy?
4. Were there any potentially harmful environmental exposures during the pregnancy: to hormones, drugs (prescription, over-the-counter, and those frequently abused), cigarettes, alcohol, chemicals, fumes (at work and at home), heat (hot tubs, saunas, and fever), or radiation?

Explore these last issues carefully and delicately, and document them. Modern society is preoccupied with the role of environmental factors as a cause of birth defects, and misconceptions regarding the relationships between environmental exposures and congenital anomalies are common. For example, we know that diagnostic radiography hardly ever involves exposure to doses high enough to cause anomalies. Because inquiries about such procedures, although they are important, may increase parental anxiety and guilt about such exposures, be prepared to inform the families about these issues when you ask these questions.

Key Point

Remember: Few agents are proven teratogens, although equally few have been proved safe.

LABOR AND DELIVERY HISTORY

When asking about the labor and delivery, keep several other points in mind. Although breech delivery occurs in 3% to 4% of pregnancies, it is more common in many syndromes. Breech presentation may be caused by the fetus's inability to move into the correct position, and it may indicate in utero that CNS damage is causing fetal motor weakness. Similarly, a difficult birth and asphyxia may not be the cause of a child's problems but the result of them. For example, it is now well established that cerebral palsy, which is often attributed to obstetric difficulties and perinatal asphyxia, is due in most instances to fetal abnormalities that long antedated delivery.

Although the anomalies found on physical examination may help substantiate the diagnosis—which may have medicolegal implications—historic data also may help.

Key Point

Asking about such historical data as the onset, strength, and frequency of fetal movements helps bolster a diagnosis of congenital neuromuscular abnormalities.

Fetal movement is usually felt at 16 weeks' gestation. Although the amount of movement is variable and the mother's perceptions are subjective, fetal movement is normally strong enough at some point to hurt the mother and to be visible to the father. An experienced mother can compare the strength and frequency of fetal movement in one pregnancy to that in previous pregnancies. Feeble, rare, or unusual movements or lack of change in fetal position may indicate neuromuscular dysfunction or fetal constraint, in which case congenital contractures or positional deformations might be expected. In the evaluation of an asphyxiated dysmorphic newborn, a history of abnormal movements may help distinguish the effects of congenital neuromuscular abnormalities from those of intrapartum events.

FAMILY HISTORY

The first step in taking the family history is to make the family feel comfortable. It does not help much to ask the parents whether there are any inherited disorders in the family, because that question presumes they understand genetics, effectively asking them to make diagnoses. Also, inquiring about similarly affected individuals in the family may increase the parents' feelings of guilt and anxiety.

I prefer to begin by asking questions about the parents themselves. Because at this point any chronic or pregnancy-related health problems have been discussed, now is the time to ask about the parents' ages at the time of the child's birth. Advanced maternal age (generally held to be more than 35 years) is associated with a higher risk for chromosomal abnormalities (*aneuploidies*), whereas advanced paternal age may be associated with a higher risk for new dominant mutations (and therefore disorders such as achondroplasia).

Key Point

A woman 35 years old has a 1 in 200 risk of having a chromosomally abnormal child; the risk rises to 1 in 65 at 40 years, and 1 in 20 at 45 years.

Next, ask about previous pregnancies. Were there any spontaneous abortions, stillbirths, or problems in conceiving? Recurrent pregnancy loss (multiple miscarriages) as well as stillbirth, particularly of a malformed child, is often a clue to a familial chromosome rearrangement. Although about 50% of spontaneous abortions occurring in the first trimester involve chromosomal anomalies, most occur sporadically. However, in about 5% of couples who have experienced three or more spontaneous abortions, a chromosomal rearrangement is found in one of the partners.

Sketch out the family pedigree, covering, in general, three generations. Using the details of pedigree construction and the appropriate pedigree symbols (found in any introductory genetics textbook), begin with the parents, recording each pregnancy and the outcome (including stillbirths and miscarriages) in chronologic order, from eldest to youngest, from left to right. The easiest way to stay organized is to begin in the middle of the page.

The convention in drawing a pedigree is that the male partner is drawn on the left. Circles are used to designate females, squares are used for males, and diamonds are used when the sex is not known. Affected individuals are indicated by solid figures, carriers by half-shaded figures. Deceased individuals are shown by a diagonal line through the symbol. Horizontal lines represent matings, and a double one is used for consanguineous matings. Vertical lines denote offspring. Indicate the *proband*, the child you are assessing, with an arrow pointing to the pedigree symbol. Take note not only of full siblings of the proband but also of half-siblings from any previous union of either parent.

Record the four grandparents, their other children (i.e., the parents' siblings) and, finally, the child's first cousins (the children of the parents' siblings). Then document the health of each individual. Note the age of all those living and the date and age at death of deceased family members. An example is shown in Figure 5–1.

Next, determine whether there is any consanguinity. Remember that the risk of both autosomal recessive and multifactorial conditions rises when the parents are consanguineous. Start by directly asking the parents whether their families are related to each other (by blood). You might phrase the question by asking one parent, "Is anyone in your family related to anyone in your partner's family?" This question may not lead to the correct answer, however. As I record the pedigree, I note last names, maiden names, and birthplaces that may raise the possibility of consanguinity. In people who come from small communities, parents are often unaware of consanguinity; it can help to know whether both parents' families come from the same community and whether any family names appear on both sides of the family. When there is consanguinity, a pedigree usually illustrates the relationship more clearly than trying to describe it (e.g., "the parents are third cousins once removed").

Obtain the family's ethnic background, because that information may provide valuable clues to a diagnosis. Certain disorders occur at higher frequency among par-

ticular ethnic groups, and some are virtually limited to a specific group. The carrier frequency for Tay-Sachs disease among Jews of Eastern European descent, for example, is 10 times higher than in the general population. Italians, Greeks, and others of Mediterranean descent are at higher risk for carrying a gene for β-thalassemia; families of Asian descent may carry a gene for α-thalassemia. Approximately 8% of North American blacks carry the sickle cell gene.

Before completing the family history, I ask specifically about any instances in the extended family of multiple miscarriages, stillbirths, infertility, neonatal deaths (especially unexplained ones), birth defects, or mental retardation. Because the words *mental retardation* have an emotional impact, it is often better to ask whether anyone in the family has had "learning problems" or "schooling difficulties." A history of multiple males in the mother's family affected with mental retardation may suggest the fragile X syndrome; this is the most common genetic cause of mental retardation, and its diagnosis can have important implications for genetic counseling. Testing using cytogenetic and molecular studies can be triggered by the recognition of a pedigree pattern suggesting X-linked inheritance.

Ask about any conditions that run in the family, and also about anomalies similar to those in the child. When the situation warrants, examine the parents and other relatives to uncover evidence of similar but perhaps more subtle manifestations of the same disorder.

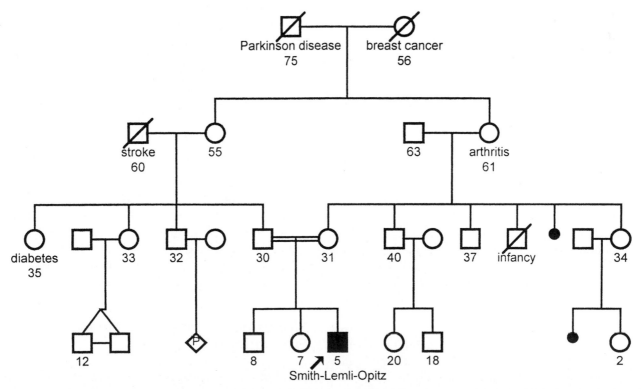

Figure 5–1 A sample pedigree from a consanguineous family of a child with Smith-Lemli-Opitz syndrome (child indicated by *arrow* and *solid square*). See text for explanation of symbols.

GROWTH AND DEVELOPMENT HISTORY

Although *congenital* means "present at birth," some congenital anomalies may not become evident and detectable, or may not be evaluated, until later in life. Obviously in such cases, the history of the present illness must include a description of the evolution of the child's problems, their evaluation and management, and information about the child's growth and development.

Similarly, developmental delay may become apparent only gradually, as the child grows. Because accurate diagnosis of a syndrome may have important implications for prognosis, the timing of the child's achievement of specific developmental milestones may add important diagnostic information.

Key Point

Developmental delay is always an indication for a morphologic examination, because 42% of patients with idiopathic mental retardation have three or more malformations, of which 80% are minor.

If the child's development seems to have proceeded normally for a time, followed by a deterioration of development, the cause of the problem may be a neurodegenerative process rather than a structural brain malformation. Understanding progressive changes in appearance, growth patterns, and behavior makes clear the general nature of the underlying process.

APPROACH TO THE PHYSICAL EXAMINATION

What Is Normal?

The most difficult aspect of the physical examination, especially for a dysmorphology examination, is learning what is "normal." It has become apparent, with the deciphering of the human genome, that there is actually no such thing as a completely normal individual. Indeed, it has been suggested (only slightly facetiously) that a normal person is someone who has not yet been adequately investigated. Remember that genetics is the study of human variation, and a wide range of variation exists for each characteristic considered "normal." It takes experience to appreciate dysmorphic features and to know where normal variation ends and minor abnormality begins. The more normal infants you examine, the more comfortable you will feel about making this distinction. The computer programs mentioned earlier, such as POSSUM,[2] include a CD-ROM with thousands of photographs of dysmorphic features; they are also often helpful in helping you gain an appreciation of the range and description of these features.

Consider the appearance of both parents when trying to determine whether a particular feature is unusual. As mentioned, ethnic background can be important. For example, before concluding that a particular child's upslanting palpebral fissures and epicanthal folds are dysmorphic, ask whether the parent not present at the examination is of Asian descent; if the answer is yes, these features are to be expected. If the child's father is not present, ask the mother whether she has a photograph of him with her. Similarly, if a parent says "Jeffrey looks just like his Uncle Steven did when he was that age," do not just accept the statement; ask to see both old and recent photographs of Uncle Steven. Perusing the family photograph album, looking especially at old baby pictures, can be rewarding; it helps establish rapport with the family and is a nonthreatening way to compare the child's features with those of other family members.

Do not be fooled, however. Even when a child shares certain features with a parent, sibling, or a parent's sibling, do not exclude the possibility that these are minor abnormalities. The parent may simply have an undiagnosed, milder form of the same autosomal dominant syndrome.

If all the grandparents agree that the child does not take after either side of the family, however, take a closer look at the baby. A child's dysmorphic features may be quite subtle and not immediately distinctive. More often, however, the dysmorphic child's appearance is *clearly different* from that of other (unaffected) family members.

Nevertheless, it is also important to bear in mind the considerable variability of syndromes and genetic disorders. Often, even within the same family, two affected individuals may have quite different manifestations. Sometimes, the particular features observed in another affected family member may help you establish the diagnosis if these features are absent in the child. Just as you need to appreciate the range of normal variation, you must also recognize the variability of these disorders. Although obvious, distinctive features may make the diagnosis of a particular syndrome easy, those features may be rare, even in an affected child. There may be more common features that are more likely to be found. For example, *heterochromia iridis* (a difference in color of the iris in the two eyes) may be a distinctive feature allowing the diagnosis of Waardenburg syndrome, but telecanthus, lateral displacement of the inner canthi (see later and Fig. 5–2), is seen more frequently.

Two Basic Techniques of Physical Examination

Morphologic physical examinations are approached either qualitatively and descriptively (the "gestalt" technique) or quantitatively and analytically. The qualitative

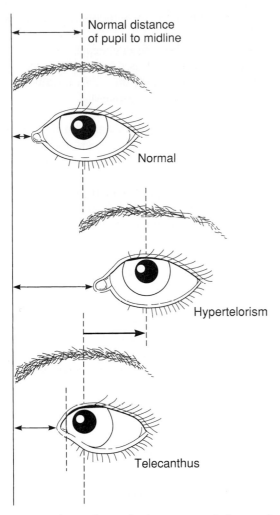

Normal distance
of pupil to midline

Normal

Hypertelorism

Telecanthus

Figure 5–2 In *hypertelorism* (wide spacing of the eyes), the interpupillary distance is increased. When the inner canthi are laterally displaced but the interpupillary distance is normal, the eyes falsely appear widely spaced; this feature is called *telecanthus.* In *hypotelorism (not shown)*, the interpupillary distance is decreased.

school holds, for example, that the eyes should be described as widely set if they appear so; the quantitative school requires that the distance between such eyes be measured and compared with normal standards.

DESCRIBING VISUAL OBSERVATIONS: QUALITATIVE VERSUS QUANTITATIVE TECHNIQUES

The Qualitative Approach

The qualitative approach applies to individual characteristics and also to the child's general appearance, which may be immediately identifiable as representing a specific syndrome. Sometimes a "quickie" diagnosis is possible on the basis of total pattern ("gestalt"), although you generally need to establish a diagnosis by evaluating each feature, both quantitatively and descriptively. It takes some time to become comfortable describing the

particular configuration of different characteristics accurately. For example, a child's face can be described as coarse or elfin; as prematurely aged or expressionless; as round, square, or triangular; as long, flat, or asymmetric. If I describe a child's face as elfin, does that description mean the same thing to me as it does to someone else? If someone else reads that a child was diagnosed as having a syndrome called leprechaunism and that his facies were described as elfin, they might envision a cute, cherubic-looking child, but the face in this disorder is just the opposite; the emaciated children with this syndrome actually have grotesque features.

Key Point

When words fail, one solution is to document visual observations with a photograph—a true example of a case in which one picture is worth a thousand words. A photograph allows others to see exactly what the physician has observed and enables the physician to document changes that may occur with time.

When describing findings, be detailed and specific. Instead of stating that the child has only four fingers, for example, state explicitly whether the thumb is absent or whether the second and third fingers appear fused. When deciding on descriptions, consider questions such as the following:

1. Do the eyes appear deeply set because they are microphthalmic or because the supraorbital ridges are prominent?
2. Are the eyes prominent because the orbits are shallow, or is the problem exophthalmos, or are the lids retracted?

With accurate descriptions, extensive measurement and quantitation may not be necessary.

The Quantitative Approach

Measurements allow (1) comparison with normal values and (2) objective evaluation of a particular feature, free of observer bias. The eyes, for example, may *appear* to be widely set, but when the appropriate measurements are made, it may be clear that they are not. A flat nasal bridge and epicanthal folds may make the eyes seem more widely spaced than they really are.

COMBINING APPROACHES

Combining the qualitative and quantitative approaches yields the best results. Some traits can be described more accurately, whereas others lend themselves better to being measured. "Standard" measurements often do not allow for familial or ethnic variations or permit correction for the effects of deviation in other features. Sometimes a "gestalt" impression may be preferable to any measurement. An example of the problem with the quantitative approach can be seen in the following scenario:

In a child whose head is small, are the eyes normally placed? If the child's head circumference is below the 3rd percentile, should the interpupillary distance also be less than the 3rd percentile, or should it be at the mean (50th percentile) or somewhere between the two? Here, a "gestalt" impression may be preferable to measurement.

Combining the two approaches can compensate for the limitations of the individual method.

The Physical Examination

Murphy's law dictates that the infant you most want to examine carefully and completely is also the one who is the most difficult to examine. Sooner or later, you will be called to the neonatal intensive care unit to see a baby suspected of having a "syndrome." You will find yourself looking down into an incubator at what you can only assume to be a baby … stocking cap over the head to prevent heat loss, eyes bandaged to protect against phototherapy lights, nose obscured by a nasogastric tube, mouth filled by an endotracheal tube held in place by several yards of tape, chest covered with monitor electrodes, umbilical artery line in place, one arm taped to an arm board with an intravenous line in place and the other restrained, and the genitalia completely covered by a urine collector. You may be lucky to be able to measure the length of the child's philtrum!

Key Point

As complete an examination as possible is needed to diagnose the specific nature of a child's problem, a critical issue in making treatment decisions. For example, deciding that a newborn boy has trisomy 18 may have tremendous relevance in a decision whether he should undergo heroic cardiac surgery.

GENERAL ASSESSMENT

Examine as much as possible at the time, returning later if necessary. Begin the evaluation with some general assessments of the child, as listed here, and then proceed methodically from the head down to the feet.

General Assessment Questions

1. Note the height, weight, and head circumference. Are they appropriate? Plot measurements on appropriate growth charts.
2. Is one of these measurements discordant with the others?
3. Is the child obese or cachectic?
4. If the child is short, is the short stature proportionate? If not, this is an instant clue to underlying skeletal dysplasia.
5. If the child's stature is disproportionate, is the abnormality due to shortening of the limbs or the trunk? Measuring arm span and determining upper-to-lower-segment ratios may help sort this out.
6. If the limbs are short, which portion of the limb is more affected? Achondroplasia, for example, manifests as shortening of the proximal bones of the extremities.
7. Are there any asymmetries of body size, shape, or function? Always compare one side of the body with the other.
8. Observe the posture, responsiveness, and level of activity. Are they appropriate for age?
9. Does the child have an unusual cry?
10. Does the child have an unusual odor? A dysmorphic child may have a metabolic disorder.

SPECIFIC ASSESSMENTS

Head

Key Point

Palpable bony ridges over the suture lines suggest premature craniosynostosis. A large fontanel may be seen in hypothyroidism. A "third" fontanel is seen in children with Down syndrome. The child with Down syndrome typically has a brachycephalic skull—round, with a short anteroposterior length and a flat occiput—whereas the child with trisomy 18 typically has a prominent occiput.

Examine the face as a whole, then inspect the individual components. What is the complete gestalt? What aspect of the face is most unusual? Measure the circumference, and note the shape of the head. In the examination of a newborn, molding and edema may make evaluation of the shape difficult, and a second examination may be necessary. Examine the head from different angles to look for asymmetries. Note the size and position of the fontanels as well as the presence of overlapping, ridged, or widely split sutures.

Scalp

The scalp hair pattern is established by the 18th week of gestation and reflects the stretching of the scalp due to underlying brain growth. Abnormal hair patterns suggest prenatally determined underlying abnormalities of the brain. A low posterior hairline may be due to a short or webbed neck and occurs in Turner and Noonan syndromes. Scalp defects are seen in trisomy 13. The hair itself may provide a diagnostic clue. It is kinky in Menkes syndrome, coarse in the mucopolysaccharidoses, sparse in the ectodermal dysplasias, and hypopigmented in albinism. A white forelock, seen in Waardenburg syndrome, calls for a hearing assessment because affected individuals may experience deafness.

Eyes

Although the eyelids of a newborn are frequently edematous, their careful examination is important. Start with the set of the eyes. Are they deeply set or prominent? Note the size and slant of the palpebral fissures. Is there hypotelorism or hypertelorism? These findings may be part of a total pattern of midline facial maldevelopment that may accompany similar brain abnormalities. Holoprosencephaly may be found with hypotelorism; absence of the corpus callosum may be found on computed tomography in a child with hypertelorism. Distinguish hypertelorism from telecanthus (see Fig. 5–2) and from a flat nasal bridge and epicanthal folds. Standards for the normal values for inter canthal and interpupillary distances may be found in various reference sources.[1, 4]

Beyond the lids, look at the globe itself: cornea, iris, lens, sclera, retina. The number of potential abnormalities of the eyes and orbits, including those in the eyebrows, lids, and lashes, is enormous; many of them are listed in Table 5–1. An ophthalmology consultation can be very helpful in dysmorphologic diagnosis.

Ears

Because the ear has a complex origin, it is subject to a wide variation in position, size, and structure and is almost as individual as fingerprints. Assessing ear position and rotation is often extremely subjective and imprecise. A scrupulous examination technique is required to conclude that a child has "low-set" ears. The ears must be examined at an appropriate angle. If examined from the front with the child's neck extended, the ears will appear low. If the ears are examined from the side, assessment of their set is subjectively influenced by its relation to the vertex above and the chin and shoulder below; in infants, in whom the mandible and neck are small in relation to the head, this often results in an incorrect judgment of low-set ears. The ears also appear low set if (1) the head shape and size are unusual, (2) the helix is poorly developed, (3) the mandible is particularly small, or (4) frequently, no matter the angle from which the ears are examined, they are rotated posteriorly.

The best way to assess the set of the ears is to examine the child from the front, with the child's head held erect and the eyes facing forward. Then draw an imaginary line between the two inner canthi of the eyes and extend it around the head. The superior attachment of the pinna of the ear should be at or above that line (Fig. 5–3).

Table 5–1 OCULAR FINDINGS IN DYSMORPHOLOGY

Feature	Conditions to Watch for	
Orbits (the set of the eyes)	Hypotelorism/hypertelorism	Prominent/deeply set eyes
	Palpebral fissures: size and slant (up, down)	Prominent/flat supraorbital ridges
Eyebrows	High arched	Thick
	Synophrys (eyebrows that meet in the middle)	Thin
	Medial flare	Absent
Eyelashes	Long	Absent
Eyelids	Absent or fused	Ptosis
	Epicanthal folds	Epicanthus inversus
	Telecanthus	Coloboma or dermoid
Globe	Anophthalmia	Microphthalmos
Cornea	Corneal clouding	Microcornea
Lens	Cataract	Dislocated lens
	Stellate pattern	
Iris	Aniridia	Brushfield spots
	Coloboma	Lisch nodules
	Heterochromia	
Sclerae	Blue sclerae	Telangiectasis
Retina	Albinism	Optic atrophy
	Pigmentary changes	Coloboma
	Cheerry-red spot	Detachment
Motility	Nystagmus	Strabismus

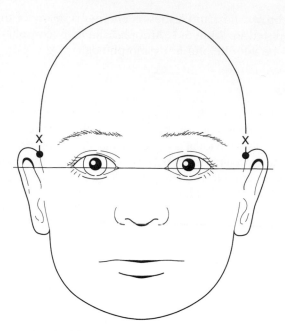

Figure 5–3 Method for determining the position (set) of the ears.

Next, note the size and shape of the ears. Interestingly, the right ear is often slightly larger than the left. Examine the preauricular region carefully for tags, pits, and fistulas (Fig. 5–4). These findings can be important clues to other abnormalities, especially to those involving the branchial arches and often to hearing deficits.

Key Point

Evaluate any patient with malformations involving the external ear for deafness and for kidney and urinary tract abnormalities.

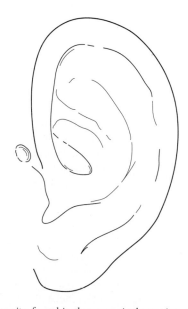

Figure 5–4 Ear pits, found in the preauricular region, may be important clues to other abnormalities.

The shape of the ear is often distinctive in various syndromes and should be compared with the photographs in the standard reference texts. Examine the earlobe for the diagonal creases that are commonly found in patients with the Beckwith-Wiedemann syndrome. Some authorities allege that such creases are found at higher frequency in patients with coronary artery disease. Individuals with Beckwith-Wiedemann syndrome also have punched-out grooves on the backs of the auricles.

Nose and Mouth

Evaluation of the nose, mouth, palate, tongue, and chin is more subjective. The nasal bridge may be low or prominent; the tip may be downturned, flat, broad, bulbous, or narrow. It may even be bifid in cases of frontonasal dysplasia. The nares may be upturned (anteverted) in many syndromes. In the neonate with respiratory distress, always check for choanal atresia.

Examination of the mouth begins with the lips. The philtrum is often flat and featureless in fetal alcohol syndrome. Clefts of the upper lip may occur with or without cleft palate and may be unilateral or bilateral. They are rarely in the midline, but midline cleft of the lip may be a clue to midline CNS abnormalities such as holoprosencephaly. Clefts of the lip may extend up to involve the nostril and may extend through the maxilla.

An important part of the evaluation of the child with a cleft lip, with or without cleft palate, is to examine both the child's and the parents' lower lips for lip pits (Fig. 5–5). The van der Woude syndrome is an autosomal dominant syndrome in which a parent may have only the lip pits but his or her child may have the syndrome's full expression with clefts of the lip, palate, or both. The parents of such a child face a risk as high as 50% of having another affected child, whereas parents

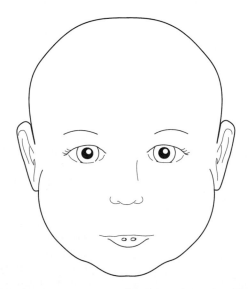

Figure 5–5 Lip pits are important physical signs in the evaluation of a family with cleft lip.

whose child has only an isolated cleft lip have only a 3% to 5% risk of recurrence.

Note the size of the mouth and the shape of the lips. Examine the palate for posterior clefts, which are frequently missed. Use palpation and inspection. A V-shaped cleft warrants a search for other anomalies, because it results from fusion arrest of the palatal shelves rather than from interference with closure by the tongue, as seen with a U-shaped cleft. The latter may be observed with micrognathia in the Pierre Robin syndrome. If you note an apparently enlarged tongue, consider whether it is truly large or whether the jaw is small. Is it really large or merely prominent because it is protruding? Remember that the mandible is normally slightly recessed in newborns.

Key Point

The finding of a bifid uvula is important; although it represents a subtle form of a cleft palate, it may be associated with a submucous cleft of the palate.

Note any gingival hyperplasia or oral frenula, and the state of the teeth. Record the presence or absence of teeth, spacing and arrangement, timing of eruption (premature or delayed), size, structure, and color, which may provide clues to the state of the enamel. Consider ectodermal dysplasias in a child whose teeth are delayed in eruption, few, or abnormal in shape (cone-shaped).

Neck and Chest

Examine the child's neck for branchial cleft sinuses and cysts, webbing and redundant skin folds, a short neck, and torticollis. Because torticollis often develops as a result of intrauterine crowding, it is frequently associated with congenital hip dislocation.

When examining the chest, note its size, that is, measure the chest circumference and shape, and consider the following questions:

1. Is it small, bell-shaped, or "shieldlike"?
2. Is there pectus excavatum or pectus carinatum?
3. Is the sternum short, as seen in trisomy 18?
4. Are the nipples normally spaced or widely spaced? Normal standards are available for comparison.[1]
5. Are there any accessory nipples? These are often overlooked, because they can be found anywhere along the "milk line," which runs from the normal nipple position down toward the inguinal ligament.
6. Are the clavicles absent or hypoplastic, as in cleidocranial dysostosis?
7. Are there any asymmetries that suggest hypoplasia of the pectoralis muscles, as are seen in the Poland syndrome (in which a unilateral defect of the pectoralis muscle accompanies syndactyly of the hand on the same side)?

A thorough cardiac examination is, of course, imperative.

Abdomen

Note whether the abdomen is protuberant or scaphoid. Are there any abdominal wall defects? Distinguish an omphalocele from gastroschisis and from an umbilical hernia. An omphalocele protrudes at the umbilical cord insertion site and is covered only by a sac of amnion. An umbilical hernia protrudes at the same site, but it is covered with skin and subcutaneous tissue. *Gastroschisis* is a defect in the abdominal wall, not at the umbilical cord insertion site, that occurs as a sporadic isolated defect, whereas an omphalocele carries a high risk of associated anomalies or chromosomal abnormalities. Is any organomegaly present? Are there any unusual masses?

Take a moment to examine the umbilicus and, in the neonate, the cord and its vessels. A short umbilical cord suggests poor fetal movements that have not stretched the cord. Infants with a short umbilical cord should be watched for neurodevelopmental problems. Other anomalies should also be considered when a single umbilical artery is found. "Contemplating the navel" helps identify the unusual umbilical shapes seen in many syndromes, such as Aarskog, Rieger, and Robinow syndromes.

Back

Examine the back for kyphosis, scoliosis, and lordosis. A neural tube defect may be obvious, but do not neglect subtle abnormalities, such as sacral dimples that may accompany sinuses; hair tufts; and other overlying cutaneous changes such as pigmentation, hemangiomas, and lipomas. Note the position and patency of the anus. An anteriorly placed anus is often associated with constipation.

Ambiguous Genitalia

The parents' first question on the birth of their child is likely to be "Is it a boy or girl?" They expect an immediate, definitive answer. Ambiguity of the genitalia makes this determination difficult (see Chapter 4), and how you handle this issue from the beginning is critical.

Key Point

The finding of ambiguous genitalia constitutes a genetic emergency.

Parents of a child with ambiguous genitalia should be told that their baby was born with genitalia that are not yet fully developed, making it impossible to tell at that moment whether the baby is a girl or a boy. They should be told that studies and consultations will be performed immediately to determine the nature of the problem. It is important that all health care personnel involved with the family are consistent in their counseling and that no one makes "snap" predictions. The parents should be advised to delay the naming and sex assignment of the baby until the necessary tests are completed to allow a firm gender assignment. They should be encouraged to see the baby and examine the genitalia with the physician. Ultimately, consultation with a team that may include an endocrinologist, geneticist, urologist, and plastic surgeon is necessary for appropriate gender assignment and case management. Reassure the parents that whatever the final diagnosis, surgical procedures can be performed to complete the process of development of the genitalia to allow appropriate sexual functioning.

The most important physical finding is the presence or absence of palpable gonads. Gonads that are palpable in the inguinal canal or labioscrotal folds are nearly always testes, and the infant is a biologic male; the possibility of a virilized female is excluded. Any infant with ambiguous genitalia and without palpable gonads must be presumed to be a female with salt-losing congenital adrenal hyperplasia, a potentially life-threatening condition, until proved otherwise.

Next, examine the phallus. If the phallus has a urethral opening at or near the tip, it is more likely to be a penis. The size of the phallus may be important in determining the sex of rearing. Genital abnormalities range in a spectrum from clitoromegaly in a female to hypospadias, micropenis, and cryptorchidism in a male.

Abnormalities of the Genitalia in Older Children

Key Point

Abnormalities of the genitalia in older children are also important indications of potential problems. They may signify endocrine (often hypothalamic or pituitary) dysfunction or urinary tract maldevelopment.

A variety of syndromes are associated with genital hypoplasia, including the Prader-Willi and Bardet-Biedl syndromes. An affected male has a micropenis and an underdeveloped scrotum. Scrotal abnormalities may be part of various syndromes, such as the "shawl scrotum" seen in the Aarskog syndrome (in which the scrotum appears bifid, with the scrotal fold extending around the base of the penis in a manner resembling a shawl around the neck). In the female, absence or hypoplasia

of the labia minora and hypoplasia of the clitoris may be found. The detection of genital abnormalities should arouse suspicion of urinary tract anomalies.

Limbs

Examination of the limbs is another critical component of the physical examination for abnormalities. Almost 25% of minor anomalies are found in the hands. A good place for the physician to begin limb examination is to count the baby's fingers and toes. Failure to notice polydactyly can be embarrassing, so look carefully. The extra digit may be on the thumb side (*preaxial polydactyly*) or on the little finger side (*postaxial polydactyly*). In some infants with polydactyly, the supernumerary digit can appear only as a tiny nubbin of tissue (inappropriately named "skin tag") at the base of the little finger. These nubbins are just as significant as full extra digits with bones. If they have been removed previously (e.g., in the neonatal period by suture ligation), the only evidence of the polydactyly may be the presence of a tiny stellate scar opposite the base of the little finger. Postaxial polydactyly is a relatively common, autosomal dominant feature, particularly in black people.

Observe whether the digits are fused (*syndactyly*), short (*brachydactyly*), or long and spindly like a spider's legs (*arachnodactyly*). Are they restricted in their ability to extend (*camptodactyly*), or hyperextensible? Is the little finger short? It should extend to the distal flexion crease of the fourth finger. Does the little finger have a single flexion crease, or is it incurving (*clinodactyly*) (Fig. 5–6)? The incurving fifth finger represents hypoplasia of the middle phalanx, perhaps the most common physical sign associated with chromosomal disorders.

Hypoplasia of the nails may be a mild form of limb reduction and is seen in the fetal hydantoin syndrome. Look at the thumbs. Are they unusually broad, finger-like or proximally placed, hypoplastic or absent, or

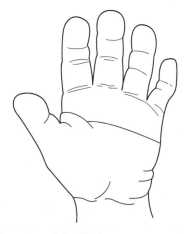

Figure 5–6 Incurving of the fifth finger, termed *clinodactyly*, results from hypoplasia of the middle phalanx. Note that this child with Down syndrome has only a single flexion crease of the fifth finger and a single transverse palmar crease.

triphalangeal? Is the hand held in a clenched fist with the second finger overlapping the third and the fifth overlapping the fourth? This latter finding is seen in trisomy 18 and occasionally trisomy 13 as well as in the Smith-Lemli-Opitz and Pena-Shokeir syndromes. Are any of the metacarpals short? Shortening is apparent as a short knuckle and is seen typically in Turner syndrome and in pseudohypoparathyroidism. Is there dorsal swelling of the hands or feet? This swelling may be the only sign of Turner syndrome in the neonate, and it is often transient. If it is missed or ignored, a major diagnostic clue may be neglected.

Note the palmar flexion creases (see Fig. 5–6). A transverse crease, either single or a bridging of two creases, reflects a short palm. A single palmar crease is found unilaterally in 4% of the normal population, bilaterally in 1% of the normal population (twice as often in males as in females), and in about 50% of children with Down syndrome.

A thumb held adducted in the palm, often referred to as a "cortical thumb," may be a sign of CNS damage from birth asphyxia, but if you observe that a web of skin has formed, tethering the thumb, you can be sure that the defect is prenatal in origin. This finding can have important medicolegal implications.

More formal measurements of the hands and digits and careful analysis of dermatoglyphics can be performed. Although these evaluations are beyond the scope of this chapter, details may be found in dysmorphology reference books.[1, 4]

Dermatoglyphic abnormalities also can be present on the feet. A wide space between the first two toes would accommodate an extra digit. A common finding is syndactyly of the second and third toes, often a familial trait but also seen in Smith-Lemli-Opitz syndrome. When examining the feet, look for a prominent calcaneus or "rocker-bottom" foot, which may be seen in trisomy 18, as may many forms of clubfoot.

Note the length and mobility of the limbs. Is there joint hypermobility or contracture? Are any of the other joints webbed, indicating long-standing contracture? Are there joint dislocations? Are the limbs short? The fingertips should reach to the upper thigh if the upper extremities are of normal length. If they are short, is the shortening due to limb reduction defect (are there congenital amputations?) or dwarfism? Is there disproportion? Which segments are involved? Are there any missing bones? Many syndromes feature radial aplasia or hypoplasia or patellar hypoplasia.

Skin

Examine the skin with the child unclothed. You may note diffuse skin changes, such as thin, thick, coarse, elastic, or lax skin, or localized changes such as hemangiomas, nevi, café au lait spots, or hypopigmented macules (see Fig. 4–24). The last two features are among the important cutaneous findings in the phakomatoses, such as neurofibromatosis and tuberous sclerosis. Examination with a Wood ultraviolet lamp, which makes depigmented lesions more obvious, is often helpful. There may be other abnormalities of pigmentation, ichthyosis, or photosensitivity. Besides the scalp hair and nails, remember that body hair and sweat glands are skin appendages, and they may also be affected in the child with an ectodermal dysplasia. Readers interested in more detail may read one of several excellent reference works on the genodermatoses.[5]

SUMMARY

Although geneticists have an increasingly sophisticated armamentarium of diagnostic tests, ranging from microdeletion chromosome analysis using fluorescence in situ hybridization, to gas chromatography–mass spectrometry for organic acid analysis, and to molecular (DNA) analysis, diagnosis of the child with structural anomalies is still based primarily on the history and physical examination. Special laboratory or imaging studies may be indicated in particular circumstances. Perhaps in the future we will uncover the molecular basis of many more individual defects and syndromes, but until we do, the clinical approach remains the essence of diagnostic dysmorphology.

REFERENCES

1. Jones KL: Smith's Recognizable Patterns of Human Malformation, 5th ed. Philadelphia, WB Saunders, 1997.
2. POSSUM (Pictures of Standard Syndromes and Undiagnosed Malformations). Available from Murdoch Childrens Research Institute, Royal Children's Hospital, Flemington Road, Parkville, Victoria, Australia, 3052.
3. Winter R, Baraitser M: London Dysmorphology Database. Oxford, Oxford University Press, 2000.
4. Hall JG, Froster-Iskenius UG, Allanson JE: Handbook of Normal Physical Measurements. Oxford, Oxford University Press, 1989.
5. Spitz JL: Genodermatoses: A Full-Color Clinical Guide to Genetic Skin Disorders. Philadelphia, Williams & Wilkins, 1995.

SUGGESTED READINGS

Cohen MM Jr: The Child with Multiple Birth Defects, 2nd ed. Oxford, Oxford University Press, 1997.
Goodman RM, Gorlin RJ: The Malformed Infant and Child. New York, Oxford University Press, 1983.
Gorlin RJ, Cohen MM Jr, Levin LS: Syndromes of the Head and Neck, 3rd ed. New York, Oxford University Press, 1990.

chapter 6

Developmental Assessment

SARAH SHEA

A comprehensive pediatric history must include an evaluation of the child's development and behavior. In most cases, such an evaluation can take the form of "developmental surveillance," by which you incorporate screening questions in the general history and observe the child in the office before, during, and after the physical examination. For some children, direct assessment of developmental skills is indicated.

Parents appreciate an opportunity to discuss concerns about their child's behavior. Direct developmental assessment of a child lets you interact with the child in a way that is not intimidating and allows you to observe the child's behavior firsthand.

OBTAINING THE HISTORY

Developmental Surveillance

If concerns about development or behavior are not presenting complaints and if the child is not thought to be at high risk for problems in these areas, simply incorporating questions about development and behavior in the general history is an excellent method of first-level screening. General questions for this purpose are suggested in the remainder of this section. Alternatively, you may choose to use a structured tool such as the PEDS[1] (Parents' Evaluation of Developmental Status) or The Rourke Baby Record,[2] which has a section on development. If you obtain information suggesting direct assessment of development is needed, you can proceed to that assessment later.

Unless such a structured tool is being used, it works best to routinely include sections on development and behavior in the functional inquiry. I emphasize this point because these areas are often forgotten, primarily by physicians who have not made them an automatic part of the history. (I am one of the many who organize the functional inquiry in a head-to-toe fashion and have found it helpful to visualize these areas of investigation as floating around the head.)

Do not forget the importance of the general or open-ended question! My favorite way to find out how parents perceive their child's behavior is, in fact, to say, "Tell me about your child's behavior." Alternatively, you might ask, "Do you or does anyone else have any concerns about your child's behavior?"

For a child who is attending daycare or school, supplement these questions by asking specifically about the child's behavior in those settings. If parents express concern about the child's behavior but have difficulty being specific, try suggesting that they describe everyday situations, such as mealtime, bedtime, or shopping expeditions. Ask, too, about the approach to discipline in the family.

Surveillance questions about development should also be very general at first, such as "Do you have concerns about how your child is learning and developing?" Always ask how a school-aged child is doing in school. In this case, however, I would caution you against simply asking, "How is he doing in school?" My experience has been that the answer is often "Fine," even when the child is having difficulties. It is better to ask specifically what grade the child is in and whether he or she has repeated any grades or has required any additional help for schoolwork.

Other sections of the functional inquiry are obviously very relevant to the area of development, particularly those that touch on vision, hearing, and neurologic symptoms. Information learned elsewhere in the history sometimes suggests the need to look closely at development and behavior, such as evidence of abnormal growth patterns, chronic illness, nutritional deficiency, or medication use. For the child with asthma, for example, you should ask how many days the child has missed from school and whether the parents have observed any behavioral side effects of the therapies used. Learning more about the child's behavior pattern improves your management of such chronic illnesses. Asking questions about behavior provides the opportunity to discuss how the child and family are coping.

It is traditional to ask about developmental milestones in the past medical history. I do not find this terribly useful except in children in whom a developmental problem is suspected. In such children, questions about developmental milestones can provide helpful data about the pattern of development. I suggest emphasizing current levels of development rather than past ones in the functional inquiry. I would go back to ask, for example, at what age a child walked independently or talked only if I had uncovered concerns about development. Precise recall of many of these milestones is difficult for parents, particularly several years after the fact or in families with multiple children. Recollection is fairly reliable for the age at which a child walked independently, but for other milestones, it generally is not.

For preschool children, ask one or two screening questions in each key area of development: gross motor, fine motor–adaptive, personal-social, and receptive and expressive language. The milestones indicated in Tables 6–1 and 6–2 provide some suggestions. If you are pressed for time, I recommend that you ask about language function and personal-social skills, because you will generally have an opportunity to observe the child's gross motor and fine motor skills during the physical examination.

More Detailed Developmental Assessment

For the child for whom there are developmental or behavioral concerns, a more complete history and a direct screening or assessment are needed. Note that behavioral and developmental problems often go hand in hand. If you have a concern in one area, it is always wise to evaluate the other thoroughly.

Your goals are to answer the following questions:

1. What is this child's current level of development?
2. Is his or her development symmetric—that is, are skills developing at the same rate in each of the key areas—gross motor, fine motor–adaptive, language, and personal-social?
3. How does this child's development compare with that of his or her peers? Is his or her development in the "normal" range?
4. What has been the pattern of developmental progress? Has development occurred at a steady rate? Is there any evidence of regression?
5. What is this child's behavior pattern? Are there abnormalities of behavior that suggest a specific diagnosis, such as autistic spectrum disorder or attention deficit hyperactivity disorder (ADHD)?

Additional History-Taking

You can glean information about the child's current level of functioning through the history obtained from the parents and through direct observation and testing. You may supplement it with reports from teachers, psychol-

ogists, speech-language therapists, and so on. If you intend to use a standardized developmental screen or assessment tool, save your detailed questions until you have administered the test. For example, several questions on the Denver Development Screening Test II (DDST II) can be answered through parental report. If you are not proceeding with an immediate assessment or the evaluation does not include parental report, you will want to ask more detailed questions about the child's development. The information listed in Tables 6–1 and 6–2 is suggested as a starting point. (I find it is essential to match what I learn from the parents' history with what I observe on direct assessment; doing so helps me interpret the child's performance better.)

Most parents' reports about their child's current developmental skills and their ability to identify developmental problems are quite accurate, although there are exceptions. Discrepancies between reports and observations of performance may arise if the informant is not the child's regular caretaker or is not a good observer. For example, foster parents who have not had a child with them for a long time; an ill, depressed, or substance-abusing parent; or a parent who has had little recent contact with the child may not be good sources for observations about the child's performance. Some parents overinterpret their child's language ability or overreport developmental skills as a coping mechanism, although this behavior is not common.

Patterns of Developmental Abnormality

It is important to distinguish the child who has *always* shown developmental delay from the one who began normally and has subsequently slowed or regressed. The latter pattern may indicate the need for assessment for conditions such as metabolic disorders, neurodegenerative diseases, autistic spectrum disorder, and seizures. In such cases, a review of past acquisition of skills and earlier milestones is helpful. I encourage families to consult the child's baby book for accurate information.

Family History

Developmental and behavioral problems can run in families. If you suspect a developmental problem in the child, *ask specifically* about the early development and educational level of other members of the immediate family rather than simply asking, "Did anyone in the family have learning problems?" If parents or other family members left school early, find out why. Ask whether those individuals had to repeat any grades and about their current reading and mathematical abilities. This information is important not only for understanding the child's risk factors but also for future management.

Text continued on page 99

Table 6-1 DEVELOPMENTAL MILESTONES: INFANT AND TODDLER-PRESCHOOLER

Age Group	Gross Motor	Fine Motor Adaptive	Personal-Social	Language (Receptive and Expressive)
Infant				
0–4 weeks	Prone: knees come up under abdomen Prone: can rotate head to side In ventral suspension (see Fig. 6–10): head held down Supine: head usually to the side; tonic neck reflex position predominates	Hands fisted, thumb in fist Visual following from side to midline (90-degree arc)	Regards human faces with interest	Responds to sound (bell): quiets briefly if active, startles or blinks if quiet Cries
2 months	Prone: knees no longer under abdomen (frog position) Prone: lifts head to 45 degrees briefly In ventral suspension: head held erect briefly (bobbing) Supine: head kept in mid position briefly	Hands open most of the time Follows past the midline (>90-degree arc) Follows object moved vertically when supine	Smiles responsively Face expressive	Coos Increases vocalization when spoken to Vocalizes with single vowel sounds (ah, uh)
3 months	Prone: lifts head to 45 degrees for sustained period In ventral suspension: head up above level of body. In sitting position: head mostly steady, occasional bob only Supine: head in mid position predominantly	Hands open Hands together in midline, plays with own fingers Holds placed object actively Looks at object placed in hand Looks promptly at objects in midline Follows visually in 180-degree arc and in circular pattern	Anticipates feeding Enjoys watching own hands Smiles spontaneously	Chuckles
4 months	Prone: head up 90 degrees on extended arms Bears weight briefly on extended legs Rolls front to back Downward parachute response emerges In ventral suspension: head and legs held up Sitting position: head steady but slightly forward	Reach and grasp begin Brings toys to mouth Looks at objects in hand	Excited when toys presented Anticipates feeding by opening mouth Pats bottle while fed Smiles and vocalizes at self in mirror	Laughs out loud Shows excitement with voice inflection and breathing Increases vocalizations to toys and people
5 months	Supine: lifts legs high Sitting: head erect and steady When pulled to sit, no head lag May roll back to front	Can hold 1-inch cube Holds two objects simultaneously if placed in hands	Mouths objects Distinguishes strangers from family	Vocalizes with growls Lateralizes to sound Two-syllable vocalizations (ah-goo)

Table continued on following page

93

Table 6-1 DEVELOPMENTAL MILESTONES: INFANT AND TODDLER-PRESCHOOLER—CONT'D

Age Group	Gross Motor	Fine Motor Adaptive	Personal-Social	Language (Receptive and Expressive)
Infant—cont'd				
6 months	When pulled to sit, assists by lifting head Pivots in prone position Sits leaning forward on arms Bears full weight on legs if held standing Anterior propping response emerges Asymmetric tonic neck reflex fully inhibited	Reaches for toys with one-hand approach and grasp Palmar grasp of the cube Reaches after dropped toy Has object permanence (looks for dropped yarn)	Takes solids well without tongue thrust Pushes adult hand away to reject Plays with feet in supine Pats at mirror image Displeased when toys removed	Increasing babble Expresses displeasure with noncrying sounds
7 months	Bounces when held standing Sits erect for brief periods Assumes crawling position	Radial palmar grasp of 1-inch cube Radial raking grasp of raisin (Fig. 6–12B) Reaches and grasps first one cube, then second cube with other hand; maintains grasp on both Smooth transfer Bangs toys on table surface Actively shakes rattle	Brings feet to mouth in supine play Bites and chews on toys Persists to obtain toys out of reach Indicates when full during feeding by closing mouth Anticipates being picked up by raising arms	Beginning of consonant sounds in vocalization (da, ba, ga) Plays peek-a-boo "Mum-Mum" heard with crying Imitates sounds: cough, clicking tongue, "raspberry"
8 months	Sits steadily on hard surface for 10 minutes In sitting, leans forward to reach and re-erects Lateral protection response in sitting emerges Stands holding rail if placed in position	Obtains raisin or pellet with scissor grasp of thumb and finger Removes cube from inside cup	Holds own bottle Drinks from cup held for baby Finger feeds	Understands "no" when strongly spoken Responds to name when called (turns)
9 months	Sits indefinitely on hard surface Gets to sitting position Pulls to stand Reciprocal crawl Forward parachute response present	Explores pellet with index finger	Imitates tricks such as waving Dressing: straightens arm through sleeve when started	"Mama" or "dada" nonspecifically Responds to "no" regardless of tone
10 months	Cruises using two hands on rail or furniture Lets self down from stand with partial control Posterior propping response present	Smooth thumb-finger grasp of small objects Grasps bell by handle Waves bell, explores bell clapper with other hand Bangs two cubes together in imitation	Imitates three nursery tricks (modeled). Examples: pat-a-cake, waving, "so big"	Performs one trick on verbal command alone ("Play pat-a-cake," "Do peek-a-boo," "Wave bye-bye") One word with meaning ("dada")
11 months	Stands momentarily Walks with one hand held	Places cube in cup in imitation but will not release Picks up cup to discover hidden toy (visual memory)	Hands over toy on request with accompanying hand-out gesture Lifts feet to assist dressing	Increased vocabulary

Toddler-Preschooler

Age	Gross Motor	Fine Motor/Adaptive	Personal-Social	Language
12 months	Walks a few steps Stands independently well Creeps upstairs Climbs into small chair and sits	Prefers small objects (e.g., raisin) to larger one (bottle) when presented simultaneously Neat overhand pincer grasp (Fig. 6–12A) Helps turn book pages Releases ball with good throw Unwraps toy hidden in paper Places cubes in cup with release Places raisin or candy pellet in bottle Imitates scribbling	Hugs doll or animal Throws away toys in play or to refuse Gestures for wants Cooperative ball play	Three nursery tricks to verbal request Looks at named object One word besides "mama" and "dada"
15 months	Walks well Creeps downstairs backward Climbs onto furniture to reach things Throws the ball while standing without falling Walks up steps with one hand held Gets to standing without support	Towers two or three 1-inch cubes Scribbles spontaneously Dumps pellet from bottle in imitation Places round block in formboard puzzle (Fig. 6–5) Uses spoon but spills much due to lateral rotation	Leaves food dishes on tray during feeding Attempts to use spoon Helps remove clothing	Seeks help through gestures Four or five words Gestures to indicate wants
18 months	Walks pulling toys or carrying object	Towers three to four cubes Turns two or three book pages at a time Completes form board puzzle after demonstration	Feeds self with spoon without rotation Imitates domestic activities Removes simple garments	Follow simple directional commands ("Give it to Mommy") Points to one to four body parts
21 months	Runs well Walks up and down stairs holding rail Kicks a large ball with demonstration	Towers five or six cubes Completes three-piece formboard without demonstration Aligns three blocks in imitation of train design (Fig. 6–13)	Requests food and drink Uses fork Identifies self in mirror Helps in simple household tasks (putting toys away)	20 to 50 words Combines two words Echoes (repeats words said immediately afterward) Names at least one picture in book Points to pictures on request Points to four to six body parts Follows associative commands ("Give the ball to Mommy," "Put the block on the table")
24 months	Jumps with both feet from floor Jumps off the step Kicks a ball on request Throws the ball overhand	Threads shoelace through hole Turns doorknobs Towers of six to seven cubes Does formboard forward and reverse without difficulty (Figs. 6–5 and 6–6) Imitates vertical stroke and circular scribble Aligns four blocks to imitate train design (Fig. 6–13)	Feeds self with little spilling May indicate toileting needs Enjoys parallel play Washes and dries hands Puts on simple garment Steers toys well	Three-word sentences At least 50 words Names at least one body part Points to seven body parts Uses personal pronouns (me/you/I) Fills in missing word in familiar nursery rhymes or songs

Table continued on following page

Table 6-1 DEVELOPMENTAL MILESTONES: INFANT AND TODDLER-PRESCHOOLER—CONT'D

Age Group	Gross Motor	Fine Motor Adaptive	Personal-Social	Language (Receptive and Expressive)
Toddler-Preschooler—cont'd				
30 months	Alternates feet going upstairs Stands briefly on one foot (1 sec)	Towers of eight to nine cubes Turns single book pages Smooth manipulation of 10 raisins into glass bottle in less than 30 sec (dominant hand) Exact imitation of five-block train design (Fig. 6-13) Imitates horizontal stroke and imitates circle in drawing	Attention span 5 min Toileting accomplished but requires help for wiping Puts on shoes (incorrect feet) Pulls up pants if started Finds armholes correctly Claps or stamps to music Names self in mirror	Multiple-word sentences Carries tune Refers to self as "I" Names multiple body parts Names many familiar objects or pictures Points to pictures of objects described by use ("Show me what we eat with," "Show me what you play with") Discriminates "big" versus "little" ("Give me the big block") Uses plurals
36 months	Pedals tricycle Broad jumps Stands on one foot (2 sec) Alternates feet going downstairs	Tower of 10 cubes 10 pellets in bottle in <25 sec Holds crayon in fingers Attempts to cut with scissors Imitates three-block bridge design (Fig. 6-14) Copies vertical stroke Copies horizontal stroke Copies circle Matches five geometric shapes in puzzle (Fig. 6-7)	Toilet training—goes to toilet without prompt Takes turns Plays interactive games (hide and seek) Dresses with supervision	Gives first and last name Gives own gender ("Are you a boy or a girl?") Recites nursery rhyme or song Understands action agents ("What flies?" "What roars?")
48 months	Balances on one foot (5 sec) Hops on one foot	Builds bridge from model (not imitated) (Fig. 6-14) Imitates a five-block gate design (Fig. 6-15) Copies cross Picks longer of two lines Traces diamond shape	Buttons up Dresses without supervision	Separates easily. Correctly answers comprehension questions ("What do you do when you are cold? tired? hungry?") Understands prepositions (under/on/behind/in front of) Points to colors on request (red/blue/yellow/green) Give opposites Counts three objects correctly Asks questions

Table 6-2 DEVELOPMENTAL MILESTONES: SCHOOL-AGED CHILD

Gross Motor Skills	Children should be able to (1) do a smooth forward heel-toe gait easily by age 6, (2) balance on one foot for 10 seconds or longer by age 5, and (3) skip, alternating their feet, at age 5
Fine Motor Adaptive	By age 5, children should be able to (1), hold a pencil in a mature tripod pencil grasp and (2) cut along a line with fairly good accuracy

Age	Language (Receptive and Expressive)	Visual Motor Skills	Immediate Auditory Memory	Reading	Math
5 years (primary grade or kindergarten)	Defines words by use (e.g., ball, lake, hat) ("What is a ball?" "You throw it") Indicates understanding of concepts by pointing to appropriate pictures or lining up blocks to indicate knowledge of: center, widest, nearest, forward, first, beginning	Copies a square and triangle (no demonstration) Can draw a man: includes six to eight items Copies five-block gate design without demonstration (Fig. 6–15) Prints letters (may copy)	Repeats four digits	Recites alphabet in order Names upper- and lowercase letters May read simple words: see, dog, stop, no Reads own name	Understands concept of one-half Identifies coins Counts (with one-to-one correspondence) up to 10 objects
6 years (grade 1)	Sentence structure is usually grammatically correct Few if any articulation errors Defines words by use, category, composition (e.g., orange, envelope, puddle) Knows right from left Understands yesterday versus tomorrow, more versus less, several versus few, most versus least Can state differences ("How are a bird and a dog different?")	Copies a triangle and Union Jack (Fig. 6–4) Can draw a man: 8 to 10 items, including two-dimensional arms and legs and fingers as details Copies a 10-block "stairs" design (Fig. 6–16)		Reads one-syllable words such as cat, was, ball, blue Can give initial consonant sounds on request By end of grade 1, can read simple sentences: "The little girl saw the brown dog"	Can do simple addition and simple subtraction with numbers less than 10 (2 + 3 = 5; 7 – 3 = 4). May require blocks or fingers to assist in this Counts up to 20 objects Tells time by the hour Understands values of nickel, dime, penny

Table continued on following page

Table 6-2 DEVELOPMENTAL MILESTONES: SCHOOL-AGED CHILD—CONT'D

Age					
7 years (grade 2)	Defines words: football, tiger. Can state similarities and differences ("How are an apple and a peach alike?")	Printing is legible. Only occasional letter reversals, if any. Can copy a Union Jack design (Fig. 6-4) and diamond shape. Ties shoelaces. Can draw a person; includes 14 items and includes clothing	Repeats five digits	Reads words such as hide, across, road, happen, hope, only, could	Counts by 2's. Counts by 100's. Adds two-digit numbers without carrying. Subtracts two-digit numbers not requiring borrowing
8 years (grade 3)	Defines words such as eyelash, tap, roars, Mars. Recites days of the week in order. States similarities and differences ("How are a baseball and an orange similar, and how are they different?")	May begin to learn cursive writing. Can draw a person; includes 15 items. Copies shapes, such as circle, diamond, Swiss cross (Fig. 6-4)	Repeats five digits forward. Repeats three digits in reverse	Reads words such as forest, station, reward, empty, desire, ocean. Can read many two-syllable words	Counts by 5's. Counts by 10's. Can do complex addition (carrying), such as $24 + 79$. Complex subtraction (borrowing), such as $52 - 35$. Simple multiplication, such as $3 \times 4 = 12$
9 years (grade 4)	Understands absurdities in sentences: ("The man's feet are so big that he has to pull his pants over his head")	Can copy a cylinder (Fig. 6-4). Can draw a man with 20 items, including five fingers on each hand	Repeats five digits forward. Repeats four digits in reverse order	Can read some three- and four-syllable words. Can read the following words: timid, delicious, understood, silence, develop, anger. Can alphabetize	Understands fractions. May do two-digit multiplication (12×24). May do simple division (note that school systems vary considerably with respect to the math curriculum)
10 years (grade 5)	Understands the meaning of words such as curiosity, grief, surprise	Can draw a person with more than 20 items, including details such as nostrils, two-dimensional lips, knees and elbows, clothing details	Can recite six digits forward and four in reverse	Can read the following words: promptly, region, common, generally, gracious, applause, marriage, obedient, future	May be able to add and subtract with fractions; do simple and complex multiplication, division, decimals, estimating (curricula vary)

At least 20% of parents have difficulty reading material given to them by physicians! If parents mention reading problems, I like to ask whether they can read a newspaper without difficulty, which indicates a reading level at the late elementary or early junior high level. If they cannot do that, I establish whether they can read simpler text, such as road signs or food product labels.

When children have developmental problems, it is important to ask specifically about consanguinity.

Social History

To understand a child's risk factors for developmental problems, you need to know as much as you can about his or her environment. I like to find out how a child spends his or her days, including the details of child care arrangements, amount of television viewing, the toys he or she plays with, and how much time the child spends sleeping or in a crib, playpen, or stroller. I also ask about any family involvement with social agencies, parent support groups, and intervention resources such as speech/language pathology, occupational therapy, physiotherapy, psychology, and early intervention programs.

Behavior Problems

If behavioral problems are the presenting complaints or concerns about behavior are revealed during the functional inquiry, you will need more details. It helps to record specific examples of difficult behaviors. Find out how the child functions in different settings—at home, at school, with other caretakers, and with one parent or the other.

Behavior problems take many forms. Parents may be concerned about a specific issue, such as sleeping behavior, feeding behavior, or aggression. Alternatively, they may be worried about a child's general tendency toward noncompliance, hyperactivity, or poor social adjustment.

In children whose development is delayed, especially those with language delay, it is particularly important to ask about behavioral patterns suggestive of an autistic spectrum disorder (described in the Diagnostic and Statistical Manual of Mental Disorders, 4th edition [DSM IV],[3] in the section on Pervasive Developmental Disorders). There is controversy about the prevalence of autistic spectrum disorders. Most authorities believe that the full spectrum manifests in at least 1 in every 500 children. Children with this behavior pattern show impairment in the following three key areas:

Social interactions: They may show a marked lack of awareness of the existence or feelings of others, poor eye contact, abnormal social play, difficulty developing peer friendships, impaired imitation skills, etc.

Unusual pattern of development of communication: Such children may experience delays in acquisition of speech along with abnormal nonverbal communication. There may also be unusual use of language, such as *echolalia* (the repeating of words or phrases), or difficulty sustaining conversation.

Abnormal repertoire of activities: Children with an autistic spectrum disorder may have restricted interests or play. They may be preoccupied with certain activities, such as gazing at lights or spinning, and may appear to use their senses in unusual ways, such as looking at things with the peripheral vision or needing to smell or taste objects. It may be difficult to detach such children from activities. They may have stereotyped body movements, such as repetitive hand flapping or jumping. They may be distressed over changes in routine or in the environment.

Such patterns are usually associated with delays in one or more areas of development. Recognize that in these children, development may be uneven, and there may be areas of strength that make the initial picture confusing.

A condition with even higher prevalence is ADHD, estimated to occur in 2% to 5% of children. (Some authors suggest a prevalence as high as 10%!) The full diagnostic criteria for this disorder, as with the pervasive developmental disorders, can be found in the DSM IV.[3] The characteristics generally can be divided into three areas: behaviors suggestive of inattention, of hyperactivity, and of impulsivity. Problems may manifest in the academic situation with poor persistence at tasks, easy distractibility, and disorganization. They may manifest in home and play situations as well. The behaviors can include poor social skills, difficulty waiting (e.g., interrupting conversations), and a high level of physical activity. There are no specific diagnostic tests for ADHD, and the criteria for diagnosis are based on consensus or convention.

While obtaining the history, keep an eye on the child. Observation gives valuable insights into the youngster's behavior and development.

If a child's behavior pattern suggests the possible diagnosis of ADHD, I recommend that you use a checklist based on the DSM IV[3] or one of the standardized questionnaires designed to help look at concerns about these behaviors.

It is crucial that information be obtained directly from teachers about any child who has behavior problems in school, including those suggestive of ADHD. Parental observations of behaviors of inattention or hyperactivity have been shown to be quite sensitive to detection of such problems but are not sufficiently specific to be used in isolation.

You need to ask as well about problems suggesting conditions that are often comorbid with ADHD. Oppositional-defiant or conduct disorders, learning problems, depression, substance abuse, poor self-esteem, enuresis, encopresis, and tic disorders are all more common in children with ADHD. Like other developmental and behavioral problems, ADHD often runs in families, and I emphasize again the importance of taking a complete family history for ADHD and its comorbidities in relatives.

> **Key Point**
>
> A child can be negatively affected by discussions about development and behavior, particularly if they are unflattering. *Consider carefully whether the child should sit outside the room during this kind of discussion.*

APPROACH TO DEVELOPMENTAL ASSESSMENT

Essential Equipment

Besides the usual medical paraphernalia, you need specific materials to perform a developmental assessment. Most important, you need a copy of the appropriate screening tests and tables of age-appropriate milestones on which to base both questions and testing. These items are essential. There is no need to memorize endless lists of milestones; rather, keep handy copies of a screening test or of Tables 6–1 and 6–2 in this chapter. I also recommend keeping a list of the milestones for primitive reflexes and protective responses of infants, because these are difficult to memorize.

The choice of assessment battery depends on your specific goals. An instrument such as the DDST II can provide a general sense of whether a child is performing within the expected age range. Such screening tests are designed to indicate whether a child needs further developmental assessment with more detailed methods. The DDST II should never be used to produce a developmental quotient, a "developmental level," or a diagnosis; thus, you cannot perform a DDST II and then state that a child "shows language skills at a 12-month level according to the DDST II."

> **Key Point**
>
> Whatever screening or assessment test you use, be thoroughly familiar with its scoring criteria and interpretation. Read the test manual entirely before proceeding.[4–8]

Additional Materials

All the DDST II materials are included in the kit, except paper and pencils. To use the techniques recommended here, you also need the following items:

1. Safety scissors
2. 20 1-inch blocks, with one larger but otherwise identical block
3. 12-oz nontransparent cup (Fig. 6–1)
4. Two picture vocabulary cards illustrating a spoon, ball, shoe, dog, cup, house, car, and clock (Figs. 6–2 and 6–3)
5. A cardboard-style book with simple pictures of common household objects and toys (no more than four pictures per page)
6. Cards on which have been drawn a circle, cross, square, triangle, Union Jack–like design, diamond, Swiss cross, and cylinder (Fig. 6–4)
7. A small glass bottle
8. Some small (roughly ¼-inch) candies to be used as pellets for fine motor manipulation
9. A formboard puzzle with removable geometric blocks of a color contrasting with the base (Figs. 6–5 and 6–6)
10. A five-shape matching puzzle card, 11 × 5 inches, with five red, flat shapes pasted on it, and forms, all red, matching exactly the shapes on the card: circle, 2-inch diameter; square, 2-inch sides; triangle, 2⅝-inch sides; semicircle, 3¼-inch diameter; cross, 2⅞-inch long with arms ¹⁵⁄₁₆-inch wide (Fig. 6–7)

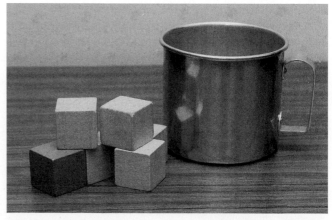

Figure 6–1 Testing materials. A nontransparent cup and 1-inch block.

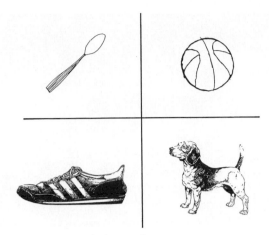

Figure 6–2 Picture vocabulary card.

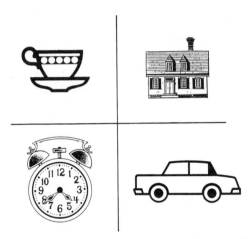

Figure 6–3 Another picture vocabulary card. Only one card at a time should be shown to the child.

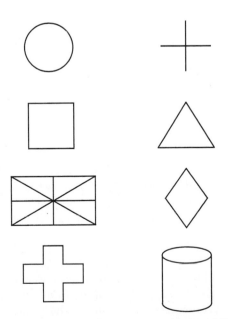

Figure 6–4 Geometric figures for testing visual-motor skills.

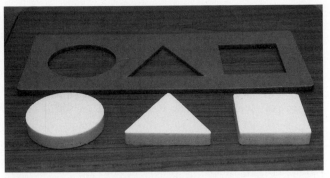

Figure 6–5 Formboard puzzle in "forward" (matched) position. (Figures were made by following instructions given in the Revised Gesell Developmental Schedules.[8])

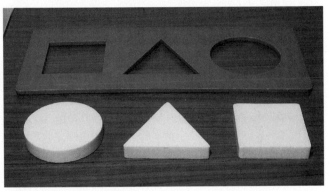

Figure 6–6 Formboard puzzle in reversed (unmatched) position. (Figures made following instructions in the Revised Gesell Developmental Schedules.[8])

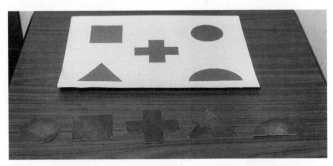

Figure 6–7 The five-shape matching puzzle. (Figures made following instructions in the Revised Gesell Developmental Schedules.[8])

Strategies to Enhance the Child's Participation

You need the child's full and active cooperation to test his or her developmental abilities. Assessment can be particularly difficult when a child is inordinately shy, hyperactive, inattentive, anxious, fearful, or oppositional or if the parents are unusually intrusive during the procedure.

SHY AND FRIGHTENED CHILDREN

You know you are in trouble when you walk into the room, introduce yourself, and the youngster immediately dives for his mother and buries his face in her lap. When this happens, you may have the urge to take refuge yourself and refuse to participate—but all is not lost. Most shy children can be won over by a gentle, nonthreatening approach. First, remove any items that the child may consider threatening, including your white coat. Medical equipment should not be hanging around your neck or protruding from your pockets (Fig. 6–8). For children in hospital, a change of environment may help. A parent counseling room or conference room offers a less threatening environment for developmental assessment.

When a child is shy or anxious, do not stare at the child or rush to coax him or her into playing. Sit, chat with the parents, take some history, and give the child a chance to get used to you. Offering some toys while you speak with the parent may help (Fig. 6–9). Items in the developmental assessment kit come in handy here. For children older than 3 years, paper and crayons work well. You can give almost anything to a younger child, provided it is neither sharp nor ingestible. Blocks, a rattle, or even a penlight will do. Many physicians carry around at least one pocket-sized toy to hand to children. These toys presumably will be retrieved at the

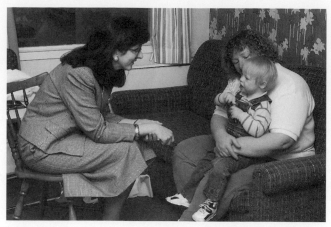

Figure 6–9 Correct way to approach the child. Use the eye-level approach and have no intimidating "appendages" in your pockets.

end of the visit—an excellent test of your negotiating skills.

Always allow or even encourage shy or anxious children to stay close to their parents at first. Maintain a gentle, friendly tone and use lots of positive verbal reinforcement. Some children, particularly hospitalized children experiencing separation from their parents or uncomfortable procedures, are genuinely frightened. For children with sufficiently developed verbal skills, clarify that you are not there to perform medical procedures ("no needles"). If a child is so frightened that you cannot carry out a good developmental assessment, you may have to try again on another occasion. If so, take a few minutes to play before leaving. This low-key interaction makes the second visit more successful.

OPPOSITIONAL CHILDREN

Some children are frankly oppositional. They make it clear that they are out to give you a hard time and will not cooperate. Such children do not appear genuinely frightened, and they may smile, particularly when they realize that they are causing frustration for the physician or their parents.

> **Key Point**
>
> Stay calm, maintain a friendly approach, and provide positive verbal and even physical reinforcement through a touch on the shoulder or the like. You may even wish to be a more concrete philanthropist and reward participation with stickers or edibles.

For developmental assessment of most younger children, it helps greatly to have the parents present. For a few, however, parental presence is the principal trigger for oppositional behavior, and such children may need to be assessed alone. Involve the parents in this deci-

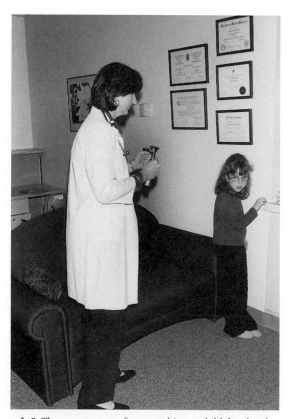

Figure 6–8 The wrong way of approaching a child for developmental assessment. Avoid medical equipment, white coats, and towering over the youngster.

sion, and be as diplomatic as possible. I usually ask, "Do you think Barry might concentrate better if he and I worked together alone for a little while?" Most parents agree to the suggestion with considerable relief. Often, the child's behavior improves when the parent leaves. You may have to weather a brief tantrum at the time of the separation, but if you wait it out calmly and then present some play activities, most children, particularly oppositional children between 3 and 5 years old, eventually cooperate.

HYPERACTIVE OR INATTENTIVE CHILDREN

Some children are hyperactive, inattentive, or both. *Hyperactivity* refers to a high level and intensity of motor activity, whereas *inattention* implies difficulty concentrating on desired tasks in the face of potentially distracting stimuli. When confronted with a physically overactive child who is nonetheless able to maintain attention, be flexible. You can ask the child questions even though he or she is jumping up and down or climbing the bookcase. Children do not need to be sitting down to carry out activities such as block design, copying, and writing, but you should note whether they are sufficiently stationary to accomplish the tasks before deciding whether their performance is at a satisfactory level.

The inattentive child needs much positive reinforcement, such as "I like the way you are working; that's a terrific job. Let's do another game." As with the oppositional child, a touch on the shoulder or a pat on the back may be in order.

Key Point

Do not give instructions or ask questions unless you have direct eye contact.

Change tasks with reasonable speed to maintain the child's interest, but make sure the child has been given enough time to accomplish each task. If the child's attention wanders, redirect it. It may help to ask the child to repeat the instruction or question before answering. You may be firm but you must never be angry with an uncooperative child. *Firm* means using a serious voice and repeating commands several times. For example, say in a serious tone, "Billy, I would like you to stop standing on your head and come back and sit down; we still have work to do." If you believe that you are truly becoming angry—especially if the anger is starting to show—it is time to retreat. Take a break, take a walk in the hallway, or simply quit for the time being.

Inattentive children work best where there are as few visual and auditory stimuli as possible. They should never be assessed in a busy room or on a hospital ward. They are also sensitive to internal distractions, such as fatigue or hunger, and their attention is usually at its best in the morning. If a child is taking medication that may interfere with the attention span (e.g., large doses of bronchodilators for asthma), the assessment should be timed to minimize such effects.

The Intrusive Parent

Sometimes attempts to assess a child's development are impeded by an intrusive parent whose understandable eagerness for the child to succeed interferes with the youngster's spontaneous responses. This can be a problem when you are testing language, because parents may inadvertently give the child visual or verbal cues. Address this problem directly. Start by saying, "Now, I'm going to be asking Maria to follow instructions to find out whether she can understand what to do from my words only. You and I both have to be careful that we don't give her any hints by using our eyes or gesturing."

A parent who continues to provide answers or clues to a child despite such warnings may be doing so out of anxiety about the child's performance. Stop the assessment and address the issue through gentle questioning. For example, ask the parent how he or she thinks the assessment is going. If the parent expresses anxiety, explain that you will be giving the child some tasks that are beyond the child's current abilities. If the parents truly are unable to divorce themselves sufficiently from the assessment, it may be best to work with the child alone.

APPROACH TO THE PHYSICAL EXAMINATION

At the time of the physical examination, simply watching the child dress and undress reveals a great deal about the youngster's motor skills and ability to follow directions.

Key Point

The physical examination should be left until last to avoid losing the child's cooperation.

In infants, primitive reflexes (Fig. 6–10), protective responses, and behavior in the prone and supine positions should be assessed after the physical examination, because the methods used to elicit them may distress the infant.

Start with the infant or child in a sitting position. Babies can sit on a parent's lap or in an infant seat that provides good support and allows both arms to be free. If a child is in the parent's lap or in a seat without a tray, improvise a table by having an assistant hold a

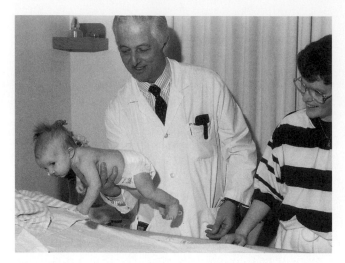

Figure 6–10 The ventral suspension maneuver. This 1-month-old baby holds the head above body level and the legs partly extended

large book in front of the baby. A highchair or other appropriate-sized chair and table can provide a good surface for testing (Fig. 6–11). Children with problems of muscle tone or motor control may be best assessed while they sit in customized seats or wheelchairs.

Direct testing of fine motor skills and problem-solving tasks such as block manipulation and coloring are generally very engaging for children. Leave language testing, particularly the parts that require a child to speak to you, until later so that the child is cooperating well before these assessments are attempted. Leave testing of gross motor skills to the very end, because those activities may get the child excited. Such testing also fits more naturally into the neurologic and general physical examination (see Chapter 13). Be flexible; a fidgety child may benefit from taking a break in the hallway to play ball or skip.

When you give the child a toy or object to manipulate, engage his or her interest in that item alone. With infants, it helps to tap the object on the table, then bring it within the baby's reach. When it is time to

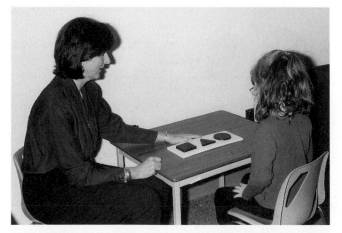

Figure 6–11 Seat the child at an appropriate-sized table for testing. Present only one task at a time, and avoid visual or auditory distractions.

switch test objects, have the next object in hand before removing the previous one, and clear the table completely before introducing it. If the child insists on clinging to the previous toy despite your gentle attempts to remove it, let him or her hold it, but find a high-interest activity and try to engage the child in it. Play with the new test object yourself, tapping it to make interesting noises, or engage the parent in the activity. With the ambulatory child, another option is to switch to a gross motor activity and quickly remove the object from sight before the youngster sits down again. Give plenty of reinforcement for effort and accomplishment. Younger children love to have their efforts rewarded with smiles, praise, or clapping.

Special Considerations

Whether to correct for gestational age when evaluating children younger than 18 months who were prematurely born is still a matter of controversy. If a child is seen at a chronologic age of 15 months but was born 3 months early, the child's corrected age is 12 months. For children with no neonatal complications, full correction may overestimate performance, especially in language and personal-social skills. Check the guidelines for the specific screening test you are using to find out whether it has correction for prematurity.

Key Point

Remember that you are looking for strengths as well as weaknesses.

Discordant development in different areas gives important information about potential problems. For example, excellent motor skills and good nonverbal problem-solving skills but delayed social and language development in a child could suggest a hearing deficit, a communication disorder, or an autistic spectrum disorder. More detailed speech and language testing and an audiogram may be in order.

Every child's performance must be interpreted against the background of the history. When performance and history are discordant, it is often because the child's cooperation could not be elicited during the assessment. Alternatively, the history may be inaccurate.

Developmental Milestones

Tables 6–1 and 6–2 list developmental milestones and skills. Although these lists do not replace more detailed developmental assessment, they do provide useful general guidelines about the typical progression of skills in children. It is my experience that parents and physicians have the greatest difficulty knowing what to expect for a child's receptive language at any given age. This is a very important area to have norms for, because delays in a child's "talking" are a common developmental concern.

For convenience, Table 6–1 is divided into two age groupings, infant (0 to 12 months) and toddler-preschooler (15 months to 48 months); Table 6–2 lists the skills for the school-aged child (5 years or older). As children reach school age, assessment of motor skills becomes less important, and the focus is more on higher cognitive functions and specific academic skills.

The following case histories illustrate assessments of an infant, a preschooler, and a school-aged child.

Case Histories

Case 1

Twelve-month-old Susan is an only child of unrelated parents who are concerned about her slow development. She is growing normally but does not walk yet. She is silent, speaks no words, and babbles little. Her mother's pregnancy was uncomplicated except for a "flulike" illness at 14 weeks. Susan was born 4 weeks early with a normal birth weight and no neonatal complications.

She smiled at 1 month, rolled from front to back at 3 months, and sat without support at 7 months. Susan babbled by 6 months of age but thereafter became increasingly quiet. Her parents had always thought that she was an alert happy baby, but lately they notice she seems to startle easily. There is no family history of developmental problems.

When asked about Susan's vision, the parents say that she can follow things normally and seems to see objects both near and far away. Her eyes have never crossed. When asked about her hearing, they report that she often startles when they walk into a room and she sees them. They wonder if she does not hear them coming. She has had two ear infections but has undergone no formal hearing testing. She has never had seizures, unusual movements, or head injuries.

Both parents work outside the home, and Susan is in daycare with three other children younger than 4 years. There are no financial, housing, or family problems.

Questioning about gross motor performance reveals that Susan can sit indefinitely and protects herself from falling. She can get herself to a sitting position, pull herself up to stand, and cruise along furniture. She crawls and can walk when both hands are held. She is starting to lift one foot up when standing if her mother is putting on or removing Susan's pants and straightens her arm through her sleeve when it is started.

During the history taking, Susan has been sitting on her mother's lap. The physician hands her two tongue depressors. She takes the first one and then the other, bangs them together, and chews on them happily. The physician begins a more detailed developmental assessment, remembering to correct for her prematurity comparing her with an average infant of 11 months. Susan imitates people when they wave their hands or clap them together (pat-a-cake), and she slaps an extended hand. Her parents say, however, that she does not do any of these on verbal request only; she seems to respond only to the gesture. She will hand a toy to her parents if they extend their hands. She can hold her bottle, drink from a cup, and feed herself crackers.

When asked about language milestones, the parents report that Susan has never imitated any sounds or syllables. Her babble has been decreasing over the past 2 months. She has never turned specifically toward a sound. Her vocalizations are largely vowel sounds of varying loudness. She laughs but does not turn when called by name and does not respond to a spoken "No."

Because Susan seems comfortable, the physician decides to sit her close to her parents at a toddler's chair and table. The physician starts by placing two blocks on the table. She immediately reaches first for one, then the other, using a thumb-finger grasp. When the physician takes two cubes and bangs them together, she immediately imitates the motions. The physician puts a cup on the table and demonstrates putting the cube into it. Susan puts her hand with the cube into the cup but does not let go of the cube and takes it back out instead. The physician removes the cup and the cubes and presents her with a small interesting toy (a 1-inch figure of an animal), engaging her interest by marching the toy along the table and then hiding it under the overturned cup. She immediately lifts up the cup to get at it. The physician lets her play with it for 30 seconds. The physician then places the toy in the middle of a thin piece of paper (tracing paper or onion skin) and twists the four edges together so that it is inside the paper. She watches the physician do this; the physician then hands her the paper. She does not unwrap the toy.

The physician removes the wrapped toy and gives her a small pellet-sized candy and glass bottle. She immediately pokes at the pellet with her index finger and picks it up with a smooth overhand pincer grasp (Fig. 6–12). The physician notices that the ulnar side of her hand rests on the table when she picks it up. The physician demonstrates putting another pellet inside the bottle, but she does not imitate the action. The physician replaces the pellet and bottle with a crayon and paper. She does not scribble. The physician demonstrates scribbling, but Susan still is not interested.

Holding a bell carefully out of her sight, the physician rings it, first quietly and then louder. She

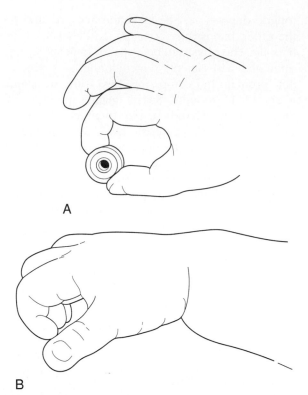

Figure 6-12 A, Overhand pincer grasp. B, Radial raking grasp.

does not respond. The physician brings the bell closer to her but still keeps it behind her and to the side while she is distracted by a toy in front of her. The physician continues to ring it loudly, but she does not turn. The physician passes the bell to Susan's father behind her back and asks him to ring the bell on her other side. She does not respond at first but when he brings it very close she seems to become alert. She spies the bell and takes it by the handle. She looks at it and pokes at the clapper but waves it only briefly.

At this point, the physician decides to proceed to the physical examination, which reveals some pigmented areas in the right optic fundus but no additional neurologic or other abnormalities. The physician tells Susan's parents that her physical examination is normal and that her development in most areas is normal for a child of her corrected age. However, the physician is concerned that both her receptive and expressive language skills are late, and the office screening test suggests possible hearing impairment. A subsequent audiogram reveals profound bilateral sensorineural hearing loss, and a consulting ophthalmologist confirms the presence of chorioretinitis, findings compatible with a prenatal infection, such as cytomegalovirus or toxoplasmosis. Susan is fitted with hearing aids and given speech and language therapy to stimulate her development. She is also referred for evaluation regarding cochlear implant surgery.

Case 2

Three-year-old Steven is brought to a physician because his daycare supervisor reports that he is hyperactive and does not seem to "fit in" with the other children. He does not participate in group activities; he wanders off and always plays alone. He will not sit during circle time and does not follow directions well. His family believed that he was fine but a little "slow." Steven was born after a normal full-term pregnancy, with normal birth weight and no neonatal complications. He had been in good general health. His mother remembers that he sat at 10 months, learned to walk at 20 months, and said his first word ("Dada") at 18 months. She is not sure when he started to put words together but thinks that it was within the past 6 months.

Steven has a 7-year-old sister who is doing well in grade 1. His mother had learning problems in school, repeating grades 1, 5, and 8. She did not complete grade 9 and received resource help for many years. She remembers being told that she walked and talked late. Steven's father has a high school education and had no learning problems.

The functional inquiry and social and personal histories are noncontributory.

While taking the preliminary history, the physician regularly observes Steven, who is sitting quietly. When offered paper and crayons, he scribbles in different colors. The physician decides it is time to review his development further by means of his mother's report. Steven is unable to pedal a tricycle, although he has tried it. He can walk up and down stairs holding the rail. His mother has seen him kick a ball and throw overhand. The physician later confirms these skills during the examination. Steven is not toilet trained. He feeds himself with a spoon and a fork and drinks from a cup. He can put on a hat and a loose sweatshirt but does not know front from back and cannot put on other garments. He likes to steer toys around and will help in simple household tasks such as emptying the dishwasher. He does not play games such as hide-and-seek or tag. He speaks mostly in single words or two-word combinations ("Mommy go"). He can name three body parts, and he refers to himself as "me" and likes to fill in missing words in songs. His mother is not sure how many words he has in his vocabulary.

At this point, the physician moves to direct play with Steven, starting by getting a fresh piece of paper and a crayon. The physician notices that Steven holds the crayon in his fist. The physician shows him a vertical line and asks him to draw one. He scribbles in a circular fashion instead. He does the same when shown how to draw a vertical or horizontal stroke or circle. The physician removes the crayon and paper and brings out the blocks. The physician shows him how to build a tower by piling

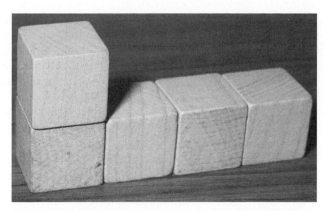

Figure 6-13 The five-block "train" design.

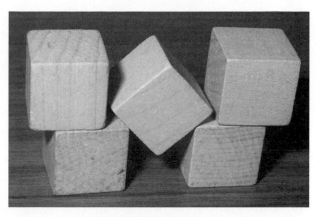

Figure 6-15 The five-block "gate" design

three blocks and then places one block down and hands him a second one, saying, "Now you build it." As the child places each block, the physician hands him the next one and praises his efforts. Steven builds a seven-block tower, and then it falls. He achieves a six-block tower on the next try.

The physician praises his efforts and removes all but five of the blocks, which the physician sets up in a train design (Fig. 6–13). The physician says, "I am going to make a train. Here is a car, here is a car, here is a car, and see, it has a little chimney on top." The physician takes the train apart and says, "Now you build me a train." Steven puts four blocks in a line. The physician asks him where the chimney is, but he does not put it on. The physician then gives him three blocks and keeps three. The physician builds a three-block bridge design (Fig. 6–14) and then asks Steven to build a bridge just like it, leaving the sample bridge standing. He is unable to complete the design.

The physician removes the blocks and gets out a three-piece formboard, placing it as shown in Figure 6–5 with the matching puzzle pieces underneath the

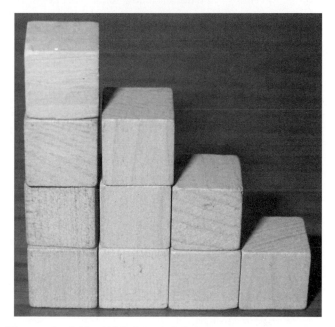

Figure 6-16 The 10-block "stairs" design

spot closest to the child. Steven promptly does the puzzle. The physician then removes the pieces and reverses the board (see Fig. 6–6). Steven immediately does the puzzle again and smiles with satisfaction. The physician removes that puzzle and gets out the five-shape geometric matching puzzle (see Fig. 6–7), showing Steven that the circle goes on top of the circle on the figure. The child, however, does not complete that puzzle.

The physician gets out a paper and child-size scissors and notices that Steven is unfamiliar with how to use the scissors. He hands them back and says, "You cut." The physician obliges him briefly, then puts out a bottle with 10 pellet candies and asks the child to put the candies in the bottle. Steven does so slowly, taking more than 30 seconds. The physician then asks him to turn pages in a book, and he turns them two or three at a time.

At this point, the physician says to Steven, "I would like to ask you some questions. Are you a boy

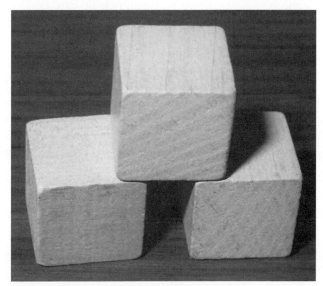

Figure 6-14 The three-block "bridge" design.

or a girl?" He responds, "Me Steven." The physician asks him what the rest of his name is, and he repeats, "Steven." The physician asks him to name demonstrated parts of the body. He names only nose and ears. The physician then asks him to point to his body parts, and he points successfully to seven. Next, the physician shows him picture vocabulary cards (see Figs. 6–2 and 6–3) and asks him to name the items shown. He names the house and the shoe but not the others. The physician names pictures and asks Steven to point them out. He points to most of them. The physician asks Steven to show "what we drink from" and to show "what we play with," but he is unable to do so. The physician asks Steven to sing "Twinkle, Twinkle, Little Star" because his mother indicates that he can do so. He carries part of the tune. He does not sing the words, but when the physician leaves out a phrase, he fills it in.

Next, the physician gets out a large and small block and asks him to hand over the big block. He does so. The physician puts the blocks back down and asks him to hand over the little block. However, this time Steven offers the big block. The physician puts the blocks down again and says, "Give me the big block," and he offers the little block. The physician decides that Steven does not really understand the difference between "big" and "little." The physician shows him the two blocks and asks what they are; he calls them "block" without pluralizing the word.

The physician then moves into the gross motor examination and leads into the neurologic examination. Steven can kick, throw overhand, and jump with both feet but cannot do a broad jump or stand on one foot. His height and weight are normal. His ears appear large, as do his hands. He has a somewhat coarse facial appearance. His testes measure 2 mL in volume with the orchidometer—slightly large for a 3-year-old boy. The remainder of the physical examination is normal.

Steven has been cooperative and attentive throughout and has not demonstrated any hyperactivity. When the physician asks his mother whether she thinks today's behavior was typical for him, she says yes.

The physician decides that Steven does not show significant hyperactivity but that he has developmental delay in all areas, functioning more like a 24-month-old child than a 36-month-old. The slight enlargement of the testes, coupled with developmental delay, are the clues to the diagnosis. The physician refers Steven for a more detailed developmental evaluation and karyotype, which confirms that he has the "fragile X" chromosomal abnormality.

Case 3

Nine-year-old Tommy is not doing well in school; he is currently repeating grade 2. After his first school year, his teacher reported that he did not learn his letters and numbers as well as the other children. Tommy was born after a normal pregnancy by cesarean section due to cephalopelvic disproportion. A review of his early milestones reveals that he walked at 10 months and used at least five words before the age of 1 year. His mother thought that he was bright in every respect before he entered school at age 6. She recalls he was never interested in ABCs or numbers or in paper and pencil work before he started school. He has never presented behavior problems. His teachers always thought that he was trying hard, yet each year, he required resource help because he was behind the other students.

Tommy is an only child. Although his father has a university-level education, he repeated three grades in the first 7 years of school and had a major problem learning to read. He is still slower at reading than his colleagues but makes up for it in his job as a technical supervisor through extra work. Tommy's mother also has a university-level education and is a nursing supervisor. She did not have any school problems, but one of her brothers required resource help throughout elementary school for reading problems. There has been much family conflict over Tommy's homework, because it is difficult for him to accomplish, and he has become resistant to doing it.

The physician has taken this part of the history with all three members of the family present. A review of Tommy's self-help skills shows that he has no difficulty with dressing or running errands. He is popular with friends and involved in swimming and scouting. At this point, the physician asks the parents to leave, wanting to do some further interviewing and assessment with Tommy alone. The physician chats initially with Tommy about his favorite activities to put him at ease. The physician starts by having him do some drawing, asking him to draw the very best picture of a man that he can. He draws a picture with more than 20 items and many details. The physician then asks him to copy the geometric shapes shown in Figure 6–4. He does so without any difficulties. He prints the letters of the alphabet in capitals with no difficulty. He has no difficulty defining the following: football, tiger, eyelash, tap, roar, Mars. He recites the days of the week in proper order and describes the similarities and differences between a baseball and an orange. He gives correct answers to the following written problems:

$$\begin{array}{cccc} 2 & 4 & 17 & 24 \\ +3 & +6 & +11 & +79 \end{array}$$

$$\begin{array}{ccc} 7 & 11 & 37 \\ -2 & -4 & -23 \end{array}$$

Tommy is unable to correctly answer "52 – 35 =" because he does not yet know borrowing. He does not yet do simple multiplication. The physician screens his immediate auditory memory by having him repeat numbers recited in a monotone at one per second. He can repeat five digits forward, and four in reverse.

The physician then moves to reading. Because it is Tommy's area of acknowledged weakness, this evaluation has been left to the end to avoid distressing him. He can read words such as cat, was, ball, and blue and can read "A little girl saw the brown dog." However, he is unable to read such words as hide, across, road, happen, hope, only, and could. He gets upset during this part of the assessment. When presented with unfamiliar words, his guesses frequently make no sense. For example, he reads hide as horse and road as river.

The neurologic and general physical examinations reveal nothing out of the ordinary, and the developmental screening shows no weakness except in reading, for which Tommy is at a grade 1 level, although he is now repeating grade 2.

Further psychological testing shows that Tommy has above-average intelligence but poor auditory analytic skills, an area of development essential for reading. He has difficulty discriminating the sounds that go into making words and using analysis of sounds in his reading. With specific instruction in this area and more reading help, Tommy begins to narrow the academic gap.

SUMMARY

Appropriate developmental screening depends principally on good history-taking and strong powers of observation. Such a "surveillance" approach rather than direct developmental assessment usually suffices. When concern is raised about a child's development or behavior, the physician may choose to directly observe developmental performance in order to better assess the child's problems. With a small collection of additional test materials, you can obtain abundant information about a child's current development. Remember that you are always looking for a child's best performance and that you must contrast his actual performance during the examination with what is described by parents or other caregivers. Development is not a static phenomenon, and current performance must also be interpreted with respect to previous and future developmental patterns.

Pediatric assessment is greatly enhanced by routine attention to behavior and development.

REFERENCES

1. Glascoe FP: Collaborating with Parents: Using Parents' Evaluation of Developmental Status to Detect and Address Developmental and Behavioral Problems. Nashville, TN, Ellsworth & Vandermeer, 1998.
2. Rourke LL, Leduc DG, Rourke JT: Rourke Baby Record 2000: Collaboration in action. Can Fam Physician 47:333–334, 2001.
3. Diagnostic and Statistical Manual of Mental Disorders, 4th ed. Washington, DC, American Psychiatric Association, 1994.
4. Frankenburg WK, Dodds JB, Archer P, et al: Denver II Screening Manual. Denver, CO, Denver Developmental Materials Inc, 1990.
5. Frankenburg WK, Dodds JB, Archer P, et al: Denver II Technical Manual. Denver, CO, Denver Developmental Materials Inc, 1990.
6. Knobloch H, Stevens F, Malone AF: Manual of Developmental Diagnosis. Philadelphia, Harper & Row, 1980.
7. Illingworth RS: Basic Developmental Screening 0–4 Years. Oxford, Blackwell Scientific Publications, 1988.
8. Knobloch H, Pasamanick B (eds): Gesell and Amatruda Developmental Diagnosis, 3rd ed. Philadelphia, JB Lippincott, 1974.

chapter 7

Examination of the Head and Neck

ALAN L. GOLDBLOOM

Successful examination of the head and neck in a young child or infant is a daunting challenge for many clinicians. In this context, "success" means that you have examined everything that you want to and have confidence in the results. If you manage to do so without causing the child to cry or resist—and thereby preventing completion of the examination—you will have attained a major milestone in the development of your clinical skills.

Observations of the general appearance of the head and neck should begin as soon as you enter the room and should continue throughout the history-taking. The hands-on examination can usually be deferred until near the end of the assessment, because this portion is more likely to make the younger child cry. Once the child is beyond the toddler years, the order of the examination is less critical; still, the situation varies from one child to another, and you must make this judgment according to your observations of the youngster's comfort level.

To complete this part of the examination, you need to use three instruments that strike terror into many children: the otoscope, the ophthalmoscope, and the dreaded tongue depressor.

Key Point

Unless you are comfortable and competent with these instruments before examining a child, your efforts may result in frustration and disappointment for both you and your patient.

Proficiency with an ophthalmoscope and otoscope requires eye-hand coordination and familiarity with the relevant anatomy. These skills improve steadily with practice. It is best to acquire your initial experience with adults; the easiest method is to examine your colleagues, who will provide instant feedback if your examination causes pain.

GENERAL OBSERVATIONS

Never lose sight of the forest for the trees. Your initial impression of a child's appearance can be extremely important. A youngster's facial expression and animation may be valuable indicators of mood, alertness, or neurologic dysfunction. You can often assess visual and auditory function more easily while a child plays than with specific attempts at hands-on examination. You can pick up important clinical clues from the quality of a baby's cry or a child's speech or from the nature of a cough. Cyanosis, pallor, and jaundice are usually readily apparent.

Initial important observations of facial features usually are made during the head and neck examination. Your "gestalt" impression of the patient's facial appearance is valuable: Does the head look proportional to the face? Is its shape abnormal? Are the right and left sides of the face symmetric, and are the ears normally placed? Are the eyes too close together or too far apart? Is the chin appropriately developed?

Sometimes a child's appearance seems unusual but you may find it difficult to define the abnormality. The ability to describe visual observations is an essential clinical skill; to be able to describe something as abnormal, you must first be familiar with the normal. In pediatrics, the range of normal for almost any physical parameter is extremely broad. When assessing a child whose appearance seems unusual, first look carefully at the parents. If there is a marked similarity in facial features, you may assume either that the apple has not fallen far from the tree or that an autosomal dominant dysmorphic syndrome may be present. For a detailed review of the dysmorphic assessment, see Chapter 5.

One word of caution—never use expressions such as *funny-looking kid,* or *FLK,* to describe any child. Such terms, which were once part of the colloquial medical lexicon, are demeaning and offensive.

APPROACH TO PHYSICAL EXAMINATION OF THE HEAD

Examining the Head

HEAD SHAPE

Children's heads come in a wide range of sizes and shapes. In adults, a thick covering of hair, often suitably styled, minimizes this phenomenon. Brain growth is the prime determinant of head size. Additional factors are genetic influence, changes in intracranial pressure, and bony abnormalities. Hydrocephalus, which increases intracranial pressure, usually causes rapid expansion of the infant's skull. In young infants, this expansion may cause the sutures to separate so that you can feel a space between the individual skull bones. *Craniosynostosis*, or premature closure of the sutures, limits the skull growth.

Each skull bone grows relatively independently and usually symmetrically. Skull growth occurs in a direction perpendicular to the suture lines. If, therefore, there is synostosis of the saggital suture, growth in skull width is prevented. As a result, compensatory overgrowth occurs in the anteroposterior axis. This process produces a long and narrow skull, described as *scaphocephalic*. If the coronal suture closes prematurely, a tall, wide head results. When a suture has closed prematurely, there is sometimes a palpable firm, bony ridge along the suture line itself; this ridge should not be confused with the overlapping sutures sometimes felt soon after birth.

The most common variant of head shape is that associated with prematurity. The "preemie head" is flattened along both temporal aspects, giving it a long, narrow appearance. Presumably this results from the inability of premature infants, unlike full-term infants, to turn their heads from side to side. For such an infant, there is always pressure on one side or the other of the head, until someone changes the infant's position. This pressure affects normal skull contour.

Newborns have pliable heads. Experienced clinicians can often tell at a glance whether an infant was delivered from an occiput anterior, occiput posterior, or breech position. Most babies are born by vertex presentation, usually occiput anterior. As they pass through the birth canal, the intense external pressures mold the head so that the occiput assumes unusual prominence. There also may be overlapping of some skull bones. The head begins to remold spontaneously in a matter of days.

When you examine a newborn's skull, carefully palpate each suture line, running your hand over the entire head. In doing so, you may discover two other abnormalities that are caused during birth. The first is *caput succedaneum*, an area of edema of the scalp usually found in the presenting part of the head. It does not follow bony landmarks and does cross suture lines. The second is a *cephalohematoma*, a subperiosteal hemorrhage usually found over the parietal bones posteriorly. When such a hemorrhage occurs bilaterally, the appearance is that of two "horns." Cephalohematomas often heal partly by subperiosteal ossification, which occurs first around the edges of the hematoma where the periosteum has been lifted away from the skull. This process often creates a palpable ridge around the base so that there seems to be a circular hole in the bone. Because the bleeding is limited by the periosteal attachments at the edges of the skull bones, these hematomas do not cross the suture lines. When you identify a cephalohematoma at the initial examination, advise the parents that the condition is usually harmless but may take several months to disappear completely.

Postnatal molding, causing asymmetry of the skull, can also occur, particularly in infants younger than 1 year. Most typically, this molding takes the form of unilateral parieto-occipital flattening, which develops because an infant preferentially lies on one side in the crib. If you ask a few detailed questions about the position of the crib in the room, you usually discover that the baby has been lying mostly on one side in order to look at the most interesting visual stimuli in the room (e.g., lights or a window) rather than the wall. Such minor asymmetry is virtually always a benign condition requiring no treatment.

HEAD MEASUREMENT

Surprisingly, head circumference is often measured inaccurately. Even slight variations in the position of the measuring tape can change the result significantly. Measure the largest circumference possible by ensuring that the tape wraps around the most prominent parts of the forehead and occiput (Fig. 7–1).

> **Key Point**
>
> It is best to take three measurements of head circumference to ensure reliable results. If you get three different measurements, your technique needs improvement.

Never begin the physical examination of an infant or toddler by measuring the head circumference. Although this procedure is neither painful nor invasive, many infants and toddlers resist it, turn their heads vigorously from side to side, and may cry. It may be best to leave the measurement to the end of your examination, and you may need a parent's help to complete the task.

The second step is to plot the measurement correctly on a standardized head circumference graph. Remember that no single value on the graph represents a "normal" head circumference. The graph simply depicts the range

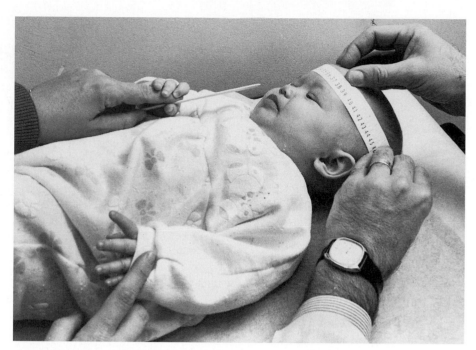

Figure 7–1 Measurement of head circumference in an infant. The tape should encircle the most prominent parts of the forehead and occiput.

of measurements observed in a normal population. The 50th percentile is no more normal than the 90th or the 10th, and by definition, head circumference in 3% of the population is above the 97th percentile, and that in another 3% is below the 3rd percentile.

Key Point

Be alert to the possibility of a problem when a head circumference measurement is at one extreme or the other.

Clinicians commonly encounter normal children with seemingly large heads. When you do so, always measure the head circumference of both parents. Head sizes, like body shapes, tend to follow familial patterns. For reasons that are unclear, it is more often the father who has a large head. If he is not present, you may learn on questioning the mother that the father always has a difficult time finding a hat that fits.

Although a single measurement of head circumference may identify significant microcephaly or macrocephaly, this variable has greater value as an indicator of growth over time. A measurement that falls on the 75th percentile may be strikingly abnormal if it represents an increase from the 25th percentile measurement obtained just 3 weeks earlier, provided that both measurements were accurate.

FONTANELS

The *fontanels* are the gaps between the bones of the infant's skull at the sites where three skull bones meet (Fig. 7–2). Palpating the anterior and posterior fontanels is a routine part of the newborn examination.

Because the posterior fontanel usually closes or is extremely small by 6 weeks of age, only the anterior fontanel remains as a useful clinical indicator beyond the newborn period. In most infants, the anterior fontanel will have closed by 18 months of age, but the potential variation in time of closure is enormous. Some are closed at 12 months, others only at 24 months. The four other fontanels, used less frequently in clinical assessment, are the two anterolateral (sphenoid) fontanels at the junction of the coronal and squamosal sutures and the two posterolateral (mastoid) fontanels at the junction of the squamosal and lambdoidal sutures.

Occasionally, a child may have extra fontanels or skull bone defects, including symmetric "holes" in the parietal bones, known as *persistent parietal foramina.* These are situated along the sagittal suture between the anterior and posterior fontanels. First observed by anthropologists in skulls from Egyptian tombs, such holes were believed to have resulted from trephining; they are now recognized as persistent parietal foramina. Anyone unfamiliar with these foramina may be alarmed on first seeing a radiograph or computed tomography scan showing a skull with two striking symmetric holes, one on either side of the sagittal suture. In fact, these are variants of normal. The so-called metopic fontanel is a widening of the metopic suture as an anterior extension of the anterior fontanel.

Most variations in fontanel size and shape are insignificant, especially if head growth follows a normal pattern. Anterior fontanels may admit no more than an adult's fingertip or they may measure several centimeters in width and length throughout infancy before closing. Persistent delays in closure or an unusually large size, particularly of the posterior fontanel, may be a clue to a pathologic delay in bone growth, as may

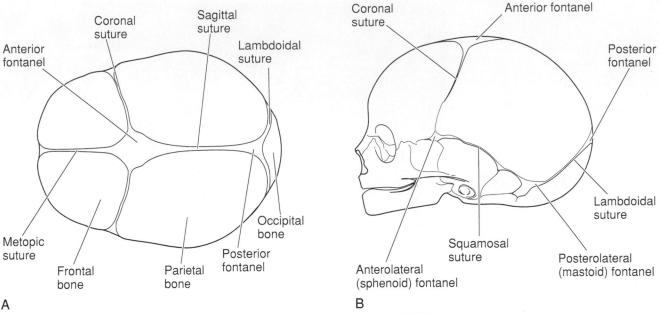

Figure 7–2 *A,* Fontanels and bones of the newborn skull, viewed from above. *B,* Lateral view of newborn skull, showing fontanels and bones.

occur, for example, in hypothyroidism. Document any observed abnormality.

Key Point

The fontanel is a useful window to the intracranial space. Perfectly normal anterior fontanels can vary enormously in size, from almost pinpoint to those that admit three fingertips. Size has relatively little to do with time of closure.

Changes in intracranial pressure, as occur with meningitis, are reflected by changes in palpable tension at the fontanel. If you place your fingers gently over the fontanel of a quiet infant, you can feel venous pulsations, which are normal. A fontanel that is tense and bulging may be a sign of increased intracranial pressure. Large normal fontanels may feel full when the baby is lying down, because cerebrospinal fluid pressure always rises in the recumbent position. Because crying also increases intracranial pressure, feel the fontanel only when the baby is calm and in an upright position to avoid the effects of hydrostatic pressure change that occur when a child is supine (Fig. 7–3). In a dehydrated infant, the fontanel may be sunken.

CRANIOTABES

The skull's ability to indent under pressure and spring back to normal contour like a Ping-Pong ball is called *craniotabes,* a normal finding in newborns, particularly along the lambdoidal suture. However, conditions that diminish bone mineralization, such as rickets, exagger-

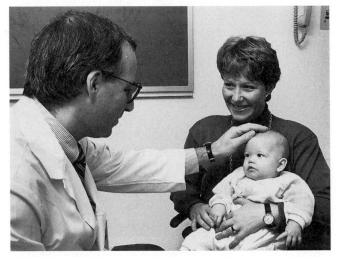

Figure 7–3 Palpation of the anterior fontanel. For best results, the infant should be upright and calm.

ate this phenomenon, causing it to persist beyond the first few months.

AUSCULTATION

Listening to the skull is occasionally valuable. Although you may hear soft bruits or flow noises in many normal children, especially if they are febrile, a harsh, loud bruit suggests the presence of an arteriovenous malformation. The best places to listen are over the vertex, the temples, and the eyeballs. Auscultation should be done routinely in any child complaining of headaches and in all children with vascular malformations over the face and head. The vast majority of bruits are normal variants, just like the innocent murmur heard on cardiac auscultation. Indeed, many skull bruits are transmitted from the heart or great vessels, so a careful cardiovascular examination is essential.

Key Point

Be suspicious of a cranial bruit that is unilateral or unusually loud.

As with skull shape, the best way to determine whether a bruit is truly abnormal is to listen to lots of heads and learn to appreciate the range of normal.

TRANSILLUMINATION

See Chapter 4 for a detailed explanation of transillumination.

HAIR

When examining the head, note any unusual features of the hair. Patchy areas of hair loss may be associated with fungal infection, twirling or pulling of the hair (also known as trichotillomania), or an idiopathic condition called alopecia areata. Twirling of the forelock may produce a characteristic frontal bald spot. A focal area of hair loss in an infant younger than 6 months usually means that the baby spent some time in a neonatal intensive care unit and undoubtedly had a scalp intravenous infusion, for which the head was shaved.

Key Point

A patch of hair loss over the occiput may occur from normal friction, or it may indicate that the infant is spending excessive time lying supine. This sign has been associated with deprivation and neglect but now seems to be occurring more frequently in normal babies as a result of recent recommendations in favor of the supine sleeping position.

Hair is extremely sparse and fine in children with ectodermal dysplasia. Patchy depigmented hair, such as a white forelock, may be seen in children with Waardenburg syndrome, which is inherited dominantly and is usually associated with deafness. In hypothyroidism, the hair becomes coarse. In Menkes syndrome (kinky hair syndrome), a degenerative neurologic condition, the hair shafts grow twisted and brittle, breaking off a few centimeters from the scalp; these abnormal hairs are called pili torti.

Be sure to examine the underlying scalp as well. The presence of hair may hide an underlying skin problem such as seborrheic dermatitis or psoriasis.

Examining the Ears

HEARING

Hearing assessment is frequently forgotten during ear examination, despite the fact that sound reception is the major function of the ear. Formal assessment of hearing has become a science in itself, and audiologists can measure hearing in infants from birth onward. Nevertheless, most examiners can use simple screening tools to determine whether a problem is likely to be present. Any child with congenital anomalies of the head and neck should be considered at risk for hearing impairment.

Infants younger than 6 weeks often react with a Moro reflex to a sudden sound or may demonstrate brief facial changes, such as blinking and opening the eyes widely. From 2 to 6 months, a baby may awaken or quiet to the sound of mother's voice or may cease activity in response to soft sounds. A baby may also turn the eyes and head in the direction of the sound source. (When testing, be sure the baby is not responding to simultaneous visual stimuli. A simple trick is to rub your thumb and forefinger together 1 to 2 inches from the infant's ear—and out of sight—as a screen for ability to hear low-level sound.) By 9 months, infants may begin to imitate specific sounds. Because a baby's mood, fatigue, and hunger state can affect responsiveness to these stimuli, it is appropriate to obtain some of this information by asking the parents about the infant's response to sound. Although absence of response to sound may indicate a possible hearing problem, it can also be a sign of an underlying neurodevelopmental problem.

As children grow, achievement of expressive language milestones (see Chapter 6) provides an indirect measure of hearing function. Any lag in language development should prompt a referral for audiologic evaluation. No child is too young to be tested.

SHAPE AND POSITION

Before using the otoscope, take a good look at the child's ears. Are both ears present and normally formed? In conditions such as Goldenhar syndrome, one ear may be absent. Are the ears in normal position? Specific criteria exist for labeling ears as "low set" (see Chapter 5). Sometimes the ears are posteriorly rotated so that the usual vertical axis of the pinna is tilted posteriorly, giving the ears the appearance of being low set; this is an optical illusion. Minor congenital anomalies of the ears are quite common and are often meaningless if they occur in the absence of other anomalies; such minor anomalies include small skin tags, pits, or fistulas that are most often located just anterior to the tragus. Gently move the pinna and tragus; tenderness with this maneuver suggests otitis externa. Also, inspect and palpate the mastoid and postauricular area, looking out especially for tenderness and enlargement of lymph nodes.

HANDLING THE OTOSCOPE

> **Key Point**
>
> The otoscope can be a strange, menacing instrument for a young child, particularly one who has had a prior painful experience with one.

The confidence and skill with which you use the otoscope are reflected in the child's cooperation. For an adequate examination, use a halogen light with a good bulb and either fully charged batteries or, even better, an AC power source. The speculum should be the largest that fits comfortably into the auditory canal. Pediatric wards and clinics are notorious for having every size available but the one you need, so it may be worthwhile to carry a personal set.

When examining toddlers and older children, explain that you are going to use the light to look into their ears, and then demonstrate that the instrument is no more than a flashlight by shining the light on their hands. Children often become interested if you shine the light in front of them and ask them to blow it out; as they blow, you deftly turn the rheostat dial to achieve the desired effect. Also, demonstrate by placing the otoscope at the entrance to your own auditory canal so that the child can see what the procedure involves, then do the same to the child.

> **Key Point**
>
> If the child is brought in because of pain in one ear, always start by examining the ear that doesn't hurt.

POSITIONING THE CHILD

Some infants or toddlers are amazingly cooperative and put up little fuss during an ear examination. The infant should never be subjected to more restraint than is absolutely necessary, although this is sometimes difficult to judge in advance. It is a frightening experience—even for a toddler—to feel out of control. Try to imagine being the same size as the child and lying on the table in the child's position, watching an enormous adult descending from above with a frightening and unfamiliar instrument. Skilled, experienced clinicians are able to examine most children without restraint or complaint, especially if children are kept in the sitting position rather than lying down.

> **Key Point**
>
> When performing an otoscopic examination, it is important to (1) try to work with youngsters at eye level rather than from above, (2) use a soft gentle voice, and (3) use a gentle touch.

Despite your best efforts, some infants will not cooperate, and in these situations, the examination becomes a two-person procedure. Not only must the baby's head be immobilized, but the hands must be kept out of the way. Parents are sometimes reluctant to immobilize the baby until they are told that appropriate positioning and holding will reduce pain and accelerate the procedure. A variety of positions work, and the extent of immobilization necessary depends on the child's age, mood, and disposition.

Sometimes, a mother can successfully hold the baby against her shoulder or chest with one hand while holding the baby's head steady with the other. Often it is easier to place the infant supine on an examining table with the parent or an assistant leaning over the infant, holding the child's arms at the sides and immobilizing both the arms and the body, while you use one hand to hold the baby's head against the mattress and the other to hold the otoscope. If you need to use both hands, for example, to curette wax out of an ear, the second person must immobilize the baby's head. Endless possibilities exist. Gentleness is the most important element in achieving a successful ear examination.

Hold the otoscope in the "forehand" or "backhand" position (i.e., with your thumb pointing either toward the light or toward the handle) (Fig. 7–4). The advantage of the latter position is that it allows the back of your hand to lie against the side of the infant's face so that if the child makes any sudden movement, your hand moves with the child's face. With this arrangement, the position of the speculum relative to the ear will not change when the baby moves, and you avoid causing pain. Many examiners use the forehand position with equal comfort, especially if they use the other hand to stabilize the baby's head.

Hold the otoscope with your right hand, using your left thumb and forefinger to grasp the pinna and gently apply traction away from the head and slightly posteriorly. This maneuver straightens the normally curved external auditory canal, enabling you to see better. Depending on your level of manual dexterity, it also may be helpful to use the third finger of your left hand to gently push the tragus anteriorly, thereby opening the auditory canal further.

> **Key Point**
>
> The most common cause of failure to visualize the eardrum is not retracting the pinna properly away from the head.

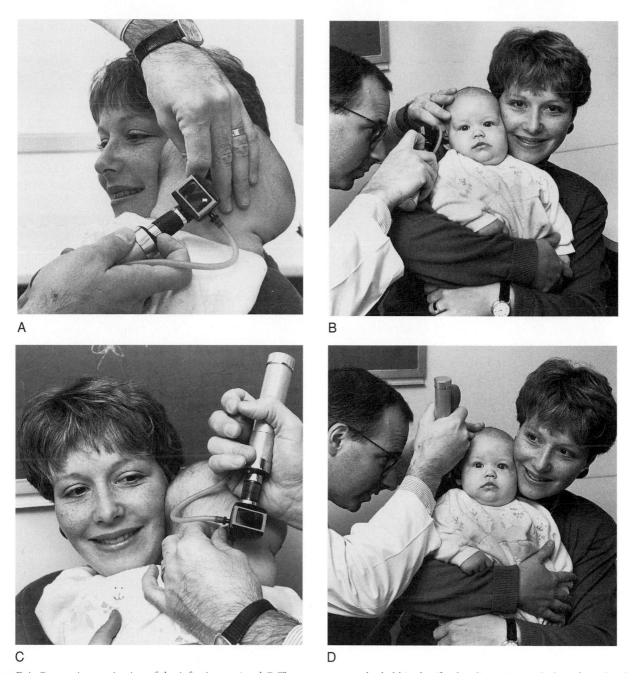

A

B

C

D

Figure 7–4 Otoscopic examination of the infant's ear. *A* and *B*, The otoscope may be held in the "forehand" position with the infant's head stabilized against the mother's face and the infant positioned over the shoulder (*A*) or facing forward (*B*). *C* and *D*, Alternatively, the otoscope may be held in the "backhand" position. Note that the back of the examiner's hand rests against the infant's head to stabilize the otoscope. The infant may face backward (*C*) or forward (*D*), whichever position seems more calming.

Observe the external auditory meatus, and gently place the tip of the otoscope there. At this point, your head is still away from the otoscope and you are not actually looking through it. Once the otoscope tip is in position at the meatus, move your head up to the otoscope and look through it, gently aiming the otoscope to see the ear canal beyond. Remember that your head should move with the otoscope as it is aimed in different directions.

Once the lumen is visible, gently advance the instrument. *Never advance it blindly*. The wall of the bony portion of the external auditory canal is exquisitely sen-

sitive, and if the child suddenly screams in pain during the examination, you are pressing too hard against the wall or inserting the speculum too far. Insertion of the otoscope is also painful if the child has any infection in the external canal—otitis externa or a furuncle. Never allow the instrument's weight to rest against the auditory canal; instead, support the otoscope fully with your hand. The ability to find and follow the lumen is acquired gradually with practice.

While advancing the otoscope, inspect the external auditory canal, looking for foreign bodies or signs of inflammation. A discharge may represent an exudate associated with an inflamed external canal (otitis externa) or may emanate from behind the eardrum if perforation has occurred. If otitis externa is suspected, swab the exudate and sniff it. *Pseudomonas* often has a characteristic sweetish odor.

Not infrequently, wax, a normal constituent of the ear canal, obstructs your view. When wax is present in only small amounts, you can see around it if you position the instrument carefully. If you cannot see the eardrum but must, there is no choice but to remove the wax (see later section on wax).

TYMPANIC MEMBRANE

The goal of this whole exercise is to see the eardrum; you may have only a few seconds in which to assess it completely, so you must be familiar with the normal architecture and appearance. Unfortunately, the otoscopic photographs in most books and atlases do little justice to the true visual appearance of the tympanic membrane (TM), so you must become familiar with the "normal range" by examining as many ears as possible.

The major visual landmarks are shown in Figure 7–5. The structure most easily identifiable is the long process (handle) of the malleus, which runs from the anterosuperior area to the drum's center, terminating in the umbo. The tympanic membrane is most concave at the umbo; therefore, the otoscope light is reflected back as a narrowed cone starting at the center and expanding in an inferoanterior direction. Although this "light reflex" cannot be relied on as a sole indicator of disease, changes in the degree of concavity or convexity of the tympanic membrane understandably produce changes in

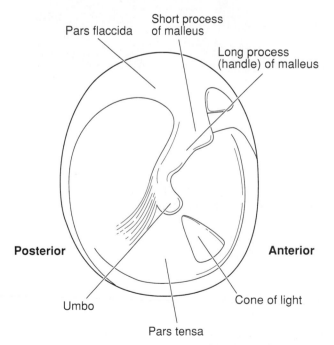

Figure 7–5 Visual landmarks of the right tympanic membrane.

the way light is reflected. Thus, if middle ear pressure is increased and the drum is bulging out, the light may be diffused so that no cone is visible at all. Look carefully at the pars flaccida, located in the anterosuperior quadrant, where the tympanic membrane is thinner because of the absence of the fibrous membrane found in the pars tensa; early inflammatory changes may be most visible in this area. The short process of the malleus is visible at the inferior border of the pars flaccida.

Pressure changes in the middle ear are best assessed with pneumatic otoscopy (see later section). With practice, however, you can learn much from visual inspection. Imagine the eardrum as a piece of plastic wrap stretched over the protuberances of the ossicles. Thus, you see the long and short processes of the malleus pushing slightly outward through this membrane without piercing it. If negative pressure develops in the middle ear, as often occurs with eustachian tube blockage or chronic effusions, the membrane is sucked inward, wrapping itself even more tightly over the bony landmarks, which then become more prominent. If middle ear pressure increases, as in acute bacterial otitis media, the tympanic membrane bulges outward and becomes convex; the bony indentations are invisible or poorly demarcated.

> **Key Point**
>
> Changes in the architecture and landmarks of the tympanic membrane are more important than color changes.

Color changes in the eardrum are notoriously unreliable, particularly in infants. Just as vascular changes cause the febrile or crying infant to appear flushed or red-faced, similar changes take place in the tympanic membrane when the baby cries—in the absence of any ear infection. Therefore, it is essential to determine whether the shape and landmarks of the tympanic membrane are normal. Too often, a child with such findings is diagnosed as having otitis media, resulting in overdiagnosis and unnecessary treatment, giving false reassurance that the cause of a fever has been found, and possibly allowing a more serious diagnosis, such as meningitis, to be overlooked.

Finally, look for more obvious abnormalities of the tympanic membrane, such as perforations, which may be caused by infection or a foreign body. Currently, the most commonly seen perforation has been surgically created, and the most common foreign body is the ventilation tube, or grommet, which protrudes through the tympanic membrane.

PNEUMATIC OTOSCOPY

Pneumatic otoscopy, a relatively simple procedure, can yield important information about middle ear pressure. It works on a simple principle. Remembering the example of the plastic wrap and the effect of changes in middle ear pressure, imagine now that the pressure changes are imposed from the *other* side of the membrane (i.e., from the external auditory canal). To perform this procedure, use an otoscope with a pneumatic bulb attachment—it is best to carry your own—and a special speculum with an expanded tip that forms an airtight seal in the external canal without the application of pressure. As an alternative, a small piece of rubber tubing placed over the tip of a standard speculum provides an excellent seal. Look through the otoscope while squeezing and releasing the rubber bulb (Fig. 7–6).

The normal tympanic membrane moves medially (away from you) when you apply external pressure by squeezing and moves laterally (toward you) when you create negative pressure by releasing the bulb. If middle ear pressure is already significantly negative and the eardrum is retracted medially, this pneumatic maneuver may produce only slight lateral motion of the drum when the bulb is released. If the middle ear pressure is abnormally positive, you may produce only slight medial movement when you apply positive pressure. If the pressure changes are significant, the drum may be immobile. Experience brings an appreciation of the nuances of these changes. As with every other aspect of the examination, you must see many eardrums move before you can recognize "slightly reduced mobility."

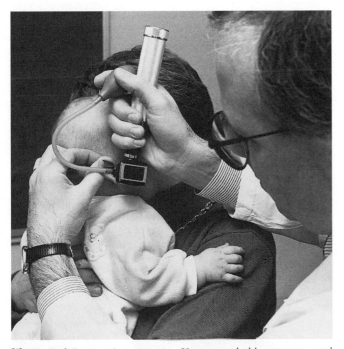

Figure 7–6 Pneumatic otoscopy. You may hold otoscope and bulb in one hand and retract the pinna with the other. Also, rest the back of your hand against the infant's head, stabilizing the otoscope. If the head moves suddenly, your hand and the otoscope will move with it.

WAX

You cannot comment on an eardrum that you cannot see adequately. Although that truth may seem self-evident, clinicians are often reluctant or too rushed to do what is necessary to provide a clear view. Wax is a perfectly normal constituent of the ear canal and, on its own, causes no harm. It becomes problematic only when it obstructs your view; then it must be removed.

Wax can be removed either by curettage or with a syringe. Children dislike both procedures, so they should be deferred until the end of the examination. The easier (and less traumatic) method is to flush out the wax with water. In most children, an ear syringe can be used, but in young infants, it is sometimes easier to use a 20-mL disposable syringe attached to butterfly tubing (with the needle cut off). The tubing can be inserted into the auditory canal for more accurate aim. Either way, this should be expected to be a messy procedure. Some towels and a kidney basin are needed to catch the water as it runs out of the ear. Be sure that the water is lukewarm. It may take multiple squirts of water to flush out the wax, and this procedure may change the appearance of the tympanic membrane. A device that produces a fine jet of water (such as a Waterpik) also may do the job effectively.

Curettage requires more skill but is usually less messy and often more effective. It requires a blunt ear curette (plastic curettes may be less traumatic than the metal variety), an otoscope, and the experience of having successfully performed this procedure on a few adults. Always begin by explaining to parents that the lining of the ear canal is very sensitive and fragile and bleeds easily when touched, much like the lining of the nose. By warning them that this procedure may cause a little bleeding, you may temper the otherwise inevitable, dismayed reaction of parents who see a bit of blood draining out of their child's ear and assume you have inadvertently performed office neuro-surgery.

Total restraint of the younger child is absolutely necessary for curettage. Because both your hands will be busy, rely on others to keep the child still. Once you see the auditory canal, carefully advance the curette so that the tip is just beyond the wax, and then pull gently backward, dragging the wax outward.

Key Point

Always perform curettage of the ear canal under direct vision.

It helps to imagine trying to roll a little ball of wax out along the wall of the canal. Surprisingly large clumps of wax can be removed in this way. You need remove only enough to provide an adequate view.

To become proficient at curettage, you must learn from an expert; you cannot learn it from this or any other book. Furthermore, you must perform it frequently to maintain your skill. Occasional curetters are more likely to produce trauma.

If wax is truly impacted and cannot be dislodged, the two following choices remain: (1) the parent may instill a few drops of an ear wax softener for a few days until cleaning becomes easy to accomplish or (2) the child can be referred to an otolaryngologist, who can attempt the procedure using an operating microscope, often with more success.

Key Point

If an ear wax softener is to be used, caution parents about some commercial brands that can cause a nasty inflammatory reaction in the ear canal, extending to the soft tissues around the ear. A gentler approach may be the instillation of a few drops of mineral oil each day until the wax is softened and can be flushed out easily.

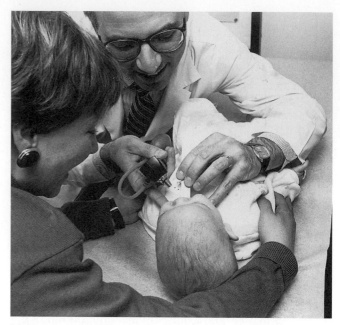

Figure 7–7 Examination of the mouth, supine position. The mother restrains the infant's arms at the sides.

Examining the Mouth

POSITION FOR EXAMINATION

Examination of the oral cavity is generally easier to master than examination of the ear, but the same principles apply when approaching the child—proper positioning, minimal restraint, and familiarity with landmarks. Most older children are cooperative, although some have a long-standing fear of the tongue depressor, a fear more pronounced in those with an exquisitely sensitive gag reflex and in those who have had a previous bad experience.

From the time a child is old enough to understand simple instructions, he or she may be able to cooperate without any restraint. This should always be the first approach, unless it is clear from the outset that the child will have no part of the procedure. As with otoscopy, show the child the flashlight or otoscope light, and begin examining the mouth *without* a tongue depressor anywhere in sight. Some children, on spotting the tongue depressor, clench their jaws tightly shut until they see you drop the wooden weapon into the garbage pail.

In some children, the soft palate rises and the tongue descends quite spontaneously when the mouth is opened, yielding a panoramic view that may even include the epiglottis. In others, it is necessary to depress the base of the tongue to see anything. This procedure rarely induces gagging if the tongue depressor is placed no further back than the anterior two thirds of the tongue. With the tongue depressor in this position, gentle, steady downward pressure is usually

enough to provide a good view of the pharynx. If you do trigger a gag reflex, you will often have lost a friend, to say nothing of the child's lunch!

With infants, cooperation is unlikely. The easiest method is to place the baby supine and ask the parent to help restrain the arms (Fig. 7–7). Beyond early infancy, the baby should be examined while sitting in the parent's lap, with the parent using one hand to restrain the child's forehead and the other to restrain the arms (Fig. 7–8).

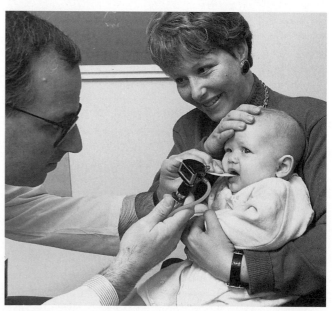

Figure 7–8 Examination of the mouth, sitting position. The mother uses one hand to restrain the infant's arms and the other to keep the head steady.

BREATH

Smell the child's breath. This can be an instructive maneuver. Young, febrile children are very susceptible to the rapid development of ketosis secondary to carbohydrate depletion and combustion of fat reserves. This is easily recognized from the sweet odor of acetone on the breath. If you do not remember the distinct acetone odor, take a sniff of a bottle of nail polish remover, and note the typical sweetish smell of acetone.

Halitosis can be associated with poor dental hygiene, oropharyngeal or gingival infection, sinusitis, and constipation—in the last case due to increased concentration of methane in the breath.

LIPS

Begin by inspecting the lips. Blue lips indicate central cyanosis, whereas a bluish discoloration in the circumoral area is more likely a peripheral vasomotor phenomenon often seen in young infants. A blister or callus in the center of the upper lip is frequently seen during the first few weeks of life, caused by friction during vigorous sucking. Midline anomalies such as cleft lips are usually readily seen.

Note specifically any signs of inflammation or cracking or any lesions such as "cold sores," which signify a herpes simplex infection. Cracking at the corners of the mouth may be associated with monilial (*Candida*) infection. Reddened patches above or below the lips or at one side of the mouth in toddlers or older children are often caused by habitual licking of the affected areas ("lip-licker's rash").

GINGIVA AND BUCCAL MUCOSA

Next, look at the gums and buccal mucosa. You can accomplish this examination even while the child clenches the teeth. Simply use the tongue depressor to move the lips away from the teeth or to retract the cheek laterally while shining a flashlight against the exposed surface. You can gain important information about the presence of any gum inflammation (gingivitis) and also detect vesicles or ulcers (canker sores) that can occur in diverse conditions. Such lesions, when in the healing phase, often appear gray-white.

Young infants may have a whitish coating on the buccal mucosa from either recently ingested milk or oral candidiasis (thrush), a common and generally harmless infection. To differentiate, try to scrape the coating off with a tongue depressor or cotton swab. If it comes off, it is milk.

TEETH

As you look at the gums, you also can see at least the external surface of the teeth. First count them, because delayed dental eruption may be a sign of general delay in skeletal development, such as occurs in hypothyroidism. The "normal" age of the first tooth eruption can be any time from intrauterine life until about 1 year; the average age is about 6 months.

Some children have poor dental enamel formation, with mottling and discoloration. This finding is often blamed on sugar in juices given by bottle and labeled "nursing bottle caries," especially when the infant is allowed to go to sleep with a bottle in his or her mouth. The condition also occurs, however, in babies with no such history and probably reflects a genetic predisposition. Tapping on the tooth's occlusive surface may be painful if there is an underlying abscess.

Dental health is often overlooked in the physical examination, yet dental abnormalities may provide clues to systemic problems. For example, children with ectodermal dysplasia often have peg-shaped teeth. Periodontal diseases may adversely affect the course of some chronic diseases, such as juvenile arthritis, nephrotic syndrome, and congenital heart disease. Therefore, the condition of teeth and gingiva deserves careful attention in all children, but especially in those with chronic illnesses.

TONGUE

To examine the tongue and all structures beyond, you must get the mouth open. Toddlers and older children often protrude their tongues on request, giving a clear view of the tongue and pharynx. If this does not work, initially place the tongue depressor on the anterior portion of the tongue, where it is not uncomfortable and will not elicit a gag. The child will readily accept this maneuver, enabling you to look around the mouth. If the child's resistance to opening the mouth is absolute, you may have no recourse but to restrain him or her and then gently but firmly force the mouth open. If the child has no teeth, it is easy to slip a tongue depressor between the gums and depress the mandible.

If most of the dentition had erupted, you may have to slide the tongue depressor between the buccal mucosa and the molars. When the stick reaches the space posterior to the last erupted molar, turn it medially and press down on the back of the tongue. The resulting gag reflex will cause the mouth to open widely and the soft palate to rise. The light should be aimed appropriately in readiness, because you will have just a second or two to visually assess all the remaining structures of the oral cavity. Actually, with experience, this procedure is rarely necessary; further, as your hands become steadied by increasing confidence, you can keep a child's mouth open by keeping the tongue depressed just a few seconds longer. If the child is an "easy vomiter," be alert for the facial expression and gurgle that warn of an impending expulsion of stomach contents. Remember that producing a gag reflex normally requires touching the posterior third of the tongue.

Key Point

The message is clear: If you have to use a tongue depressor, never start by touching the posterior third of the tongue.

Touch the tongue gently at first, and then slowly depress it with gradually increasing pressure. In many children, this provides a gag-free view of everything. If a child does gag in the process, rapidly withdraw the tongue depressor and quickly press the child's chin upward. This maneuver interrupts the gag reflex and reduces your laundry expenses.

Key Point

A *strawberry tongue*, sometimes seen with streptococcal infection or Kawasaki disease, is produced by enlargement and reddening of the papillae. The *geographic tongue* has sharply demarcated areas of differing coloration, giving the appearance of a map, a condition lacking clinical significance that represents a cyclic irregular desquamation of the tongue surface.

Consider the tongue size. Children with large tongues may have underlying dysmorphic syndromes. The enlarged tongue often protrudes from the mouth at rest (e.g., Beckwith-Wiedemann syndrome or congenital hypothyroidism). The normal tongue is wet and glistening. With dehydration, secretions tend to get more sticky and stringy and ultimately dry up. Although you should note any unusual color changes in the tongue, remember that most coating of the tongue is without significance.

Remember to examine the tongue's underside, because the floor of the mouth may be the site of retention cysts, or *ranulas*. The underside of the tongue is attached to the floor of the mouth anteriorly by the *frenulum*, a structure that, despite popular belief, has never been proved to cause speech delay or speech impediment (see Fig. 3–17). It was once popular to cut the "tongue tie" or clip the frenulum in the delivery room or as an office procedure. Any subsequent clarity of the child's speech was inevitably (and mistakenly) credited to surgical release of the frenulum.

Be sure to look as far beyond the base of the tongue as possible, remembering that anomalies such as an ectopic lingual thyroid gland can be seen in this way.

HARD PALATE AND SOFT PALATE

Looking up at the roof of the mouth, you can determine—by comparing with many normal children—whether the palate arch is high or any anomaly is present. The most common major anomaly is the cleft palate, an embryologic defect of midline development. At its most severe, a cleft is bilateral and extends anteriorly to involve the alveolar ridges and the palate itself; however, any number of variations is possible. A cleft lip may or may not accompany a cleft palate. After checking the newborn's or infant's hard palate visually for fissures or clefts, palpate it with a finger to check for the presence of a submucous cleft, a bony defect that may be covered by a mucous membrane layer. Finally, look at the soft palate and uvula. A cleft may involve only the soft palate.

Key Point

A notched or bifid uvula can occur in normal children but can also be a sign that midline facial development is incomplete. Such children should be checked carefully for a submucous cleft.

Petechiae on the soft or hard palate are often associated with streptococcal infection.

While examining the soft palate, watch it move, an important part of cranial nerve testing. Note any asymmetry of movement or deviation to one side. Asymmetric movement may be neurologic in origin or merely secondary to scarring from a past tonsillectomy. Either stimulating a gag reflex or having the patient say "aaahh" initiates elevation of the soft palate and uvula.

TONSILS

Beyond the molars along either side of the mouth, the next visible structures are two vertical webs of tissue known as the anterior and posterior tonsillar pillars. Between them, on either side of the mouth, lie the tonsils themselves. Because tonsils are composed of lymphoid tissue, they can vary tremendously in size. In a newborn, the tonsils are almost invisible. They usually increase steadily in size (a normal manifestation of generalized lymphoid hyperplasia), reaching their lifetime maximum size when the child is between 6 and 9 years old. After this age, they tend to involute, often making adult tonsils hard to identify even though they were never removed.

Tonsillar size does not necessarily reflect tonsillar health. The amazing variation in tonsillar size and appearance makes it tempting to label any given set of tonsils as abnormal. Unless your conclusion is based on very good evidence, refrain from doing so. In some children, past infection may leave the tonsils looking hypertrophied, pitted, and containing whitish "concretions" for many months. Unfortunately, the only time such tonsils are examined closely is at an office or clinic visit triggered by an acute illness or fever. A glance at these ugly tonsils may persuade a gullible examiner that "tonsillitis" is the cause of the current problem. Yet if the tonsils were viewed when the child was well, the findings might be identical, one of many reasons why tonsillitis achieved its undeserved reputation as a major cause of childhood morbidity. As one astute observer commented, "When you see big tonsils you should remove them immediately; otherwise they might disappear on their own." If the child gags during the examination, the tonsils are thrust together in the midline, often making them appear larger than they are. Even when children's tonsils "kiss" in the midline at rest, remarkably few complain of any swallowing difficulty except in the presence of acute infection.

Note the size, color, and contour of the tonsils and the presence of any exudate, vesicles, lesions, or changes in the adjacent soft tissues—namely, the soft palate, uvula, tonsillar pillars, and buccal mucosa.

Key Point

Asymmetry of the tonsils may be important in a child with a febrile illness and dysphagia, particularly if one tonsil protrudes medially enough to displace the uvula, a sign of a peritonsillar abscess.

The tonsils and tonsillar fossae are normally slightly redder than the buccal mucosa and posterior pharynx. Familiarity with this variation helps you avoid overinterpreting what may be normal redness either in healthy children or in children with febrile illnesses.

POSTERIOR PHARYNGEAL WALL

The most distant part of the view plane is the posterior pharyngeal wall. In some children, this structure is easily visible if the mouth is opened wide. In others, the base of the tongue may touch the soft palate, essentially obstructing the view. In such cases, you must rely on the gag reflex to obtain a brief glimpse.

With experience, you should be able to decide whether the posterior pharyngeal wall is truly red and inflamed. Other changes may be encountered, such as edema, lymphoid hyperplasia (small yellowish nodules giving a "bumpy" appearance to the surface), and excessive secretions. It is far better to describe what you see than to attempt to diagnose.

EPIGLOTTIS

Although examining the epiglottis is not a routine part of the head and neck assessment, be aware that the epiglottis is sometimes easily visible when you look at the posterior pharyngeal wall. In some children, the epiglottis sticks up from beyond the tongue base, appearing as a fairly thin, curved, pink structure. When infected, it looks like a red, swollen thumb sticking up.

Key Point

Do *not* attempt to view the epiglottis by manipulating the tongue or oral cavity in any way when examining a child in whom acute epiglottitis might be a diagnostic possibility; such a maneuver could result in immediate airway obstruction.

Examining the Nose

The nose can be examined quickly and fairly easily, but this examination is all too often forgotten. Look for any obvious deformity or deviation to one side. If there is nasal discharge, describe it. A particularly foul unilateral discharge is a good clue that the child may have a foreign body in the nostril. Most important, subtle signs of respiratory distress may be signified by flaring of the alae nasi. A horizontal crease across the lower part of the nose is seen in children with allergic rhinitis, who may also give the "allergic salute" by periodically rubbing the tip of the nose upward with the palms or heels of their hands (see Fig. 9–2).

To look inside the nose, use either a spring-type nasal speculum and light or a regular otoscope fitted with a large nasal speculum. Remember that although the external structures of the nose seem to run in a vertical axis relative to the face, the lumen itself runs more horizontally so that you will look more toward the occiput than toward the top of the head. Thus, it is unnecessary to have the child tilt the head backward; instead, the child can keep looking straight ahead while you push up the tip of the nose with your thumb and introduce the speculum. It is the medial wall (the septum) of each nostril that is the most sensitive to pain and the most delicate; therefore, use the speculum to push gently against the lateral wall, retracting it to see the internal structures.

As you look at the nasal turbinates and mucosa, try to determine visually whether there is any edema, pallor, inflammation, bleeding, or secretions. In epistaxis, the bleeding sites are usually seen in the lower end of the septum. Confirm that both nares are patent. Polyps may be seen as pale, boggy masses that usually occlude posteriorly.

Carefully note any other masses or findings, and indicate whether their origin can be identified specifically.

In newborns, the most important function of nasal inspection is to determine bilateral patency. In congenital choanal atresia, one or both sides may be obstructed posteriorly (see Chapter 4).

PARANASAL SINUSES

Because full development of the paranasal sinuses is an ongoing process from birth to adolescence, the examining method used for these structures depends on the child's age. The ethmoid and maxillary sinuses are present at birth but are still quite small. As they develop and become more fully aerated, they become potential sites for infection. The frontal sinuses start to develop and show signs of pneumatization between 4 and 7 years of age and rarely cause clinical problems until late childhood. The sphenoid sinuses are present at birth but are unusual sites of clinical disease during infancy and toddlerhood.

Palpation is the most direct method of sinus examination. Remember that *any* child may find pressure over the maxillary antra to be slightly painful (try it on yourself!), so be careful not to overinterpret the findings. Pushing against the medial corner of the orbit, against the side of the nasal bridge, can elicit tenderness in the ethmoid sinuses. Similarly, check the frontal sinuses by direct pressure when the child is old enough.

Remember the structures that are contiguous with each sinus. Sometimes the best clue to sinus infection is the effect it has on adjacent areas. For example, maxillary or ethmoid sinusitis may be associated with periorbital edema or cellulitis. Tooth pain may be associated with maxillary sinusitis. Also, a unilateral, persistent nasal discharge may emanate from the ostium of the maxillary sinus. Review the three-dimensional anatomy of the paranasal sinuses to understand related signs and symptoms.

SALIVARY GLANDS (PAROTID AND SUBMANDIBULAR)

For practical purposes, the parotid gland can be felt only when it is enlarged. It should not be difficult to recognize parotid enlargement if you remember the anatomy. A good portion of the gland overlaps the lateral aspect of the mandible; swelling in this area is seen as a bulge in front of the ear, often displacing the tragus.

The gland empties through the parotid duct, the orifices of which are seen on the buccal mucosa just opposite the second upper molars. This site should be checked for redness. When required by the child's clinical condition, the parotid gland and duct should be examined using bimanual palpation, with a gloved finger inside the mouth and another finger over the gland.

The other major salivary gland is the submandibular gland, whose ducts empty into the space under the tongue, just lateral to the frenulum. It may be difficult to differentiate from enlargement of the submandibular lymph nodes, which overlie the gland. The latter condition occurs more frequently.

APPROACH TO PHYSICAL EXAMINATION OF THE NECK

Examination of the neck should be a brief exercise, but it can have a high yield. In very sick children, omitting this part of the examination may have serious consequences. For example, a cardinal sign of meningitis in children beyond infancy is neck stiffness (*nuchal rigidity*), which occurs in the presence of any kind of meningeal irritation—including hemorrhage. In older children, test neck mobility by asking the child to touch the chin to the chest. In younger children or those unable to cooperate, attempt to gently flex the neck by placing a palm under the occiput and lifting. As an alternative, lift the child by placing one hand under the child's upper back, and observe whether the neck is held rigid. Depending on the severity of the symptoms, you may simply encounter increased resistance or find that the child's entire trunk and head are being lifted with this maneuver.

Full mobility of the neck not only helps rule out meningeal irritation but also reveals something about the muscular and bony integrity of the neck and cervical spine. Check all ranges of motion, including lateral rotation ("Touch your chin to your shoulder"), lateral flexion ("Touch your ear to your shoulder"), and extension ("Bend your head back and look at the ceiling"). In the younger child, it may be more useful to shine a light at various points on the ceiling and wall and ask the child to follow it with the eyes, thereby demonstrating the range of mobility of the neck.

Remember that pain on neck flexion does not necessarily mean meningeal irritation. In fact, it is far more common to see such a reaction in children with inflamed, tender lymph nodes ("swollen glands") or a sore throat (acute pharyngitis). Always ask the child to show exactly where it hurts before you assume that the pain is meningeal in origin. Children with meningitis usually have other signs that suggest serious infection.

Lymph Nodes

You can palpate the lymph nodes of the head and neck in seconds when you know where to look. The one truism about lymph nodes is that some are palpable in virtually any child more than a few months old. Total absence of palpable lymph nodes in any child beyond early infancy should prompt you to consider the possibility of an immune deficiency, such as agammaglobulinemia.

It is easiest to use both hands in one continuous sweeping motion to examine the lymph nodes. While facing the child, move both hands around to the back of the head, and feel the occipital chain, located along the hairline. Then bring your hands forward to feel the postauricular and preauricular areas before moving them down to feel the posterior and anterior cervical chains (Fig. 7–9). The nodes just below the angle of the jaw are particularly likely to be inflamed and swollen during minor respiratory infections. Moving forward, feel the submental area, and finally, check the supra-clavicular fossae.

Public awareness of cancer is such that many parents are understandably concerned about any unexpected "lumps" found in a child's neck. To be able to reassure them (and yourself) with reasonable confidence, you must familiarize yourself with the feel of "normal" nodes in most children. The classic "shotty" nodes found in the necks (and inguinal chains) of most children are pea- or marble-sized masses that are non-tender, are easily mobile, and do not appear fixed to surrounding structures. They may change little with time and may persist for years. A lymph node that enlarges with inflammation may never return to its original size, persisting as a palpable but harmless little lump. Given the frequency of minor upper respiratory tract infections, skin infections, and insect bites in young toddlers and given that the affected structures are drained by the lymph nodes of the head and neck, it is easy to understand why palpable nodes are so ubiquitous. Even nonrespiratory viral illnesses such as roseola can produce lymphadenopathy. Remember that lymphoid tissue follows a normal curve of growth and involution in children; lymph nodes, tonsils, and adenoids may attain peak size when the children are 6 to 9 years of age. If adenopathy is detected in the neck, check the other lymph node sites (axillary, epitrochlear, and inguinal) to determine whether the adenopathy is localized or generalized.

In general, nodes up to 1 cm in diameter can be considered normal if there are no other suspicious findings. In the presence of acute illness, the nodes are often tender and enlarged. Occasionally, primary infection of a lymph node (lymphadenitis) occurs, producing exquisite tenderness, some induration of surrounding tissues, and possibly some fluctuation.

Thyroid

See Chapter 16 for details of thyroid examination in infants and older children.

Trachea

The tracheal position can be assessed quickly with the child in either the supine or the upright position. The main purpose of this examination is to determine whether the mediastinal structures have been shifted to the right or to the left by an intrathoracic abnormality such as atelectasis or pneumothorax (see Fig. 9–9).

Classic Neck Anomalies

Be aware of a few classic anomalies of the neck: Neck webbing is typically seen in Turner syndrome (XO anomaly) in girls or in Noonan syndrome in boys. There may be lumps, dimples, or pits that are remnants of embryonic development. A midline neck mass that moves upward when the tongue is protruded is probably a thyroglossal duct cyst. An epithelial tract (the thyroglossal duct) may attach such remnants of embryonic migration of the thyroid gland to the base of the tongue. If the cyst becomes infected, it shows the usual signs of inflammation and may even rupture externally to form a draining sinus. A cystic mass or small opening a little more laterally on the neck may be a branchial cleft remnant, usually found just anterior to the sterno-cleidomastoid muscle.

A mass due to a fibroma within the body of the sternocleidomastoid muscle may be found in babies with congenital torticollis. In this form of "wry neck," the

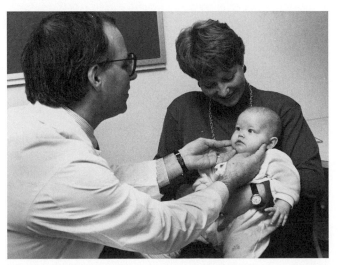

Figure 7–9 Palpation of lymph nodes in the anterior cervical chain. Note that the infant is still in the mother's lap, and the examiner maintains visual contact with the infant.

affected sternocleidomastoid is functionally shortened and has limited range of motion. The head is typically tilted toward the lesion but rotated away from it.

SUMMARY

Several recurring themes apply to virtually every aspect of the pediatric examination. First, remember the enormous range of "normal" that characterizes the pediatric population. Second, make your concern for the child's comfort and well-being apparent to the child and to anyone watching, especially the parent, every step of the way. Third, you can develop expertise in these techniques only with much practice and experience. Finally, if you are uncertain about a finding, say so in your written report; it happens to all of us.

chapter 8

Examining the Visual System in Children

G. ROBERT LAROCHE

Because vision provides almost 80% of the sensory input during the first years of life, a faulty visual system can have a major effect on a youngster's intellectual and physical development. In addition to conditions primarily affecting the eyes or parts of the visual system, many systemic diseases can manifest as ocular signs and visual symptoms, which can be important clues to a timely diagnosis.

The performance of a reliable visual assessment does not require either expensive equipment or prolonged practice. The first part of this chapter describes the normal visual system in infants and children and provides a glossary of terms used to describe the ophthalmologic findings and conditions commonly encountered. The second part comprises a description of examination techniques. Finally, some of the key questions required to evaluate particular ophthalmologic problems are described, along with the role of sequential diagnostic logic in elucidating etiologies.

NORMAL VISUAL SYSTEM IN INFANTS AND CHILDREN

Although the gross anatomy is similar at all ages, there are important differences between the young child's eye and the adult's eye. For example, the volumetric relationship between the eye and the orbit is dramatically different in children.

Key Point

The child's globe occupies a larger portion of the orbit, making it more vulnerable to injuries. The eyeball achieves 50% of its total growth during the first year of life: the corneal diameter increases from 10 to 12 mm.

In infants, the choroid gives a blue hue to the overlying thin sclera. In whites, the iris is often poorly pigmented at birth, and the final eye color may not be established until at least 8 months of age. Examination by direct ophthalmoscopy shows a baby's fundus to be pale, the macula barely visible. As the child gets older, the fundus becomes darker, the macula becoming darker than the surrounding retina. The macula then displays the easily recognized oval, bright reflection of the ophthalmoscope light, known as the *macular umbo* (Plate 8–1).

The birth process can be somewhat traumatic to the eyes. Many newborns suffer episcleral and retinal hemorrhages during vaginal delivery (see Fig. 4–14). These hemorrhages are alarming to both parents and physicians but are harmless and usually disappear within 2 weeks. At birth, the nasolacrimal duct is often blocked at its junction with the nasal mucosa under the inferior turbinate. The blockage resolves spontaneously in more than 90% of cases, although it can remain until the age of 1 year in some children, causing persistent tearing. A few affected children then need surgical treatment.

The process and rate of development of vision in infants are still not fully understood, because vision exists in several forms. Different neuronal channels carry specific visual functions, such as contrast sensitivity, orientation, movement, and hyperacuity. Each function develops at a different rate. For practical purposes, normal newborns can see a human face easily and demonstrate their visual ability by looking at it—and even following the face with eye or head movement as it passes slowly before them at close range (Fig. 8–1). A baby's ability to follow a face can be verified only when the baby is awake and alert, often just before or in the middle of a feed. This innate ability is paramount to the infant's future, because few parents fail to form an emotional attachment to a little one who looks directly at them minutes after birth. By contrast, parents

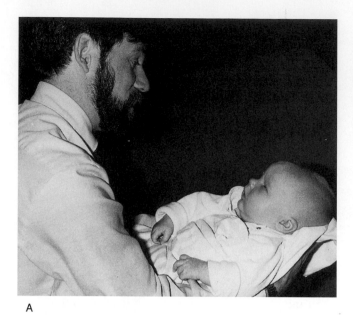
A

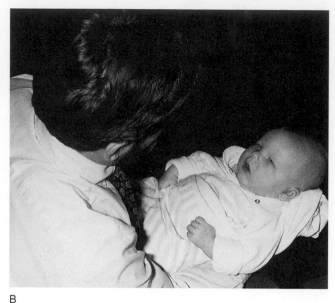
B

Figure 8–1 Face follow vision testing of a young infant. *A*, Hold the child at arm's length with the head comfortably supported. The examiner's face is lined up with the apparent direction of gaze of the child. *B*, Move your face slowly to the side, and observe the response. This 2-month-old boy now has a good "face follow"; he received his contact lenses 2 weeks after cataract surgery.

of a blind or strabismic infant, who are unable to establish the interaction that comes with normal eye contact, may have significantly greater difficulty developing the same level of emotional attachment to their offspring.

By 3 months of age, babies enjoy looking at the human mouth and eyes and at simple, colored toys. A 1-year-old toddler's vision is about half as good as the best attainable adult score. Three-year-olds can see at least 6/9 (or 20/30 in the American system) in each eye, and their visual acuity can be tested with charts specially designed for children (see section on the HOTV test). The numerical ratio 20/30 actually indicates that a 3-year-old can see at 20 ft what the average adult sees at 30 ft.

Key Point

Infants' visual fields are good in the temporal area at birth; by the age of 6 months, they are comparable with adults' visual fields.

Color vision is present from an early age. Newborns have color vision, although it is less sensitive than that of older infants. Newborns do not see faint colors well—if at all—but by 3 months of age, definite trichromatism is established; babies of this age can differentiate between red, green, and yellow.

Binocularity, which confers the ability to see in three dimensions, has been proven to exist by 3 months of age, coinciding with the time the eyes finally maintain good alignment. This finding underlines the clinical significance of any persistent deviation of the eyes after age 3 months.

Eye movements may appear irregular, "unbalanced," or disconjugate until the third month of life. Healthy newborns can display tonic movements of the eyes downward or upward. Sometimes, the eyes turn toward (*esotropia*) or away (*exotropia*) from each other.

Key Point

Remember that constant deviation of an eye in any direction or persistent "jiggling" of one or both eyes is abnormal at any age.

Pupillary movements are limited in the newborn and are almost impossible to examine thoroughly at that age. A good pupillary examination in older children demands cooperation and patience, because children can rarely stare fixedly at a distant target while an observer tries to evaluate their pupils by shining a bright light in them. The children look either at the light or anywhere else and change their accommodation continuously, keeping their pupillary diameter in constant flux and possibly preventing adequate assessment of light-induced responses.

Accommodation in the newborn is limited. From a practical viewpoint, consider the newborn's focus as "stuck" at an adult arm's length. Within a few months after birth, focus improves, and the child's accommodative amplitude soon reaches remarkable proportions. A 5-year-old, for example, can clearly see a plane in the sky, then switch in a fraction of a second to look with great intensity at the details of a tiny spider close at hand. Unfortunately, this marvelous accommodative ability does not last forever.

DEFINITION OF TERMS

As an aid to diagnosis, this section contains a brief glossary of diagnostic terms that summarize the features to look for in children with eye problems. Table 8–1 and Figure 8–2 show the tools for examination of the eyes; Table 8–2 lists definitions and acronyms.

Amblyopia: Decreased vision in one or both eyes once no detectable or residual uncorrected organic or optical anomaly remains. Reversible if treated early enough (well before 9 years of age). Severe if it develops early, as when it is caused by congenital cataract or congenital ptosis. Occlusion amblyopia can occur if treatment such as patching of the sound (good) eye is too prolonged.

Blindness: Legal blindness is defined as vision of 6/60 (20/200) or less. Most assistance agencies for visually handicapped children use 6/24 (20/70) as the maximum vision cutoff for registration for their services. The leading causes of blindness vary dramatically in different regions of the world. Malnutrition, onchocerciasis, and trachoma are the culprits in many developing countries, whereas macular degeneration, glaucoma, diabetic retinopathy, amblyopia, trauma, and corneal herpes are responsible in developed countries. Eye injuries by BB guns are a leading cause of trau-

Table 8–1 EQUIPMENT NEEDED TO PERFORM AN ADEQUATE PEDIATRIC EYE EXAMINATION

Essential (see Fig. 8–2)
Your face (preferably without glasses)
Direct ophthalmoscope
Other portable focal source of light (otoscope is good)
Red open-faced rubber nipple (to stick on top of focal light source for a bright red object)
HOTV vision kit with tape for eye occlusion
Tropicamide (1%) short-acting mydriatic (weak cycloplegic) drops

Ancillary
Optokinetic nystagmus strip (a necktie with stripes will do)
Fluorescein strips with loupes and cobalt-blue light
Food (or a nursing mother)

matic blindness in North American children; many medical professional groups have proposed that these guns be regulated by legislation. Amblyopia, with a prevalence rate of 4% to 5%, is a significant cause of monocular blindness. Genetic diseases (involving mainly the optic nerve and retina), birth injury, and

Table 8–2 OPHTHALMOLOGIC SHORTHAND*

Abbreviation/Acronym	Definition
Alt.	Alternating strabismus. In almost all cases of strabismus, fixation (use of the eye to look at something) is with at least one eye at a time. If there is equal vision, the eyes will "alternate" fixation
APD	Afferent pupillary defect
CD	Corneal diameter
C/D ratio	Cup/disc ratio (cup size can be enlarged in glaucoma)
CL	Contact lens
Comit.	Comitant
E	Esophoria. The eye turns in only when there is interference with binocular vision (as with covering).
ET	Esotropia. One eye is turned in spontaneously
E(T)	Intermittent esotropia. The eye turns in only occasionally
IOL	Intra-ocular lens
IOP	Intra-ocular pressure
OD	Oculus dexter (Latin); right eye (English)
OS	Oculus sinister (Latin); left eye (English)
OU	Oculus uterque (Latin); each eye (English)
PERLA	Pupils equally reactive to light and accommodation
SLE	Slit-lamp examination
VA cc	Visual acuity with correction (with glasses or contact lens[es])
VA sc	Visual acuity without correction
X	Exophoria
XT	Exotropia. One eye turns out (exodeviation).
X(T)	Intermittent exotropia. The eye turns out only occasionally.

* For example, a diagnosis of strabismus could be written: Alt. Comit. X(T). This would mean: alternating comitant intermittent exotropia.

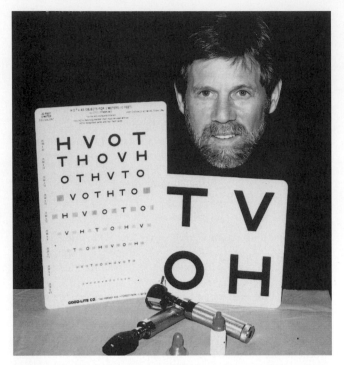

Figure 8–2 Equipment for evaluating the visual system in children: your face, ophthalmoscope, otoscope, red nipple, visual acuity test kit, short-acting mydriatic (tropicamide 1%).

congenital defects (cataracts are the most common) are important causes of blindness in North American children, as are retinitis pigmentosa and albinism. With increasing survival of very low birth weight infants, both retinopathy of prematurity (ROP) and optic nerve atrophy are making a comeback as significant causes of visual loss in children.

Cataracts: An important cause of *leukocoria* ("white pupil," from the Greek; see Plate 8–5). Causes of pediatric cataracts include congenital rubella, metabolic disorders, and chromosomal anomalies. Cataracts can be secondary to ocular inflammations (uveitis) or accompanied by other ocular malformations. Many idiopathic cataracts are sporadic, but some are genetic. Some systemically administered medications cause cataracts. Steroids are common culprits, which can cause glaucoma as well. Amblyopia in a child with a cataract is severe; therefore cataracts in infants need immediate attention. Postoperative optical correction may require the use of contact lenses in infants, although intraocular lenses are becoming more popular in children older than 2 years.

Coloboma: A defect of closure of the embryonic fissure of the eye; hence, its inferonasal location in the eye. In mild form, only the iris is involved; in more severe cases, the choroid and the optic nerve can be involved (Plate 8–2). With optic nerve involvement, central nervous system (CNS) midline defects should be suspected, as in optic nerve hypoplasia (see definition of this term).

Epicanthal fold (pseudostrabismus): Skin folds hiding nasal sclera. When the child looks sideways, the

appearance of a misalignment can be dramatic. This is so-called pseudostrabismus (see Plate 7–11*C*).

Esophoria and esotropia: Forms of strabismus in which the eyes deviate toward the nose. One eye is often the "preferred" one, implying a strong possibility of amblyopia in the non-preferred eye. Alternating fixation suggests that vision in the two eyes may be equal. The visual inferences from the fixation pattern apply to all forms of strabismus. Some esotropias, due to accommodative factors, are amenable to optical treatment (i.e., glasses). Most cases of esodeviation are partially accommodative and require a combined treatment with glasses and surgical correction. A *tropia* is a strabismus present at the time of the observation, whereas a *phoria* is a "tendency" toward a particular type of strabismus. A phoria can be seen only when the eyes do not fuse or are prevented from doing so (e.g., by a patch over one eye). Fatigue or daydreaming can elicit a phoria as well.

Glaucoma (infantile or congenital): A rare but important ocular disease often manifesting as tearing and photophobia (an inability to tolerate normal daylight). Can be mistaken for lacrimal duct obstruction, but the photophobia and increased corneal size help make the correct diagnosis. Treatment is urgent and often surgical. Amblyopia is also associated.

Head tilt: Abnormal head positions can be induced by a large array of conditions, many of them ocular. Typical is the compensatory head tilt seen in a fourth cranial (trochlear) nerve palsy, assumed to avoid diplopia and keep the eyes together. Without the tilt, the eyes show a vertical strabismus and the patient sees double (Fig. 8–3*A*).

Head turn: An abnormal head position taken when reading or looking at a small visual target. Caused typically by either a sixth cranial nerve (abducens) palsy or nystagmus. In the former, the turn is used to avoid horizontal diplopia (Fig. 8–3*B*); in the latter, the turn

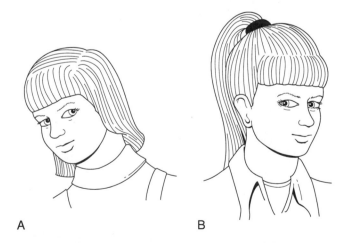

A   B

Figure 8–3 Abnormal head postures. *A*, Tilt to the right in a fourth cranial (trochlear) nerve palsy. *B*, Child turns head to the left to avoid diplopia caused by a left sixth cranial nerve palsy (the patient turns the head toward the side of the palsy).

improves vision by reducing nystagmic oscillations (null position).

Hemangioma (orbital, capillary): Benign congenital tumors that grow rapidly when a child is between 1 and 6 months of age but tend to regress spontaneously later. May cause severe amblyopia by pupillary obstruction, high astigmatism, or both. Early treatment is essential for the preservation of vision. Steroid injection of the tumor, systemic treatment, glasses, and patching of the sound eye may all be necessary (Plate 8–3).

Hyperphoria, hypophoria, hypertropia, hypotropia: Vertical ocular deviations.

Hyphema: Bleeding into the eye's anterior chamber (Plate 8–4). A trauma severe enough to cause a hyphema can involve other eye structures, leading to retinal detachment or injuring the trabecular meshwork of the iridocorneal angle and thereby causing glaucoma. Hyphema is the principal diagnosis in one third of eye traumas and a major cause of ocular morbidity in children. Hyphemas rebleed in 6% of cases within 5 days of onset, causing further complications, but rebleeding can possibly be prevented by decreased physical activity and, in selected cases, systemic antifibrinolytics.

Laceration (cornea or globe): A cut through the protective shell of the eye. Suspect a laceration if there is a history of trauma with a sharp object (a forceful blunt impact can also rupture the globe). Do not try to pry the lids open; doing so might expel the contents of the globe. Repair of a simple laceration of the cornea can be followed by astigmatism, an amblyogenic factor necessitating further intensive treatment including contact lenses and patching.

Lacrimal duct obstruction (congenital): Benign but included in the differential diagnosis with congenital glaucoma. Resolves spontaneously in 90% of children by age 12 months, rarely thereafter.

Leukocoria: A white pupil. This finding has major clinical implications. The differential diagnosis includes retinoblastoma and cataract. Delaying treatment of the former leads to death; delaying treatment of cataract causes permanent loss of vision (Plate 8–5).

Lymphangioma: Another cause of ptosis, proptosis, or both; a diffuse benign tumor of the orbit that often bleeds internally. Almost impossible to resect completely in childhood, it is a cause of astigmatism and amblyopia (Fig. 8–4).

Myelinated nerve fiber layer: Abnormal presence of myelin around the superficial nerve fibers of the retina near the optic disc. It can be so extensive that the pupillary red reflex can be made to appear white (leukocoria). The vision is generally normal except when the macula is heavily involved (Plate 8–6).

Nystagmus: This is a descriptive term for "jiggly," "unstable," "wiggly," or "trembling" eyes. In up to 90% of cases, an ophthalmic cause can be identified. It is mainly found when vision has been poor since early in

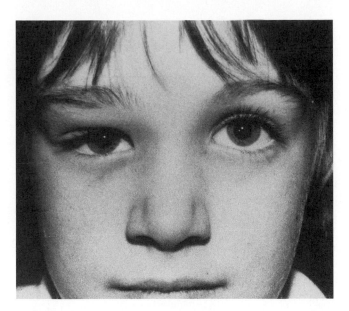

Figure 8–4 Lymphangioma of the right orbit with poor vision due to astigmatism caused by the mass effect of the lesion on the shape of the eye.

life. Most causes are "sensory," affecting the anterior visual pathway; the causes can be retinal (cone dystrophy, early retinitis pigmentosa, or congenital retinal toxoplasmosis scar), neuronal (optic nerve anomalies or early dystrophies), ectodermal (various forms of albinism), or even optical (cataract or corneal anomalies). In nystagmus, the type of movement is often not indicative of any particular cause.

Ophthalmia neonatorum: In North America, neonatal ophthalmia was once principally caused by gonorrheal infection; Now, the most common causative organism is *Chlamydia trachomatis. Staphylococcus pyogenes* may cause outbreaks of conjunctivitis in newborn nurseries. Transient chemical conjunctivitis normally occurs after 1% silver nitrate prophylaxis in the newborn. There is continuing debate over the best agent for prophylaxis of gonococcal and chlamydial ophthalmia neonatorum.

Optic nerve hypoplasia: A common cause of congenital blindness in children. Often misdiagnosed as optic atrophy because secondary nystagmus (sensory) makes the hypoplasia difficult to visualize. The optic nerve head (disc) is smaller than normal (Plate 8–7). Look for central nervous system midline defects, including the involvement of the hypothalamic-pituitary axis with accompanying growth hormone deficiency (see Chapter 16).

Palsies (sixth, third, and fourth cranial nerves): The extraocular muscles are innervated by various cranial nerves: the superior oblique by the fourth cranial nerve (also called the trochlear); the lateral rectus by the sixth cranial nerve; and all the others by the oculomotor nerve, the third cranial nerve, which also innervates the pupil and the ciliary body for accommodation. Any injury to these nerves induces a strabismus, the angle of which varies according to the direction of gaze—an incomitant strabismus. Typically, a head turn is seen in sixth nerve palsy and lid ptosis in third nerve palsy. Fourth cranial nerve palsy (trochlear) causes an ipsilateral hyperdeviation and a contralateral head tilt (see Fig. 8–3).

Periorbital cellulitis: Any inflammation around the orbit is cause for concern, and the differential diagnosis should include rhabdomyosarcoma (see later). When the orbital content is involved, ocular motility is decreased and the patient is at imminent risk of loss of vision. *Haemophilus influenzae* meningitis is an early complication in children younger than 5 years. Periorbital cellulitis is most often associated with ethmoiditis in children who do not have a clear history of skin trauma or infection around the eye, and both computed tomography scanning and magnetic resonance imaging are invaluable for a clear evaluation of the best therapeutic regimen. This condition is less common in areas of the world where *Haemophilus influenzae* B vaccine is used. Most cases of periorbital cellulitis require systemic antibiotic therapy (Plate 8–8).

Persistent hyperplastic primary vitreous (PHPV): PHPV is the presence of a unilateral dense residual vascularized glial frond of tissue that originates from the optic nerve disc and projects toward the back of the lens. It is the first tissue present in the eye required to initiate the growth of the lens. In PHPV, the lens is abnormal and cataractous, causing a leukocoria; the differential diagnosis of leukocoria includes other forms of cataract and retinoblastoma. PHPV is associated with microphthalmos and cataract. The vessels in the back of the lens can bleed, inducing a very rare but diagnostic hemorrhagic cataract. PHPV is a progressive malformation that requires early surgery to save the eye and possibly restore its vision (Fig. 8–5).

Plexiform neurofibroma: A type of hamartomatous formation found in neurofibromatosis. In the orbit, it is accompanied by sphenoid bone defects with herniation of the contents of the anterior fossa into the orbital cavity. This condition may or may not cause visual problems, such as strabismus, astigmatism, and optic nerve dysfunction (Fig. 8–6).

Refractive amblyopia: Amblyopia is caused by the blurred image of a poorly focused eye (hyperopia, myopia, or astigmatism). This condition is found most commonly in 3- to 4-year-olds.

Retinitis pigmentosa: A generic term describing a variety of retinal degenerations, including choroidal degenerations, diseases of either type of photoreceptors, and syndromes involving other organ systems (e.g., Laurence-Moon-Biedl and Alström syndromes in which progressive retinal degeneration is associated with obesity and other systemic dysfunctions). Most patients with retinitis pigmentosa experience a severe visual deficit at an early age (Plate 8–9).

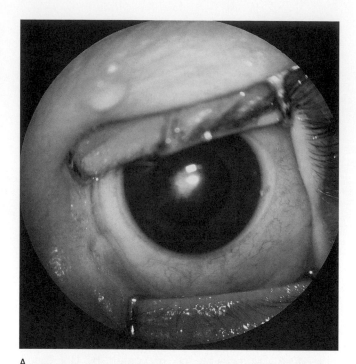

A

B

Figure 8–5 Persistent hyperplastic primary vitreous is a cause of cataract. *A,* Vessels can sometimes be seen in the lens; they can bleed. *B,* The fibrotic nature of the vascular membrane present behind the lens (the hyperplastic primary vitreous) causes traction of the ciliary processes, which become visible once the pupil is dilated.

Retinoblastoma: The most important cause of unilateral or bilateral leukocoria. Occurs in 1 in 15,000 births. Often also present with a strabismus or a red eye. The gene for this condition is located on the long arm of chromosome 13. Retinoblastoma is most curable if diagnosed early. Later death from a second malignancy is a major concern in bilateral and autosomal dominant familial cases (Plate 8–10).

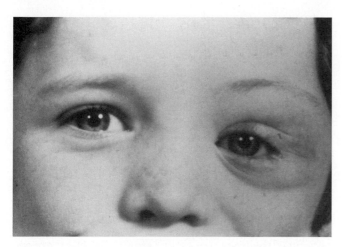

Figure 8–6 Plexiform neurofibroma of the left upper orbit. Such a hamartoma most often displaces the eye down, but in this case, the neurofibroma has not induced any strabismus; the corneal light reflexes are symmetric. Note the fullness of both upper and, to a smaller extent, lower lids.

Retinopathy of prematurity (ROP): A proliferative (abnormal vessels and glial tissue) disease of the retina in small premature babies, ROP can lead to blindness through scarring and tractional retinal detachment. In such rare advanced untreated cases, ROP can be the cause of leukocoria in smaller eyes. The growing incidence of this condition parallels the improving salvage rate for low-birth-weight infants. Eighty percent of cases of ROP resolve alone. New, early, aggressive detection and treatment protocols are designed to prevent scarring and preserve vision.

Rhabdomyosarcoma: A very aggressive malignancy of embryonal muscle tissue found in the orbit. It must be differentiated from orbital cellulitis (see earlier). Manifests as an acute red swollen eye. It is curable with irradiation and chemotherapy, which preserve vision in 80% of cases.

Strabismus: Any deviation of the eyes away from their common alignment toward the object of regard. The misalignment can be horizontal, vertical, or torsional. A *comitant strabismus* measures the same in all positions of gaze and normally excludes a paralytic or myogenic cause for the deviation.

TORSCH lesions (ocular): TORSCH is an acronym for congenital *t*oxoplasmosis, *r*ubella, *s*yphilis, *c*ytomegalovirus, and *h*erpes simplex. Shared ocular features of these syndromes include cataract (leukocoria) and abnormal retina.

Toxocara canis: Larvae of the canine Ascarididae, which may be picked up by children from dog feces and dirt, may cause major ocular disease. The ocular involvement is often asymptomatic, being detected as a leukocoria. Mostly 3- to 5-year-olds are affected. Blindness (one eye only) may be caused by retinal traction secondary to the scarring induced by the dead larvae lodged in the posterior uvea. The vitreous inflammation, followed by retinal detachment, causes the appearance of leukocoria. Only very early treatment with systemic steroids may offer potential benefit.

Uveitis: Inflammation of the uvea. In children, uveitis often occurs in the monoarticular or pauciarticular forms of chronic rheumatoid arthritis—a term now more frequently used in pediatric practice than "juvenile rheumatoid arthritis"—most often in girls 4 to 6 years old who test seronegative for rheumatoid factor, seropositive for antinuclear antibody, and seronegative for human leukocyte antigen B27. The inflammation is usually chronic, indolent, and bilateral. Blindness may occur because of cataract, glaucoma, or corneal disease. The eye stays white, without redness until the end-stage of the disease. The only possible clinical screening that can be performed between slit-lamp examinations involves a pupillary examination that can be taught to the parents (Fig. 8–7). The examination is difficult in dark-eyed individuals but can be enhanced by dilating the pupils (during a lively conversation at the supper table or by pharmacologic means at the physician's office).

OBTAINING THE HISTORY

Getting the child's cooperation is so critical for evaluation of the visual system that it is sometimes useful to postpone most of the history-taking until after the eye examination. Your initial efforts should succeed in getting the youngster interested in new "visual" toys and games that you will be introducing during brief playful moments. As you examine the child, elicit details from the parents about the relevant background issues—family history, pregnancy, perinatal events, developmental milestones. Also elicit general impressions from the parents about the child's visual abilities. The other history details needed depend on the initial complaint and your findings.

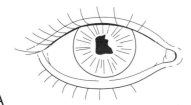

A

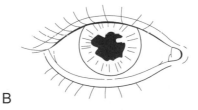

B

Figure 8–7 *A,* Pupillary anomalies in chronic uveitis of juvenile rheumatoid arthritis. They are caused by inflammatory adhesions (synechiae) between the iris and the lens. *B,* The anomalies are best seen when the pupil is dilated.

APPROACH TO THE PHYSICAL EXAMINATION

General Observation

In ophthalmology more than in any other specialty, observation is the most important technique to master; let the child show you the nature of the problem. It may seem impossible to evaluate a child's visual system when you are faced with a pair of tightly closed eyelids. Often, you can achieve success only by resisting the temptation to touch, probe, or test.

Key Point

Your face is the most available and reliable target to confirm some form of vision in children.

BEHAVIOR

Does the child walk in the examination area or run into things, or is the child wheelchair bound? Do you observe any eye gouging or poking (a form of mechanical retinal self-stimulation characteristic of blind children)?

HEAD POSITION

Is the youngster's head held straight up or down? There is no advantage to the child in holding the head up when there is no vision. Also, photophobic children avoid the light by hiding from it, holding their heads down. While looking at a visually demanding target such as a small picture, does the child's head turn sideways to prevent diplopia (double vision) because of an extraocular muscle paresis or to stabilize the eyes (nystagmus)? Does the head tilt to alleviate diplopia, as in superior oblique weakness, or seem to fall forward (chin down) or backward (chin up) as in certain types of strabismus, or to see better from under a droopy lid?

FACIAL FEATURES

Is the child's face symmetric and normal-looking or dysmorphic, suggesting the possibility of a syndrome? Does the child's nose appear wide at the base (epicanthal folds), giving the impression that the eyes are turned in, especially when the child looks sideways?

Ocular Observations

OPEN VERSUS CLOSED EYES

Are the child's eyes open, or are they closed because of *photophobia* (an inability to tolerate normal daylight)? Does only one eye close in bright light or while outdoors because of an outward turn (exotropia)? To get a sleepy baby to open the eyes spontaneously indoors, gently blow air in the baby's face or tickle a foot. If this fails, hold the baby and perform a few rotations in either direction to stimulate oculovestibular responses (see later for details of the "spinning" technique). Does the child have droopy lids or obvious bulging of the tissues over and around the eyes? Are the lids moving up and down during feeding, as in the Marcus Gunn oculotrigeminal dyskinesia?

TEARING EYES

Are the tears clear or replaced by thick discharge (indicating infection)? Is there photophobia (indicating corneal disease or congenital glaucoma)?

RED EYES

Is the redness more pronounced in the cul-de-sac and at the lid margin, as in blepharoconjunctivitis? Or is it pink all over, as in viral conjunctivitis? Is it more intense around the cornea where it meets the sclera (limbus), as in corneal diseases and intraocular inflammations (Fig. 8–8)? Is there a preauricular node, a sign of a lymphadenopathy associated with a conjunctival infection?

BIGGER THAN NORMAL EYES

Eyes appear larger than normal in congenital glaucoma (the cornea is bigger). A baby's cornea should not appear bigger than an adult's. To help make the comparison, have an adult hold the baby sitting forward on his or her lap, with both facing you. Have them put their faces close to each other so that the two pairs of eyes are in proximity. Comparison is easy with mothers and babies in a "cheek-to-cheek" position or with the baby's head just below one parent's chin (Fig. 8–9).

CLOUDY EYES

The cornea may be cloudy in congenital glaucoma, in congenital corneal malformations, or in rare storage diseases (mucopolysaccharidoses).

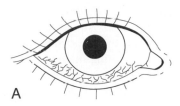

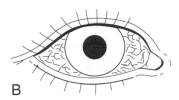

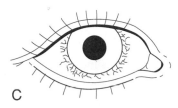

Figure 8–8 Distribution of maximum redness in three common causes of red or pink eye. *A*, Margin of the lower lid with inferior conjunctiva in blepharoconjunctivitis (often caused by *Staphylococcus*). *B*, Overall redness, the classic viral pink eye (often caused by an adenovirus). *C*, Limbal or circumcorneal redness, the so-called ciliary flush of corneal or intraocular inflammation (typically in corneal erosions or ulcers, or in acute anterior uveitis, which is rarely seen in children).

JITTERY EYES

Nystagmus (jiggling, wiggling, trembling, instability of the eyes) can be due to any of several causes, includ-

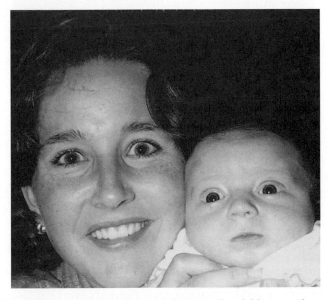

Figure 8–9 Assessment of corneal diameter. The child's corneal size is compared with the mother's.

ing intracranial tumors, cataracts, and retinal diseases, or may be idiopathic and purely motor.

PROTRUDING EYES

Proptosis is rarely equal in both eyes. By looking from above the child's forehead, you can confirm your suspicion of a true proptosis. Exophthalmos (its other name) is often an ominous sign of either severe infection, neoplasm, or severe malformation in the orbital region.

DEMONSTRATING CORNEAL LIGHT REFLEXES

A normal shiny cornea shows a neat, crisp light reflection when a light source is aimed at it. You can see the reflection almost in the center of the child's pupils when both eyes are looking at the same light source, held between you and the child at 25 cm. If the corneal light reflexes are not positioned symmetrically, assume that both eyes are not looking at the light (Fig. 8–10). Judging the position of the light reflexes requires practice; the reflex is neither highly specific nor terribly sensitive for detecting slight degrees of eye misalignment (strabismus), but it is a good start.

It is also useful to show parents what a "pseudostrabismus" really is: a common pediatric nondisease that often concerns parents and physicians unnecessarily. It is usually seen in children with broad flat nasal bridges and epicanthic folds. When the child looks to one side

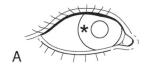 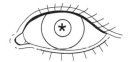

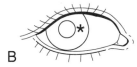 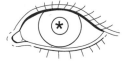

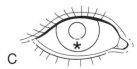 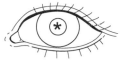

Figure 8–10 Corneal light reflexes in esotropia (*A*), exotropia (*B*), and hypertropia (*C*).

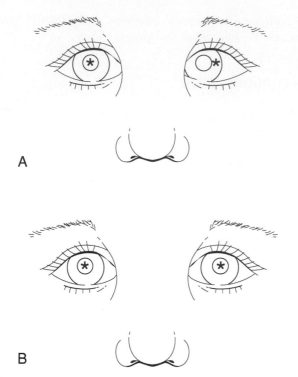

Figure 8–11 Comparison of the corneal light reflexes in esotropia (*A*) and epicanthal folds (so-called pseudostrabismus) (*B*).

or the other, the nasally turned eye becomes partly hidden under the epicanthic fold, creating a false impression of strabismus—an optical illusion (Fig. 8–11 and Plate 8–11). The eyes look turned-in because of the asymmetry of scleral show. You can show the true alignment with the corneal light reflexes. The corneal light reflexes can be quickly evaluated with the ophthalmoscope at the same time as the pupillary red reflexes (described later), but an otoscope light is a better choice for a more careful evaluation of a deviation.

If you establish that there is a true strabismus, it is not worthwhile to try to determine how large or how small it is. The strong suspicion of genuine strabismus is what counts. Evaluate whether the angle of strabismus (the asymmetry between the corneal reflexes) is the same in different fields of gaze as you observe the child while he or she is looking around the room. This will indicate whether the strabismus is comitant or incomitant. If one or more extraocular muscles do not work properly (whatever the cause), the degree of strabismus varies with the direction of gaze; this is called *incomitance*. Unlike a comitant strabismus, an incomitant strabismus has serious implications until proven otherwise.

FINDING PUPILLARY RED REFLEXES

Take the few seconds required to verify the presence of a pupillary red reflex in each eye for every young patient,

whether or not the youngster has an eye problem. Evaluating the quality and symmetry of the pupillary red reflections, known as the Brückner test, is universally considered a valid screening method for detecting visual anomalies in children 6 months and older.

Remember those family Halloween party color photographs taken with a cheap flash camera, in which everyone looks at the camera flash and appears in the photograph with big red eyes? Look for the same effect when examining infants and children for the red reflex (Plate 8–12). Demonstration of the red reflexes requires the following conditions and instruments:

1. A room darkened slightly to dilate the child's pupils and enhance the red reflexes.
2. A light source aimed at the examined eyes that allows you to visualize its reflection from the fundus (i.e., a direct ophthalmoscope).
3. Absence of optical obstructions between you and the child's choroid (behind the normal retina).
4. A child with normal eyes.

Set your direct ophthalmoscope at the widest beam setting. Turn the wheel until you see the patient's eyes clearly, staying a good foot (30 cm) away from the child to prevent both unexpected uncooperative behaviors and accommodative pupillary constriction. Aim the beam so that it illuminates both pupils, and observe (Fig. 8–12). The first observation should confirm normal or abnormal corneal light reflexes. In newborns, this may be the only chance to combine observations of corneal and pupillary light reflexes, at least in the primary position (eyes looking straight ahead).

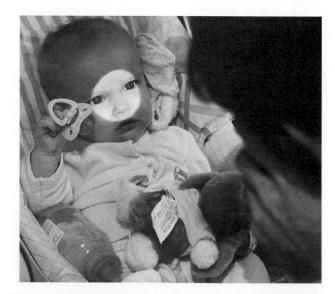

Figure 8–12 How to elicit the pupillary red reflexes. Make sure the child is comfortable in his or her own environment (with his or her own things). Position yourself about 2 feet (0.66 m) away, with the widest beam of the ophthalmoscope encompassing both pupils. Rotate the lenses of the instrument until the child's eyes are in focus. You can assess the corneal and the pupillary red reflexes at the same occasion (Brückner test). Looking just above the ophthalmoscope sometimes enables you to see the corneal light reflexes more clearly.

In whites, the pupillary red reflexes should be orange and equally bright; in more darkly pigmented races, including Native Americans and some Asians, the orange is less bright. Anything else is abnormal.

Abnormal red reflexes could be caused by problems such as opacified cornea (as in Hurler syndrome, a mucopolysaccharidosis); cataract (opacity of the lens); or retinoblastoma, a potentially lethal retinal malignancy. Mild asymmetry of brightness between the reflexes is produced by large refractive errors and by various degrees of strabismus. Normal red reflexes are shown in Plate 8–11.

Knowing how to assess the pupillary red reflexes (and remembering to do it) can sometimes mean the difference between life and death for your young patient.

SPECIFIC EXAMINATION TECHNIQUES

Additional specific techniques can help establish a reasonable diagnosis; they are described here.

Testing Visual Acuity

FACE FOLLOW TEST

From birth onward, infants prefer looking at the human face to looking at other objects. Take advantage of this preference when you want a child to look at something. Following are some points to remember:

1. A child who looks at you can see you.
2. To the child of 6 months or older, the contrast of white teeth surrounded by darker lips adds a compelling detail to the face as a preferred visual target.
3. Conversely, wearing glasses can interfere with the face follow test. So, remember to smile and take your glasses off.

TESTING FOR OPTOKINETIC NYSTAGMUS

Optokinetic nystagmus (OKN) describes the eye movements produced when a succession of relatively slow-moving targets, maneuvered in the same direction over a short time, is presented to the child. The eye movements have (1) a slow phase, corresponding to pursuit of a target, followed immediately by (2) a quick, jerky fast movement (*saccade*) that rapidly returns the eyes to a subsequent target as it appears in a more central part of the visual field after the preceding target has moved away. This cycle repeats continually as long as sequential targets are presented.

Elicit OKN in newborns or young infants by showing a series of black-and-white vertical stripes mounted on a slowly but steadily moving cloth. Be sure the

newborn is awake and alert with eyes open before you begin the test. For older children, replace the stripes with cartoon characters.

> **Key Point**
>
> If the child sees the OKN stripes, his or her eyes will move, so this is a good vision test for youngsters who cannot or will not talk.

Simple black-and-white stripes work well, but red-and-white stripes work even better (Fig. 8–13). You can also use an inexpensive striped necktie.

It is even possible to quantify vision with OKN using an array of OKN targets with stripes of different widths. Some early research on vision testing in nonverbal subjects was based on the principle that when the stripes are placed too close together, OKN stops.

TESTING FOR FIXATION BEHAVIOR

While the face follow and OKN tests are used mainly to assess visual capability, the "central steady maintain fixation" (CSMF) method is used to assess one eye at a time, hence to compare one eye with the other. Used routinely in infants with strabismus, this technique evaluates the fixation behavior pattern. Cover the child's eye with a finger, the parent's hand, or, if all else fails and you do not mind risking the loss of the child's cooperation for the day, a patch (see the section on the

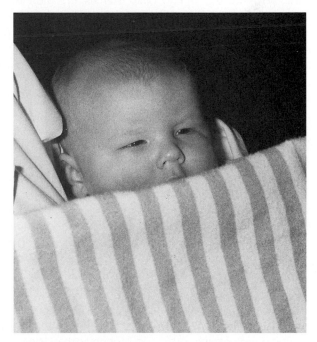

Figure 8–13 Using optokinetic nystagmus in an infant to confirm the presence of some vision. A cloth of red-and-white bands (here, a hospital receiving blanket) is positioned 1 ft (30 cm) in front of the child and then moved sideways at a speed of about 1 ft/2 sec.

cover test). Show the uncovered eye an interesting visual target, and assess the response by answering the following questions:

1. Is fixation central (i.e., does the eye appear lined up with the target)?
2. Is fixation steady (stable eye)?
3. Is fixation maintained (i.e., when the cover is taken away from the other eye, does the tested eye remain fixed on the target)?

The last component, maintaining fixation, really compares the two eyes. If vision is better in the covered eye, it will pick up fixation vision preferentially when it is uncovered. The child is unlikely to maintain fixation with the weaker eye. Often, the poorer eye shows some unsteadiness or even some paracentral fixation. The child's behavior is also different (see section on the cover test).

TESTING VISUAL ACUITY USING HOTV

HOTV, the standard test for visual acuity in children older than 3 years of age, derives its name from the four optotypes (characters; H, O, T, and V shapes) used in the test. It has definite advantages over use of the Snellen chart, the standard vision chart used for adults at the physician's office, because it does not require the child to know how to read. Its advantage over the Illiterate E test is that it does not test the ability to differentiate between right and left. Indeed, the HOTV test optotypes are symmetric from left to right. In the Illiterate E vision chart, the letter E is presented in all four cardinal directions: up, down, left, and right. The child signals the difference between left and right by pointing when giving the correct answer, a requirement greatly limiting the reliability of this test in many children younger than 6 years.

For the HOTV test, the child is given a plastic board with the four letters on it and is simply asked to point out on the board the letter shown by the examiner on a typical visual acuity-type card hung on the wall. Performed at a distance of 10 ft (3 m) for better compliance in younger children, the test is widely available; its components are standardized for the 3-m distance and are made of durable plastic. Every clinic or office should have this test kit to measure vision (Fig. 8–14). Newer versions are available with a decreasing space between letters proportional with the decreasing letter size; this feature maintains the crowding aspect of the test, important in testing for amblyopia.

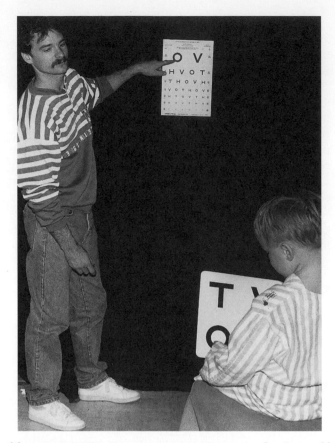

Figure 8–14 HOTV vision measurement. You can teach a 3-year-old the pointing game in less than 1 minute. Conduct the test with the child positioned a distance of 10 ft (3 m) from a typical visual-acuity card designed for that distance and mounted on the wall. Point to a letter on the card, and ask the child to point out the same letter on his or her letter board.

COMMON QUESTIONS ASKED ABOUT VISUAL ACUITY ASSESSMENT

Should each eye be tested singly or both eyes at the same time? Let the child first use both eyes. Children are upset if they are not allowed to look at things with their good eye (see sections on CSMF and cover tests). In testing both eyes at once, you may observe important phenomena: abnormal head positions, head movements, tearing, and blinking. Perform a quick check to confirm any suspicion of a bad eye. Assess the vision of the bad eye before testing the good one, making sure the occluded eye is well covered. Use an adhesive patch to prevent peeking.

Should near vision be tested? The reading cards are poorly standardized, so leave this assessment for the adults who must be tested for presbyopia.

Assessing Extraocular Movements and Looking for Incomitance

SPINNING

The vestibular system has a major influence on eye movements. "Spinning" a child stimulates the vestibular ocular movement, especially if you observe the corneal light reflexes carefully.

TWISTING THE HEAD

As a last resort, while the child looks at you, hold the top of his or her head and turn it quickly, first to one side then the other (Fig. 8–17). This maneuver may upset the child a little, but it allows assessment, through the vestibular system, of the activity of the horizontal muscles. Perform this movement vertically to assess the vertical muscles (superior and inferior rectus muscles, innervated by the third cranial nerve).

Key Point

Incomitant strabismus, which changes with different gazes, indicates an effector problem: from the brainstem to the muscles. It is, therefore, a sign of significant disease.

Assessing Visual Fields

Assessing visual fields in children is not as daunting or difficult as it might seem. In most situations, you can tell the child to "look for the wiggly fingers." Instead of asking a child to fix on a stationary target while you check the peripheral field, as is done with adults, ask the child to look for a more exciting target, as follows (Fig. 8–18):

1. Sit 2.5 ft (75 cm) in front of the child, with your eyes at the same level as the child's.
2. Ask the youngster to look at your nose.
3. Now, extend both arms in opposite quadrants.
4. Wiggle two fingers on only one hand, and ask the child to find the wiggly fingers. The child may just look at them or may even try to grab your hand.
5. Repeat step 4 with your other hand.

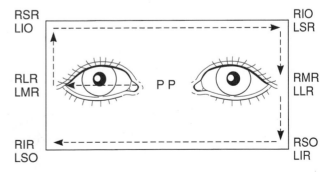

Figure 8–16 The frame used to evaluate comitance of a strabismus. A slow continuous movement of the dim fixating light along an imaginary "frame" around the patient's eyes allows the assessment of all 12 extraocular muscles. LIO, left inferior oblique; LIR, left inferior rectus; LLR; left lateral rectus; LMR, left medial rectus; LSO, left superior oblique; LSR, left superior rectus; PP, primary position; RIO, right inferior oblique; RIR, right inferior rectus; RLR, right lateral rectus; RMR, right medial rectus; RSR, right superior rectus; RSO, right superior oblique.

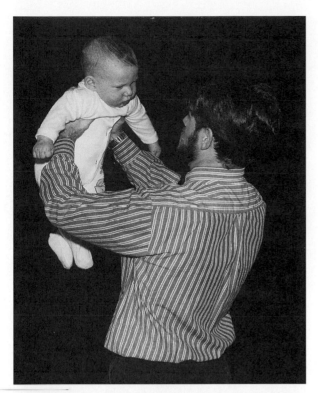

Figure 8–15 Spinning the baby to evaluate extraocular motility. Note the 30-degree-forward inclination of the baby's head, which is performed to achieve maximum stimulation of the horizontal semicircular canals. This ensures a good response of the horizontal recti. A half turn in each direction is often sufficient to generate good movement of the eyes.

system, which in turn stimulates the extraocular muscles. This method is used mainly for testing infants. To do it effectively and appreciate what is actually going on with the child's eyes, you must hold the child up in the air, facing you and tipped slightly forward, with his or her head a few inches away from yours (Fig. 8–15); watch the child's eyes as you turn yourself and the child around, first in one direction (two or three turns), then in the other direction. The baby's eyes should deviate in the direction of the turn. With this technique, not only will the youngster open his or her eyes but also the horizontal deviation of the child's eyes will allow you to assess simultaneously the medial (third cranial nerve) and lateral (sixth cranial nerve) rectus muscles of both eyes. One word of caution: Do not take too long to spin the child. After a few seconds, the surprise that prompts the child's eyes to open can change to unhappiness at being suspended in the middle of nowhere and spinning dangerously in the arms of a stranger.

THE FRAME

Have an older child follow an object of interest (e.g., a red nipple placed on top of a turned-on otoscope) to the four corners of an imaginary frame around the face. This technique tests all of the extraocular muscles (Fig. 8–16). You can readily detect any anomaly of

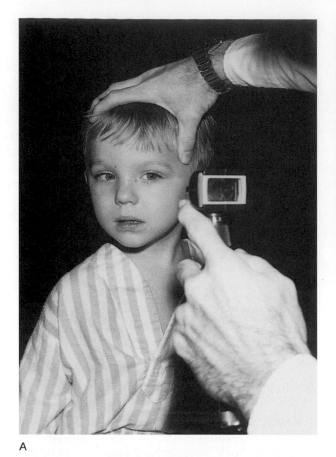

A

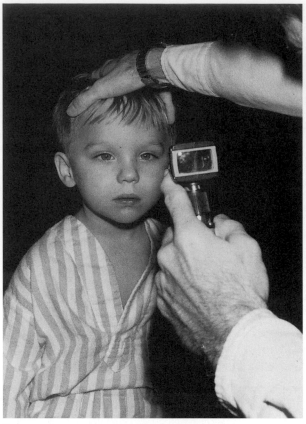

B

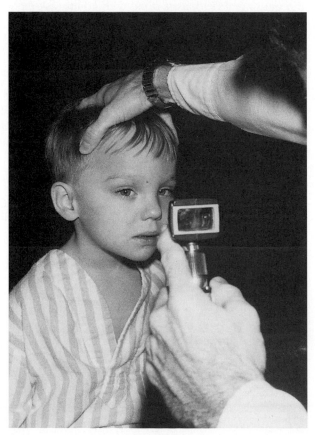

C

Figure 8–17 *A* through *C*, Twisting the child's head to evaluate horizontal ocular movements. This is a last-resort effort to find out whether an eye can adduct (turn toward the nose by the action of the medial rectus) or abduct (turn in the opposite direction by the action of the lateral rectus). Use a dimmed light source to assess the corneal light reflexes and as a fixation target. Both the fixation and the vestibular stimulation generated by actively moving the head help produce changes of position of the eyes as the head is rotated.

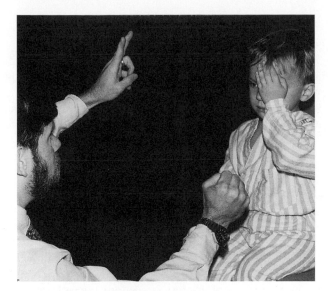

Figure 8–18 Testing visual fields. While the child looks at your face, ask him or her to tell you how many fingers you are holding up. Two opposite quadrants are assessed at the same time, one eye at a time. Make sure the child's hand is well apposed to the nose to prevent peeking.

Two variations of this technique can be used, depending on the child's age. If the child is too young to play the wiggly finger game, just watch the youngster's eyes as you introduce into the peripheral fields either your hands (as just described) or an interesting target (a bright, small silent toy or a familiar face) from behind the child's head. With an older child, do not wiggle your fingers; instead, present various combinations of numbers of extended fingers on both hands simultaneously and in opposite fields of each eye. Ask the youngster to tell you the total number of fingers shown or to count the fingers in each hand while he or she looks at your nose. Assessing two opposite quad-

rants at the same time enables you to examine all four quadrants of each eye very quickly.

These tests for visual field assessment are qualitative only, but they can be very useful in many situations. For example, after brain injury, a young boy keeps banging into things. Has he lost his balance, is he having absence seizures, is he careless because of some personality change, or does he have a recognizable visual field defect? Visual field assessment can help determine the cause.

Cover Test for Strabismus and Vision

With the child's attention on an object placed nearby or person of interest placed straight ahead, look for shifts of the eyes as you cover one of them. Movement may occur only as you remove the cover or may be seen in only one eye. The responses depend on the vision of each eye and the cause of the strabismus. An observable shift occurring during the cover test should confirm the impression gained during examination of the corneal light reflexes. Sometimes, however, to confirm the parent's observations, you must have the child fixate on a very distant object (e.g., through a window) to elicit a movement of the eyes on the cover test. This is characteristically the case in intermittent exotropia.

The cover test can also tell you something about vision (Fig. 8–19). If you try to cover the child's only good eye, you will be informed of that fact in more than one way: The child either cries or becomes uncooperative, or you cannot keep the eye covered because the child's eye, his or her whole head, or a quick hand moves to reestablish the vision you have just interrupted. The child will get both you and your cover out

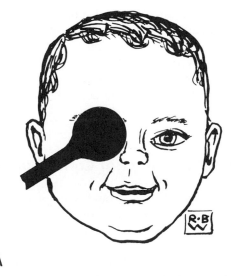

A

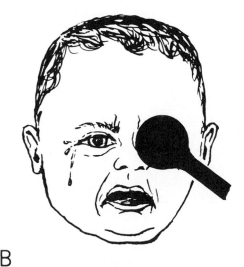

B

Figure 8–19 Cover test, used to compare the vision between the two eyes. An infant with right esotropia may not resist the cover over his deviated eye (*A*) but does protest the occlusion of the dominant eye (*B*). In this patient, poor vision of the right eye must be suspected, especially when the eye has unstable fixation. (From Von Noorden GK, Maumenee AE: Atlas of Strabismus, 4th ed. St. Louis, CV Mosby, 1983, p 65.)

of the way. Unfortunately, such a response may spell an end to the child's cooperation.

Ophthalmologists use the cover test regularly to measure the angle of strabismus. For the pediatric examination, it is sufficient to confirm the existence of a strabismus and to help compare the vision in the two eyes.

Funduscopy in Children

Funduscopy should be reserved for last, right before the child leaves the examining room, unless corneal staining is indicated (see next section). Funduscopy is sometimes a frustrating experience for both the examiner and the child. If you really suspect an abnormality, dilate the pupil to see what you are looking for. Use a short-acting cycloplegic, such as tropicamide 1%, putting one drop in each eye. Pupillary dilation is achieved within at least 20 minutes in most children; it may take a little longer in children with darkly pigmented eyes. The easiest way to put drops in the eyes is to have the patient lie supine with the eyes closed. You then put the drop in the inner canthus (corner of the eye) and ask, or wait, for the child to open the eyes. Instantly, the drops are in, and nobody has had to fight—at least until the next time, when the child may remember your method.

Most young children will not hold their eye still while you try to locate some familiar landmark, such as the disc or a blood vessel. The solution is for you to stay still, let the child's eye do the moving, and let your eye do the looking. The chances of finding something are far better if you are not moving while you search. Because the other secret of funduscopic success is good old practice (for which there is no reasonable substitute), try to examine the fundi in most infants and children with each complete physical examination. Funduscopy will become progressively easier for you.

You should make the following three important observations as part of the funduscopy:

1. Evaluate whether the red pupillary reflex is equal in all four fundus quadrants. You can accomplish this goal without having to obtain a perfect focus on the retina; perform the examination at a distance of 25 cm (10 to 12 inches) from the child.
2. Once the fundus is in focus, make sure you can see a normal foveolar reflex. Invite the child to look at your "little magic light." Sometimes the child's curiosity prompts him or her to do this anyway when you come close with the direct ophthalmoscope. One problem is that shining the light on the fovea stimulates the pupillary light response maximally (constriction) and may make viewing of the fundus difficult. Do not despair: The sharp bright foveolar reflection of the ophthalmoscope is easy to see.

3. Visualize at least part of a well-demarcated temporal edge of the disc as it passes by.

An even, red pupil indicates an attached retina with no major inflammatory or tumor process. Good fixation plus a sharp foveolar reflex eliminates an organic cause of poor vision, especially if the optic nerve looks normal. Most optic nerve diseases in the child involve the temporal half early in their evolution.

Lacrimal Sac Examination

In cases of lacrimal duct obstruction, the most important way to eliminate recurrent infections and also, according to some, a good way to help spontaneous resolution of the problem, is to know how to empty the lacrimal sac of its mucopurulent secretions. The technique is simple and is actually the best way to examine the lacrimal system to confirm a blockage. Minimal knowledge of the anatomy is required: Simply palpate the bony depression behind the insertion of the inner canthal ligament on the medial orbital rim. The best place to start is on yourself, as follows:

1. Find the small, hard bump in the inner corner of your eye with the index finger of your hand on the same side.
2. Roll your finger posteriorly to feel a small depression where the end of a small cotton-tipped swab could fit.

The next step is to do the same in a normal newborn to realize the difference in size. Finally, try it in a patient with a presumed blocked tear duct (Fig. 8–20). You will discover that (1) it is difficult to feel the depression, and (2) while you roll your finger, a significant amount of secretion will appear in the child's eye. The latter finding is proof of a blocked tear duct, whereas the fullness of the tissues on palpation was the dilated lacrimal sac waiting to be drained. All you have to do now is to show the parents how to do the "finger roll," which by the way is *not* a massage.

Corneal Staining (for Corneal Injuries)

When indicated, you should attempt corneal staining before using cycloplegic drops to prepare for fundus examination. However, the procedural problems are twofold. First, the staining dye stings a bit, which could end the child's previous amiability. Second, when fluorescein staining is indicated (e.g., as with corneal erosion or a foreign body), there is usually photophobia and discomfort, which may make it impossible to induce the child to open the lids.

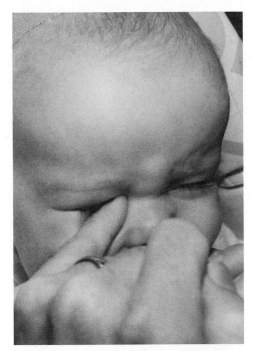

A

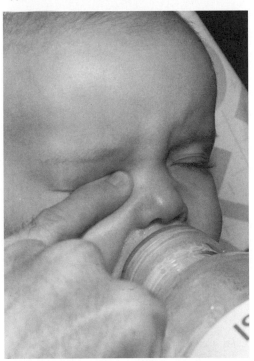

B

Figure 8–20 *A*, Lacrimal sac drainage, recommended to be performed once a day, uses slow but firm pressure applied by rotating the finger posterior to the lacrimal crest. Parents should locate their own sac before trying the procedure on the child. *B*, Wrong way to drain the sac; the finger used (index) is too big, the position of the finger is too anterior, and the pressure is applied to the side of the nose.

Figure 8–21 illustrates the procedure for corneal staining, in which a fluorescein paper strip, moistened with a couple of drops of ocular irrigation fluid, is applied at the lower lid margin of the open eye.

APPLYING SEQUENTIAL LOGIC TO ASSESS CHILDREN'S EYES

The following five different clinical situations illustrate how to apply sequential logical assessment to common specific visual problems. Table 8–3 lists the main examination techniques to be used in each age group.

Case Histories

Case 1: Nystagmus
Nystagmus is frequently overlooked despite the fact that it is the most common presenting sign of debilitating, genetically determined ocular conditions. The presenting complaint is most often "wiggly eyes" (Fig. 8–22). See Table 8–4 for aspects to consider, and the questions to ask, for a child with nystagmus. The first and most important question to answer is whether the vision is good. If the vision is good, relax. The child most likely has idiopathic motor nystagmus, usually an early-onset (3 months) hereditary condition with only moderate visual deficit.

If the child's vision is poor (found to be less than 6/30 [20/100], or evidenced by poor visual behavior), the underlying condition may carry a poor long-term visual prognosis with significant risk of recurrence in the family. Nystagmus accompanied by poor vision and photophobia usually signifies some form of cone disease. Such conditions can be

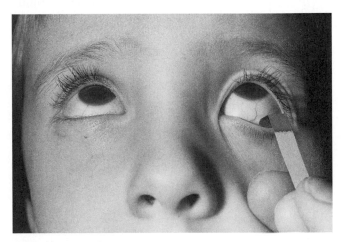

Figure 8–21 Application of a fluorescein strip. Warn the child first that you will be "tickling" the eyelashes. Instruct the child to look up, and just touch a wet paper strip of fluorescein to the edge of the lower lid. Immediately withdrawing the strip prevents an uncomfortable corneal touch when the child blinks. Use of a cobalt-blue light helps illuminate the pattern of a stained corneal epithelial defect.

Table 8–3   MAIN EXAMINATION TECHNIQUES BY AGE GROUP*

Technique	Newborn/Infant (0–1 year)	Toddler (up to 3 years)	Preschool and Older
Pupillary red reflex	Yes	Yes	Yes
Corneal light reflex	Yes	Yes	Yes
Vision	Face follow, OKN†	Cover test HOTV‡	HOTV
Ocular movement	Spin baby	Head twist	Frame
Visual fields		Wiggly fingers	Count fingers
Funduscopy	4 quadrants red reflex	4 quadrants red reflex (and temporal disc and macula clear images)	4 quadrants, temporal disc, and macula, all clear images

* See text for descriptive details.
† Not critical.
‡ Successful in very cooperative child.

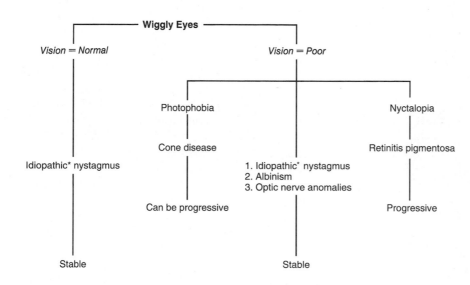

Figure 8–22 Diagnostic algorithm for a child presenting with "wiggly eyes."
*Also called "motor" nystagmus.

stable and are associated with very poor color vision. However, nystagmus plus night blindness (*nyctalopia*) probably indicates progressive retinitis pigmentosa. When neither photophobia nor nyctalopia is present in a child who has both nystagmus and poor vision, you should consider albinism, optic nerve disease, and severe idiopathic motor nystagmus as possibilities.

Table 8–4   NYSTAGMUS

Aspects to Be Considered	Questions to Ask Parents
Evidence of poor vision	Toys close to face?
	Poor eye contact?
	Poor motor development?
Photophobia	Squinting outdoors?
	Opens eyes only in semidarkness?
	Stays up all night?
	Refuses to play outside?
Nyctalopia	Cries when lights are out?
	Runs into walls at night?
	Wets the bed?
Family history	Nystagmus?
	Progressive blindness?

Key Point

In the child with nystagmus, a thorough pediatric ophthalmologic investigation is essential to establish the appropriate diagnosis, initiate genetic counseling, and provide appropriate support.

Case 2: Lid Ptosis

Lid ptosis (Fig. 8–23), which has important implications, both systemic and for vision, is often poorly understood. Unilateral or asymmetric lid ptosis has greater clinical significance than bilateral ptosis. Systemic problems or other local lid abnormalities can be seen in unilateral or intermittent ptosis. The child with ptosis often adopts a "chin-

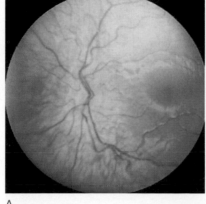
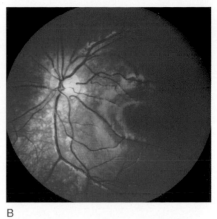

A

B

Plate 8–1 Fundi of a 6-year-old white boy. Note the excellent definition of the light reflection of the macular region by the healthy interface between vitreous and inner limiting membrane by the retina. Also, note its darker pigmentation.

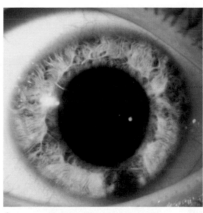
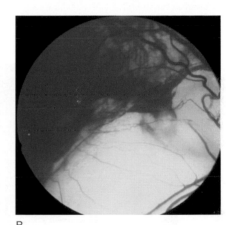

A

B

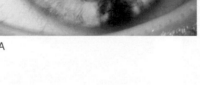

Plate 8–2 *A*, Coloboma of the stroma of the iris. *B*, Same eye shows extensive defect of the choroid, retina, and the optic disc, resulting in poor vision.

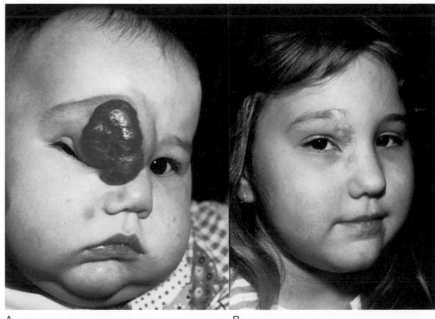

A

B

Plate 8–3 Capillary hemangioma involving the upper nasal orbit. *A*, The head turn represents the child's attempt to preserve binocular vision. There is evidence of some vision in the obstructed eye. *B*, Six years later, the tumor has all but disappeared spontaneously. Vision was maintained through intensive, prolonged amblyopia treatment.

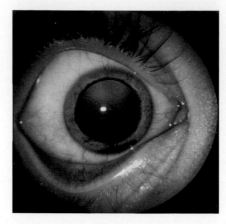

Plate 8–4 Hyphema can produce a visible level of blood in the anterior chamber. The blood is not visible if the patient is lying supine, because blood has not had a chance to settle, or if there are too few red blood cells in the aqueous to precipitate (a microscopic hyphema). Therefore, have the child supine with head up at 45 degrees for 15 to 20 minutes. Visualization of a microscopic hyphema requires a slit-lamp examination.

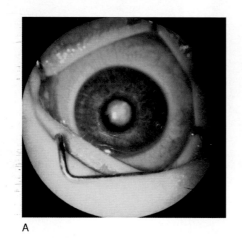

A

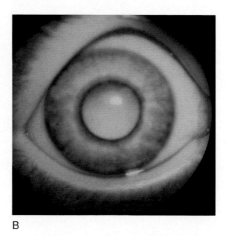

B

Plate 8–5 Leukocoria. *A,* Congenital nuclear cataract. Here, fluorescein is staining the tear film. *B,* Retinoblastoma with extensive invasion of the vitreous cavity. Note the yellowish tinge of the opacity in retinoblastoma.

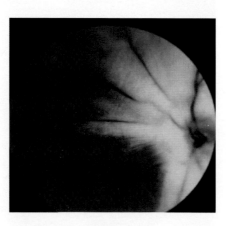

Plate 8–6 Myelinated nerve fiber layer. Abnormal presence of myelin around the ganglion cell fibers of the inner surface of the retina gives the white color with the feathery edges seen here. It is most frequently continuous with the margin of the optic nerve head (disc).

Plate 8–7 Optic nerve comparison. *A*, Normal-sized optic nerve head with normal coloration. *B*, Optic nerve hypoplasia (ONH) with some pallor. Note the relatively large size of the blood vessels at the surface of the disc. The amount of visual deficit is impossible to predict from the appearance of the disc. The disc is the inner circle of the two seen on the photograph; hence the term, double-ring sign of ONH.

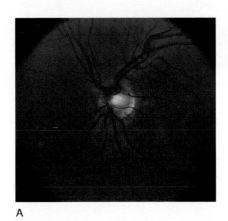

A

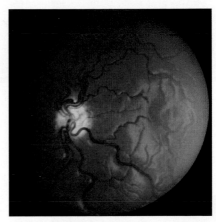

B

Plate 8–8 Periorbital cellulitis is a rapid-onset inflammation of the tissues around the eye. It can involve the orbital tissues with rapid spread to the cavernous sinus and may be life threatening.

Plate 8–9 Retinitis pigmentosa (RP) manifests the typical "bone spicule" pattern of pigment. These typical retinal lesions are rarely seen in children. Even with far-advanced retinal degeneration and severe visual deficit, this patient with Laurence-Moon-Biedl syndrome shows few pigment clumps. Instead, the overall retinal background looks "dirty," and the vessels have become very tenuous. The optic disc is pale and has taken on a waxy appearance. The crisp, shiny reflections of the retinal surface are lost.

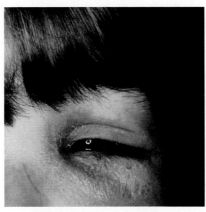

Plate 8–8

Plate 8–9

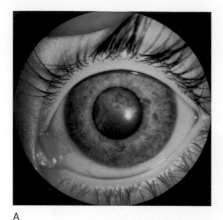

A

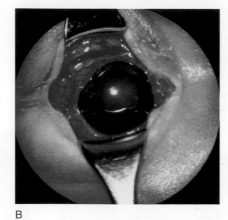

B

Plate 8–10 Retinoblastoma is lethal; watch for it. Leukocoria can be (*A*) pink with visible wavy vessels if the retina has been pushed (detached) forward, close behind the lens, or (*B*) associated with a red eye caused by raised intraocular pressure due to the closure of the iridocorneal angle.

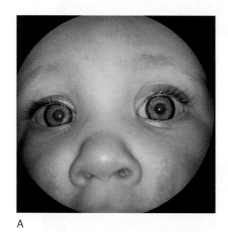

A

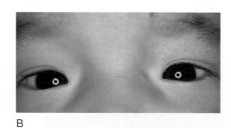

B

Plate 8–11 Pupillary red reflexes. *A*, Normal reflexes in an 8-month-old white baby with straight eyes. *B*, Pseudostrabismus showing lack of sclera nasal to the cornea, giving the impression of an esotropia. Corneal light reflexes are nevertheless central.

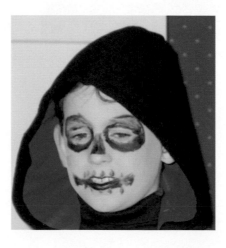

Plate 8–12 Pupillary red reflexes inadvertently produced with an automatic flash camera.

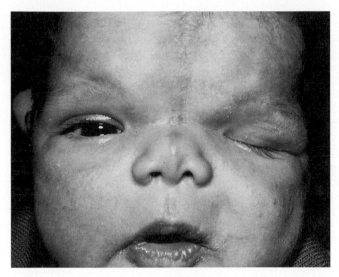

Figure 8–23 Lid ptosis in a 1-month-old infant. The ptotic (droopy) lid completely obstructs the eye, making this condition an emergency. Failure to open the lid would result in a deep deprivation amblyopia of severity equal to or worse than that caused by a congenital cataract.

up" position, freeing the pupil to allow binocular vision.

The presenting complaint is most often "droopy lid," for which Figure 8–24 presents a diagnostic algorithm. Also see Table 8–5 for aspects to consider, and questions to ask, for a child with ptosis. The most important question is whether the ptosis is constant. If the ptosis is constant, involving one or both eyes, vision is at risk, and early intervention is required to allow normal visual development in the obstructed eye. This situation is comparable with that of the child with congenital cataract, in which severe visual deprivation prevents establishment of the normal neuronal organization of vision.

The lid's appearance helps identify local tumors, such as hemangiomas, whereas a good neurologic examination, including assessment of ocular motility, often gives clues to rarer congenital "misfirings," such as Marcus Gunn oculotrigeminal dyskinesia (jaw-winking phenomenon; Fig. 8–25), myasthenia gravis, and even mitochondrial diseases.

Always remember the possibility of deep amblyopia, even in cases of partial ptosis, because partial ptosis is often accompanied by a significant degree of astigmatism in the affected eye, which in turn usually causes amblyopia. Only prompt treatment, including surgery, can restore vision.

Case 3: Epiphora

Tearing, or epiphora, is the most common of ocular complaints, and the causes are innumerable, from a hysterical emotional reaction to a splash of a destructive alkali in the eyes. Figure 8–26 presents a diagnostic algorithm for a child presenting with tearing eyes. In young children, the differential diagnosis is often somewhere between a chronic conjunctivitis and the dreaded (albeit extremely rare) blinding infantile glaucoma or a potentially devastating herpes simplex keratitis.

See Table 8–6 for aspects to consider, and questions to ask, for a child with epiphora. The most important question to ask is whether there is photophobia. Equally important is assessment of corneal size, which you accomplish by comparing the child's cornea with those of the parent on whose lap the child sits (facing you). An adult cornea has a horizontal diameter of 12 mm; anything bigger in a child is abnormal. Therefore, if an infant presents with teary eyes, photophobia, and enlarged cornea, the diagnosis is most certainly infantile glaucoma, a potentially blinding but treatable disease. The

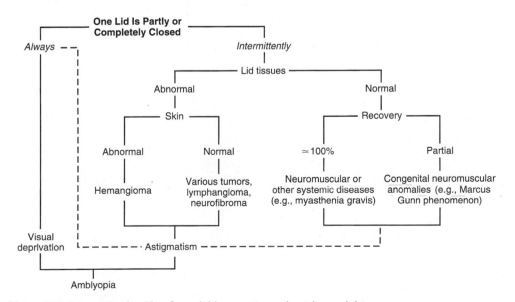

Figure 8–24 Diagnostic algorithm for a child presenting with a "droopy lid."

Table 8–5   PTOSIS

Aspects to Be Considered	Questions to Ask Parents
Hematoma	History of trauma?
Plexiform neurofibroma (see Fig. 8–6)	Birthmarks?
	Plexiform neurofibroma in the family?
Jaw-winking phenomenon (see Fig. 8–25)	Ptosis improves with drinking, sucking, and/or chewing?
Hemangioma (capillary) (see Plate 8–12)	Abnormal lid?
	Bluer when crying?
Lymphangioma (see Fig. 8–4)	Increase in size with colds?
	Increase in size after trauma?
Third cranial nerve palsy (ophthalmoplegia)	Little voluntary eye movement of one eye?
Acquired third cranial nerve palsy	Diplopia when lid open?
Third cranial nerve palsy and aberrant regeneration	Lid movements with attempted eye movements?
Myasthenia gravis	Ptosis gets worse intermittently in the afternoon?
Myasthenia, mitochondrial diseases	Poor gag reflex and/or poor feeding?
	Progressive weakness during the day?

disease can be unilateral in the early stages (i.e., one cornea is enlarged).

A teary eye with photophobia and normal corneal size could be caused by a corneal erosion, a foreign body, or herpetic keratitis. Fluorescein staining of the cornea is absolutely essential to detect an erosion. If both eyes are involved, ask whether anyone might have thrown sand, dirt, or even lime at the child. Obviously, in cases involving lime, immediate copious and prolonged irrigation can save the child's sight. The typical story in a child with herpes keratitis is that of a nonresponsive uni-

lateral conjunctivitis and teary eye with photophobia that remains after more than 7 days of topical antibiotic treatment. A photophobic teary eye can also be a sign of uveitis, although most uveitic eyes in children are asymptomatic.

Key Point

Photophobia and tearing are signs of serious eye disease when present together. Have the patient seen promptly by an ophthalmologist!

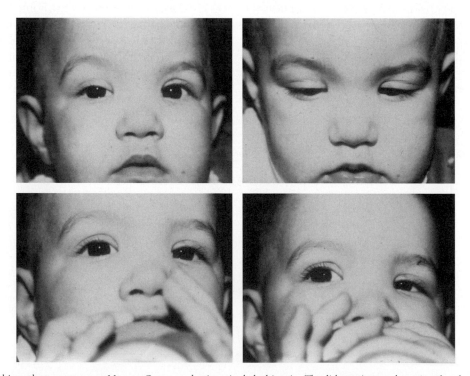

Figure 8–25 Jaw-winking phenomenon, or Marcus Gunn oculotrigeminal dyskinesia. The lid ptosis may be missed unless the jaw is made to move by sucking or chewing. The lateral movement of the mandible by the pterygoid muscle is accompanied by the elevation of the lid. In this case, when the jaw is moved to the left, the right lid goes up. This condition results from a congenital "misfiring" in the brainstem between motor cranial nerve V and cranial nerve III.

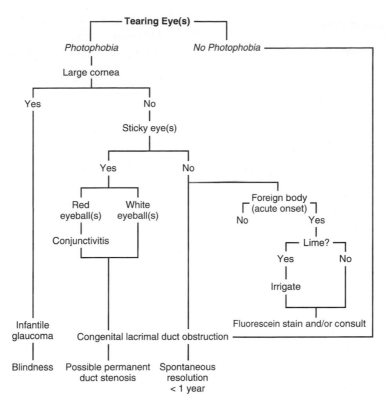

Figure 8–26 Diagnostic algorithm for a child presenting with tearing eyes.

A teary eye that has been present since birth, without photophobia but with secretions causing sticky lids, is most often due to a congenitally blocked tear duct. Without recurrent significant conjunctivitis, this problem can be monitored until spontaneous resolution occurs, which happens in 90% of the children before 1 year of age. Daily drainage (once per day) of the lacrimal sac greatly reduces the rate of recurrent infections. Control of recurrent infections is important to prevent damage to the lacrimal drainage system. Antibiotics are rarely needed; when they are indicated, any of the broad-spectrum antibiotic eye ointments is adequate for a 5-day, three-times-a-day treatment regimen. If infection recurs often, surgery (probing) is indicated.

Table 8–6 EPIPHORA

Aspects to Be Considered	Questions to Ask Parents
Blocked tear ducts	Two eyes first, then one only?
	Worse with colds?
Congenital glaucoma	Photophobia?
	Constant tearing?
	Big eyes?

Case 4: Strabismus

Because it is so common, strabismus is probably the subject most extensively covered in texts on children's eye problems.

> **Key Point**
>
> Strabismus can signal several serious conditions and is never outgrown.

Parents commonly complain that the child's eyes "do not look straight." Figure 8–27 presents a diagnostic algorithm for this situation. Also, see Table 8–7 for aspects to consider, and questions to ask, for a child with strabismus. Immediately decide whether the corneal light reflections are normal. If they are normal in the primary position (looking straight ahead), check whether they are normal in other positions of gaze. An incomitant strabismus, which may show only in certain positions of the eyes and may or may not be present in the primary position, must be identified promptly. The cause of strabismus may be paralytic, restrictive, myogenic, or mechanical.

If the corneal light reflections are abnormal in the primary position, evaluate the comitance of the deviation and establish the alteration of deviation. Does the child alternate the eye with which he or she fixes the target? If a child presents with an alternating stra-

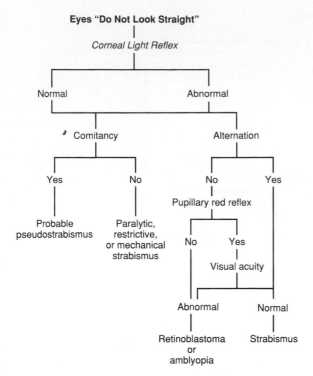

Figure 8–27 Diagnostic algorithm for a child presenting with eyes that "do not look straight."

bismus, chances are that his or her vision is equal in the two eyes. Evaluation of the strabismus may raise suspicion of poor vision. Such a finding has great clinical importance and may lead to an etiologic diagnosis. For example, absence of a normal red reflex in the deviating eye can be a sign of a retinoblastoma or cataract.

Case 5: Leukocoria

Although strabismus is a common condition with potentially major systemic implications and with obvious direct effects on visual function, leukocoria is an uncommon but ominous sign. The presenting complaint is most often an eye(s) or pupil(s) that "does not look right," for which Figure 8–28 presents a diagnostic algorithm.

Key Point

When a child presents with a white pupil, immediately define the state of the pupillary light reflexes, deciding whether they are present at all in either eye and, if so, whether they are symmetric.

Absence of a pupillary light reflex is significant and can be caused by corneal or choroidal lesions or anything in between. A white or gray-white reflex, termed leukocoria, is caused by lesions dense and close enough to the crystalline lens to reflect most of the penetrating light. Cataracts and retinoblastoma are two classic examples. See Table 8–8 for aspects to consider, and questions to ask, for a child with leukocoria.

Asymmetric gray (dark) reflexes are equally or more ominous, because they indicate bilateral disease. Symmetric orange light reflexes, bright and uniform throughout the pupil, are normal for whites; symmetric gray reflexes, uniform throughout the pupil, are normal for dark-skinned people. Anything else may be abnormal.

Table 8–7   STRABISMUS

Aspects to Be Considered	Questions to Ask
Intermittent esotropia	Worse when looking up close?
Intermittent exotropia	Worse when looking outside?
Large exophoria or esophoria	Worse when tired?
Migrainous ophthalmoplegia (third or fourth cranial nerve palsy)	Onset after a bad headache?
Idiopathic sixth cranial nerve palsy	Onset after a cold?
Rare congenital sixth cranial nerve palsy	Onset at birth?
"Congenital esotropia" (early-onset infantile)	Onset at about 3 months of age?
Accommodative esotropia	Onset at about 3 years of age?
Intracranial process with sixth and fourth cranial nerve involvement	Accompanied with or preceded by a chronic headache?
Onset of deviation (according to parents)	Ask the child to show you what he or she sees (diplopia signifies neurologic cause).
	Inspect the family photo album for corneal light reflexes and abnormal head posture.

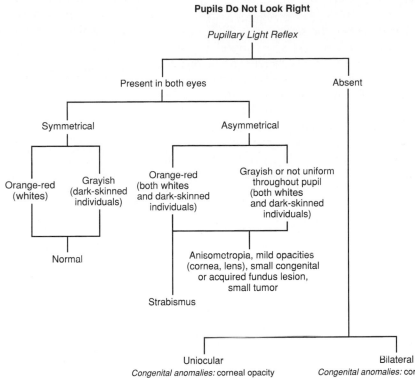

Figure 8–28 Diagnostic algorithm for a child presenting with pupils that "do not look right."

Table 8–8 LEUKOCORIA

Aspects to Be Considered	Questions to Ask
Localized lesion of the posterior pole, retinoblastoma	Intermittent?
	Seen only at certain angles?
Toxocara canis (visceral larva migrans), retinal toxoplasmosis	Family pet (puppy or kitten).
	Youngster likely to put dirt in the mouth (2–4 years)?
Cataract, big posterior coloboma	Onset at birth or very soon after?
Retinoblastoma	Onset about $1\frac{1}{2}$ years old?
	Family history?
Toxocara canis (visceral larva migrans)	Age 2–4 years: close encounter with a puppy?
Cataract, retinal detachment	History of recent eye trauma?
Sarcoid or *Candida* vitritis	Sick child?
Uveitis with cataract and glaucoma	Arthritis?
Cataract	Maternal rubella?
	Child on steroids?
	Trauma?
	Diabetes?
	Storage disease?
	Chromosome anomalies?
	Family history?
Retinopathy of prematurity; formerly called retrolental fibroplasia	Prematurity with low-birth-weight and use of respirator?

SUMMARY

This chapter has described the simple steps necessary to evaluate not only the eyes but also some important visual functions in children. Study of this chapter should enable you to include in your standard pediatric examination skills some simple, effective, and quick means of examining children's eyes and vision with the aid of basic equipment. However, the value of simple observation cannot be overemphasized, in addition to the knowledge of the following "golden rules": (1) a constant deviation or persistent jiggling of the eyes is abnormal at any age,

(2) an abnormal pupillary reflex represents a retinoblastoma until proven otherwise, and (3) photophobia is always a sign of serious ocular disease.

SUGGESTED READINGS

Berson FG (ed): Ophthalmology Study Guide for Students and Practitioners of Medicine, 5th ed. San Francisco, The American Academy of Ophthalmology, 1987.

Taylor D, Hoyt C. Practical Paediatric Ophthalmology. Oxford, Blackwell Science, 1997, pp 13–22.

Von Noorden GK, Maumenee AE: Atlas of Strabismus, 4th ed. St. Louis, CV Mosby, 1983, p 65.

chapter 9

Evaluating the Child's Respiratory System

DANIEL M. HUGHES

Most children's respiratory problems can be diagnosed with confidence by the time the history and physical examination are completed. Even when a specific diagnosis is not immediately clear, there are usually enough clues to allow you to narrow the possibilities to a manageable few. The anatomic-physiologic relationships of the respiratory system are readily revealed through symptoms and signs.

Understanding the origin and mechanism of abnormal respiratory sounds (e.g., stridor or wheeze) helps localize the site of an airway obstruction even if you have not yet pinpointed its cause. For children who require further investigations, a limited number of procedures, such as chest radiographs, pulmonary function tests, blood gas analyses, measurement of sweat chloride levels, and cultures, will clarify their problems. Immunology studies, bronchoscopy and biopsy, and further imaging studies are required less often.

Besides providing essential information about the child's complaints, the process of history-taking helps establish a good rapport with the family. This support is usually important when dealing with children with recurrent or chronic respiratory problems, such as asthma or cystic fibrosis; it is essential for successful management.

Relevant details from the functional inquiry often clarify the diagnosis and uncover other problems that need attention, such as allergic rhinitis or atopic eczema in a child with asthma. The physical examination usually confirms the suspicions aroused by a good history; occasionally, it reveals no abnormalities, and management must then be based largely on history.

Key Point

Evaluating the respiratory system involves much more than examining the chest. Important clues are often located far from the thorax (e.g., finger clubbing is associated with chronic pulmonary disease).

Resist the temptation to lead with your stethoscope. Auscultation is only a small part of respiratory examination, and it is often left to the last unless the child is uncooperative. Other aspects of physical examination often make the auscultatory findings more easily interpretable; for example, finding decreased breath sounds over the left hemithorax can have different meanings depending on whether the trachea is midline, pulled to the left, or pushed to the right.

OBTAINING THE HISTORY

Taking a respiratory history from the parents is appropriate in very young children, but try to involve older children in the interview whenever possible, because they can provide valuable information about their symptoms. For instance, a child with asthma often admits to cough and shortness of breath resulting from physical activity at school, symptoms often not appreciated by the parents.

When asked for the chief complaint, parents may respond with either a specific diagnosis or a symptom, often cough, wheeze, shortness of breath, noisy breathing, or recurrent respiratory tract infections. Their diagnosis may be correct, but it must be confirmed by a detailed history and a complete physical examination. A missed diagnosis, such as inhalation of a foreign body or unrecognized cystic fibrosis, can have significant implications for the child.

Parents must understand your terminology, and you must understand theirs (see Chapter 1). What parents describe as a wheeze may, in fact, be stridor. What you call asthma may mean something much more alarming to parents. Do not assume that parents understand what is meant by terms such as *wheeze*. Be prepared to imitate a wheeze, stridor, or whoop or to ask the parents to imitate the sound they are trying to describe.

Establishing whether the child makes the sound on inspiration or expiration may seem easy to you, but many parents have difficulty making that distinction.

Some parents have difficulty recalling the circumstances or triggers that cause or aggravate their child's respiratory symptoms. This is frequently the situation in the child with asthma. Have a prepared list of common asthma triggers on hand to help them (Fig. 9–1).

Each symptom should be probed until it has been characterized well with respect to timing, aggravating and relieving factors, and associated features. Establish whether the symptoms are *acute* (less than 3 weeks' duration), *long-standing* or *chronic* (more than 3 months' duration), or *recurrent* (symptom-free intervals of at least 2 weeks' duration).

These answers help narrow the diagnostic possibilities when dealing with stridor or wheezing. To narrow the diagnostic possibilities further, try to relate symptoms to each other: cough and stridor; cough and wheeze; and cough, wheeze, sputum, and failure to thrive.

Before completing the history, ask the parents and child what *they* see as the major problem. Parents occasionally bring up concerns they did not mention earlier in the interview. Likewise, do not assume that their concerns are the same as yours—often they are surprisingly different.

Chief Complaints

Cough, wheeze, and recurrent infections are the most common complaints arising from respiratory diseases, although parents of younger children may complain that their child has noisy breathing. To characterize the main complaint, you must consider the child's age, duration of the symptom, timing, aggravating and relieving factors, and the effect of previously prescribed medications.

Begin the history-taking for young children by asking about details of the pregnancy and birth. A history of maternal infections, drug use, cigarette smoking, and any problems during labor and delivery should be sought. The baby's gestational age, birth weight, Apgar score, and need for resuscitation, oxygen, or assisted ventilation should be documented. Difficulty establishing feedings, episodes of apnea, or any evidence of respiratory distress in the neonatal period may set the stage for respiratory problems later in infancy. Dating the onset of symptoms can help; the closer to birth, the more likely that they are due to a congenital disorder. If the child appeared well early in life, ask how old the child was when the complaint began.

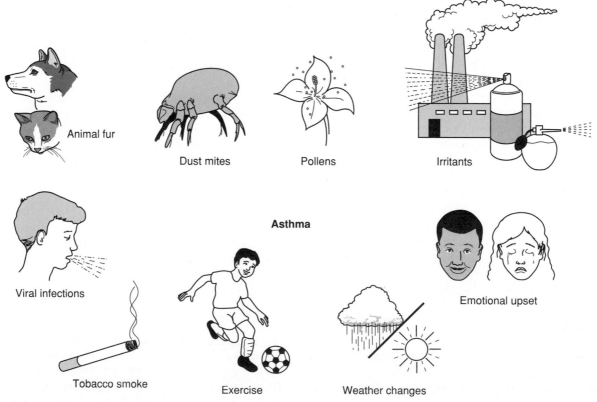

Figure 9–1 The common triggers of asthma.

The following sections describe some common complaints and the important questions to ask about them during the history-taking.

COUGH

Whether cough is the principal or a secondary complaint, obtain as much information as possible about it. Is it dry or loose? At what time of the day or night does it occur? What triggers, aggravates, and relieves it? Coughing associated with sputum production is always a serious complaint in a child. Remember that infants, younger children, and some older children cannot or will not spit but swallow their sputum. Try to establish the color, volume, odor, and viscosity of the sputum and the presence or absence of blood. In infants, it is always important to establish whether a cough is associated with feeding and whether there is associated choking or spluttering, which may occur in children with gastroesophageal reflux, a tracheoesophageal fistula, or swallowing incoordination. Short, dry, or loud honking coughs that occur only when the child is awake and that are associated with parental anxiety but show no evidence of underlying respiratory disease should suggest a nervous (habitual) or psychogenic cough. Such coughs may last for weeks or months and can be difficult to treat.

Although it is generally agreed that postnasal drip can cause a "throat-clearing" type of cough, particularly at night, it is doubtful that this process can cause a troublesome chronic daytime cough in children. It is more likely that a similar pathologic process affects the nose, sinuses, and tracheobronchial tree, such as that occurring in children with asthma, allergic rhinitis, and sinusitis.

NOISY BREATHING

The nonspecific complaint of "noisy breathing" can usually be narrowed down to one of five specific possibilities—snoring, stridor, wheezing, grunting, or rattly breathing (see the section on physical examination elsewhere in this chapter). Many parents and some physicians make the mistake of believing that noisy breathing indicates chest (bronchopulmonary) problems, whereas in many infants and children, the noise originates in the nose, nasopharynx, or upper airway.

RECURRENT RESPIRATORY INFECTIONS ("COLDS")

You should obtain a full description of a typical episode, establishing whether there was an infectious contact, fever, rhinorrhea, earache, sore throat, facial pain, headache, or lymphadenopathy. A cough associated with wheeze, chest pain, or shortness of breath suggests lower respiratory tract involvement. Ask about the response to previous treatment, but understand that some parents are convinced that viral respiratory tract infections have responded to antibiotic therapy.

Remember, parents vary considerably in their tolerance for recurrent respiratory infections in their children. They may be unaware that the average preschooler can have six to eight such infections per year, the majority occurring during the winter months, making it seem that one infection has run into the next. When a youngster is an only child, he or she may have lacked the opportunity to pick up respiratory illnesses from siblings before starting daycare, nursery school, or kindergarten. For such children, the first year in a group setting often results in an above-average number of infections.

Key Point

In the evaluation of the child with recurrent respiratory illnesses, it is important to assess the extent of exposure (number of contacts) both at home and in group settings, such as daycare.

Finally, what parents describe as a "cold" may or may not represent viral respiratory infection. Wheezing episodes are often preceded by 24 to 48 hours of nasal congestion and cough, and although these symptoms may be due to a viral infection that initiates wheeze after a day or two, they occasionally represent the "prewheezing" manifestations of an allergic response to an inhaled allergen.

CHEST PAIN

Chest pain in children is not uncommon, especially in adolescents, but as an isolated complaint, it is usually a benign phenomenon. When chest pain is accompanied by other symptoms and signs, the diagnosis may be obvious, as in the chest pain from coughing in a child with asthma. When the underlying diagnosis is less clear, remember that organic chest pain can arise from a limited number of anatomic structures (chest wall, myocardium, pericardium, esophagus, or pleura). Questions that ferret out the site of origin often bring rewards.

In teenagers, chest pain is often traced to minor transient chest wall problems that do not affect general health. Sometimes a little chest wall tenderness can be demonstrated on pressure. Many teenagers who complain of chest pain report sudden recurrent pain that lasts only a few seconds or minutes. Typically, the pain "catches them" if they try to take a deep breath. Many of us have experienced these ourselves. They appear to be due to transient involuntary spasm of intercostal muscles, possibly analogous to nocturnal leg cramps ("growing pains") or to the sudden "foot-in-a-knot" cramps that many adults experience, especially at night. In costochondritis (Tietze syndrome), also a relatively benign condition, localized tenderness may be found (with or without swelling) over one of the costochondral junctions.

Key Point

Laboratory investigations, electrocardiograms, and imaging procedures are uniformly unhelpful in the child with chest pain unless directed by solid historical or physical evidence of abnormality.

A teenager's chest pain is often a psychosomatic complaint reflecting anxiety generated by some major family life event, such as a relative's myocardial infarction or malignant disease. It is essential to ask teenagers who complain of chest pain whether they are worried that it might be serious. For example, you might ask, "Some people with chest pain are worried that it might be something serious—how about you?" Always ask about serious illness among family or friends.

Key Point

Chest pain in teenagers is rarely due to serious disease. Brief, transient chest pain may be due to intercostal muscle spasm, the so-called precordial catch syndrome.

SHORTNESS OF BREATH (DYSPNEA)

Shortness of breath rarely occurs in isolation. Associated signs of infection may suggest pneumonia, pleural effusion, or bronchitis. Accompanying pain may suggest pneumothorax, rib fractures from trauma, or pleurisy.

HYPERVENTILATION

Hyperventilation is a common symptom in adolescents, seen more often in girls. The child may complain, "I can't catch my breath," "I can't get enough air," "I have trouble breathing," or even "I have wheezing." You can also detect hyperventilation by specifically questioning teenagers who present with other anxiety-related complaints.

When you suspect that a teenager may be hyperventilating, ask whether he or she has ever had any problem with swallowing. Sometimes the teenager will reveal often sensing a "lump" in the throat and having difficulty swallowing (the so-called globus hystericus).

Other features that sometimes are associated with such psychosomatic complaints are dilated pupils or, for unexplained reasons, absent or highly suppressed gag reflex, such that a tongue depressor can practically touch the epiglottis without eliciting a gag.

Inquire about events leading up to the hyperventilation, and be aware that some adolescents with asthma have acute episodes of dyspnea triggered by vigorous exercise or sports, leading to anxiety and subsequent hyperventilation.

CHOKING ASSOCIATED WITH FOREIGN BODIES

Ask whether the child has a history of putting foreign objects in the nose or of choking or coughing while having access to peanuts or small objects.

Previous Hospitalization

Record the dates and circumstances of previous hospitalizations and treatment. Try to determine whether the hospitalizations resulted from failed medical management at home and whether the parents have sufficient information and the tools required to reduce the frequency of future hospitalizations.

Medications

It is not enough simply to list the medications given to a child. Dosages and timing of administration are essential information. Try to distinguish between the medication regimen the child is supposed to be following and what the child actually takes, remembering that compliance with regularly prescribed medications in children is very poor. Ask, "Many children have trouble remembering to take their medications—does this ever happen to you?" If the child replies in the affirmative, ask, "How many times a week do you remember to take your medications?"

For patients using home nebulizers, record details of how the medications and diluent are mixed and administered. Inquire about the particular devices being used to deliver aerosol medications and the technique used (open-mouth versus closed-mouth technique when using metered aerosols). Ask about side effects from medications. Some children experience side effects from "normal" therapeutic doses of bronchodilators.

Key Point

It is not sufficient to simply ask whether the child's technique with a particular device is satisfactory. Observing the child using the device is essential.

Immunizations

Inquire whether the child has received influenza or pneumococcal vaccines.

Smoking

Ask who smokes in the child's environment and how much. The history of smoke exposure applies not only to the home and the family car but also to friends and relatives who visit the home and visits to relatives or friends in their homes. Does smoke exposure aggravate the respiratory symptoms? Ask the child how he or she feels when exposed to smoke. Parents who smoke often say their child does not have respiratory symptoms when exposed to their cigarette smoking, but the child may tell quite a different story. Remember, children as young as 10 years may smoke cigarettes; always ask about this possibility out of parents' hearing.

Environmental Factors

Ask about the effects of exposure to specific home environments and inhalants—moldy basements, dusty areas, sprays, perfumes, and substances the parents may use in their occupations that can trigger symptoms. Ask about symptoms from exposure to grass, trees, and pollens; to dust and chalkboard dust at school; and to pets at home or in the homes of family or friends. Regularly recurring symptoms during a particular season may provide the essential tip-off to allergies, for example, symptoms from trees in spring, grass in summer, and ragweed in autumn. Symptoms occurring at school can occasionally be difficult to sort out, to the frustration of many parents.

Family History

A history of similarly affected family members not only helps the diagnostic process, as in asthma or cystic fibrosis, but also offers some understanding of the family's experience with the disease. A family may seem overly worried about a child's asthma until you discover that an uncle died during an asthma attack.

Pets

List all pets with which the child comes into contact, both inside and outside the home. Ask whether the child has any symptoms with such exposures, and describe examples of symptoms, such as itchy eyes or nose. Not infrequently, a child admits to symptoms from exposure to a neighbor's or relative's pet but not to his or her own pet.

Key Point

Parents sometimes neglect to mention a pet that does not come into the house, such as an outdoor cat or dog, or they overlook exposure at neighbors' or relatives' homes or at school (e.g., the pet rabbit or guinea pig in the nursery school classroom).

Exercise-Related Symptoms

The relationship between increased physical activity and respiratory symptoms is important. Toddlers with asthma often cough when they are excited or when they are tickled. Ask about symptoms associated with normal activities, such as running or bike riding, or during school recess or sports participation, and, particularly, during cooler weather in the fall and winter. Rather than asking parents whether their child has symptoms during gym class in school, ask the child what happens when he or she runs around the gym at school. Sometimes, the previously undiagnosed asthmatic patient replies, "I cough." For older children, the type of exercise that triggers symptoms is important. Activities such as cross-country running, soccer, competitive basketball, hockey, and ice skating, which do not allow for a rest period, can often aggravate asthma, particularly if carried out in cold, dry air. Ask children previously diagnosed as asthmatic whether they take any medication before, during, or after exercise. If so, does it prevent or reduce the symptoms?

School Absenteeism

Parents may underestimate or overestimate the amount of school time a child misses for respiratory symptoms. Brief absences are often forgotten. Checking the school records may give you a more accurate picture. Ask the parents to obtain the information or, with their permission, contact the school.

Allergies

When eliciting the history of allergies, distinguish between unequivocal clinical reactions to specific allergens and the results of allergy skin testing. When parents volunteer a list of items to which the child is allergic, they are often merely reiterating reported positive results of previous skin tests, which may or may not reflect clinical hypersensitivity. Ask the parents whether they have noticed symptoms whenever the child is exposed to any of the items that gave positive skin test responses. Ask about cough, wheeze, symptoms of allergic rhinitis or conjunctivitis, laryngeal edema, and hives.

Allergic Rhinitis

Because many parents are unfamiliar with the terms *allergic rhinitis* and *hay fever,* ask instead about itchy nose, runny nose, the classic "allergic salute" (repeatedly rubbing the tip of the itchy nose with the palm or back of the hand) (Fig. 9–2), or fits of sneezing. Establish whether any of these symptoms occur seasonally or year-round. Elicit the specific factors triggering these symptoms and what treatments have been tried.

Ear, Nose, and Throat

Recurrent otitis media, chronic otitis media with effusion, and sinus involvement often appear with respiratory symptoms in allergic children and in children with ciliary dysfunction or immunoglobulin deficiencies. Ask about snoring and mouth breathing. Curiously, adults are much less tolerant of snoring in children than in themselves or their spouses!

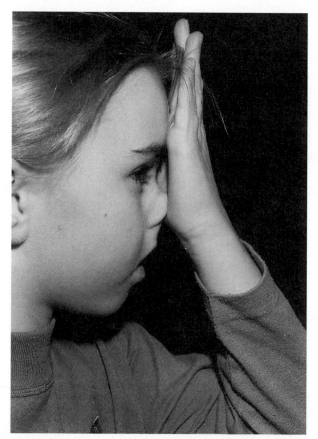

Figure 9–2 The "allergic salute." The child repeatedly rubs the tip of the itchy nose with the palm or back of the hand.

Eczema

Parents are usually aware of overt eczema, but they forget dry skin or small patches of eczema, particularly dry skin behind the ears in the atopic child. List past treatments for this problem.

Croup

Croup is a viral infection of the larynx, trachea, and bronchi. If parents are unfamiliar with the term *croup,* they will usually recognize the symptom pattern, which consists of a harsh, barking cough and hoarse voice occurring at night, sometimes preceded by 1 or 2 days of upper respiratory symptoms (coryza). Spasmodic or recurrent croup occasionally occurs without any obvious preceding respiratory infection. The previously well child suddenly awakens during the night with a harsh cough, hoarse voice, and inspiratory stridor. Symptoms often improve in a cool, moist atmosphere but may recur over the next few nights. Some children continue to have recurring bouts during early childhood and later develop asthma.

Gastrointestinal Symptoms

Ask whether the child eats poorly or is ravenous. Has there been normal weight gain, weight loss, or failure to thrive? Inquire about previous growth measurements, and determine the growth pattern. Ask about swallowing difficulties (such as choking while eating or drinking) and symptoms of gastroesophageal reflux, as well as rectal prolapse (an important clue to cystic fibrosis), abdominal pain, stool frequency, and the appearance and odor of stools. A child with oily, foul-smelling stools and failure to gain weight satisfactorily despite a huge appetite usually has cystic fibrosis.

> **Key Point**
>
> When parents report that their child tastes salty when kissed, the youngster must be investigated for cystic fibrosis.

Unusual Infections

Always note unusual or persistent infections; for example, a history of *Pseudomonas* cultured from the sputum may suggest a diagnosis of cystic fibrosis. Pay attention to recurrent infections involving the ear, nose, and throat; skin; or respiratory tract and to troublesome abscesses, which may suggest an underlying immunologic deficit. Ask about previous immunizations and any unusual reactions to them.

Family Attributes

The summary of the respiratory history should also include details on the family's beliefs about and knowledge of the diagnosis of the child's problems. Try to determine family strengths, weaknesses, and coping abilities, and inquire about financial resources and employment. Exercise caution when inquiring into such sensitive areas, particularly when meeting a family for the first time. The success or failure of future management of the child's problems may depend on the sensitivity you demonstrate and the rapport you establish during this part of the evaluation.

APPROACH TO THE PHYSICAL EXAMINATION

Begin the physical examination with observations as you take the history, before formally examining child; watch for the allergic salute, and listen for noisy breathing and the quality of the child's cough.

A complete examination of an infant or toddler's respiratory system is often best accomplished with the child sitting in the parent's lap (Fig. 9–3). For older children and teenagers, having them sit on an examining table is best. Although the order of the examination is not crucial, it should be complete. Forgetting to examine for clubbing or to listen to the child's cough are major omissions. Use a pediatric stethoscope for infants, because the diaphragm and bell of an adult stethoscope are often too large.

Many aspects of respiratory examination and findings in a child resemble those in the adult. Some of the important differences are as follows:

1. Normal respiratory rates are faster in infants and children (Table 9–1).

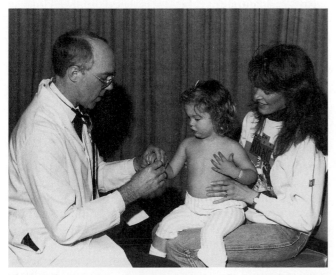

Figure 9–3 Most of the physical examination of a young child is best accomplished with the youngster sitting on the parent's lap.

Table 9-1 NORMAL AWAKE RESPIRATORY RATES IN CHILDREN

Age (years)	Respiratory Rate (breaths/min)
0–1	25–40
1–5	20–30
5–10	15–25
10–16	15–20

2. Compliance of the younger child's chest wall is markedly greater, as amply demonstrated in the indrawing associated with croup and bronchiolitis.
3. Respiratory sounds (noises) are readily transmitted to the child's thorax from the upper airway; indeed, the air-filled thoracic cage acts as an amplifier for breath sounds.

Cyanosis

Examine the skin of the extremities, tongue, and mucous membranes for cyanosis, and distinguish between peripheral cyanosis and central cyanosis. Central cyanosis indicates cardiorespiratory disease. Because it occurs at different levels of arterial oxygen saturation according to the amount of total hemoglobin present, central cyanosis is not a reliable early sign of hypoxemia.

Nasal Flaring

You can easily overlook flaring of the alae nasi if you do not look for it specifically. It is a nonspecific but important sign of respiratory distress, probably reflecting increased work of breathing and dyspnea.

Ears, Nose, and Throat

A detailed examination may uncover serous otitis media, allergic shiners, inflamed nasal mucosa in the allergic child, or, rarely, nasal polyps in a child with cystic fibrosis.

Use of Accessory Muscles

When airway obstruction or pulmonary disease is present, the child uses accessory muscles, mainly the sternocleidomastoids, scalenes, and abdominal muscles, to aid respiration.

Retractions

When present in children, retractions usually involve soft tissue (suprasternal, supraclavicular, or intercostal) but can be in the lower sternum in younger children and infants with compliant chest walls. Retractions result from differences between intrathoracic and atmospheric pressures in airway obstruction or from increased lung stiffness. Subcostal or lower costal retraction, either of acute onset or chronic, is usually associated with flattening of the diaphragm due to air trapping and pulmonary hyperinflation. When it contracts, the flattened diaphragm pulls on the chest wall at the site of its attachments, creating a groove.

Chest Wall Shape and Deformity

Observe whether the chest configuration is abnormal (Figs. 9–4 to 9–6); remember that infants' chests are rounder than those of older children because of the more horizontal position of the ribs. Chronic, diffuse, small airway obstruction with air trapping produces an abnormally rounded or "barrel-shaped" chest with a greater anteroposterior diameter (see Fig. 9–4). This finding is often associated with subcostal or lower costal indrawing. Note bony thoracic deformities, such as *pectus excavatum* (funnel chest) (see Fig. 9–5) or

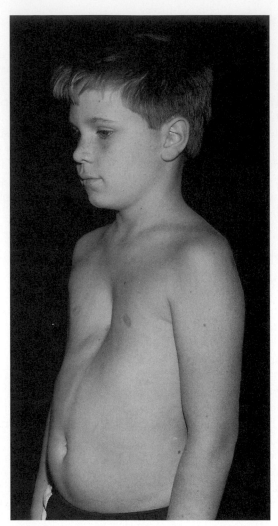

Figure 9–5 Pectus excavatum (funnel chest). For most children, this is a purely cosmetic problem.

pectus carinatum (pigeon breast) (see Fig. 9–6). As an isolated finding, pectus excavatum is seldom associated with any respiratory abnormalities. In some cases, pectus carinatum may be an isolated finding, but in other cases, it may signal a chronic cardiorespiratory problem. Occasionally, other chest wall deformities are found, either congenital or resulting from thoracic surgery.

Chest-Abdominal Movement

Carefully observe chest movement from the child's side to confirm that the two sides move equally. By observing a child's breathing with the youngster in both a standing and a supine position, you can easily see the relative contributions of chest and abdomen during respiration. Children have more abdominal movement during respiration than adults.

During sleep, further changes occur in the activity of respiratory muscles. During rapid eye movement (REM) sleep, there is intercostal muscle inhibition and, occa-

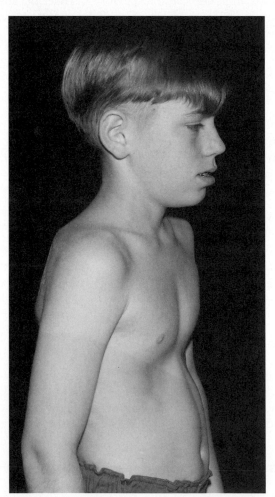

Figure 9–4 Increased anteroposterior diameter ("barrel chest") and lower costal retraction in a child with poorly controlled asthma.

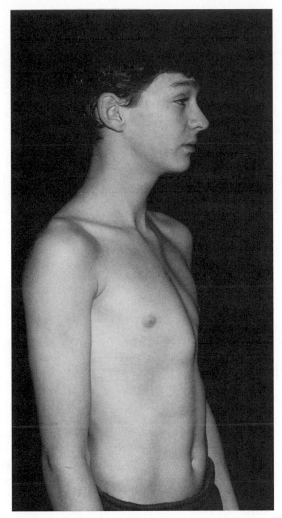

Figure 9–6 Pectus carinatum (pigeon-breast deformity) is usually not associated with cardiopulmonary disease.

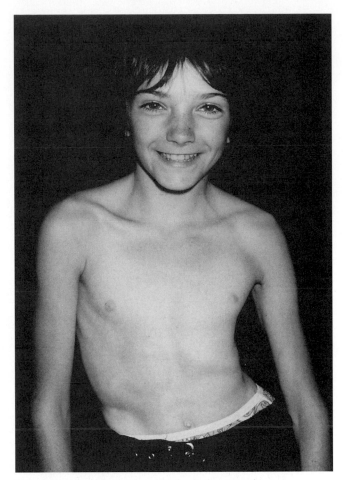

Figure 9–7 Distortion of thoracic shape due to scoliosis.

sionally, some paradoxical movement of the chest and abdomen, which is particularly noticeable in children with obstructive sleep apnea.

Kyphoscoliosis

Look at the spine's configuration. Marked scoliosis affects the shape of the thoracic cage and may impede pulmonary function (Fig. 9–7).

Respiratory Rate

An abnormally fast or slow respiratory rate may reflect a disturbance in the respiratory or cardiovascular system or in the central nervous system (CNS) control of breathing. Measure the respiratory rate by counting *for a full minute.* (See Table 9–1 for normal values at different ages.)

Depth of Respiration

Deep breathing (hyperpnea) and shallow breathing (hypopnea) are appreciated easily if pronounced but can be missed if subtle.

Ease of Respiration

Estimate the ease of respiration by observing whether the child appears short of breath (*dyspneic*), is distressed when lying supine (*orthopneic*), has retractions of soft tissue or sternum, has flaring of the alae nasi, or uses accessory muscles of respiration. Labored respiratory efforts reflect the increased work of the respiratory muscles and often are caused by airway obstruction.

Rhythm of Respiration

Although several abnormal respiratory rhythms can reflect CNS disturbances, note particularly the presence of sleep apnea, and distinguish between central and obstructive types (this distinction requires observation while the child is asleep). *Central apnea* occurs when there is no airflow and no apparent respiratory effort.

In *obstructive apnea*, airflow may be completely or partially reduced in association with vigorous inspiratory efforts and paradoxical movements of the rib cage and abdomen.

The duration of apnea considered to be abnormal varies with age. Apnea lasting up to 20 seconds is normal in premature infants, whereas shorter apneic periods may be significant in the older child. The diagnosis of obstructive sleep apnea syndrome should be considered in a child with partial or complete airway obstruction during sleep, which manifests as snoring and sleep disturbance, is associated with documented hypoxemia and hypercarbia, and results in failure to thrive, cor pulmonale, or neurobehavioral disturbance. Periodic breathing in infants, particularly premature babies, consists of two apneic periods of 3 seconds or more within 20 seconds of each other.

Finger Clubbing

Inspect the lateral aspect of the finger and the angle formed at the skin-nail junction on the dorsal surface of the terminal phalanx. Finger clubbing (Fig. 9–8) results from a proliferation of nail bed tissue that raises the nail's base. Gross clubbing is obvious, but subtle degrees of clubbing are easily missed. Clubbing is seen in children with cystic fibrosis, but it also can occur in other respiratory, cardiac, and gastrointestinal disorders.

Key Point

Always conduct a careful search for serious disease in the child with clubbing.

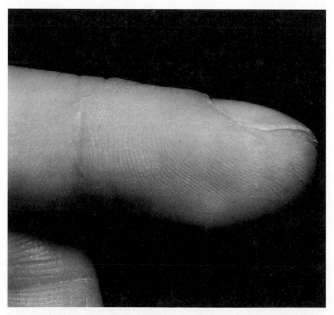

Figure 9–8 A mild but significant degree of finger clubbing. Inspection must be made from the lateral aspect of the fingers.

Cough

Familiarize yourself with the characteristics of different types of cough, and become adept at describing the cough. Characterizing the sound of a child's cough is a neglected aspect of the physical examination. If the child has not coughed during the examination, ask the child to do so. Gently pressing on the trachea in the suprasternal notch sometimes elicits a cough in a younger child.

Table 9–2 lists some common and some not so common respiratory illnesses and the kinds of cough associated with them.

Noisy Breathing

Pay careful attention to any sounds emitted by the child while he or she breathes. See Table 9–3 for a full description of these sounds.

Palpation

POSITION OF THE TRACHEA

Using two fingers when examining older children and one finger for younger children, you can accurately assess the position of the trachea in the suprasternal notch (Fig. 9–9). Tracheal shift indicates that the mediastinum has shifted, signifying either change in volume or pressure in one hemithorax. The mediastinum can be either pushed or pulled to one side, depending on the location and nature of the abnormality. Other aspects of the physical examination usually shed light on the underlying problem, so do not rush to order imaging studies when you detect tracheal shift.

CHEST EXPANSION

It is seldom necessary to estimate chest expansion in children by palpation because this parameter can usually be approximated visually.

VOCAL FREMITUS

Palpating for vocal fremitus over an area of consolidation is easier in adults, but it also can be done in older children.

PULSUS PARADOXUS

Pulsus paradoxus describes the fluctuation in systemic arterial pressure that occurs with normal respiration.

Table 9-2   ILLNESSES AND ASSOCIATED COUGHS

Illnesses	Cough	Comments
Bronchitis	Initially dry; after a few days, may become loose and rattling	Produces small amount of sputum that is usually swallowed. Occasionally, sputum is thick and yellow, but this finding does not always indicate secondary infection
Asthma	Classic cough is dry, "tight"; occasionally wheezy	Some children produce abundant secretions with wet cough. May be spasmodic, occur mainly at night, and be associated with vomiting. Throat clearing that parents believe to be a habit may be early manifestation of asthma. Wet asthma cough can mimic cystic fibrosis cough.
Croup (acute laryngotracheo-bronchitis)	Sounds like the "bark" of a seal	Sudden onset; child goes to bed well or with slight cold; often associated with an inspiratory stridor and hoarse voice
Pertussis	Spasmodic, choking, repetitive cough with no inspiration during coughing spasm	Associated eye tearing, profuse secretions, facial suffusion; spasm punctuated by sudden crowing inspiration (the "whoop") or vomiting
Pulmonary inhalation	May be dry or loose; often associated with lower airway obstructions	More commonly heard in children with swallowing incoordination or developmental delay. Can be similar to cough of asthma, bronchitis, or bronchiolitis
Chlamydia pneumoniae pneumonia	Typically paroxysmal, dry, and staccato (short inspiration between cough), unlike pertussis	Usually occurs in young infants
Tracheomalacia	Has loud characteristic brassy or vibratory sound, reflecting its tracheal origin	When associated with coarse inspiratory and expiratory stridor, or an inspiratory stridor and an expiratory wheeze, the cough virtually pinpoints the diagnosis
Psychogenic	Uncommon, but not rare, cough; sounds like the loud "honk" of a Canadian goose	Remarkably, this cough never occurs during sleep

Table 9-3   RESPIRATORY NOISES

Noise	Quality	Comments
Snoring	Inspiratory noise of irregular quality	Produced by partial obstruction of the upper respiratory tract, usually in the region of the naso-oropharynx
Stridor	Continuous, usually harsh inspiratory sound	Caused by extrathoracic airway obstruction; may be heard on expiration if obstruction is in the subglottic area or trachea, where the sound resembles a wheeze
Wheeze	Continuous sound with musical quality heard mainly during expiration; often a shorter sound on inspiration	Indicates intrathoracic airway obstruction; results from dynamic compression of large central airways from either peripheral or central airway obstruction
Grunting	Episodic, short expiratory sound	Caused by partial closure of glottis during expiration
Rattly breathing	Coarse, irregular sound heard mainly during inspiration; rattles can be felt through hands placed on the chest	Indicates secretions in trachea or major bronchi

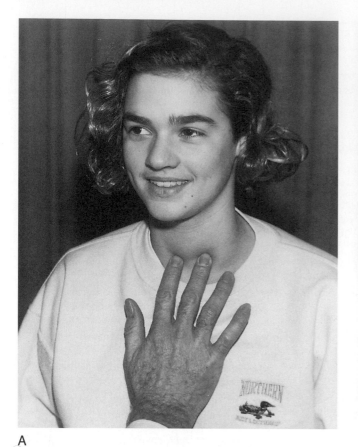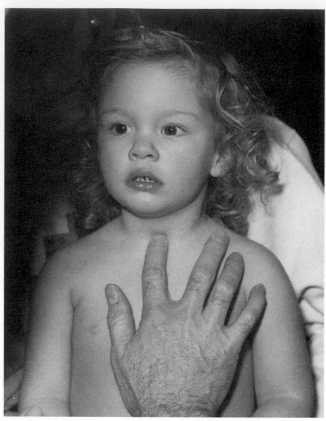

Figure 9–9 Palpating tracheal position. Use two fingers in older children (*A*), one in younger children.

Arterial pressure falls during inspiration and rises in expiration because of the effect of right ventricular preload and the greater force required by the left ventricle to maintain the previous arterial pressure (left ventricular afterload). Using a blood pressure cuff and stethoscope, note the difference in systolic blood pressure between the pressure at which the sporadic faint pulse sounds are first heard and the pressure at which all the sounds are first heard.

It is often difficult and usually unnecessary to try to correlate the pulse sounds with the phase of respiration, particularly in a tachypneic child. In most normal children, the pulsus paradoxus is less than 5 mm Hg. Severe airway obstruction, pericardial effusion, or constriction can cause pulsus paradoxus of greater than 20 mm Hg. Inspiratory retractions and use of accessory muscles are obvious when airway obstruction is this severe.

SUBCUTANEOUS EMPHYSEMA

The presence of subcutaneous air over the chest wall or up into the neck, felt as a crackling under the skin on palpation of the neck or chest, indicates an air leak and is usually associated with pneumomediastinum, which can be confirmed by chest radiograph. Pneumothorax may or may not be present but should be investigated because of its potential seriousness.

Percussion

In children, as in adults, use chest percussion to detect dull, flat, or hyperresonant areas and to locate the liver's position and size. An area of consolidation may sound dull to percussion; a pleural effusion, flat; and a hyperinflated area, hyperresonant. Asymmetric findings on percussion are more obvious because a normal hemithorax can be compared with the abnormal side. With time and experience, you will find that the normal percussion note in the child becomes more familiar and that you can more readily detect subtle changes. Useful percussion of the chest in infants and young children calls for much lighter percussion than is used in older children or adults. In younger individuals, as much or more can be learned from the "feel" of the percussion note as from its audible sound.

The chest radiograph has replaced percussion for precise location of the position and size of the heart, but percussion is still useful for detecting the upper and lower liver margins to determine whether a child has true hepatomegaly or whether the liver has simply been pushed downward by a hyperinflated lung.

Auscultation

Auscultation over each segment of both lungs is neither practical nor necessary in most circumstances. You should know the surface anatomy of the pulmonary lobes and listen over each one (Fig. 9–10).

Mostly, auscultation is performed with the stethoscope diaphragm because breath sounds tend to be higher pitched than heart sounds.

Always compare the two sides of the chest during auscultation, characterize the breath sounds, and then listen for adventitious sounds. Determine whether the breath sounds are normal, increased, or decreased in intensity, and describe their quality. Always note any asymmetric differences. The closer the stethoscope is to a larger airway, the more audible and tubular the note will be; these are differences that are best appreciated by listening during expiration. The bronchial breath

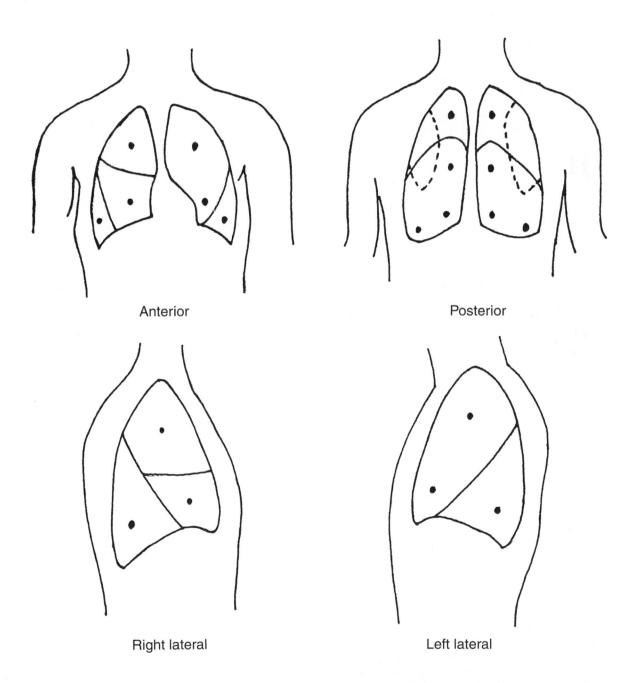

Anterior   Posterior

Right lateral   Left lateral

Figure 9–10 Surface anatomy of the pulmonary lobes and suggested auscultation sites (indicated by *solid circles*).

Table 9-4 BREATH SOUNDS

Sound	Quality	Comments
Tracheal	"Tubular," high-pitched	Heard during inspiration and expiration
Vesicular	Softer, lower-pitched	Heard in axillary area and lung bases; heard on inspiration and little heard on expiration
Bronchovesicular	Slightly higher pitched than vesicular breath sounds	Heard mainly on inspiration, but an early low-pitched note may be heard on expiration
Bronchial	Have a tubular quality that is less pronounced than in tracheal breath sounds	Heard on inspiration and expiration

sounds heard over an area of consolidation or atelectasis illustrate the improved transmission of sound through solid or airless tissue (Table 9–4). Note any adventitious or "extra" sounds, using the descriptions in Table 9–5.

Key Point

A child's vocalization can often be clearly heard when the stethoscope is placed over an area of consolidation or atelectasis.

Differentiating Extrathoracic from Intrathoracic Airway Obstruction

Localizing an obstruction site in the respiratory tract can be both challenging and rewarding in children (Fig. 9–11). You must remember that although the airway extends from the nose to the bronchioles, the anatomic site of an obstruction can be determined through the use of the following simple clinical guidelines:

1. Extrathoracic (i.e., upper respiratory tract) obstructions are associated with inspiratory stridor, and intrathoracic obstructions are associated with expiratory wheeze.
2. Stridor is mainly an inspiratory sound, whereas wheeze is an expiratory sound. Holding the bell end of the stethoscope about 1 inch (2.5 cm) from the child's mouth can help you distinguish between these sounds (Fig. 9–12).
3. Predominantly suprasternal and lower sternal retractions usually suggest extrathoracic obstruction.
4. Stridor and hoarseness indicate an obstruction in the larynx; when they are associated with a cough, the trachea is involved.
5. Stridor that worsens over weeks or months suggests a progressive airway obstruction.
6. Subcostal or lower costal retractions and an increased anteroposterior diameter of the chest reflect air trapping and a flattened diaphragm resulting from small airway obstruction.
7. A high-pitched monophonic wheeze that is heard mainly over one hemithorax usually indicates an obstruction in a single larger airway.

Table 9-5 ADVENTITIOUS SOUNDS IN THE CHEST

Sound	Description	Comments
Crackles/crepitations (formerly known as rales)	Short, crackling, nonmusical sounds heard on inspiration or expiration	Fine inspiratory crackles due to alveolar or bronchiolar disease, which has allowed collapse of the peripheral airway, leading to a crackle as it gradually opens and a thin film of fluid bursts. Coarser inspiratory or expiratory crackles may arise from air bubbling through mucus in larger airways, the auscultatory finding in a child with rattly breathing.
Wheezes	Continuous musical, usually expiratory sounds produced by air moving past obstruction or narrowing airway	Distinguishing between high-pitched (sibilant) and low-pitched (sonorous) wheezes is probably unnecessary because it may reflect differences only in flow rates. Wheezes arise from larger bronchi because air velocity in smaller airways is too slow to produce a musical sound
Friction rub	Harsh grating sound synchronous with respiration, indicating friction on movement between the two layers of pleura	Usually easily distinguished from a pericardial friction rub

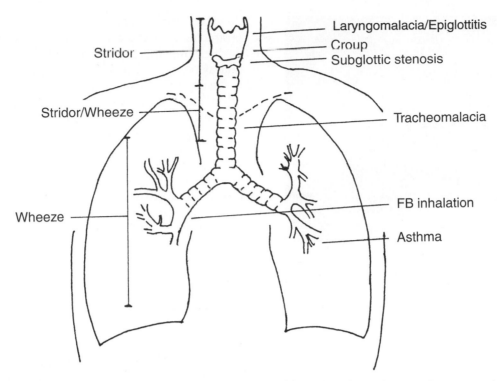

Figure 9–11 The common sites of upper (extrathoracic) airway obstruction and lower (intrathoracic) airway obstruction and examples of each.

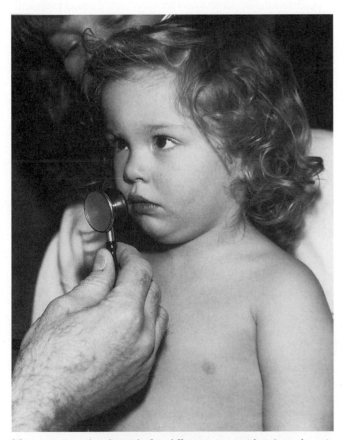

Figure 9–12 A handy trick for differentiating stridor (extrathoracic airway obstruction) from wheeze (intrathoracic obstruction). This maneuver should precede auscultation of the chest, because it helps differentiate abnormal bronchopulmonary noises from transmitted and amplified upper airway noise.

8. The symptoms must be identified as being either acute or chronic so that the diagnostic possibilities may be narrowed. Nocturnal onset of acute stridor with a barky cough and hoarse voice is most likely croup, whereas chronic stridor from early infancy in an otherwise healthy child usually indicates laryngomalacia and less often signifies congenital subglottic stenosis or some other anomaly in the region of the larynx or upper trachea.

TRACHEOMALACIA AND LARYNGOMALACIA

Tracheomalacia is a term used when a portion of the trachea is unusually soft (Fig. 9–13). Tracheomalacia usually occurs in children with esophageal atresia and tracheoesophageal fistula, but it also can arise secondary to a vascular compression, usually by an anomalous artery. Tracheomalacia can also occur without any associated abnormality. The soft area of the trachea is more collapsible and causes a rather coarse inspiratory stridor. A vibratory expiratory stridor, or occasionally a wheeze, is often heard in these patients. When the child coughs, the more easily collapsible soft area of the trachea generates a loud, brassy sound—best described as the "supermarket cough" because the parents remark that their child receives immediate attention from other shoppers when they hear the loud, harsh cough. Full evaluation, including fluoroscopy and

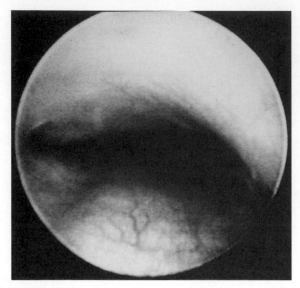

Figure 9–13 Bronchoscopic view of the trachea in a child with tracheomalacia.

bronchoscopy, is usually required to establish the exact nature of the disorder and to guide management. A loud vibratory cough without stridor or any other associated symptoms is occasionally heard in some older children and is of no clinical significance.

Tracheomalacia and laryngomalacia are sometimes confused, but the distinction can be made easily on clinical grounds. *Laryngomalacia* (infantile larynx, congenital laryngeal stridor) is the most common cause of chronic stridor in infancy. It is a supraglottic airway obstruction resulting from laxity of the soft tissue above the vocal cords (in the aryepiglottic folds), which fall inward on inspiration, partially obstructing the airway. Noisy stridor ("crowing") develops soon after birth, but by 12 to 18 months, the noise disappears. There is no associated cough, feeding difficulty, or failure to thrive.

Because laryngomalacia is an extrathoracic airway obstruction, the characteristic feature is a variable high-pitched crowing inspiratory stridor that many parents find alarming, at least initially. Typically, the loudness of the stridor varies with the baby's position: it worsens when he or she is supine and with upper respiratory infections and improves when he or she is prone. There may be some associated sternal retraction, but the infant is rarely distressed.

Direct examination of the larynx is required only in the presence of atypical features (Fig. 9–14). In most cases, the only treatment required for laryngomalacia is reassuring the parents about the condition's benign, self-limited nature. Because laryngomalacia and tracheomalacia are quite distinct in both origin and clinical presentation, the use of the term *laryngotracheomalacia* is inappropriate.

Key Point

Obstructions in the thoracic inlet can be difficult to sort out because they may manifest as stridor, wheeze, or both.

Case Histories

Although complete and detailed history and physical examination are recommended in most situations, you can sometimes make the diagnosis from a brief evaluation, avoiding intrusions that might be detrimental to the child.

Case 1

Six-year-old Bobby's parents have noticed his nasal stuffiness and difficulty breathing through the nose for almost a year. Nasal decongestants and several courses of antibiotics have not helped. There is

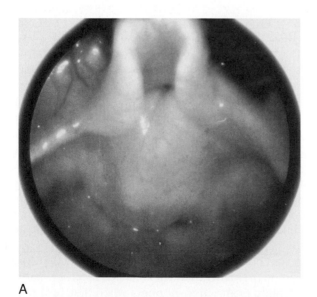

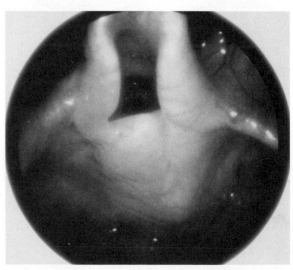

A   B

Figure 9–14 Endoscopic appearance of the laryngeal opening on inspiration *(A)* and expiration *(B)* in a child with laryngomalacia. On inspiration, the unusually soft structures collapse inward to partially obstruct the airway.

rarely any nasal discharge and no history of allergies. The parents are convinced that if Bobby could only learn to blow his nose properly, he would be well. Physical examination reveals an obese boy (both parents are obese) with a large nasal polyp in his right nostril. Subsequent investigations, including a sweat test, lead to a diagnosis of cystic fibrosis (CF). CF genetic mutation testing reveals that Bobby has a less common CF mutation associated with pancreatic sufficiency, explaining why he did not have the classic CF presentation.

Key Point

Because more than 1000 mutations cause cystic fibrosis, the clinical presentations can be variable, and the index of suspicion must be high. Children with nasal polyps should be investigated for CF.

Sometimes the parents' observations of physical signs are critical to the diagnosis. This issue is especially important in respiratory problems that occur during sleep.

Case 2

Four-year-old Jennifer's parents are worried about her noisy breathing during sleep. For the past year, Jennifer has been snoring at night, but her parents have also noticed that her snoring seems to stop suddenly at times, and they interpret this as a cessation of breathing. When they rush to awaken her, she seems fine. During the day, apart from being a mouth breather, she lacks specific respiratory symptoms. For the past 6 months, Jennifer has been sleeping in her parents' bed because they fear they will not get to her in time to arouse her. Jennifer's physical examination is entirely normal, except that she does have moderately enlarged tonsils and breathes through her mouth.

The key to the correct diagnosis is either to observe Jennifer during sleep or to ask the parents to do so after telling them what to look for (with the bedroom lights on).

Key Point

The important information to be sought is whether any movements of the chest or abdomen occur when the child appears to have stopped breathing.

Parents often equate "not breathing" with "not hearing any breath sounds." The child with obstructive sleep apnea may make few or no breath sounds during an obstructive episode, but her chest and abdomen usually move as she tries to inspire through a transiently obstructed upper airway. These obstructive episodes usually occur in a cyclical fashion, with each apneic

period culminating in an arousal associated with many snoring noises and, occasionally, body movements. By contrast, in apnea of central origin (seen mainly in small infants), respiratory movements cease. Understandably, obstructive sleep apnea creates anxiety in the family, which can be reduced considerably by appropriate discussion and explanation once the nature of the problem is established. The presence of an intercom between the parents' bedroom and the child's may be a marker of such anxiety. In a few instances, removing the tonsils and adenoids may be required to alleviate the problem.

It is important to remember that a child may have two respiratory diagnoses, a situation occasionally causing confusion.

Case 3

Nine-year-old William has had asthma for the past 7 years, which is usually controlled with a simple medication regimen. This autumn, his cough has been particularly difficult to control, and despite several courses of oral steroids and extra bronchodilators, he continues to have troublesome coughing and vomiting, especially at night. Further questioning reveals that William's cough is spasmodic in nature and is associated with facial suffusion and tearing. During the evaluation, when asked to cough, William demonstrates his "new" cough, leaving little doubt that he has whooping cough in addition to the asthma. In William's case, a more thorough respiratory history had a significant impact not only on his subsequent management but also on the explanations given to his parents.

SUMMARY

A thorough history and physical examination of the child's respiratory system is a rewarding diagnostic exercise. Allowing sufficient time for the history-taking not only enables you to narrow the diagnostic possibilities but also permits a better understanding of the child, the family, and their concerns. This process reveals the family's knowledge about the problem or disease and influences future management.

The physical examination should not be limited to the respiratory system or the chest, because important clues may be missed—finger clubbing, eczema, nasal polyps, or evidence of failure to thrive. Likewise, examination of the chest should never be limited to auscultation. The assessment of noisy breathing in the young child can be aided by an understanding of stridor and wheeze and their origins. It will then be obvious why the child with asthma does not present with stridor and the infant with laryngomalacia does not wheeze. When auscultating the chest, in addition to noting the presence of adventitious sounds, describe the breath sounds, their quality, and whether they are asymmetric. The physical examination of a child with a cough is not complete unless you have heard and characterized the cough. Remember that the physical examination of some children with a respiratory illness may reveal no abnormalities, making a detailed history crucial.

If you determine that further investigation is needed, performing a systematic and complete clinical assessment should allow you to be highly selective in your choice of tests.

SUGGESTED READINGS

Forgacs P: Lung Sounds. London, Bailliere Tindall, 1978. (A small but classic reference on lung sounds that explains the terminology.)

Phelan PD, Olinsky A, Robertson CF: Respiratory Illness in Children, 4th ed. Oxford, Blackwell Scientific Publications, 1994. (A practical, readable text on the common respiratory problems in children. Particularly useful for sorting out noisy breathing.)

chapter 10

Cardiovascular Assessment of Infants and Children

DOUGLAS L. ROY

Before the era of cardiac catheterization, echocardiography, nuclear studies, and computerization, few cardiac assessment aids were available to supplement the physician's eyes, hands, and ears. Today, some patients are examined by echocardiography even before a thorough bedside appraisal has been performed. Such misuse of modern technology can escalate medical costs in patients whose problems might be resolved easily at the bedside with a good clinical assessment. A systematic approach helps you develop the skills and confidence that will allow you to make correct decisions for most children without indiscriminate use of "high-tech" procedures.

CLASSIFICATION OF HEART DISEASE IN CHILDREN

Heart disease in children may be divided into the following categories:

Congenital: This category can be further divided into (1) structural cardiac changes present at birth (i.e., ventricular septal defect [VSD]) and (2) genetic tendencies, which lead to overt changes that develop after birth (i.e., cardiomyopathy).

Acquired: Almost any disease process that affects adults can occur in children. Processes such as neoplasia, cardiac infection, metabolic and endocrine abnormalities, and autoimmune disorders may occur in the child. Rheumatic fever, now uncommon in North America, is still prevalent in South America and occurs more commonly in children. Thus, in approaching the cardiovascular examination of the child, you should be aware not only of the variations of normal but also of the wide spectrum of diseases that may occur.

Because disease states may surface at different times during childhood, and because the cardiovascular system changes with age, physical examination of the cardiovascular system is described separately in this chapter for three age groups: the infant, the 3-year-old child, and the teenager.

EXAMINING THE INFANT AND YOUNG CHILD

The most common heart lesion in newborns and older infants is congenital heart disease. Less common conditions are persistent pulmonary hypertension, asphyxia, and symptomatic cardiac arrhythmia.

Of every 1000 live births, approximately 13 infants are born with a congenital cardiovascular anomaly. Congenital heart lesions may be divided naturally into the following three groups:

- Obstructive lesions cause pressure overload (aortic stenosis, coarctation of the aorta, and pulmonary stenosis).
- Left-to-right shunts cause volume overload (VSD, atrial septal defect [ASD], and patent ductus arteriosus).
- Cyanotic lesions produce central cyanosis (tetralogy of Fallot, transposition of the great arteries, and tricuspid atresia).

The three most common clinical presentations are (1) a murmur, (2) cyanosis, and (3) respiratory difficulty.

Always interpret clinical findings in terms of the underlying hemodynamic disturbance, as described in the following discussions of clinical manifestations.

Respiratory Distress

When a newborn or a young infant is in respiratory distress, do not assume that the underlying problem is primarily respiratory. A child whose problem is primarily cardiac may present with pulmonary infection.

For our purposes, two types of respiratory distress can be defined, (1) *tachypnea*, or abnormally rapid respirations, and (2) *dyspnea*, or difficult breathing.

Cyanotic heart lesions or lesions involving low cardiac output may be associated with a compensatory rapid respiratory rate, particularly on exertion, because of diminished peripheral oxygenation. When left ventricular failure results in a high end-diastolic pressure in the left ventricle and elevated pulmonary venous pressure, the early clinical manifestations, such as easy fatigue, result from low cardiac output. Increased pulmonary venous pressure causes greater stiffness of the pulmonary vessels and transudation of fluid into the interstitial tissue, making the lungs less compliant. The child works harder to breathe. Wet, stiff lungs are very susceptible to secondary infection; respirations become rapid, the accessory muscles come into use, and *subcostal indrawing* is observed.

Fatigue, Excessive Perspiration, and Poor Weight Gain

In young infants, metabolic demands are usually greatest during feedings. The infant with poor peripheral oxygenation due to low cardiac output therefore tires easily during feeding, the equivalent of exercise in older children. Because of fatigue, the infant is unable to take a full feeding. In addition, rapid respiration diminishes the time available for swallowing. This combination of factors results in failure to gain weight. In the baby with a large left-to-right shunt, the process is exaggerated by the higher caloric needs of an overworked myocardium. Increased sympathetic activity causes excessive perspiration—often a valuable diagnostic feature.

Key Point

When a young baby tires rapidly, sweats during feedings, and has subcostal indrawing, always think of the possibility of congestive heart failure.

Squatting

Parents of children with certain cyanotic heart defects, especially tetralogy of Fallot, may offer the observation that when their youngster tires, he or she assumes a squatting position. Squatting helps increase systemic oxygen saturation by decreasing the amount of right-to-left shunting.

Central Cyanosis

Central cyanosis is caused by increased deoxyhemoglobin content (>5 g/dL), reducing oxygen available for delivery to the tissues. By various compensatory mechanisms, the fetus lives happily in utero, despite a low oxygen saturation (65%). Even when a congenital anomaly such as transposition of the great arteries is present, birth weight is usually normal.

Hypoxic Spells

Hypoxic spells typically occur in children with cyanotic congenital heart disease that involves stenosis of the infundibulum of the right ventricular outflow tract and a VSD, classically known as tetralogy of Fallot. A typical spell is characterized by a sudden increase in intensity of the cyanosis, at times in association with loss of consciousness. This clinical phenomenon is caused by infundibular muscle tissue contraction, which further restricts right ventricular outflow and increases right-to-left shunting.

Key Point

Not all instances of central cyanosis are attributable to the heart; it may also be seen in certain types of pulmonary disease, when abnormal hemoglobin is present at birth, or with acute methemoglobinemia at any age.

Angina

Angina is rare but not unknown in infants and children; it can occur in severe aortic stenosis, or possibly in pulmonary stenosis, because of associated myocardial ischemia. Angina also may occur with very rapid paroxysmal tachycardias and has been recognized in infants with an aberrant left coronary artery.

Peripheral Edema

Infants and young children differ strikingly from adults in the development of peripheral edema in congestive heart failure. Pretibial and presacral edema are *late* developments in a child with congestive circulatory failure, apparently because of a difference in tissue turgor. When peripheral edema due to heart failure does develop in an infant, it first appears periorbitally and is usually preceded by other manifestations, such as tachypnea, tachycardia, dyspnea, and liver enlargement.

Orthopnea

Unlike with adults, orthopnea is not obvious in the infant with heart failure, even when tachypnea, dyspnea, hepatomegaly, and the radiographic findings of pulmonary edema are present. In the adult, orthopnea is a symptom; in the infant, it is a sign.

Age of Onset

SIGNIFICANCE OF THE AGE OF ONSET OF CONGESTIVE HEART FAILURE

The clinical significance of the age of onset of congestive heart failure is as follows:

1. If a child becomes symptomatic because of congenital heart disease, there is a 95% probability that the symptoms will develop before the age of 3 months and usually before 2 months.
2. Heart failure is rarely present at birth, because the fetal circulation is in parallel and there are communications between the two sides; when there is obstruction on one side, blood flows easily to the other. Because the fetal lungs are collapsed, increased pulmonary blood flow does not occur in utero.
3. Heart failure that develops during the first week of life, especially in the first 3 days, is usually due to an obstructive lesion or to persistent pulmonary hypertension.
4. Heart failure that develops 4 to 6 weeks after birth is invariably due to left-to-right shunting through a defect (volume overload). Pulmonary resistance is high at birth, and although a communication may exist between the two circulations, little left-to-right shunting occurs. Pulmonary resistance usually reaches its nadir by 4 weeks of age, allowing left-to-right shunting to reach a maximum.

Key Point

When an infant presents at age 6 weeks with respiratory distress, it may not be pneumonia.

5. If heart failure develops after age 3 months, look for causes other than anomalies, such as myocarditis, cardiomyopathy, and paroxysmal tachycardia.

SIGNIFICANCE OF AGE OF ONSET OF CYANOSIS

Central cyanosis due to congenital heart disease may be present at birth or may appear first when the ductus arteriosus closes off, usually by 5 days after birth. In tetralogy of Fallot, it may develop later (2 months older) when the infundibular stenosis becomes more

severe, increasing the volume of right-to-left shunting. Because the murmur of infundibular pulmonary stenosis greatly resembles that of a VSD, the newborn infant presenting with what appears to be VSD just could have tetralogy of Fallot.

OBTAINING THE HISTORY

Incidence and Family History

In a study in the Maritime Provinces of Canada, a region where the level of patient care was considered high (i.e., an area with a medical school and readily available specialist consultation), the incidence of congenital heart lesions was found to be 12.2 per 1000 live births.[1]

Consanguinity is a significant causative factor in congenital heart disease, but the tendency varies between families and with the type of heart lesion. Reports exist of as many as three children of the same parents being affected with ventricular septal defect, patent ductus arteriosus, and aortic stenosis. These are exceptions, however, as the tendency for a congenital heart lesion to occur when one parent has a congenital heart lesion (usually the same lesion) is only slightly increased (2% to 3%). The genetic tendency for a congenital heart lesion also exists in siblings. The author has observed an instance in which brothers with normal hearts each had a child with tricuspid atresia. In certain syndromes or hereditary disorders, however, the genetic tendency for recurrence is high. In Marfan syndrome, the disease is inherited as an autosomal dominant gene.

In summary, a search for evidence of congenital heart disease in the family is important. However, when there is a history of congenital heart disease in one parent, or in a previous child, counseling is best done by a geneticist.

Prenatal History

Because the cause of congenital heart disease is multifactorial, known contributory factors should be sought in the prenatal history, including (1) exposure to drugs (lithium, hydantoin, thalidomide), (2) excessive alcohol intake, (3) possible rubella in the first trimester (check the mother's rubella immunization status), (4) maternal diabetes (which bestows a higher risk of congenital heart malformations), and (5) exposure to radiation. In most instances, however, no specific contributory factors can be identified.

History of Delivery

An important but infrequent cardiovascular problem in newborns is persistent pulmonary hypertension, which may cause central cyanosis, myocardial dysfunction, or both. This condition is often preceded by a difficult delivery and meconium aspiration. It is unlikely to occur after an uncomplicated delivery. Clinical differentiation of pulmonary hypertension from congenital heart disease may be difficult and usually requires cardiac ultrasonography. It is important to elicit a history of prematurity, because patency of the ductus arteriosus is common in premature infants.

APPROACH TO PHYSICAL EXAMINATION OF THE INFANT

Because infants and children have an unfortunate habit of not always cooperating ideally, you need to organize a thorough agenda for the cardiovascular examination but also to stay flexible. Do what can be done when the opportunity arises. Begin by assessing the child's physical development and looking for dysmorphic features, using a systematic approach (see Chapter 5).

Five percent of congenital heart lesions are associated with a chromosomal disorder, and many nonchromosomal dysmorphic syndromes have an associated cardiac lesion. A child with a cleft palate, for example, has a 20% possibility of having a congenital heart lesion.

The infant is usually most comfortable on the parent's lap during the examination. Do not undress the baby right away. The baby usually allows you to examine the palmar creases and to check the nail beds and muscle tone without much protest. After this, feel the brachial pulses for rate, rhythm, and volume, the last being the most important. Feel this pulse in every baby you examine to learn the difference between normal and abnormal. An abnormally full pulse suggests patent ductus arteriosus or aortic insufficiency; a shallow slow rising pulse suggests left ventricular outflow tract obstruction. Do not feel for the femoral pulses yet.

Because the most pressing clinical problems are congestive circulatory failure and cyanosis, decide early in the examination whether central cyanosis is present. Because this determination is not always easy, you may find an experienced nurse's opinion invaluable. Many normal newborns have a deep plethoric appearance as a result of transiently high hemoglobin concentrations, particularly if the obstetrician was slow in clamping the umbilical cord. Plethora is not as obvious in the mucous membranes, so look carefully in the baby's mouth. Deep pressure on the skin may help, because the blanched area does not "pink up" as quickly in central cyanosis. Many normal infants exhibit a generalized mottling, particularly after being bathed (see Fig. 4–2); this is called *cutis marmorata* (literally, "marbled skin"). Observe the effect of crying. Invariably, central cyanosis due to cardiac disease

increases during crying, but do not make the baby cry until after you have listened to the heart.

It is important to be certain of the presence of cyanosis; this determination may require a second examination. When you are examining a child in the hospital, measuring the blood oxygen saturation will help greatly, as may observing the effect of breathing 100% oxygen. Finally, remember that cyanosis can occur in only one part of the body; the lower body may show cyanosis while the upper part remains pink. This condition can occur with an aortic preductal coarctation or persistent pulmonary hypertension when there is associated right-to-left shunting through a patent ductus arteriosus.

Clinical Manifestations of Heart Failure

When low cardiac output and high pulmonary venous pressure cause sufficient hemodynamic disturbance to produce clinical manifestations, cardiac enlargement is invariably present. Whether the disturbance involves primarily the left or the right ventricle, the left side of the thorax is prominent anteriorly (Fig. 10–1). This prominence may not be evident in the first month of life, but it certainly will be by 3 months. When respiratory distress due to heart failure has been present for 2 months or longer, the greater diaphragmatic contractions during respiration may produce a sulcus in the

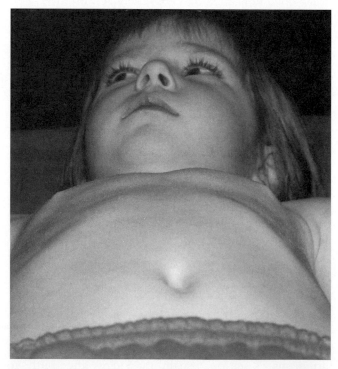

Figure 10–1 Prominence of the left side of the chest in a 3-year-old with ventricular septal defect and moderate left-to-right shunt that is causing enlargement of both left and right ventricles.

lower thorax, with outward flaring of the inferior rib cage edge. Therefore, look for a sulcus, left-sided chest prominence, abnormal movement, increased respiratory rate, and subcostal indrawing.

Key Point

Remember that young infants normally have abdominal breathing, so you must be certain that you are not simply observing normal chest-abdominal movement. Also, be sure that the indrawing is not restricted to the midline, as occurs in pectus excavatum. True subcostal indrawing is abnormal, usually signifying stiffness of the lungs from either cardiac or pulmonary causes. In contrast to adults, examination of the jugular venous pulse is useless in young children.

Palpation

Now lay your prewarmed hand very gently on the chest, remembering that the heart may not be in its normal position. With the tips of the first and second fingers of your right hand, depress the thorax just left of the xiphoid process (Fig. 10–2). Your fingertips are now lying on the right ventricle. A faint impulse is allowable, but if the heart is enlarged, a definite forceful movement will be present. Perform this maneuver repeatedly in normal infants, and you will soon be able to tell the difference between normal and abnormal. This distinction will help you make a quick decision about whether the 6-week-old baby who presents with respiratory distress has a cardiac or a respiratory problem.

Key Point

Except in the rare instance in which the baby has a dilated cardiomyopathy, if the respiratory distress is due to heart failure, a prominent pulsation is evident. It is that simple.

Now depress the thorax in the apical area. Prominence of the apical impulse is diagnostically less helpful in infants, except in rare instances such as in tricuspid atresia, in which the right ventricle is hypoplastic. Then palpate in the second interspace at the left sternal border, where a prominent pulmonary artery pulsation may be elicited. Finally, place one index finger carefully in the suprasternal notch (Fig. 10–3), searching first for an abnormal pulsation and then for a thrill. Then work in the opposite direction, searching for thrills and palpable sounds. At this point, you should have made a reasonable appraisal of cardiac dynamics.

Key Point

If you cannot palpate increased heart action and the pulses are of normal volume, the child does not have a serious hemodynamic disturbance.

Liver Size and Position

Whether you are right- or left-handed, stand or sit on the baby's right side to palpate for the liver. Use the tip of your right thumb, and begin well down in the right

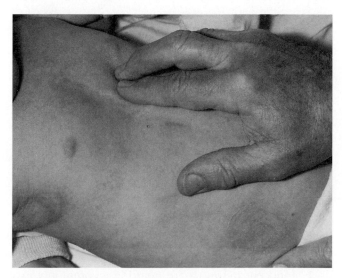

Figure 10–2 Press on the precordium to the left of the xiphoid process with first and second digits of your right hand to detect enlargement of the right ventricle.

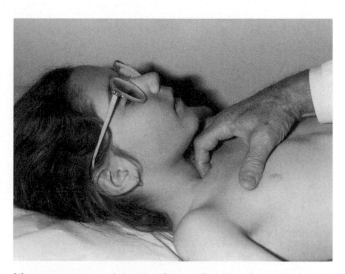

Figure 10–3 Insert the index finger of your right hand deep in the suprasternal notch, searching first for pulsation and then for a thrill.

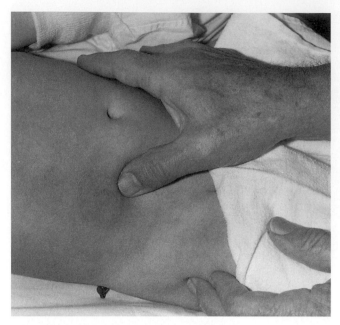

Figure 10–4 Palpate the liver with movement of the tip of the thumb inward and cephalad, begining low in the right lower quadrant of the abdomen.

lower quadrant of the abdomen, pressing inward and upward (Fig. 10–4). If the baby has just been fed, do not press very deeply. If the liver edge is soft, its margin may be difficult to detect; nevertheless, if the liver is enlarged, you should appreciate a sense of resistance as your thumb tip moves superiorly. If the edge is indefinite, use soft percussion, tapping the second digit of your left hand with the second digit of your right hand, beginning low in the right lower quadrant and placing the second digit of your left hand parallel to the liver edge (Fig. 10–5). You should be able to sense the

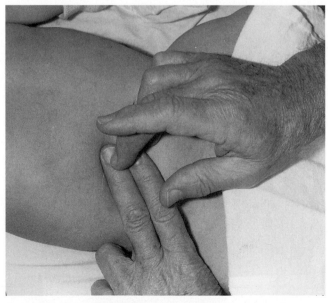

Figure 10–5 Percuss for the liver edge, using soft percussion with the second digit of your right hand on the second digit of your left hand, which has been positioned parallel to the liver edge.

change in percussion note signifying the liver edge. Except in the presence of pulmonary hyperinflation, the liver edge normally should not be more than 1 to 2 cm below the costal margin.

> **Key Point**
>
> If there is heart failure, there will be liver enlargement; therefore, if you find the heart action to be increased and the liver enlarged to palpation, you can be sure that the baby has a serious cardiac problem, even before you have applied the stethoscope.

Finally, remember that the liver can be ectopic (on the left side or up in the thorax).

Auscultation

You need all the acoustic help you can get during cardiac auscultation, so be sure to turn off radios and televisions, close the door, and get everything and everyone as quiet as possible. Cardiac auscultation is not easy, even in older cooperative patients, but coping with a restless baby with rapid cardiac and respiratory rates in a noisy nursery is a real trial. Giving the child a bottle or pacifier may help. Nursery stethoscopes are frequently of poor quality, so use a good one.

Remember that the two main determinants of auscultatory proficiency are (1) the fit of the earpieces and (2) the quality of the gray matter between them. Recognition of normal splitting of the second heart sound is often impossible when the heart rate is rapid. You should, however, be able to assess the *intensity* of the second sound. Its intensity increases in the presence of pulmonary hypertension or when the aorta is anteriorly placed, as in transposition of the great vessels. Occasionally, an ejection sound can be appreciated, which is an abnormal finding. Listen over the back for the murmur of coarctation and to both sides of the skull for the bruit of an intracranial arteriovenous malformation.

> **Key Point**
>
> Breath sounds often interfere with the interpretation of heart sounds; however, most babies will cease breathing for a few seconds after you administer a surreptitious puff in the face.

The following list contains a few dogmatic but valuable generalizations concerning auscultatory findings in young infants:

1. Innocent murmurs are heard less commonly in neonates, so if you hear a murmur, take it seriously, particularly if it is not musical.

2. If you note a loud coarse systolic murmur in the first 3 days of life, the baby has some type of obstruction.

3. The murmur of a VSD is often not present in the first week of life.

4. Frequently, the murmur of the patent ductus arteriosus is not continuous in the first week of life and may be loudest at the left sternal border in the third and fourth interspaces—not its point of maximal intensity in later life.

5. Occasionally, a long, high-pitched, blowing, "organic-sounding," systolic murmur is encountered, heard maximally in the axillae. Common in prematures, it also can be heard in full-term babies with an increased stroke volume. This murmur arises in the peripheral pulmonary arteries and is usually innocent. If such a murmur persists in an infant older than 2 months, consult a cardiologist.

6. A murmur that has the same characteristics as described in No. 5 but is heard only in the left axilla and in the back could well be due to aortic coarctation.

Case History

An account of my experience with an actual patient may help you appreciate the importance of these manifestations:

While attending a clinic in another hospital, I was asked to see an 8-week-old infant. The working diagnosis was pneumonia, and the baby had a history of failure to gain weight. I was alone during the examination. The infant had obvious Down syndrome. I reminded myself that 70% of patients with Down syndrome have a congenital heart condition.

The baby was in obvious respiratory distress with subcostal indrawing, which could have been due to either pneumonia or heart failure. The left side of the precordium was prominent but not beyond normal limits. I placed my prewarmed hand on the left side of the precordium and detected a *marked* increase in the heart action—unquestionably abnormal. Palpation of the liver detected resistance down into the pelvis, but on close examination, I could palpate the edge, deep in the pelvis.

"How could anyone miss this?" I asked myself. On auscultation, however, I detected no murmurs!

This situation, of course, can happen when pressures and resistances in the right side of the heart are increased, as in heart failure, so that velocity of left-to-right shunting, one of the causes of murmurs, is decreased. The absence of heart murmurs possibly accounted for the missed diagnosis of congestive heart failure.

The diagnosis of cardiac disease was made through palpation of the precordium and was confirmed by the finding of gross hepatomegaly, which was so marked that it had been missed by previous examiners.

This case is a prime example of the importance of simple bedside procedures.

Palpating the Pulses

Palpation of the pulses calls for gentleness, persistence, and patience, so make yourself comfortable before you begin. First, palpate for femoral pulsations. Remove the diaper. Many babies do not appreciate having their groins manipulated and may cry, urinate, or both. Femoral pulses are particularly difficult to appreciate in obese babies; do not rush into a diagnosis of coarctation of the aorta if you have difficulty feeling them. If the femoral pulses are not palpable in an asthenic baby, there is cause for concern (see Fig. 4–20). Now palpate both brachial pulses. If you can detect good brachial pulses and you are certain that the femoral pulses are absent or greatly depressed, listen to the heart before measuring the blood pressure and upsetting the baby. Listen particularly for a high-pitched blowing systolic murmur, best heard anteriorly below the left clavicle and well heard in the left axilla and back, medial to the scapula.

Key Point

Check also for wide splitting of the first heart sound at the apex; the second component of the split sound probably indicates the presence of a bicuspid aortic valve, which accompanies aortic coarctation in 75% of cases.

Blood Pressure

Although it is difficult to accomplish, an attempt must be made to measure the systemic blood pressure. The normal systolic blood pressure of an infant is between 60 and 80 mm Hg in both the arm and the leg (Table 10–1). The four methods of measuring blood pressure are (1) auscultatory, (2) palpatory, (3) visual (flush), and (4) Doppler.

All methods require the use of an inflatable cuff. The first decision is to choose the size of the cuff, the size being of great importance because the pressure measured involves occlusion of the arterial pulse—the brachial arterial pulse when the arm is used. If the cuff used is too small, greater pressure must be used to obliterate the pulse, and the blood pressure measured

Table 10-1 NORMAL VALUES OF PULSE AND BLOOD PRESSURE IN FIRST YEAR OF LIFE

	Pulse Rate (beats/min)			Blood Pressure (mm Hg)	
Age Group	Lower Limits of Normal	Average	Upper Limits of Normal	Systolic	Diastolic
Premature	80	120	170	60 (50–75)	35 (30–45)
Neonate	80	120	170	75 (60–90)	45 (40–60)
1–12 mo	90	120	180	90 (75–100)	60 (50–70)

From Moller JH, Neal WA: Heart Disease in Infancy. New York, Appleton-Century-Crofts, 1981.

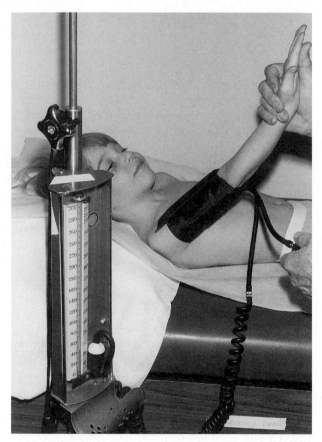

Figure 10–6 Supinate the patient's hand and elevate the arm before expanding the sphygmomanometer cuff. This maneuver positions the radial artery properly and eliminates the auscultatory gap.

will be artifactually high. Use a cuff that covers almost the full extent of the upper arm, with the elbow bent. Always have a full selection of cuff sizes available.

For all methods, first supinate the child's arm to make the radial artery easily accessible. Apply the cuff, elevate the arm, and *then* inflate the cuff. Prior elevation of the arm (or opening and closing the hand) prevents the *auscultatory gap* phenomenon (Fig. 10–6). If this procedure is not followed, when you inflate the cuff and listen for Korotkoff sounds, as you decrease the pressure in the cuff, you may hear a

sound appear, then disappear, and reappear as the pressure is further decreased. This phenomenon, the auscultatory gap, is due to increased vascular resistance distal to the cuff.

The conventional method is the auscultatory method. The edge of the diaphragm of the warm stethoscope is placed under the inferior edge of the cuff and the cuff is inflated. Listen for the Korotkoff sounds as the cuff pressure is decreased, watching the mercury level (or the needle in an aneroid sphygmomanometer) as you listen. The first sound heard denotes the systolic level. As the cuff pressure is decreased further, an abrupt change in the intensity of the sound may be heard. If this change is detected, it is recorded as the diastolic level. Continue decreasing the cuff pressure, recording the disappearance of Korotkoff sounds, which is recorded as the diastolic level if no intensity change has been detected. Usually two or three recordings are made, elevating the arm before each attempt.

It may be impossible to measure the blood pressure by the auscultatory method—usually when a baby does not cooperate. The palpatory method is then attempted. Prior elevation of the arm is not required. The radial artery pulse is palpated and the cuff elevated until the pulse disappears. The cuff pressure is then decreased, and the level of systolic pressure is estimated by the time of the reappearance of the pulse. Only the systolic pressure can be measured by this method.

The flush method also measures systolic pressure only and unfortunately requires two persons. Using both hands on the child's upraised arm, express all the blood from the arm and have the second person inflate the cuff. One person watches the arm, the other the sphygmomanometer. As the cuff pressure is decreased, the person watching the arm indicates verbally the moment at which the flush occurs while the other person records the manometer level.

Blood pressure measurement with Doppler equipment is much easier, as no auscultation is required. Unfortunately, the equipment is not always available, and the choice of cuffs is frequently limited.

One way or another, a reliable blood pressure measurement *must* be obtained. If you suspect an aortic coarctation (high arm pressure, absence of femoral pulses, murmur), repeat the procedure in the thigh, using a blood pressure cuff of appropriately larger size. In my experience, so-called radial-femoral pulse delay is a useless sign in infants with a rapid heart rate. It is easy to say that such a delay is present when one knows in advance that the diagnosis is aortic coarctation. It is better to rely on comparison of pulse volumes and blood pressure measurements.

After listening to the infant's back and finishing the general examination, you may have to make the baby cry, so advise the parents of your intention. Gently flicking the bottom of the foot usually does the trick, but at times a surreptitious pinch or two of the big toe (the "dermal compression test") is required. While the baby cries, look for central cyanosis. Remember that central cyanosis occurs in any baby with prolonged breath-holding. If there is purplish discoloration of the mucous membranes inside the mouth while the baby cries vigorously, the infant probably has a serious problem. Discoloration of the buccal mucous membranes may be the one and only clinical finding in transposition of the great arteries, a potentially lethal disorder if not diagnosed early. If you have any doubts about this diagnosis, consult a cardiologist as soon as possible.

EXAMINING THE 3- TO 5-YEAR-OLD CHILD

By the time a child is 3 to 5 years old, lesions causing cyanosis or congestive heart failure will be revealed. The spectrum of disease in toddlers and young children includes congenital lesions that have been overlooked, such as ASD, small VSD, bicuspid aortic valve, and acquired cardiac disorders—pericarditis, myocarditis, cardiac manifestations of hereditary muscular and neuromuscular diseases, rhythm disturbances, and other rare disorders. By far the most common problem clinicians face is the interpretation of heart sounds and murmurs, especially the systolic murmur.

Heart Sounds and Murmurs

HEART SOUNDS

The heart sounds are conveniently numbered S_1 through S_4. S_1 and S_2 are sounds of valve closure, the first caused by mitral and tricuspid closure, the second by aortic and pulmonary valve closure. Each heart valve makes a sound on both closing and opening. *The sound that occurs with opening is not heard in health.* When there are four valves and systole and diastole, the

concept is confusing. You must remember that in health, blood does not move during the period when pressure is building (mitral and tricuspid) or falling (aortic and pulmonary). These are the periods of isometric contraction and relaxation. In the systolic events of left ventricle contraction, mitral regurgitation begins immediately with closure of the mitral valve as left ventricular pressure immediately exceeds left atrial pressure. Regurgitation begins immediately (with S_1), and an early systolic regurgitant murmur is heard. Meanwhile, as pressure builds in the left ventricle, the aortic valve opens, ejection begins to occur, and the ejection murmur takes place, beginning a short period after S_1, and a midsystolic ejection murmur evolves. Therefore, the regurgitant murmur begins *with* the preceding sound, but the murmur of obstruction or excessive flow begins *after* the preceding sound. If you can comprehend this process, you are well on the way to understanding cardiac auscultation.

Memorize these two facts:

1. The left-sided valves close before the right-sided valves.
2. Left-sided valve closures are much louder. The right-sided valve can be heard closing only when the stethoscope is positioned directly over it on the chest.

The mechanism of production of the S_3 and S_4 is in question. They probably are due to the deceleration of blood at the end of early (third) and late (fourth) rapid filling phases of the ventricles. Although the exact mechanism of the third and fourth heart sounds is poorly understood, S_3 is usually related to high flows and S_4 reflects a poorly compliant ventricle. Third sounds are normal in children with hyperdynamic circulations and thin chest walls but are usually abnormal in patients older than 30 years, when the ravages of age have lowered stroke volume and increased body mass. Audible fourth sounds are always abnormal. S_3 and S_4 occur in the ventricles and are low-pitched. They are heard loudest over the ventricle in which they occur, and are best heard with the bell of the stethoscope.

Use of the terms *clicks* and *snaps* is a continual source of confusion. Valve opening is quiet in health and signals the end of the period of isovolemic contraction, or relaxation.

> **Key Point**
>
> When a sound is heard at the time of the opening of any heart valve, there is a problem.

A sound heard at the time of opening of the pulmonary or aortic valve is called an *ejection click*; when mitral or tricuspid opening is heard, the term *opening snap* is used. The *clicks* signal the beginning of ejection

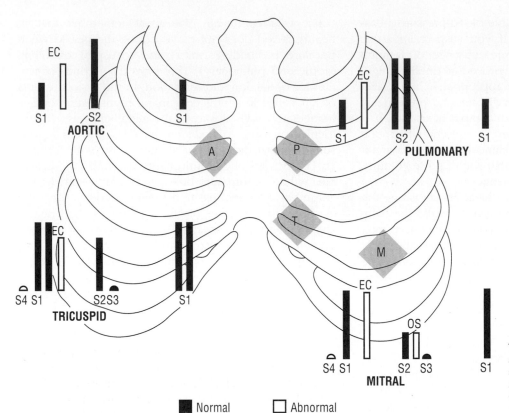

Normal   Abnormal

Figure 10–7 Normal and abnormal sounds in the four conventional auscultation areas: A, aortic; P, pulmonary; T, tricuspid; M, mitral. EC, ejection click; OS, opening snap.

into a dilated great vessel; the *snaps* signal the commencement of diastolic flow into the ventricle. Both are always high-pitched and are loudest over their respective valves, except the aortic click, which is usually well heard at the apex. The pulmonary ejection click is unique, in that it is loudest during expiration. The only hope of identifying these sounds is a thorough working knowledge of normal and of what to expect to hear in a normal infant or child when you place a stethoscope on a particular area of the chest. The normal and abnormal sounds for each listening area are shown in Figure 10–7.

Key Point

It is essential to follow a constant, systematic procedure for listening to heart sounds and murmurs in all children. *Never* auscultate the heart through clothing. The examination is difficult enough without such interference.

First, listen exclusively to the individual heart sounds (understanding in advance what is normal). Then listen, equally systematically, to the murmurs. Here is a brief summary of normal sounds as heard with the child supine:

At the apex, you should hear a single first, a single second, and possibly a third sound. The first and second sounds are high-pitched, and the first is usually louder. The third sound is heard best with the bell of the stethoscope.

At the tricuspid area, the first sound may be closely split, and the second sound is single. You may hear a third heart sound.

In the pulmonary area, the first sound is usually single. The second sound is split in inspiration and may be closely split or single in expiration.

At the aortic area, both the first and second sounds are single, and aortic closure is usually louder.

If sounds other than these are heard, the child may well have a cardiac problem. Remember that these are the findings with the patient supine. The intensity of the first heart sound varies with atrioventricular (AV) conduction time (the interval between the onset of P wave and R wave [PR interval]). When the PR interval is prolonged, the valve leaflets may have almost closed when the ventricle contracts. Accordingly, the first sound is faint or absent; this pattern can occur in normal individuals who have a long PR interval. Usually, if the patient stands up, the PR interval shortens, and the first sound increases to fairly normal intensity. There are occasions in which there is beat-to-beat variation in intensity of the first sound. This variation occurs in AV dissociation, as in complete heart block, in which there is beat-to-beat variation in the PR interval, a useful sign in differentiating complete AV block from sinus bradycardia.

Gallop Rhythm

Gallop rhythm is a misleading term, because "gallop" generally is thought to signify a problem, which it does not. It is better to speak of a *triple rhythm* and of the sound that causes the tripling. There are several types of tripling, only some of which signify a problem. If the triple rhythm is rapid, there is a gallop cadence, which should still be described as tripling. A first sound, second sound, and prominent third sound would constitute tripling, as would a fourth sound, first sound, and second sound, or a first sound, ejection click, and second sound. The type of tripling commonly called "gallop rhythm" occurs when the third and fourth heart sounds "sum" in the presence of tachycardia, which may or may not be pathologic. In infants with a physiologically long PR interval and tachycardia, summation tripling can be normal; presence of a pathologic third sound or fourth sound and tachycardia, however, would be abnormal. Because tripling can be normal or abnormal, you must try to identify the sound that causes the tripling.

Midsystolic Click

The sound that does not fit any of the preceding descriptions and is usually best heard in the midcardiac area is the sound of mitral valve prolapse—the midsystolic click. Usually heard in midsystole, this sound may be a single click or a series of clicks. It is caused by prolapse of the mitral valve or portions of it into the left atrium. Frequently associated with a deficiency of tone in connective tissue, these midsystolic clicks occur most often in tall asthenic individuals, more commonly females. It is best heard with the patient standing and leaning forward. A midsystolic click can also cause a triple rhythm; until you have heard such a click two or three times, it may be confusing. Variation in intensity from moment to moment is also characteristic.

MURMURS

Heart murmurs are caused either by turbulence in blood or by tissue vibration. Conventionally, they are classified according to their timing as *systolic* (occurring between the first and second sounds), *diastolic* (between the second sound and the first sound), or *continuous* (present continuously throughout the cardiac cycle). The last term also includes the murmur that begins in systole, passes through the second sound, and ends in diastole.

Systolic Murmurs

Systolic murmurs also are classified according to their dynamic mechanism, of which there are four types:

1. Regurgitation (backward flow of blood).
2. Obstruction to forward flow.
3. Vibration of tissue, which occurs in the normal heart when forceful contraction causes the tissue to vibrate and in an abnormal heart when a

substance such as calcium is present and is made to vibrate even by normal blood flow.
4. Excessive flow, which implies that the volume of blood is too large for a normal orifice or vessel.

Ask yourself which mechanism is operating whenever you hear a systolic murmur.

Regurgitant Murmurs

There is a general tendency to use the terms regurgitation and *insufficiency* synonymously. The term *insufficiency* is a poor one. For example, the valve may be insufficient in its ability to open properly; thus, valve stenosis could also be classified as insufficient.

Backward blood flow through a valve is regurgitation. Blood that regurgitates does not have to wait for the aortic or pulmonary valve to open; thus, turbulence may begin during the period of isovolemic contraction, commencing with the first heart sound, continuing through systole, and concluding with the second heart sound. Typically, these murmurs are pansystolic. In each of the three conditions associated with systolic regurgitation, the pressure gradient between the two chambers is high. A high-pressure gradient is associated with a high-velocity jet, which causes shedding of small vortices or eddies. Although the murmur is traditionally described as high-pitched, it is in fact of medium pitch, in the middle range of our hearing (400 to 550 Hz), but it is relatively high-pitched as most murmurs go. It sounds like a breath sound and may be blowing or harsh, like tracheal breathing. Neophyte auscultators invariably mistake breath sounds as low-pitched because of their soft quality; they are not.

> ### Key Point
>
> When a murmur sounds like a breath sound, it is not an innocent murmur.

The three hemodynamic disturbances associated with systolic regurgitant murmurs are (1) VSD, (2) mitral regurgitation, and (3) tricuspid regurgitation. These abnormalities share a common hemodynamic feature; each is associated with a high systolic pressure gradient. For example, in mitral regurgitation, left ventricular pressure is 100 mm Hg and left atrial pressure only 5 mm Hg. In small VSDs, the regurgitant murmur may be cut off in late systole as the septum contracts; therefore, the murmur begins with the first sound but ends before the second sound, and is thus early systolic to midsystolic in timing.

Generally, regurgitant murmurs are heard loudest over the chamber in which they originate. Thus, the murmur of mitral regurgitation is heard loudest at the apex and radiates toward the axilla. The murmur of VSD is heard best along the left sternal border, over the right ventricular area. The murmur of tricuspid regurgitation is unique, in that it is more intense during inspiration because of increased right ventricular filling. It is helpful to emphasize there is just no innocent murmur that sounds like a regurgitant murmur. If it sounds like a breath sound, harsh or blowing, of any degree of intensity, it is organic and signifies regurgitation of blood.

Obstructive Murmurs

All obstructive murmurs are organic. The turbulence caused by obstruction has eddies of large but varying size, and vortex shedding is associated with a large amount of energy. Therefore, obstructive murmurs are coarse and loud. Because the turbulence occurs during forward flow, it must wait for the aortic and pulmonary valves to open, and there is a pause between the first heart sound and the beginning of the murmur. The velocity and volume of blood passing through the valve is greatest toward the center of systole, so the murmur will be loudest at this time, creating a crescendo-decrescendo, "diamond-shaped" or "kite-shaped" type of murmur.

These loud coarse murmurs generally occur over the pulmonary or aortic valve. Unfortunately, there is the occasional exception. The murmur of aortic coarctation tends to be higher in pitch but is heard in a different area, being maximal high in the precordium, in the left axilla, and over the left side of the back. Occasionally, obstructions occur in the midventricle, in which case the murmur also tends to be more highly pitched and may be difficult to differentiate from a regurgitant murmur. Generally speaking, obstructive murmurs are recognized easily as being organic from their intensity and coarseness, and they tend to radiate in the direction of blood flow, where the vortex shedding process is occurring. Hence, the murmur caused by aortic stenosis is well heard over the carotid arteries.

Vibratory Murmurs

Vibratory murmurs are murmurs of musical quality. They have harmonics. The innocent vibratory murmur found in children was described first in 1909 by Still,[2] who likened it to the "twanging of string." Vibratory murmurs arise in tissue, and because tissue vibrates in harmonics, these murmurs are unlike any others. Nevertheless, the musical quality is difficult for some examiners to appreciate. A medium-pitched musical murmur would sound like a hum, whereas one with high-pitched components would sound like a seagull's cry. Because vibration occurs in tissue, it often transmits in the same tissue plane. Thus, a vibratory murmur arising in the left ventricular outflow tract will transmit through the left ventricular tissue toward the apex or through the aortic wall up toward the aortic listening area.

The innocent vibratory systolic murmur heard commonly in children probably results from a high stroke volume being ejected forcefully, causing tissue in the left ventricle to vibrate. It is heard maximally in expiration and is usually best heard midway between the left sternal border and the apex. Merely detecting a musical quality of the murmur in children means that the chances that the murmur is innocent are high (Fig. 10–8). When calcium is deposited in a heart valve, the resultant murmur is not just musical; it has high-pitched components. Occasionally, in children who have a perimembranous VSD, the murmur may have a similar high-pitched component, possibly caused by vibration of the membranous portion of the septum.

Key Point

A musical murmur in a child is almost invariably innocent. If it hums, it is not organic.

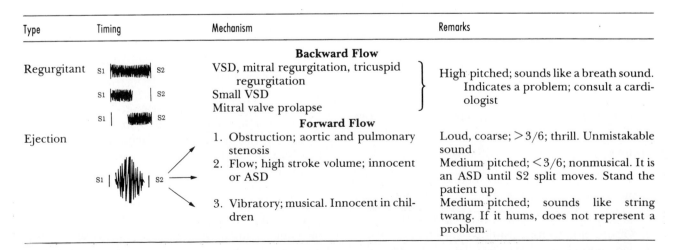

Type	Timing	Mechanism	Remarks
		Backward Flow	
Regurgitant	S1 ▮▮▮▮ S2	VSD, mitral regurgitation, tricuspid regurgitation	High pitched; sounds like a breath sound. Indicates a problem; consult a cardiologist
	S1 ▮▮ S2	Small VSD	
	S1 ▮▮ S2	Mitral valve prolapse	
		Forward Flow	
Ejection	S1 ▮ S2	1. Obstruction; aortic and pulmonary stenosis	Loud, coarse; >3/6; thrill. Unmistakable sound
		2. Flow; high stroke volume; innocent or ASD	Medium pitched; <3/6; nonmusical. It is an ASD until S2 split moves. Stand the patient up
		3. Vibratory; musical. Innocent in children	Medium pitched; sounds like string twang. If it hums, does not represent a problem

Figure 10–8 Systolic murmurs. ASD, atrial septal defect; VSD, ventricular septal defect.

Flow Murmurs

Flow murmurs are generated by the turbulence associated with an increased stroke volume. Systolic flow murmurs occur in the outflow tract of either the left or right ventricle and accordingly are usually heard maximally at the left or right sternal border in the second interspace. A flow murmur at the left sternal border is probably occurring in the pulmonary artery and is almost never loud enough to be associated with a thrill. Flow murmurs heard at the right sternal border may be associated with a short, coarse, low-pitched sound over the carotid artery. Flow murmurs are usually associated with other evidence of a high stroke volume. Invariably, when the patient with such a murmur is examined in a standing position, the systolic flow murmur greatly diminishes in intensity or totally disappears, because of the decrease in stroke volume that occurs in the standing position.

The characteristics of the second sound become extremely important in the interpretation of the significance of flow murmurs. Unfortunately, the mechanism of an ASD murmur, which is actually a flow murmur arising in the right ventricular outflow tract, is similar to that of the innocent functional flow murmur heard in normal individuals, and the two murmurs may be indistinguishable on auscultation. The key distinguishing feature is the characteristic fixed splitting of the second sound that occurs with most ASDs. When listening for the second heart sound, apply the diaphragm of the stethoscope over the second interspace at the left sternal border (with the patient supine). In the normal child, the split of the second sound widens with inspiration as a result of increasing right ventricular stroke volume and longer ventricular contraction. With expiration, the split narrows but may not close entirely. In the common form of ASD, blood ejected from the right ventricle is constant in volume in both inspiration and expiration; hence, splitting of the second sound is fixed, meaning that it does not change with respiratory phase. If you have difficulty hearing normal movement of the split of the second sound, sit the child up; movement of the split may be sluggish in the supine position. Other features (easily palpable right ventricular impulse, mid-diastolic murmur in tricuspid area) may help in the diagnosis of ASD.

Key Point

A nonmusical ejection systolic murmur in the pulmonary listening area and fixed splitting of the second sound signify ASD. A systolic murmur cannot be ignored until you are certain that the components of the second sound are moving normally.

Innocent murmurs are common. A murmur may be heard on careful auscultation in as many as 40% of 3- to 4 year-old children. Such innocent murmurs include the vibratory murmur, the flow murmur with a normal second sound, the carotid bruit, and the venous hum. It is important to know these murmurs well, because any health care system can tolerate only a limited number of cardiology consultations for innocent murmurs.

Diastolic Murmurs

Diastolic murmurs are organic, with rare exceptions, such as the mid-diastolic flow murmur that may occur with marked sinus bradycardia. Velocity of flow in diastole differs from systole; it is maximum early in diastole with the opening of the AV valves and then late in diastole with atrial contraction. These flow velocities influence the timing of diastolic murmurs, but generally speaking, diastolic murmurs are classified much like systolic murmurs and may be early, beginning with the second sound, mid, or mid to late. Yet, when a murmur is only late diastolic in timing, we term it *presystolic*. The term *pandiastolic* is never used. The mechanisms are the same, and the murmurs that are produced are therefore regurgitant, obstructive, flow, or vibratory.

Regurgitant diastolic murmurs imply either aortic or pulmonary valve regurgitation. Like regurgitant systolic murmur, the murmur begins with the closure of that portion of the second heart sound caused by the closure of either the pulmonary or aortic valve. The murmur of aortic regurgitation is high-pitched, because of the high pressure gradient between the aorta and the left ventricle in diastole, and is heard maximally along the left sternal border, where the turbulence is occurring. The murmur of pulmonary regurgitation with normal pulmonary artery pressure is low-pitched because of the low pressure gradient; it is heard in the same area as the aortic regurgitation murmur. When the child has pulmonary hypertension, the murmur, known as the Graham-Steell murmur, is of high pitch, because of the high pressure gradient between the pulmonary artery and the right ventricle in diastole.

Obstructive murmurs are caused by mitral or tricuspid stenosis, uncommon congenital heart lesions. In areas where rheumatic fever is still endemic, this murmur may be encountered when an older child has mitral stenosis associated with chronic rheumatic carditis. Decrescendo-crescendo in shape related to flow velocity, the murmur is low-pitched, and it does not begin until the mitral valve opens; therefore, there is a pause between the second sound and the start of the murmur.

With mitral valve stenosis, the murmur occurs in the left ventricle and is loudest at the apex. Frequently, only the late diastolic portion of the murmur is present, in which case it is presystolic in timing. Students commonly identify this murmur improperly, believing it to be systolic. There is just no systolic murmur maximal at the apex that is low-pitched and rumbling.

A diastolic *flow murmur* occurs with lesions such as VSD, ASD, and mitral or tricuspid regurgitation. Its presence indicates that flow volume across the AV valve is at least twice normal. Mid-diastolic in timing, of short duration, and medium in pitch, this flow murmur is heard maximally in either the apical or tricuspid area, depending on which valve generates the turbulence. As noted previously, the same murmur is heard in the presence of marked bradycardia, and it is invariably present in complete AV block before the implantation of a pacemaker.

Occasionally, a vibratory or musical diastolic murmur may be heard. One example is the "cooing," early diastolic murmur of aortic regurgitation that occurs when the regurgitant jet causes bacterial endocarditis vegetations on the aortic valve to vibrate.

Many noncardiologists have difficulty eliciting diastolic murmurs because of inexperience and the relative rarity of diastolic murmurs.

Continuous Murmurs

Of the many causes of continuous murmurs, only two are of major importance. The common continuous murmur is a normal finding known as the *venous hum.* In children whose circulation is hyperkinetic, continuous turbulence is audible over the jugular veins, usually loudest in the right supraclavicular fossa. This murmur, usually heard only in the sitting or upright position, varies considerably in intensity with movement of the child's head, and its intensity may be influenced by light pressure on either jugular vein (Fig. 10–9). The turbulence may also be palpated with light pressure on the jugular vein (Fig. 10–10). With light finger pressure, a thrill may also be palpable. Occasionally, a venous hum is audible when the child is supine with the head only slightly elevated. This murmur, as common as it is, frequently confounds the examiner, who has usually forgotten the basic rule of first listening with the patient in the supine position.

The other important continuous murmur is that of a patent ductus arteriosus. It is heard maximally on the left side of the thorax, usually just below the clavicle, or between the left sternal border and the midclavicular line in the second interspace. In the child older than 1 month whose pulmonary artery pressure is not elevated, the patent ductus murmur has the same continuous timing as the venous hum but peaks in intensity earlier, at the time of the second heart sound, when the pressure gradient between aorta and pulmonary artery is the greatest. In contrast to the venous hum, it is well heard in the supine position. Flow through a patent ductus arteriosus of average size increases aortic runoff and left ventricular stroke volume. Accordingly, the pulse is bounding, and

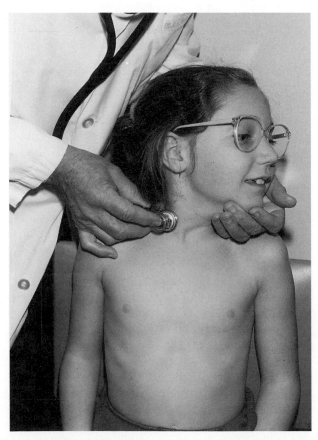

Figure 10–9 The intensity of a venous hum may be enhanced by lateral positioning of the head.

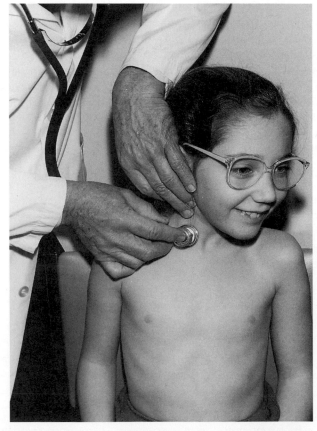

Figure 10–10 Pressure on the jugular vein influences the intensity of a venous hum, and with very light pressure, a thrill may be detected.

left ventricular activity (only the left) is readily palpable. If either of these findings is present, be sure to search particularly for a patent ductus murmur. This murmur has been variously described as having a "machinery" or "train-in-a-tunnel" quality. An inexperienced examiner hears only the loudest part of the murmur, often missing its decrescendo diastolic component.

Rarely, a continuous murmur with the characteristics of a patent ductus arteriosus murmur is heard in another location over the precordium (e.g., in a coronary AV fistula, in which it is best heard along the lower left sternal border).

Other Systolic Murmurs

Two murmurs that deserve individual attention are the cardiorespiratory murmur and the murmur of mitral valve prolapse.

The *cardiorespiratory murmur* is frequently missed because it generally does not occur in the conventional listening stations. It tends to be loudest in the midclavicular line in the third interspace on either side of the chest, more often on the right. Occasionally, it is also heard in the back. Characteristically, there are three successive systolic blowing murmurs that occur in the middle and late inspiration phases. They are entirely absent during early inspiration and expiration. When heard loudest at the apex, the cardiorespiratory murmur may be confused with the murmur of mitral regurgitation. The cardiorespiratory murmur has no clinical significance. It is thought to be generated in a portion of lung that is "trapped" and compressed during inspiration. If the patient is cooperative and can hold his or her breath, the murmur, of course, disappears.

The "whoop" that occurs with *mitral valve prolapse* is best heard with the patient standing. It occupies the mid to late portion of systole and may be exceedingly loud, sometimes being audible without a stethoscope. Whoops are usually evanescent, being loud at one time and absent at another. When a colleague performing cardiac auscultation says excitedly, "You just have to come and hear this," it usually turns out to be this whoop. The patient is usually tall and asthenic and frequently has a thoracic bony abnormality, such as pectus excavatum. No other murmur sounds like it.

You may find this clinical tidbit interesting: Mitral valve prolapse may be familial and due to a congenital connective tissue defect. I recall a case in which two sisters had mitral valve prolapse, and at times, either sister could have a whoop loud enough that it could be heard by the other sister across the room. When one sister had the noise, the other sister would say "You're whooping!"

The mitral regurgitation that may accompany mitral valve prolapse may not have a whooping quality. Instead, it may have only the blowing quality of mitral regurgitation from any cause. It will be mid to late in timing, however, at least in its mild form.

Pericarditis and Mediastinal Emphysema

Two other auscultatory findings of significance are the pericardial friction rub of pericarditis and the mediastinal crunch of mediastinal emphysema.

Pericardial friction occurs most frequently after operation in patients undergoing cardiac surgery—the so-called postpericardiotomy syndrome, which characteristically appears 3 to 6 weeks after operation. When detected without relation to cardiac surgery, it may be a sign associated with pericarditis from any cause, but usually viral. Most clinicians identify a friction rub easily because of its characteristic scratchy quality. Pericardial rubs may be heard anywhere on the left side of the chest but are usually best heard along the sternal border. Contrary to earlier teaching, their presence bears little or no relation to the amount of effusion within the pericardium. They generally have three phases, related to atrial filling, ventricular ejection, and the rapid phase of ventricular filling, giving them a characteristic "cha-cha-cha" cadence.

The *mediastinal crunch*, once heard, is also characteristic. It has much the same quality as pericardial friction, and although it may have a to-and-fro rhythm, it does not have a three-phase cadence. More often, the rhythm of mediastinal crunch is chaotic, sometimes systolic and sometimes phasic with respiration. It may occur independently or after chest injury. On two occasions, I have elicited this sign in the cardiac intensive care unit, in patients undergoing ventilation. In each case, after hearing the crunch and surreptitiously palpating interstitial emphysema in the neck (which is frequently present in ventilated patients), I turned to the intensivists and said, "Turn down your pressure, folks." Two cases of "red faces" caused by poor bedside skills.

Auscultation Technique for Murmurs

Having evaluated the heart sounds in each area, you can now begin to listen to the intervals, starting at the apex with the patient supine. Begin with the stethoscope diaphragm, because most troubling murmurs are in the medium- to high-pitched range. Listen to systole. A murmur in systole at the apex is not necessarily loudest in this area, so track the murmur with the stethoscope to its point of maximal intensity. While listening, attempt to answer the following questions:

1. Over which chamber or vessel is the stethoscope lying?
2. Is the murmur related to the first heart sound? Listen particularly for its quality and pitch.
3. What is the intensity of the murmur (grade 1 to 6)?

> **Key Point**
>
> Grade 1 is the faintest murmur that you can imagine. At grade 4, an associated thrill is felt, whereas a grade 6 murmur is so intense it does not require a stethoscope to be heard.

Let us suppose that the murmur has been described as pansystolic, of grade 3/6 intensity, and high-pitched with a harsh blowing quality, and as heard maximally at the fifth left interspace in the anterior axillary line. This is the description of mitral regurgitation. Remember that if any apical systolic murmur is pansystolic in timing, it should be identified automatically as organic. Then listen to diastole at the apex. Listen carefully to the "nothings"—the areas initially perceived to be silent.

Then move the stethoscope to the tricuspid area, and listen first to systole and then again to diastole. Suppose that you hear a murmur in systole, but as you track it to its point of maximum intensity, it is loudest at the left sternal border in the second interspace. Is it regurgitant or ejection? If it is not pansystolic and if it does not sound like a breath sound, it is probably ejection. Is it caused by obstruction, flow, or vibration? If it is not low-pitched and coarse, it is not obstructive. Listen for a musical component. If there is no musical component, the murmur is not vibratory. Thus, by exclusion, it is a flow murmur, either innocent or due to ASD.

You should now listen to the second heart sound again. If splitting is "fixed," the child probably has ASD. Do not be satisfied with this conclusion, however. Listen also to diastole. If the child has ASD, there probably is a mid-diastolic flow murmur at the left sternal border in the fourth space. If the split in the second sound moves nicely, ASD is not present. Stand the child up; if the murmur disappears, you can conclude that the murmur is innocent. In this situation, other signs of a high-output state are probably present. In this manner, proceed with auscultation at each listening area, listening to both systole and diastole.

Auscultation of the heart is a difficult skill to acquire. To become proficient requires many hours of listening to hearts. So take advantage of every opportunity you have to listen to a heart. Despite best intentions, most students do not hear enough hearts to acquire a high level of auscultatory skill. You are thus encouraged to use more modern methods to improve your skills. One is the use of an interactive cardiac auscultation CD-ROM (four of which are currently available), which contains many surrogate patients for your education.

APPROACH TO PHYSICAL EXAMINATION OF THE CHILD

The order of the examination does not differ greatly from that of the infant, except for a different emphasis on certain aspects. The first challenge is persuading your young patient to cooperate. If cooperation is in doubt, start with the child on the parent's lap.

> **Key Point**
>
> If the youngster appears likely to cry, auscultate first, even if this is not the ideal way to begin a cardiovascular examination.

If the youngster is happy to lie on an examining table, stand on the child's right side. Observe his or her body habitus, and look closely for dysmorphic features. Does the child have a marfanoid habitus? Is there pectus excavatum? Is the voice hoarse—could it be Williams syndrome—or does the child simply look like a normal healthy active (perhaps physiologically hyperkinetic) 3-year-old?

Observation

Observe the child's chest. Is the left side abnormally prominent? Are there abnormal pulsations? A safe way to begin the hands-on part of the examination is by gently picking up the child's hand. Are the palmar creases normal? Is there clubbing? Look at the fingertips from the side (Figs. 10–11 and 10–12). Clubbing can occasionally be normal and may occur in noncardiovascular diseases. Are the fingers of normal length and number? Is there clinodactyly? Dorsiflex the fingers and wrist. Is tone normal?

Taking the Pulses

Start with the brachial pulse, not the radial. The closer to the heart the pulse is felt, the truer its quality. Using

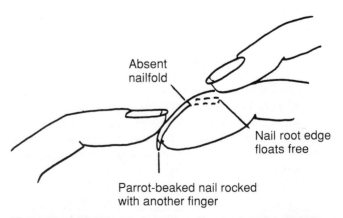

Absent nailfold

Nail root edge floats free

Parrot-beaked nail rocked with another finger

Figure 10–11 Clubbing is best seen if you view the digit from the side. The earliest sign is diminution of the angle between the nail root and the skin. (From Constant J: Bedside Cardiology, 5th ed. Hagerstown, MD, Lippincott Williams & Wilkins, 1999.)

the first and second digits of your right hand, palpate the brachial artery, just above the antecubital fossa (Fig. 10–13). In the older child it may be preferable to support the child's right arm with your left, using your right thumb to palpate the pulse. The important questions are as follows:

1. What is the pulse volume (pulse pressure)?
2. Is the rise normal (slow, fast, smooth)?
3. Is the fall-off normal?
4. What is the blood pressure?

If the pulse volume seems to have increased, check for a water-hammer pulse by elevating the child's arm and encircling the upper arm with one hand (Fig. 10–14). A pulse of normal volume is not usually felt with this maneuver. Now "dissect" the pulse by analyzing the upstroke and downstroke.

If the pulse volume is increased, the child has a hyperkinetic circulation, aortic insufficiency, or a patent ductus arteriosus. In such a patient, when blood pressure is measured, the pulse pressure is increased, and when the chest is palpated, the heart action is increased. The pulse quality reflects the manner in which blood leaves the heart and the resistance it meets in the periphery. Now palpate the femoral pulse; if it is of good volume, aortic coarctation is not present. If it is absent or is distinctly smaller in volume than the brachial pulse, the blood pressures in the arms and legs must be carefully measured. As previously mentioned, radial-femoral pulse delay is difficult to elicit (Fig. 10–15), and if aortic regurgitation accompanies coarctation, such a delay is not present.

The clinical conditions described in the following sections can be appreciated as alterations in pulse volume.

PULSUS PARADOXUS

The normal systolic blood pressure may decrease as much as 8 mm Hg during average inspiration, and more during a deep inspiration. When the decrease is greater

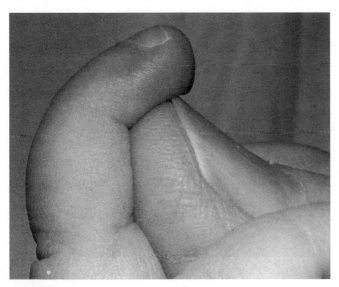

Figure 10–12 Early clubbing in a 7-month-old child with cyanotic congenital heart disease. The nail root–skin angle has been flattened, and the tip of the finger is shiny.

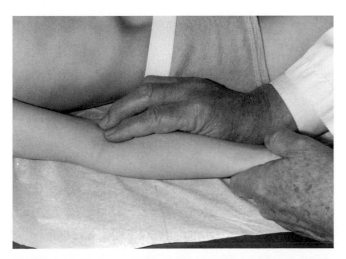

Figure 10–13 The brachial pulse, which is used to assess the quality of the pulse, is palpated with the first two digits of the right hand.

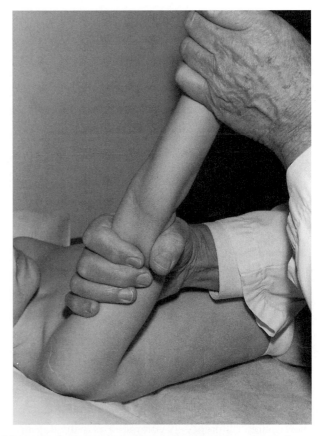

Figure 10–14 To examine for a collapsing pulse, elevate the arm and encircle the upper arm with your examining hand. This sign may be present in patent ductus arteriosus, aortic regurgitation, or hyperkinetic circulation.

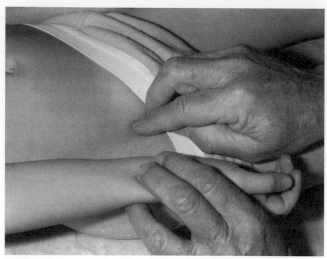

Figure 10–15 In coarctation of the aorta, the initial portion (the percussion wave) of the femoral pulse may be absent, causing so-called radiofemoral delay. Search for this sign with the radial and femoral pulses in juxtaposition.

than 8 mm Hg during average inspiration, the condition is termed *pulsus paradoxus*. It is an exaggeration of a normal phenomenon and not, as the name suggests, a paradox. Its presence usually indicates that cardiac tamponade is present.

Check for pulsus paradoxus as follows:

1. Ask the supine child to breath normally.
2. Elevate the arm (to avoid the auscultatory gap), then inflate the cuff.
3. While observing respiration, gradually decrease the cuff pressure and note the level at which all Korotkoff sounds are heard (point A).
4. Gradually increase the cuff pressure until no Korotkoff sounds are heard (point B).
5. The difference between point A and point B represents the difference in inspiratory and expiratory systolic blood pressures. Excesses greater than 8 mm Hg indicate the level of "paradox."

In patients with asthma or emphysema, the difference between inspiratory and expiratory systolic blood pressures is increased. You must take care in interpreting results of this procedure in such patients.

PULSUS ALTERNANS

Pulsus alternans is seen infrequently in children and, when present, is invariably associated with myocardial failure. It is present when regular alternating pulses have a perceptible difference in volume. The palpating finger cannot perceive a systolic pressure difference of less than 20 mm Hg, and careful observations must be made when you are recording the blood pressure in the patient with

Table 10-2   ACCEPTABLE HEART RATES IN INFANTS AND CHILDREN

Age	Resting Pulse Rates (Beats/Min)		
	Awake	*Asleep*	*Exercise/Fever*
Newborn	100–180	80–160	<220
1 wk–3 mo	100–220	80–200	<220
3 mo–2 yr	80–150	70–120	<200
2–10 yr	70–110	60–90	<200
>10 yr	55–90	50–90	<200

this sign. As the cuff pressure is being decreased, a systolic pressure is first encountered of only the alternate Korotkoff sounds. For example, if the blood pressure is 120 mm Hg systolic with a regular rate of 50 beats/min, a regular rate of 100 beats/min is encountered as the cuff pressure is lowered further, at which time the blood pressure is 95 mm Hg or possibly lower. The presence of left ventricular hypertension (aortic stenosis, systemic hypertension) increases the likelihood of eliciting this sign.

PULSUS BISFERIENS

Pulsus bisferiens is an ancient term describing the perceptible notch in the pulse wave that is detectable when a child has significant obstruction and regurgitation of the aortic valve.

SINUS ARRHYTHMIA

The normal pulse rate varies with the child's age and activity state; this phenomenon is called *sinus arrhythmia*. The range of normal for resting pulse rates in children older than 2 years is listed in Table 10–2.

> **Key Point**
>
> It is abnormal for a child *not* to have sinus arrhythmia.

At times, sinus arrhythmia may be so marked that it is impossible to differentiate from frequent extrasystoles or atrial fibrillation, and an electrocardiogram may be required.

BRADYCARDIA

If a child's pulse rate is less than 60 beats/min, complete AV block may be present. Differentiation of this condition from sinus bradycardia is usually possible at the bedside. Checking the jugular pulse is normally of little value in this age group; however, in the patient with bradycardia and possible AV block, look for cannon A waves. This procedure is performed with the child in the sitting or semirecumbent position and the head inclined to one side. When auscultating, check for varying intensity of the first heart sound, which is caused by the varying position of the AV valves at the beginning of ventricular contraction. Also observe the effect of exercise on the child's pulse rate. In complete AV block, only a small increase occurs. An innocent murmur is frequently seen in association with bradycardia because of the increased stroke volume.

Palpation of the Chest and Abdomen

A 3-year-old child is unlikely to have heart failure; nevertheless, try to identify the liver edge. If the liver edge is 2 cm or more below the costal margin, look for clinical evidence of pulmonary air trapping (which may be pushing the diaphragm and liver downward), and percuss the top of the liver.

Gently lay a warm hand on the apical area, and palpate the apical impulse. It is quick and diffuse, spilling over to the area left of the sternum in the fourth and fifth spaces. You are now palpating the left and right ventricles as they eject greater volumes of blood. If the child is quite active and pulse volume is increased, this finding is normal. If you palpate an apical impulse that is exclusively apical and is forceful and sustained, there is a problem. Palpate the area to the left of the sternum in the third and fourth spaces, searching for a right ventricular impulse. A diffuse quick impulse would be expected in ASD, for example.

When palpating the thorax for ventricular dynamics, remember the following facts:

1. The ventricle that is volume overloaded is easily palpable, and the impulse is diffuse and abrupt.
2. The pressure-loaded ventricle is palpable only if the overload is severe (and usually chronic), and the impulse is forceful and sustained.

Now palpate the second left interspace at the sternal border, using your first and second digits. If an impulse is present, an organic lesion is probably present, and there is pathologic dilatation of the pulmonary artery as a result of increased flow or pressure. Then palpate the suprasternal notch by inserting your index finger as deeply as possible. If the previous findings suggest a hyperkinetic circulation, an impulse normally can be palpated here. A marked, visible impulse at the suprasternal notch signifies increased flow in the aortic arch that is probably organic, and you should search specifically for patent ductus arteriosus or aortic insufficiency during auscultation.

Now palpate in the reverse direction, searching for a thrill. Begin in the suprasternal notch. A thrill may be

Table 10-3   THE HYPERKINETIC CIRCULATION

Physically active
Bounding pulses
Supine position
  Hyperkinetic precordium
  Pulsation in the sternal notch
  Wide pulse pressure
  Wide but moving split of S$_2$
  Third heart sound
  Musical systolic ejection murmur, grade 2–3/6 intensity, left sternal border to apex, loudest in expiration
  Nonmusical ejection systolic murmur, second interspace, left or right sternal border
Carotid bruit (Fig. 10–16)
Intracranial bruits
Standing position
  Venous hum present
  S$_3$ disappears
  Nonmusical systolic murmur disappears
  Vibratory systolic murmur diminishes

present here even in minor degrees of obstruction in the left ventricular outflow tract. Then palpate for a thrill in the conventional areas; whatever you can feel you will also be able to hear, only better. However, appreciation of a thrill does help to classify murmurs. If you palpate a thrill, an organic process is certainly present, and you will hear a loud murmur, grade 4 to 6 in intensity.

Auscultation

After palpation of the chest and abdomen, it is time to auscultate. Organize your approach. Innocent murmurs are a major problem to the physician, partly because murmurs are often considered in isolation.

Key Point

The innocent murmur is almost always encountered in the presence of a hyperkinetic circulation, which is usually physiologic.

The hyperkinesis in the hyperkinetic circulation syndrome is not restricted to the cardiovascular system, and the child usually is quite physically active. The details of this syndrome are listed in Table 10–3 (Fig. 10–16). If most of these features are not present in the child diagnosed as having an innocent murmur, question the diagnosis. Unfortunately, innocent murmurs and organic murmurs can coexist. Even in the child with all the features of a hyperkinetic circulation, if the murmur sounds like a breath sound, it is abnormal. Ejection clicks are organic in any setting.

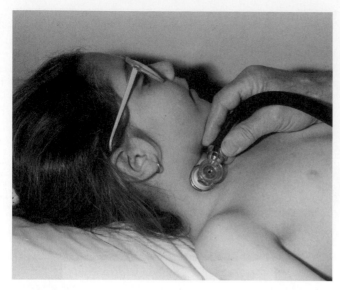

Figure 10–16 Eliciting a carotid bruit. Other findings of hyperkinetic circulation are usually present, and there is no thrill in the suprasternal notch. The murmur of aortic stenosis is also well heard over the right carotid artery, but a thrill is usually present in the suprasternal notch.

EXAMINING THE TEENAGER

Organic symptoms originating in the cardiovascular system are uncommon in teenagers who have no preexisting cardiac disease. Atypical chest pain is a common complaint in teenagers. (It is usually of sharp quality, of short duration, and unrelated to exercise.) When a parent or close relative has had angina or a recent myocardial infarction, the teenager may complain of similar distress. Providing adequate reassurance for the patient and the family usually requires no more than a good history and a physical examination; occasionally, it does demand further investigation, such as electrocardiography, exercise testing, or Holter monitoring. Even in the presence of congenital abnormalities of the coronary arteries, angina is rare in a teenager. A more likely clinical presentation of cardiovascular disease is syncope, which may or may not have a primary cardiovascular cause.

Key Point

The patient presenting with a marfanoid habitus, or with true Marfan syndrome and chest pain, requires close attention, because such individuals are subject to dilatation of the ascending aorta and dissecting aneurysm.

Patients with a marfanoid habitus must undergo chest radiography and cardiac ultrasonography. A family history of sudden death at an early age is also an indication for more thorough investigation, because familial aortic dissection may occur without any obvious connective tissue disorder. Consider hypertrophic cardiomyopathy if the history reveals this familial trait.

Symptoms Requiring Attention

Symptoms in teenagers that require special attention are syncope and nonrotatory "dizziness," which may be cardiac in origin. Cardiac syncope can occur at any age, but other causes of syncope are far more common in teenagers, the most common being vasovagal syncope, or "fainting."

Syncopal episodes are often preceded by symptoms such as weakness, sweating, and nausea, which can last for a few seconds or 1 to 2 minutes. The subsequent period of unconsciousness usually lasts no more than 2 or 3 minutes. On regaining consciousness, the child usually recognizes his or her environment almost immediately. Vasovagal syncope is usually innocent. It is more common in girls, and often one of the parents has a history of a tendency to faint.

The following two features of the history are critical in a teenager with syncope:

1. Syncope that occurs without warning (a drop) is almost always of cardiac origin.
2. Cardiac syncope may also be of gradual onset.

Although most syncopes are not caused by disease states, it is important to know the types of cardiac conditions that may cause syncope, so you can ask the appropriate questions and look for the relevant physical signs. Possible causes of syncope are as follows:

- Aortic stenosis (severe)
- Hypertrophic cardiomyopathy
- Atrial myxoma
- Pulmonary hypertension
- Long QT syndromes (familial or nonfamilial)
- Ventricular ectopic beats and normal QT interval
- Supraventricular tachycardias with very rapid ventricular rate
- Complete AV block (congenital or acquired)
- Sick sinus syndrome (bradycardia-tachycardia syndrome)

Key Point

A good history is imperative, because no abnormality may be found on physical examination and the next episode may be fatal.

A "drop" indicates urgent cardiac consultation, as does a patient with cardiac dysrhythmia and "spells." Exercise and emotional outbursts are common triggering factors. During the wait for cardiac consultation, the most appropriate investigative procedure is 24-hour Holter monitor.

A presentation that is more or less limited to teenagers is something I call the "excel syndrome," observed in adolescents who possess an intense desire to excel. The typical patient is female and 14 to 15 years of age and may complain of easy fatigue, headache, atypical chest pain, or, possibly, inability to breathe deeply. The cardiovascular findings can be dramatic. Tachycardia and systolic hypertension, possibly as high as 170 mm Hg, are present. The brachial pulse is bounding, and the heart action is hyperdynamic. A systolic ejection murmur, frequently coarse and nonmusical, is present in the pulmonary and aortic areas and may be as loud as grade 3/6 in intensity. A third sound and carotid bruit are frequently present. If an electrocardiogram is performed, nonspecific ST-segment and T-wave changes may be seen, further complicating the picture.

Have the patient with such findings stand. Invariably, the auscultatory findings disappear. On questioning, you often find that academically, the patient is first or second in her class. Ongoing observations of the blood pressure are required, but only as a basis for reassuring the patient and family that no serious problem exists. The normal range of systolic and diastolic blood pressures at different ages is shown in Figure 10–17.

SUMMARY

A good clinical assessment can spare many children with cardiovascular complaints from unnecessary or inappropriate investigative procedures. The key element is a systematic approach that always interprets each symptom and sign in terms of the underlying hemodynamic disturbance. Recognition of the characteristic manifestations peculiar to congestive heart failure in early infancy is paramount. Thereafter, the first clinical issue is often to decide whether clinical findings are normal or abnormal, hemodynamically significant or otherwise. Of special importance is determining the presence or absence of central cyanosis. As in other types of pediatric physical assessment, a keen observer can learn much from hands-off examination. This chapter has reviewed several "tricks of the trade" for conducting a successful cardiovascular assessment without antagonizing the child. Some people may believe that it is an impossible task to learn much about cardiac auscultation by reading about it; it is not. Before laying a stethoscope on anyone's precordium, the physician must have a crystal-clear concept of what to listen for as well as what each sound means. The importance of listening with the child supine cannot be overstressed.

As stated previously, cardiac auscultation is a difficult skill to acquire and only a minority of medical students graduate with the ability to differentiate normal from abnormal heart sounds.[5]

Accordingly, the management of a systolic murmur detected in a child presents a problem that is compounded by present-day time constraints on routine physical examination by the family physician. Although the clinical characteristics (e.g., vibratory and musical quality, normally moving split of S2, and features of a hyperdynamic circulation) are so archetypal, and their presence so common (50% of normal children),[6] their management still may be difficult. To refer every child with a heart murmur for an echocardiogram should be unnecessary and represents a significant financial stress on the health system. Primary care physicians are strongly encouraged to further their skills in cardiac auscultation. Reading a chapter such as this is of limited value, except to highlight the existence of this deficit. The real answer lies in the auscultation of many hearts. Today, this can be accomplished by examining "surrogate hearts," as in tapes or compact disks. Irrespective of the examiner's level of confidence, when further parental reassurance is required, referral to a specialist is recommended rather than sending the child for echocardiography.[7]

REFERENCES

1. Roy DL, McIntyre L, Human DG, et al: Trends in the prevalence of congenital heart disease: Comprehensive observations over a 24-year period in a defined region of Canada. Can J Cardiol 10:821–826, 1994.
2. Still GF: Common Disorders and Diseases of Childhood. London, Frowde, Hodder, & Stoughton, 1909.
3. Engle WD: Blood pressure in the very low birth weight neonate. Early Hum Dev 62:97–130, 2001.
4. Moller JH, Neal WA: Heart Disease in Infancy. New York, Appleton-Century-Crofts, 1981.
5. Mangione S, Nieman IZ: Cardiac auscultatory skills of internal medicine and family practice trainees: A comparison of diagnostic proficiency. JAMA 278:717–722, 1997.
6. Keith J, Rowe RD, Vlad P: Heart Disease in Infancy and Childhood, 2nd ed. New York, Macmillan, 1967, p 29.
7. Pelech AN: Evaluation of the pediatric patient with a heart murmur. Ped Clin N Am 46:167–188, 1999.

SUGGESTED READINGS

Constant J: Bedside Cardiology, 4th ed. Boston, Little, Brown, 1993.
Park MK: Pediatric Cardiology for Practitioners, 4th ed. St. Louis, Mosby, 2002.
Park MK: The Pediatric Cardiology Handbook. St. Louis, Mosby–Year Book, 1991.

Blood Pressure Levels for the 90th and 95th Percentiles of Blood Pressure for Girls Aged 1 to 17 Years by Percentiles of Height

Age (Yr)	Blood Pressure Percentile*	Systolic Blood Pressure by Percentile of Height, mm Hg†							Diastolic Blood Pressure by Percentile of Height, mm Hg†						
		5%	10%	25%	50%	75%	90%	95%	5%	10%	25%	50%	75%	90%	95%
1	90th	97	98	99	100	102	103	104	53	53	53	54	55	56	56
	95th	101	102	103	104	105	107	107	57	57	57	58	59	60	60
2	90th	99	99	100	102	103	104	105	57	57	58	58	59	60	61
	95th	102	103	104	105	107	108	109	61	61	62	62	63	64	65
3	90th	100	100	102	103	104	105	106	61	61	61	62	63	63	64
	95th	104	104	105	107	108	109	110	65	65	65	66	67	67	68
4	90th	101	102	103	104	106	107	108	63	63	64	65	65	66	67
	95th	105	106	107	108	109	111	111	67	67	68	69	69	70	71
5	90th	103	103	104	106	107	108	109	65	66	66	67	68	65	69
	95th	107	107	108	110	111	112	113	69	70	70	71	72	72	73
6	90th	104	105	106	107	109	110	111	67	68	68	69	69	70	71
	95th	108	109	110	111	112	114	114	71	72	72	73	73	74	75
7	90th	106	107	108	109	110	112	112	69	69	69	70	71	72	72
	95th	110	110	112	113	114	115	116	73	73	73	74	75	76	76
8	90th	108	109	110	111	112	113	114	70	70	71	71	72	73	74
	95th	112	112	113	115	116	117	118	74	74	75	75	76	77	78
9	90th	110	110	112	113	114	115	116	71	72	72	73	74	74	75
	95th	114	114	115	117	118	119	120	75	76	76	77	78	78	79
10	90th	112	112	114	115	116	117	118	73	73	73	74	75	76	76
	95th	116	116	117	119	120	121	122	77	77	77	78	79	80	80
11	90th	114	114	116	117	118	119	120	74	74	75	75	76	77	77
	95th	118	118	119	121	122	123	124	78	78	79	79	80	81	81
12	90th	116	116	118	119	120	121	122	75	75	76	76	77	78	78
	95th	120	120	121	123	124	125	126	79	79	80	80	81	82	82
13	90th	118	118	119	121	122	123	124	76	76	77	78	78	79	80
	95th	121	122	123	125	126	127	128	80	80	81	82	82	83	84
14	90th	119	120	121	122	124	125	126	77	77	78	79	79	80	81
	95th	123	124	125	126	128	129	130	81	81	82	83	83	84	85
15	90th	121	121	122	124	125	126	127	78	78	79	79	80	81	82
	95th	124	125	126	128	129	130	131	82	82	83	83	84	85	86
16	90th	122	122	123	125	126	127	128	79	79	79	80	81	82	82
	95th	125	126	127	128	130	131	132	83	83	83	84	85	86	86
17	90th	122	123	124	125	126	128	128	79	79	79	80	81	82	82
	95th	126	126	127	129	130	131	132	83	83	83	84	85	86	86

A *Blood pressure percentile was determined by a single reading.
†Height percentile was determined by standard growth curves.

Blood Pressure Levels for the 90th and 95th Percentiles of Blood Pressure for Boys Aged 1 to 17 Years by Percentiles of Height

Age (Yr)	Blood Pressure Percentile*	Systolic Blood Pressure by Percentile of Height, mm Hg†							Diastolic Blood Pressure by Percentile of Height, mm Hg†						
		5%	10%	25%	50%	75%	90%	95%	5%	10%	25%	50%	75%	90%	95%
1	90th	94	95	97	98	100	102	102	50	51	52	53	54	54	55
	95th	98	99	101	102	104	106	106	55	55	56	57	58	59	59
2	90th	98	99	100	102	104	105	106	55	55	56	57	58	59	59
	95th	101	102	104	106	108	109	110	59	59	60	61	62	63	63
3	90th	100	101	103	105	107	108	109	59	59	60	61	63	63	63
	95th	104	105	107	109	111	112	113	63	63	64	65	66	67	67
4	90th	102	103	105	107	109	110	111	62	62	63	64	65	66	66
	95th	106	107	109	111	113	114	115	66	67	67	68	69	70	71
5	90th	104	105	106	108	110	112	112	65	65	66	67	68	69	69
	95th	108	109	110	112	114	115	116	69	70	70	71	72	73	74
6	90th	105	106	108	110	111	113	114	67	68	69	70	70	71	72
	95th	109	110	112	114	115	117	117	72	72	73	74	75	76	76
7	90th	106	107	109	111	113	114	115	69	70	71	72	72	73	74
	95th	110	111	113	115	116	118	119	74	74	75	76	77	78	78
8	90th	107	108	110	112	114	115	116	71	71	72	73	74	75	75
	95th	111	112	114	116	118	119	120	75	76	76	77	78	79	80
9	90th	109	110	112	113	115	117	117	72	73	73	74	75	76	77
	95th	113	114	116	117	119	121	121	76	77	78	79	80	80	81
10	90th	110	112	113	115	117	118	119	73	74	74	75	76	77	78
	95th	114	115	117	119	121	122	123	77	78	79	80	80	81	82
11	90th	112	113	115	117	119	120	121	74	74	75	76	77	78	78
	95th	116	117	119	121	123	124	125	78	79	79	80	81	82	83
12	90th	115	116	117	119	121	123	123	75	75	76	77	78	78	79
	95th	119	120	121	123	125	126	127	79	79	80	81	82	83	83
13	90th	117	118	120	122	124	125	126	75	76	76	77	78	79	80
	95th	121	122	124	126	128	129	130	79	80	81	82	83	83	84
14	90th	120	121	123	125	126	128	128	76	76	77	78	79	80	80
	95th	124	125	127	128	130	132	132	80	81	81	82	83	84	85
15	90th	123	124	125	127	129	131	131	77	77	78	79	80	81	81
	95th	127	128	129	131	133	134	135	81	82	83	83	84	85	86
16	90th	125	126	128	130	132	133	134	79	79	80	81	82	82	83
	95th	129	130	132	134	136	137	138	83	83	84	85	86	87	87
17	90th	128	129	131	133	134	136	136	81	81	82	83	84	85	85
	95th	132	133	135	136	138	140	140	85	85	86	87	88	89	89

B *Blood pressure percentile was determined by a single measurement.
†Height percentile was determined by standard growth curves.

Figure 10–17 *A* and *B*, Blood pressure levels for children aged 1 to 17 years. (From The Task Force on Blood Pressure Control in Children. Pediatrics 98:653-654, 1996.)

chapter 11

Clinical Evaluation of Gastrointestinal Symptoms in Children

PHILIP C. BAGNELL

Excesses in the efficiencies of managed care and the allure of impressive, yet often unnecessary, investigations can threaten our ability to be of greatest service to our patients. A carefully structured interview and physical examination always offer the largest diagnostic yield at the least cost. This chapter provides guidelines that should facilitate development of the clinical skills you need to deal effectively with most children with gastrointestinal (GI) symptoms.

THE HISTORY

Pediatric teaching is replete with admonitions for the inexperienced—for example, bilious vomiting in the very young child signifies obstructive disease until proven otherwise. An equally important caution is that if you do not understand what is wrong with a child, revisit the history. Manifestations of dysfunction and disease usually make pathophysiologic sense.

AGE ASSOCIATIONS

Pediatrics spans the spectrum from the tiny premature infant to the healthy adolescent, and sometimes beyond. Within this diverse population, the common causes of any given symptom differ significantly by age group. For example, idiopathic intussusception is uncommon in a 12-year-old child but is a reasonable possibility in a 12-month-old child who has an acute onset of severe, colicky abdominal pain. Major malformations and serious metabolic diseases usually manifest during the early months of childhood. Congenital abnormalities, such as tracheoesophageal fistula, intestinal atresia, malrotation, duplications, Meckel diverticulum, Hirschsprung disease, and

imperforate anus, must always be considered whenever you encounter a newborn or young infant with unexplained GI symptoms.

COMMON SYMPTOMS

Swallowing Difficulties

Swallowing is a complex function. Food is chewed, then transferred to the posterior pharynx where esophageal peristalsis is stimulated. The process requires neurologic coordination as well as a structurally normal esophagus. *Dysphagia* (difficulty with swallowing) may be related to food transfer to the posterior pharynx but should be considered an esophageal symptom if there is any doubt about the cause.

Key Point

When dysphagia is esophageal, the swallowed food is felt to "stick" or "catch," and the sensation occurs *after* the food has started down the esophagus.

The sensation of a lump in the throat *before* swallowing suggests a "globus sensation" rather than true dysphagia.

Dysphagia is caused by abnormal esophageal peristalsis, a motor disorder, or mechanical obstruction of the esophageal lumen. Obstruction or narrowing of the lumen may be extramural (e.g., a vascular ring), mural (e.g., mucosal disease or a stricture), or intraluminal (e.g., a swallowed foreign body). In the absence of a complete blockage, most obstructive processes result in difficulty with swallowing lumpy, solid food, but not liquids. With mild narrowing of the esophagus, solids that are minced or well chewed may not cause symptoms, whereas food that is difficult to chew may catch or stick or may simply not be swallowed.

Dysphagia for both liquids and solids suggests a primary motor problem. Fluctuating or intermittent symptoms are also more suggestive of a motor disorder. Clearing an impacted bolus by vomiting suggests an obstructive process, whereas clearing by rinsing the bolus down with water is more consistent with a motor disorder. Pain with swallowing (*odynophagia*) and heartburn (*pyrosis*) are esophageal symptoms that suggest mucosal disease, such as esophagitis.

THE INFANT

Swallowing begins in utero, shortly after the fourth month. By term, the fetus is swallowing up to one-half liter a day of amniotic fluid.

Key Point

Inability to swallow amniotic fluid, as occurs when the fetus has esophageal atresia, results in polyhydramnios.

After birth, the combination of excessive secretions from the mouth, feeding difficulties, and respiratory distress should always suggest esophageal atresia until proven otherwise. Newborn feeding problems may also be seen with other anomalies, such as choanal atresia. Being obligatory nose breathers in early life, infants with choanal atresia are unable to breathe when their mouths are sealed around a nipple during feeding.

The feeding and swallowing pattern of infants is unique. The fetus can both suck and swallow by approximately 20 weeks' gestation, but the ability to feed effectively (nutritive sucking), is not developed until approximately 34 weeks' gestation. During nutritive sucking, the infant sucks in rhythmic bursts and swallows several times during each sustained burst. This pattern requires normal muscle tone and neuromuscular coordination; anything that interferes with tone or coordination may interfere with effective feeding. Excessive maternal sedation may be transmitted to the fetus and may slow nutritive sucking for several days after delivery.

Neuromuscular diseases may also interfere with the oral and pharyngeal phases of swallowing. During these phases, the contents of the mouth are passed through the pharynx to the esophagus without reflux into the nasal cavity or respiratory tract. Neurologically handicapped children, such as those with spastic cerebral palsy, may have feeding problems related to the oropharyngeal phase of swallowing. They also may drool excessively because of their swallowing difficulties. Examination of such children may reveal an intolerance of having anything placed in the mouth (*oral hypersensitivity*), drooling, tongue thrusting, and an exaggerated gag response. Cleft palate and other anatomic abnormalities frequently cause feeding difficulties, but tongue-tie is rarely, if ever, a problem.

THE TODDLER

Infants and toddlers do not complain about swallowing difficulties; they simply refuse to eat or they gag when attempting to eat. Because food refusal for a variety of nonorganic reasons is not uncommon in toddlers, it may be a challenge to decide whether a child is really having problems swallowing (i.e., true dysphagia) or is simply being oppositional. A child may refuse to swallow simply because he or she dislikes the taste or texture of a new food. You need to take a careful history, because the toddler with true esophageal dysphagia may also spit out lumpy food without attempting to swallow. A sudden change in ability to swallow, especially with dysphagia for both liquids and solids, should always suggest the possibility of a foreign body in the esophagus, particularly in this age group.

OLDER CHILDREN AND ADOLESCENTS

Dysphagia in an older child or adolescent should suggest a disease until proven otherwise. Patients in these age groups may show dramatic anxiety associated with swallowing problems, but their dysphagia should not be considered a psychiatric symptom without careful evaluation for an organic cause.

Case History

Case 1
Rachel is an 11-year-old who was referred by her psychiatrist for assessment of swallowing difficulties. Two months earlier she had choked on a piece of meat. Thereafter, she became very fearful of swallowing and refused to swallow anything but liquids. She had always had a tiny appetite, but had no previous history of swallowing difficulties. She did, however, have a history of recurrent heartburn.

Her parents described her as being very timid. She experienced fears of being kidnapped and of having cancer. She was afraid to swallow and was worried about losing weight. Her psychiatrist was treating her for an anxiety disorder but was concerned that she might have other problems.

Rachel was born at 28 weeks' gestation and weighed 1219 g (2 lb 10 oz) at birth. Her neonatal course was complicated by respiratory distress syndrome. After discharge from the neonatal intensive care unit, her weight and height remained below the third percentile but increased parallel with the third percentile. Her development was normal, and she did well in school.

On examination, she was thin, tiny, and prepubertal. Her height age was 7.5 years, and her weight age 5.75 years. She was very apprehensive, but general physical findings were normal.

Because of her dysphagia, the physician requested a barium swallow study. This procedure demonstrated an esophageal stricture, 2 to 3 cm long at the junction of the middle and distal thirds of the esophagus (Fig. 11–1). A small hiatal hernia was also visualized. At gastroscopy, the pediatric gastroscope could not be advanced through the stricture. The stricture was dilated. Biopsy specimens from the distal esophagus had features consistent with chronic esophagitis.

After the esophageal dilatation, Rachel's reflux esophagitis was treated medically. She also continued with psychotherapy. Helping Rachel gain the confidence to swallow solids took several weeks, but she then did well. She initially required several more esophageal dilations, but has not needed such a procedure for the past couple of years. Her anxiety symptoms have not correlated with the waxing and waning of her esophageal symptoms.

Comment. Adolescents may have anxiety secondary to dysphagia, and both may quickly disappear once the dysphagia resolves. As Rachel's case demonstrates, organic and psychiatric diseases are not mutually exclusive. Her anxiety may have been worse when she had dysphagia, but she had both primary esophageal disease and a primary psychiatric diagnosis. Dysphagia requires evaluation.

Regurgitated gastric contents, heartburn, and dysphagia suggest a diagnosis of gastroesophageal reflux disease (GERD), with esophagitis as a complication of the reflux. When dysphagia is associated with regurgitation of non-acid esophageal contents, one has to consider the possibility of *achalasia*. In achalasia, there is absence of effective peristalsis and pooling of swallowed food in the distal esophagus because of failure of the lower esophageal sphincter to relax. The esophagus empties poorly, and food accumulates in the dilated, atonic distal esophagus.

Vomiting

Vomiting is a complex, forceful act that is usually associated with nausea and retching. Regurgitation can be quite forceful but is usually a less forceful act in which gastric contents roll out with little effort and no nausea. Regurgitation in the young child is common and is most often the symptomatic manifestation of gastroesophageal reflux (GER).

Because vomiting is common in children, you must assess it in the clinical context in which it occurs. Is the child febrile? Is vomiting the major symptom (e.g., as in pyloric stenosis), one component of other GI symptoms (e.g., as in acute gastroenteritis), or associated with other systemic symptoms (e.g., as in acute pyelonephritis)? What is vomited? Gastric acid causes milk or formula to curdle and smell sour. Bilious vomiting suggests bowel obstruction in the younger child, but emesis may also become bilious after an hour or two of forceful retching and vomiting. Feculent vomiting indicates either distal small bowel obstruction or large bowel obstruction with an incompetent ileocecal valve. Emesis containing food eaten 12 hours earlier suggests there is a significant delay in gastric emptying. Blood in the emesis may come from an inflamed or torn mucosal surface, from variceal bleeding, or from the arterial bleeding of a duodenal ulcer. A "coffee grounds" appearance to the emesis indicates digestion of blood by gastric acid.

What is the relationship between pain and vomiting? In most acute surgical conditions, the pain usually starts

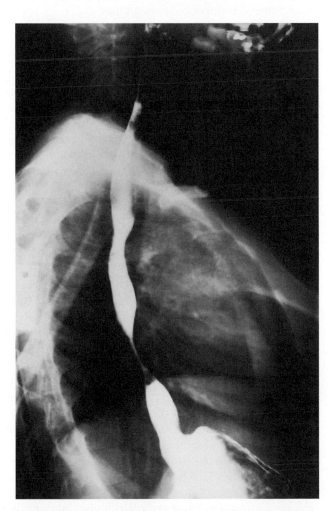

Figure 11–1 Barium swallow examination demonstrating a 2- to 3-cm long smooth tapering stricture at the junction of the middle and distal thirds of the esophagus.

before the vomiting. With high bowel obstruction, crampy central pain is quickly followed by vomiting, but the farther the site of obstruction is along the intestine, the longer the interval between the start of pain and the onset of vomiting. Intussusception may cause vomiting early in the course of the illness, but the vomiting is usually related to the severity of the pain and occurs before there is a significant obstructive component. With nonsurgical diseases, such as an acute gastroenteritis, vomiting starts before pain.

INFANTS

Most babies regurgitate small amounts of soured or curdled milk after feedings, and they do so with little effort and no warning. Half of all healthy 2-month-old infants regurgitate some gastric contents almost every day, sometimes after almost every feeding. If the regurgitated gastric contents are not streaked with bile or blood, the regurgitation is effortless, and the infant is otherwise healthy, GER is the most likely cause.

Key Point

Because virtually all infants spit up occasionally, it may be difficult to determine where normal blends into abnormal. No investigation is needed, however, in the healthy, growing infant who simply regurgitates between feedings but has no other symptoms.

Although most neurologically normal babies with GER do well with little intervention, neurologically impaired infants require more attention. Such infants not infrequently experience complications secondary to GER. Complications are uncommon in neurologically normal children.

Infants born with congenital abnormalities of the GI tract often demonstrate symptoms during the first week of life. Bile-stained emesis, failure to pass meconium in the first 24 hours, and abdominal distention in the newborn strongly suggest obstruction, which should be assumed until proven otherwise. Necrotizing enterocolitis, the most common acquired GI emergency in neonatal intensive care units, should be suspected when a premature or low-birth-weight baby starts to feed poorly and has abdominal distention, blood in stools, and bile-stained emesis.

TODDLERS

Most vomiting in toddlers is caused by infection. Acute febrile illnesses, including ear infection, streptococcal sore throat, and urinary tract infection, are all common causes of vomiting. GI infections are also common in toddlers, causing both vomiting and diarrhea. Not all congenital anomalies of the GI tract manifest in infancy, and recurrent episodes of vomiting with abdominal pain should suggest the possibility of recurrent obstruction.

OLDER CHILDREN

Cyclic vomiting is a unique childhood syndrome. Affected children, who are otherwise healthy, have recurrent episodes of vomiting often associated with abdominal pain. The vomiting episodes start without warning, commonly in the early hours of the morning. Vomiting is usually forceful and may cause dehydration. Recurrent vomiting may persist for hours or days. The children recover spontaneously but may have recurrent attacks at regular intervals. Conduct the history-taking and physical examination so as to consider a differential diagnosis including migraine, intermittent bowel obstruction, metabolic disease, and even recurrent urinary tract obstruction. Of the children with a defined cause for cyclic vomiting, most have migraine, and many later develop classic migraine.

Abdominal Pain

Visceral pain is the most common type of abdominal pain in childhood (Table 11–1). Because the abdominal viscera receive sensory afferent nerves from both sides of the spinal cord, visceral pain is a poorly localized, midline pain that is felt in the area corresponding to the dermatome from which the affected organ receives its nerve supply. For example, small bowel pain is felt in the periumbilical region. If autonomic nervous system activity accompanies visceral pain, dizziness, sweating, nausea, vomiting, and pallor may also occur. With more intense stimulation, and usually with an inflammatory component, visceral pain may be referred. *Referred pain* is felt some distance from the diseased organ but in areas that are supplied by somatic nerves entering the spinal cord at the same neurosegment that supplies the organ causing the pain. Referred pain suggests organic disease and is unlikely to be seen with functional bowel disease.

Unlike visceral pain, *parietal pain* is steady and well localized. It is caused by inflammation of the parietal peritoneum and is felt at the point of irritation. Because movement increases peritoneal irritation and pain, children with parietal peritoneal pain walk slowly, ease themselves from one position to another, and move as little as possible. This behavior is in sharp contrast with the restlessness, bending, and twisting of the child having recurrent episodes of colicky visceral pain. With localized peritonitis, there is also an involuntary protective spasm of the abdominal muscles in the region of

Table 11–1   LOCATION OF VISCERAL ABDOMINAL PAIN

Organ	Site of Pain	Site of Referred Pain
Esophagus	Substernal	Mid-back
Stomach	Epigastric	
Duodenum	Epigastric, right upper abdomen	Back
Small intestine	Mid-abdomen in broad periumbilical area	—
Distal ileum	Mid-abdomen, right lower quadrant	—
Colon	Lower mid-abdomen	—
Rectum	Lower back (sacral area)	—
Gallbladder, common bile duct	Epigastric, right upper quadrant	Right scapular region between scapulae; right shoulder
Pancreas	Epigastric	Mid-back and also left shoulder if diaphragm is irritated
Liver	Right upper quadrant, epigastric	—
Spleen	Left upper quadrant	Left shoulder

the pain. Parietal pain always indicates significant intra-abdominal disease.

Examination of children with parietal pain must be gentle. Listen for the presence or absence of bowel sounds, and while doing so, use your stethoscope to gain an appreciation of the level of abdominal tenderness, as described in Chapter 12. Gently palpate the abdomen, and note areas of tenderness, guarding, and fullness. There is no indication for assessment of rebound tenderness, which gives no information that cannot be obtained by gentle, careful palpation or gentle percussion. When a diagnosis is not suggested by the abdominal examination, a rectal examination is indicated to further assess for peritoneal irritation or an abdominal or pelvic fullness.

INFANTS

When infants cry, they are often believed to have abdominal pain. When crying is recurrent, the infant is said to have colic. Although the term *infantile colic* was probably used because of the suspected similarity of its symptoms to symptoms of intestinal colic, it does not have any pathophysiologic implication. The cause of

infantile colic is unknown. It is a syndrome of recurrent, intense, and inconsolable crying in otherwise healthy infants. Most infants with "colic" are free of symptoms during the day but have recurrent evening episodes of crying. However, normal, healthy infants also cry for prolonged periods, most commonly in the evening, and it may be difficult to define the boundaries of normal for these children. The problem is compounded by the wide variability in parental tolerance for crying.

Key Point

Studies suggest that the average amount of crying in normal infants increases from 2 hours a day at 2 weeks to a maximum of 3 hours daily at 6 weeks and that by 3 months of age, normal infants cry for an hour or less each day.

Colic should be diagnosed on the basis of a typical history and normal physical findings. Minimal criteria have been suggested as the "rule of threes"—vigorous crying for at least 3 hours a day and at least 3 days a week. With a very atypical history of "colic," you must inquire about other causes of irritability and pain. Is the baby febrile or ill? Are there other symptoms? Is the crying related to handling? Does it occur in certain settings, but not in others? There is an understandable temptation to overuse the diagnosis of colic. Acute onset of crying in an infant with no past history of colic, however, should not be dismissed simply as colic.

Acute episodes of severe abdominal pain in the infant always call for urgent assessment. Middle to late infancy is the peak age for intussusception, with two thirds of all cases occurring in the first year of life. *Intussusception* is the telescoping of a proximal segment of bowel (usually the distal ileum) into the distal segment. The onset is sudden. Typically, the infant screams with pain, draws up both legs, and cannot be settled. Because the intussusceptum lodges in the distal bowel segment, the entrapment causes vascular obstruction with engorgement and mucosal swelling. Eventually, blood and mucus ooze from the entrapped bowel and are passed through the rectum. At this stage, the bowel becomes obstructed, and the intussusceptum becomes ischemic and gangrenous if the process is not reversed. Examination of the infant is almost impossible during episodes of pain, but between episodes, the baby may sleep or become quiet enough to be examined. Typical findings in ileocolic intussusception are a flat right lower quadrant and a palpable, sausage-shaped mass in the right upper quadrant, either in the region of the hepatic flexure or more distally along the course of the colon. It is unusual, however, to be able to examine children with intussusception adequately, and early diagnosis is based mostly on the assessment that the infant has had an acute onset of severe colicky abdominal pain.

CHILDREN AND ADOLESCENTS

The combination of crampy, intermittent abdominal pain, joint pain, and a purpuric rash should suggest Henoch-Schönlein purpura (HSP). Once the rash appears, diagnosis usually is not difficult. The rash is purpuric and is located mainly on the buttocks and lower extremities. Abdominal pain may be severe and may lead to laparotomy if HSP is not suspected. This scenario is most likely to happen when the abdominal pain precedes the development of the rash and joint symptoms, making early diagnosis difficult. GI complications, including intussusception and intestinal perforation, may occur with HSP, but fortunately are seen in fewer than 5% of cases. HSP is a clinical diagnosis, as there is no defining diagnostic test.

Recurrent abdominal pain (RAP) in healthy children is a common problem in primary care. It is almost 40 years since Apley's initial studies on school children with RAP, but much of our approach to such children still reflects his influence. Although not completely satisfactory, his definition of a *recurrent* process—with pain severe enough to interfere with activity and at least three recurrent episodes over a 3-month period—identified the criteria *disability, chronicity,* and *recurrence.* When free of pain, which is most of the time, affected children are healthy. RAP is one of the functional bowel diseases of childhood, and the clinical spectrum extends from self-limiting, almost trivial problems to significant disability and chronic inability to function effectively.

The history must provide the basis for diagnosis and management. Children with RAP look healthy, and physical findings are normal. When asked, the children usually point to the umbilicus as the site of pain. This pain does not interfere with sleep. Nausea, pallor, vomiting, and dizziness suggest secondary autonomic nervous system activity. There are usually surprisingly few symptoms to link the pain to GI function. Rarely, if ever, can a single, specific cause for the pain be identified, and the causes are probably multifactorial. Some children have pain on weekdays only, correlating with school attendance, or pain on weekends only, in situations in which separation or divorce requires a child to spend the week with one parent and the weekend with the other. The history should document associations between the pain and events in the child's life.

Key Point

Psychogenic causes should always be diagnosed on positive grounds, not simply because there is no evidence of organic disease.

Although our terminology is confusing, it is important to remember that a diagnosis of *functional abdominal pain* includes, but is not synonymous with, *psychogenic pain.*

There should be no hesitancy in making a diagnosis of functional abdominal pain on the basis of a careful history, a complete physical examination, and minimal investigation. Because the management of children with functional abdominal pain is rarely specific and often requires changes in coping skills and behavior, you must seek to understand, through the history and your observations, the family's personalities, interactions, strengths, and weaknesses. RAP is obviously a heterogeneous disorder, but the 40 years of experience since Apley's study have shown that careful clinical assessment and a conservative approach to management have served affected children well.

RAP is one of several functional GI disorders commonly seen during the early school years. The *functional GI disorders* are defined as chronic or recurrent GI symptoms that cannot be explained by structural or biochemical abnormalities. They are classified according to the organ of origin and may include symptoms that appear to be referable to the esophagus, stomach, biliary tract, small bowel, or colon.

Key Point

In preadolescents, one of the most common functional bowel disorders is functional constipation, which is often associated with abdominal pain.

During later childhood and adolescence, irritable bowel syndrome is the functional bowel disorder most often associated with constipation and abdominal pain. The functional abdominal pains of childhood usually fit into one of the three following groups:

Nonspecific abdominal pain: As described previously, a pain pattern most commonly seen during the early school years. The pain is poorly described and is most often centrally located in the periumbilical area. There may be headache, dizziness, nausea, and excessive fatigue, but few other symptoms. The children look healthy, and the physical examination is normal.

Dyspepsia: A poorly descriptive, one-word term for several combinations of upper GI symptoms. Heartburn, early satiety, pain associated with eating, and belching are some of the symptoms that might suggest an upper GI tract origin. *Functional dyspepsia* implies that the symptoms are not secondary to GER, *Helicobacter* gastritis, or other acid-pepsin disease.

Irritable bowel syndrome: The combination of abdominal pain with altered bowel habits, often

---

Table 11–2   CRITERIA FOR DIAGNOSIS OF IRRITABLE BOWEL SYNDROME

1. Abdominal pain that is relieved by defecation or is associated with a change in the consistency or frequency of stool.
2. A variable pattern of defecation at least 25% of the time with at least three of the following findings:
   - Altered stool frequency
   - Altered stool form (constipation, diarrhea)
   - Straining, urgency, feeling of incomplete evacuation
   - Passage of mucus with stool
   - Feeling of abdominal distention, bloating

---

with a sensation of bloating, is consistent with a diagnosis of irritable bowel (Table 11–2).

EXAMINATION OF THE ABDOMEN FOR ABDOMINAL PAIN

Inspection

The abdomen changes in size and shape as the child grows, being prominent in the newborn and becoming flatter during the early school years. Marked distention with a shiny appearance to the skin is abnormal at any age. Air, fluid, or solid tissue enlargement may cause abdominal distention. A very flat or scaphoid abdomen, particularly in the newborn, raises the possibility that something is missing, as when abdominal contents are located in the thorax with a congenital diaphragmatic hernia. Occasionally, an ileocecal intussusception also causes the right lower quadrant to appear "empty."

Auscultation

The bowel sounds of normal peristalsis are heard easily at all ages. Air enters the stomach with the first cry, reaching the ileum by 2 hours of age and the rectum by 3 to 4 hours. In general, you should record the bowel sounds as present or absent. Normal sounds are greater in frequency and volume with any process that increases peristaltic activity, such as eating. The continuous bowel sounds of hyperactive peristalsis may be heard with acute gastroenteritis or lactose intolerance. High-pitched, loud, tinkling rushes indicate an obstructive process. Absence of bowel sounds after 5 minutes of listening suggests a paralytic ileus, but no diagnosis should be established or excluded on the basis of bowel sounds alone.

Palpation

The child should be relaxed and supine with the head slightly flexed, the arms at the sides, and the knees flexed. Rest your warmed, entire palm on as much abdominal surface as possible. Palpation requires gentle flexion of your hand at the metacarpophalangeal joints. Avoid poking and tickling, and always begin with light palpation to avoid causing pain. Explore tenderness gently. Determine its site and severity as well as any associated muscle guarding. Localized tenderness with involuntary guarding is a sign of peritoneal irritation. The presence of voluntary guarding does not exclude peritoneal irritation; it simply makes evaluation more difficult. Testing for rebound tenderness is unnecessary. The same information can be obtained with gentle percussion and without hurting the child.

Gastrointestinal Bleeding

Children may vomit blood (*hematemesis*), pass blood per rectum (*hematochezia*), or present with iron deficiency because of occult blood loss. Hematemesis may be bright red or may be dark and resemble coffee grounds. Hematemesis may result from swallowed blood or come from an upper GI bleeding site proximal to the ligament of Treitz. Rectal bleeding, however, may originate anywhere in the GI tract.

Hematochezia is the passage of bright red or maroon blood per rectum, either alone or mixed with stool. It results from either small bowel or colonic bleeding. The extent of color change from the bright red appearance of fresh blood roughly correlates with the volume of the bleed and the time it takes for blood to pass from the bleeding site to the anal canal. Anal canal bleeding is bright red; proximal colonic bleeding is darker; and small bowel bleeding is usually dark red or maroon.

Color alone is often not a reliable guide to the site of bleeding. *Melena* is the passage of black, tarry-looking stool. For blood to become black and tarry, at least 60 to 100 mL must be lost, and then sufficient time must pass for the hemoglobin to be degraded in the GI tract. As a rule, melena indicates an upper GI bleed. An acute upper GI bleed is the usual cause of the combination of hematemesis and melena. Occult bleeding may come from any level of the GI tract. With occult bleeding, the stool color is normal. A number of medications may alter the color of stools. Iron, charcoal, bismuth preparations, and licorice may cause a stool to appear black, but not usually shiny or sticky; beets, Kool-Aid, food dyes, and some medications may give stools a red color that looks like hematochezia. A stool specimen should be tested for occult blood.

INFANTS

Blood in the GI tract of the healthy newborn is most often maternal in origin. The blood may have been swallowed in the birth canal or during breast-feeding. Babies may swallow a surprising amount of blood while breast-feeding and either have hematemesis or pass altered blood per rectum. Adult hemoglobin denatures on exposure to alkali but fetal hemoglobin does not, so mixing the blood with alkali (Apt-Downey test) determines whether it is of maternal or fetal origin.

The infant with bleeding from multiple sites, including the GI tract, may have hemorrhagic disease of the newborn due to vitamin K deficiency, and the history should explore maternal medications, such as anticonvulsant and antituberculous drugs, as well as whether the infant received parenteral vitamin K at birth. A sick infant with hematochezia, abdominal distention, and bilious vomiting may have a GI emergency, such as necrotizing enterocolitis or midgut volvulus. With either disease, a distended, tender abdomen suggests peritonitis and an urgent situation. Esophagitis secondary to GER may cause hematemesis in the sick neonate.

Key Point

Beyond the newborn period, anal fissures are the most common cause of hematochezia in healthy infants.

Infants with anal fissures cry with the discomfort of bowel movements and pass small stools with bright red blood streaks on the surface. Careful examination with good light may reveal a midline linear crack or tear in the skin of the anal canal. Bright blood mixed through loose stools suggests a bleeding site above the rectum and is most often inflammatory in origin; there are usually leukocytes in the stools as well. Noninfectious colitis in infants may be allergic in origin. Infants with allergic colitis have frequent bowel movements and blood-streaked, loose stools.

Cow's milk protein may damage the small bowel mucosa, and the infant may present with silent, chronic occult blood loss secondary to the enteropathy. Infants with cow's milk–induced enteropathy are not symptomatic, appear well nourished, and are often believed to be healthy, but they gradually experience severe iron deficiency. Because of the gradual nature of this process, such an infant may not come to medical attention until the hemoglobin concentration has dropped to less than 8 to 9 g/dL (Fig. 11–2). Infants with cow's milk protein enteropathy do not have colitis.

YOUNG CHILDREN

Blood streaking in emesis may be secondary to an episode of forceful vomiting. This symptom is not uncommon and is usually transient and self-limiting once the vomiting stops. In the child with massive hematemesis and few, if any, associated symptoms, bleeding from

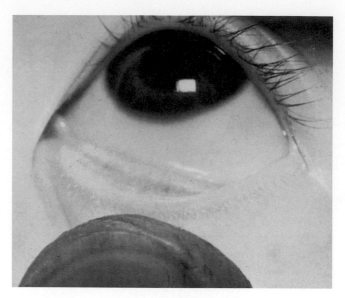

Figure 11–2 Pallor in a 9-month-old with hemoglobin of 8 g/dL. Note the marked pallor when compared with the normal color of the examiner's thumb. His parents did not notice the gradual development of pallor, which is not unusual. There was a history of large intake of evaporated milk formula with almost no solid food intake. His anemia resolved with removal of cow's milk from the diet and supplementation with iron. Anemia associated with cow's milk–induced enteropathy often will not resolve with iron supplements unless cow's milk is stopped.

esophageal varices is the most likely cause. Although uncommon, extrahepatic portal hypertension is the most likely cause of bleeding from esophageal varices in early childhood. More than half the children with extrahepatic portal hypertension bleed from varices before age 5 years. On physical examination, the presence of splenomegaly and of dilated veins over the upper abdomen suggests portal hypertension, whereas a firm or large liver, ascites, edema, and clubbing would indicate that portal hypertension is secondary to liver disease rather than extrahepatic.

Although hematochezia is most commonly caused by either anal fissures or infectious enterocolitis, intermittent painless bright red hematochezia and otherwise normal stools suggests a juvenile polyp. After the first year of life, juvenile polyps are one of the common causes of this type of rectal bleeding through the preteen years. In children with juvenile polyps, physical examination is normal. It is unusual for the blood loss to be significant, and the children are otherwise healthy.

Larger volumes of painless hematochezia, with the passage of what is often a massive amount of darkly colored or maroon blood, is most consistent with Meckel diverticulum or intestinal duplication. The latter is often associated with ectopic gastric or pancreatic mucosa, which may cause peptic ulceration and bleeding. Meckel diverticulum, found in 2% of the population, is the most common anomaly of the GI tract. It is also the most common cause of massive rectal bleeding in healthy children. Apart from the possibility of hemodynamic changes secondary to the acute blood loss, physical examination of a child with a Meckel diverticulum is usually normal.

Diarrhea, abdominal cramping, and low-grade fever are common symptoms in acute gastroenteritis in childhood. However, persistence of such symptoms accompanied by streaks of blood in the stools may be an early manifestation of hemolytic-uremic syndrome (HUS). Affected children may quickly experience microangiopathic hemolytic anemia, thrombocytopenia, and acute renal failure. HUS is seen most commonly after an infection with toxin-producing *Escherichia coli* O157:H7.

OLDER CHILDREN AND ADOLESCENTS

The source of hematemesis is usually suggested by the history. In the healthy child who vomits normal gastric contents one or more times before having hematemesis, the mucosal surface of the lower esophagus or cardia has probably been traumatized (Mallory-Weiss syndrome). Epistaxis or a history of recent tonsillectomy or adenoidectomy suggests swallowed blood and may provide the explanation for both hematemesis and melena. A preceding history of heartburn, with other symptoms suggesting GER, suggests esophagitis as the possible source.

Patients with peptic ulcer may present with hematemesis or melena, but most have a history of symptoms suggesting active peptic ulcer disease for months before the bleeding. Massive hematemesis with ulcer disease most often occurs when the ulcer disease develops secondary to severe illness, as in intensive care settings. Nonsteroidal anti-inflammatory drugs may cause hematemesis from localized gastritis or gastric erosions, in the absence of peptic ulcer disease. As with younger children, massive hematemesis and melena, with few other symptoms, may be the initial clinical presentation of esophageal varices.

Hematochezia and occult blood loss may result from small bowel lesions. Many of the lesions responsible for such bleeding cause no other symptoms. The physical examination, however, may provide helpful clues. The presence of multiple skin and mucous membrane telangiectases should suggest hereditary hemorrhagic telangiectasia (Osler-Weber-Rendu disease). However, typical skin lesions may not yet have appeared in younger patients with bleeding. Hypertrophy of one or more extremities with angiomas of the skin may be associated with similar vascular lesions in the small bowel. Multiple pigmented lesions on the lips and mucosal surface of the mouth are associated with multiple small intestinal hamartomatous polyps in the autosomal dominant Peutz-Jeghers syndrome. Girls with gonadal dysgenesis (Turner syndrome) may have vascular lesions of the bowel that cause bleeding.

Depending on the location of the bleeding, colonic bleeding usually produces bright or dark red hematochezia. The most common cause of colonic bleeding in older children and adolescents is inflammation—either infectious colitis or idiopathic inflammatory bowel disease. Colonic diverticulosis is not seen in children, and internal hemorrhoids are seen only with pregnancy or prolonged, severe portal hypertension.

Constipation

Constipation is the term used to describe an infrequent stool pattern, hard bowel movements, or stools that are difficult to pass.

> **Key Point**
>
> The overwhelming majority of constipated children have functional constipation, not organic disease.

Sometimes, as when a breast-fed baby simply has infrequent bowel movements, the pattern is a variant of normal. However, it may be difficult to tell whether a stool pattern is normal or abnormal. In addition to the guidelines for normal for all ages, a change in stool frequency or consistency also may be relevant, even if the "new" pattern still falls within the range of normal. When determining whether rectal function is normal, you must remember that most people, including children, usually have an empty rectum until just before passing stool. Of the organic diseases causing constipation, the one of greatest concern during the early months of life is Hirschsprung disease.

INFANTS

Infants have few social graces and usually pass stool either during or shortly after each feeding. However, at no other time in life is the normal range of stool frequency so variable as in infancy. Breast-fed infants may pass 10 or more loose stools daily but may also go as long as 7 to 10 days between normal bowel movements. The probability that the stool pattern is normal is usually decided on the basis of associated symptoms or lack thereof. If the infant is feeding well, is gaining weight, and has no vomiting or abdominal distention, careful follow-up will serve the child better than rushing to request investigations.

Straining to have a bowel movement is potentially a sign of constipation but is more likely to be a variant of normal if there are no other symptoms or findings. Some infants simply seem to take time to learn to relax the anal sphincter while straining to pass stool. Perfectly normal babies strain, become deeply flushed, and may even cry while having bowel movements. They do, however, maintain a reasonably normal stool habit and eventually learn to relax the pelvic floor while pushing. This situation is a nondisease that requires no intervention. In an infant who has constipation during the first year, the history of bowel movements during the first few days of life should always influence considerations—failure to pass meconium within the first 24 to 48 hours of life or constipation starting within the first few days of life should always raise suspicions of the possibility of Hirschsprung disease.

Physical examination is of great importance in assessing constipation in infancy. Infants with functional problems or stool patterns that are variations of normal are well nourished and grow well. They do not have abdominal distention. During examination of the anal region, you should take specific note of the appearance and position of the anus. In girls, the distance from the posterior fourchette to the anus is 30% of the distance from the posterior fourchette to the coccyx; in boys, the anus should be located halfway between the scrotum and coccyx. Anterior displacement of the rectum may be associated with constipation. *Imperforate anus* (the absence of a visible anal opening) is an anomaly that obviously requires urgent intervention.

TODDLERS

Toddlerhood is the age of the most common type of childhood functional constipation. Healthy children with normal bowel habits can experience dramatic problems with constipation around the age of toilet training. There are dozens of scenarios, but the common feature is that such a child develops an irrational fear of having a bowel movement and starts to withhold stool. This behavior can originate because the child has a painful bowel movement, is frightened by the flushing of the toilet, or is confused about what is expected. Most often, the cause is not apparent. The end result is fear and crying whenever the child experiences rectal stimulation by the normal descent of stool into the upper rectum. Instead of pushing and squatting to facilitate the passage of stool, the child visibly strains and stands erect with the pelvis pushed forward as he or she squeezes the buttocks together, tightens or crosses the legs, and uses every available muscle to prevent the passage of stool. Parents have surprisingly little understanding of the process, usually interpret the straining as pushing, and are convinced it is becoming impossible for the child to pass stool.

With longer and longer intervals between bowel movements, the diameter of the stool increases (Fig. 11–3). Eventually it becomes so large and hard that it cannot be flushed without being broken up. The chronic retention of stool eventually gives rise to the involuntary and uncontrollable seepage of small

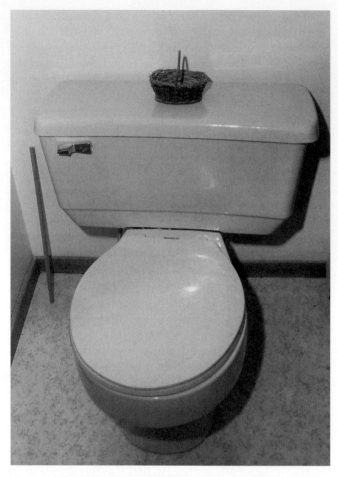

Figure 11–3 With continued holding of stool, toddlers with functional constipation pass stools of larger and larger diameter. These stools commonly plug the toilet, and it is not unusual for the family to keep a stick or a wire coathanger by the toilet to help break up the stool before flushing. Asking the leading question, "Do you keep a stick or coathanger by the toilet?" is often all that is needed to let the parents know you are familiar with the magnitude of the problem.

amounts of foul-smelling, pasty, sticky streaks of stool onto the diaper or underwear. This fecal soiling may occasionally be misinterpreted as diarrhea, particularly if the child's preceding difficulties were not noticed. Examination of such a child often reveals palpable stool in the distal colon and lower abdomen. Rectal examination confirms the presence of a large mass of stool in the anal canal. Rectal examination is rarely necessary on the initial visit, particularly when the history is typical of stool withholding and if fecal masses are palpable in the lower abdomen. However, in a child with soiling but no recognized history of constipation, the diagnosis of constipation is difficult to establish without a rectal examination or an abdominal radiograph.

ADOLESCENTS

Constipation is arbitrarily defined as fewer than three bowel movements a week, with straining or difficulty passing stool more than 25% of the time. There is, however, a great range of normal, and care must be taken to avoid overdiagnosis. Stool withholding and rectal constipation may be seen throughout the early school years but is less commonly seen in adolescence. Functional constipation in this age group is most commonly associated with some combination of abdominal pain, constipation, and a sensation of bloating as the early manifestation of irritable bowel syndrome.

Case History

Case 2

Susan, 12 years old, was referred by her primary care physician for further assessment when a large, hard mass was felt on abdominal palpation. She had not seen a physician for years but was required by the school to have a physical examination for cheerleading trials. She denied having any symptoms but on functional inquiry admitted to going to the bathroom hourly, or even more frequently, to pass small amounts of stool. She could not remember when she had last passed a large bowel movement. She denied having any soiling of her clothes but believed it would happen if she did not go to the bathroom frequently.

She had had normal bowel habits during her early childhood and no history of constipation until age 5 years. She then became constipated and started to have soiling. Her mother related the onset of constipation to the breakup of the family following her divorce. There was no follow-up of the problem, and Susan simply learned to live with it.

On physical examination, Susan looked healthy. Her weight was at the 10th percentile, and her height at the 5th percentile. Her abdomen was not distended, but palpation revealed multiple smooth masses of stool filling the abdomen from the pelvic brim to the epigastric region. An abdominal radiograph demonstrated retention of massive amounts of stool throughout the colon (Fig. 11–4).

Treatment with oral polyethylene glycol–solution facilitated evacuation of her colon. Susan was then started on mineral oil therapy. With this treatment, she began to have normal bowel habits for the first time in years.

Comment. Functional constipation during the early childhood years usually resolves with appropriate management but does not always "go away." This is an extreme, but not isolated, example of persistence of a functional problem and of its potential effect on the social development of a child.

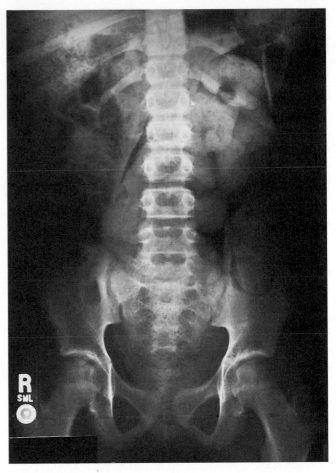

Figure 11–4 Functional constipation in a 12-year-old child. There is marked retention of stool throughout the colon. Black air shadows can be seen outlining the stool-distended rectum just medial to the pelvic brim on both sides. Onset of constipation with soiling was at 5 years of age.

RECTAL EXAMINATION FOR CONSTIPATION

Key Point

A rectal examination should be performed *only* when specifically required for diagnosis or treatment. It should not be considered a routine part of the general physical examination.

When a rectal examination is necessary, explain the procedure, and avoid surprises. Press a well-lubricated, gloved finger gently against the anal orifice, and exert pressure against one wall of the canal as you very slowly advance the fingertip. Some younger children worry about the lubricant on the glove but may be partly reassured by being allowed to touch the lubricant first. The normal rectum is empty, or nearly so. A rectum full of hard stool, particularly if the stool surface is smooth, suggests chronic retention of stool. A history of constipation with an empty rectum is unusual in children but may be seen with irritable bowel syndrome.

Diarrhea

Healthy North American adults produce 100 to 200 g of stool each day. The normal infant's stool output is 5 to 10 g per kg of body weight daily, up to the normal adult stool weight. *Diarrhea* is an increase in the daily fluid losses, and volume, of stool. The increase is usually associated with looser and more frequent stools, but greater stool frequency alone does not necessarily indicate diarrhea.

Diarrhea may be acute, chronic, or recurrent. *Acute* diarrhea is common and is most often infectious in origin. Diarrhea persisting beyond 2 weeks is arbitrarily designated *chronic*. Pathophysiologic and anatomic classifications may help with clinical problem-solving, but both have limitations and must be supplemented by knowledge of the common causes of diarrhea in each age group. The pathophysiology of diarrhea is usually based on some combination of the following three mechanisms: (1) increased secretion, (2) decreased absorption, and (3) exudation. Small bowel disease is suggested by a history of large, watery bowel movements and crampy, central abdominal pain. During episodes of small bowel diarrhea, bowel sounds are hyperactive. Large bowel diarrhea is often associated with left colon and rectal disease that produces a sense of urgency and frequent, small-volume stools. Defecation relieves the cramping, at least temporarily. Large bowel pain is referred to the lower abdomen, left lower quadrant, and, occasionally, lower back. Hematochezia with the diarrhea suggests large bowel disease.

Sudden onset of fever, vomiting, and diarrhea suggests an infectious process. In this setting, massive watery bowel movements, central abdominal pain, and vomiting are consistent with gastroenteritis, whereas smaller volume, more frequent stools, crampy lower abdominal pain, and hematochezia are more consistent with an infectious colitis. It is not unusual for a child with colitis to be symptomatic at night. If infectious diarrhea is suspected, additional history-taking should explore exposure to toddlers, foreign travel, exposure to untested water, and history of antibiotic use. Even a single dose of an antibiotic can trigger the development of pseudomembranous colitis.

INFANT

As mentioned previously, the range of normal is so wide that it is sometimes difficult to be sure that an infant actually has diarrhea. For the first 3 to 4 weeks of life, normal breast-fed infants may have as many as 10 to 12 bowel movements daily, and these may be small, seedy, and wet. In the breast-fed infant, in fact, there may be a mild degree of lactose malabsorption as a physiologic finding. Testing the stool water of a healthy breast-fed baby may reveal 0.25% to 0.50% reducing substances.

TODDLERS

Toddlers often attend daycare, do not wash their hands well, and put almost everything in their mouths. Not surprisingly, they commonly have infectious diarrheas. Most of the organisms involved cause a watery, large-volume, osmotic diarrhea that improves quickly if oral intake briefly stops. However, some bacterial infections may produce an enterocolitis, with bloody diarrhea and fever. Some toddlers do not recover from viral diarrhea as quickly as their peers or siblings. One of the more common causes of persistent postviral diarrhea is a disaccharide intolerance secondary to the mucosal damage caused by the viral illness. Affected children have watery diarrhea, central abdominal cramping, and the passage of excessive flatus with an acidic stool that excoriates their buttocks.

Failure of an acute voluminous diarrhea to subside when the child is taking absolutely nothing by mouth suggests a secretory diarrhea. These conditions are not common, but one of the secretory diarrheas to be considered in an otherwise healthy toddler with recurrent diarrhea is a laxative-induced diarrhea as a manifestation of so-called Munchausen syndrome by proxy.

Chronic diarrhea is not uncommon in toddlers. Most toddlers with chronic diarrhea are happy, healthy, and growing normally. They simply pass three to five large, mushy bowel movements daily. There is often a concern that their stool contains undigested food particles, such as whole peas, corn, and other cellulose-containing food. Because toddlers do not chew well, the appearance of this undigested food is of no clinical significance.

Key Point

Diet may play a role in *toddler diarrhea*, so you should pay particular attention to the child's juice and fluid intake. Excessive apple juice intake is a common cause, and the diarrhea may be improved or even cured simply by elimination of apple juice from the child's diet.

Physical examination is normal in children with toddler diarrhea. When chronic or recurrent diarrhea is associated with failure to thrive, a normal or increased appetite, and recurrent or chronic respiratory infections, cystic fibrosis must be considered. An abnormal stool pattern in a child with failure to thrive, abdominal cramping, and a personality change a few months after the introduction of wheat into the diet should suggest celiac disease.

ADOLESCENTS

Acute diarrhea in adolescents is most commonly infectious. Most infections are self-limiting illnesses that do not require intervention. The history should identify factors that might indicate other causes. Fever, rectal urgency, bloody diarrhea, and severe cramping relieved by defecation suggest an inflammatory process in the colon. Antibiotic use, travel, dietary history, exposure to illness, sexual activities, and information about community outbreaks are relevant parts of the history for an adolescent with acute diarrhea.

Jaundice

Jaundice is the yellow discoloration of skin, sclera, and other tissues by bilirubin. It may be difficult to detect in artificial light and is best seen in natural daylight. Gently blanching the child's skin with finger pressure also makes it easier to assess jaundice. In children and adults, the serum bilirubin level has to be greater than 2 to 3 mg/dL (34 to 51 µmol/L) before jaundice is clinically detectable. In both adults and infants, jaundice is first visible in the sclera. The toddler with yellow skin but white sclera usually has carotenemia, not jaundice. A neonate may not appear icteric until the bilirubin reaches 5 to 7 mg/dL (85 to 119 µmol/L). There is also a cephalocaudal progression of jaundice in the newborn—the head and neck are visibly jaundiced when the indirect bilirubin reaches 4 to 8 mg/dL, the upper body at 5 to 12 mg/dL, the lower body and thighs at 8 to 16 mg/dL, the arms and lower legs at 11 to 18 mg/dL, and the palms and soles at greater than 15 mg/dL. As serum bilirubin levels decline, jaundice fades, but it takes a few days for bilirubin to be released from tissues, and the child may still be visibly jaundiced at serum bilirubin levels well below the levels just listed.

The normal serum total bilirubin level is less than 1.5 to 2.0 mg/dL. Almost all the bilirubin in the serum of healthy people is indirect-reacting. Hyperbilirubinemia is classified by the pattern of elevation of the indirect (unconjugated) and direct (conjugated) levels. With indirect-reacting hyperbilirubinemia, the total serum bilirubin level is greater than 2 mg/dL and the direct-reacting component is usually less than 15% of the total. A direct-reacting bilirubin serum level greater than 2 mg/dL is considered a direct-reacting hyperbilirubinemia. Because indirect-reacting bilirubin is fat soluble but not water soluble, it may enter brain tissue, but it is not excreted in the urine. Direct-reacting bilirubin is water soluble and appears in urine when the serum level exceeds 2 mg/dL. Thus, a direct-reacting hyperbilirubinemia may be suspected when a child with jaundice has bilirubin in the urine.

Serum bilirubin levels can rise because of (1) increased production of bilirubin, as occurs with hemolysis, (2) reduced uptake of bilirubin, or (3) a decreased ability to conjugate bilirubin. Increased production, reduced uptake, and decreased conjugation all cause elevation of indirect-reacting bilirubin. Bilirubin that has been conjugated may enter the blood stream because of hepatocyte damage, defective excretion from hepatocyte to canaliculus, or obstruction to flow through the bile ducts. These conditions all cause a direct-reacting hyperbilirubinemia.

INFANT

Indirect-Reacting Hyperbilirubinemia

The placenta clears bilirubin prior to delivery, and as a result, infants are usually not jaundiced at birth. However, with a normal bilirubin production rate of 6 to 8 mg/kg/day and maturational delays in the conjugation and excretion of bilirubin, most infants have indirect-reacting hyperbilirubinemia and jaundice during the first week of life. In the full-term, healthy newborn, the bilirubin rises to a mean level of 4 to 9 mg/dL by the 3rd or 4th postnatal day and disappears by the 7th to 10th postnatal day. The premature infant has a slightly different physiologic profile, with mean serum bilirubin levels rising higher and later, to between 12 and 15 mg/dL by the 5th to 7th postnatal day and not returning to normal until the 14th day. The breast-fed infant also has a different profile, consisting of higher mean bilirubin levels during the first week of life and jaundice that may persist for weeks. The physiologic jaundice seen in most infants is always an indirect-reacting hyperbilirubinemia that develops after the first 24 hours of life. Infants with hyperbilirubinemia during the first day of life, those with severe hyperbilirubinemia (i.e., greater than 15 mg/dL), and those with a prolonged hyperbilirubinemia (i.e., present longer than 10 to 14 days) require further assessment before the process is accepted as physiologic.

Approximately 6% of infants have severe indirect-reacting hyperbilirubinemia (greater than 15 mg/dL), and half of these have a disease that requires intervention or follow-up. In most cases, the cause of jaundice is increased destruction of red blood cells. History-taking for these infants must include a review of hospital records for mother and infant blood types, the cord blood hemoglobin level, Coombs test results, and antibody titers. Polycythemia, as may occur with twin-to-twin transfusion or in the infant of a diabetic mother, may lead to an indirect-reacting hyperbilirubinemia; a review of the records for the cord hemoglobin level is helpful. Extravasated blood, as in a hematoma, may also be a source of increased bilirubin production and is usually diagnosed on physical examination. In such infants, the physical examination should be followed by examination of a blood smear to look for spherocytes (congenital spherocytosis, ABO incompatibility). Approximately 2% of healthy breast-fed infants have moderate indirect hyperbilirubinemia (serum bilirubin level 10 to 15 mg/dL) that lasts for several weeks, occasionally for months. This is a heterogeneous entity, but it appears to result from decreased bilirubin excretion secondary to factors in breast milk that inhibit hepatic conjugation of bilirubin.

Direct-Reacting Hyperbilirubinemia

A direct-reacting bilirubin level of 2 mg/dL or higher indicates disease involving the liver or the biliary tree; it is never physiologic. History of maternal illness may suggest congenital infection, and maternal prenatal records must be reviewed. Infants with severe congenital infection usually have abnormal physical findings, such as a diffuse purpuric rash, microcephaly, hepatomegaly, and splenomegaly. Metabolic diseases, such as galactosemia, hereditary fructose intolerance, and tyrosinemia, may manifest as direct-reacting jaundice and should be suspected in an infant who is feeding poorly, vomiting, or failing to thrive. Even if the infant with direct-reacting hyperbilirubinemia looks healthy and has few other symptoms, idiopathic neonatal hepatitis syndromes and biliary atresia are important considerations early in the course of the abnormality. Because early diagnosis is particularly important for infants with biliary atresia, prompt referral to a pediatrician with special expertise in pediatric liver disease is indicated even for a healthy-looking infant once it is confirmed that the infant has a direct-reacting hyperbilirubinemia of unknown cause.

OLDER CHILDREN AND ADOLESCENTS

Indirect-Reacting Hyperbilirubinemia

Gilbert syndrome, or idiopathic unconjugated hyperbilirubinemia, is the most common cause of indirect-reacting hyperbilirubinemia and jaundice in healthy adolescents. This is a benign condition that usually manifests after puberty. Affected adolescents come to medical attention either because scleral icterus is noted or because an unexplained bilirubin level is reported on a multipanel biochemistry laboratory test that was ordered for unrelated reasons. Most of the time, there are no symptoms, but some patients experience abdominal pain and fatigue. Apart from mild jaundice, physical findings are normal. The serum bilirubin level is usually less than 10 mg/dL and commonly fluctuates between 1 and 4 mg/dL. Fasting, dehydration, strenuous physical exercise, and acute illness may each cause bilirubin levels to increase temporarily. Serum transaminase, alkaline phosphatase, and γ-glutamyl transpeptidase levels are all normal in patients with Gilbert syndrome.

This benign condition may be familial, so for any patient diagnosed with the syndrome, you should inquire about family members with jaundice. Family members with Gilbert syndrome may have been given a diagnosis of hepatitis, so you should ask for details for any family history of hepatitis or chronic liver disease. Hemolytic disease may also produce a mild indirect-reacting bilirubin elevation, so a complete blood count, blood smear, and reticulocyte count are indicated in the investigation of suspected Gilbert syndrome.

Other causes of indirect-reacting hyperbilirubinemia are rare. Crigler-Najjar syndrome type 1 usually begins in the first few days of life and causes bilirubin levels to exceed 20 mg/dL. Bilirubin encephalopathy (i.e., kernicterus) is common in children with this condition. Crigler-Najjar syndrome type 2 is associated with onset of jaundice later in childhood and bilirubin levels of 5 to 20 mg/dL.

Direct-Reacting Hyperbilirubinemia

Viral hepatitis, reactions to drugs or toxins, and chronic liver diseases are the most common causes of elevations of direct-reacting bilirubin in the pediatric population. Gallstones and acute cholecystitis may be seen at any time during childhood, but the jaundice is mild and abdominal pain and vomiting are the more common presenting symptoms. In hepatocellular diseases, such as viral hepatitis and chronic hepatitis, symptoms are often nonspecific, but liver cell damage is often associated with fatigue, a sensation of "not feeling well," and a poor appetite. Nausea and vomiting may accompany the anorexia. The history-taking must include questions about exposure to crowding, conditions of poor sanitation, contact with persons who have hepatitis, and contact with other children in daycare settings. Institutionalized children are at greater risk for hepatitis A. Only 25% of acute cases of hepatitis B cause icterus, but risk factors include a household contact with chronic hepatitis B, adopted foreign children in the family, sexual activity, exposure to blood products, and intravenous drug abuse.

Fewer than one third of the patients with acute hepatitis C will be jaundiced. Risk factors for hepatitis C include exposure to blood products prior to the implementation of hepatitis C screening (1990 in the U.S.), intravenous drug abuse, sexual activity with multiple partners, and close contacts of infected individuals. Drug-associated liver disease is always a potential cause of hepatitis, and all medications, including over-the-counter agents, should be listed in the history. The potential for enhanced toxicity from drug interactions, as has been reported with alcohol abuse and acetaminophen, should be explored.

Chronic liver disease may be surprisingly silent but is usually associated with abnormal physical findings. A search for Kayser-Fleischer rings, suggesting Wilson disease, often requires an ophthalmology consultation. The child with cystic fibrosis and cirrhosis is more likely to present with complications of portal hypertension, rather than jaundice, but an increased anteroposterior chest diameter and other findings of chronic lung disease should suggest the possibility of cystic fibrosis. Prominent superficial veins over the abdominal wall indicate portal vein hypertension and may be secondary to cirrhosis, congenital hepatic fibrosis, or extrahepatic portal hypertension. Ascites, in a patient with jaundice, suggests cirrhosis.

EXAMINATION OF THE LIVER AND SPLEEN IN JAUNDICE

With gentle palpation in the right upper quadrant, you can feel the liver in all pediatric patients, from newborns to adolescents, except in extremely obese youngsters.

Key Point

The secret of palpation is to keep the examining hand still while allowing the child's respiration to move the liver or spleen down.

The lower liver edge is soft, and smooth. Firmness is a significant finding. The most reliable clinical method of assessing liver size is to measure the total span between the upper and lower liver margins. The upper margin is identified by percussion, and the lower margin by palpation. The liver span in children ranges from 6 to 10 cm in the midclavicular line (Fig. 11–5). The liver may be enlarged because of vascular congestion, storage disease, infiltration, fibrosis, or inflammation. It may be tender secondary to acute swelling with stretching of the capsule, as occurs in congestive failure and hepatitis. When cirrhosis is present, liver size varies. In the late stages of disease, the organ is often

small because of scarring and loss of parenchyma, in which case a nodular firmness of the left lobe may be appreciated in the midsternal line.

The spleen may be palpable in normal infants and children. Gentle palpation allows you to appreciate the soft spleen tip during respiration. Allow the spleen tip to move down to your hand during the child's inspiration. The spleen is normally palpable in 30% of newborns, in up to 10% of 1-year-olds, and even in 1% of 12-year-olds. Hepatosplenomegaly occurs in storage diseases, in infiltrative processes, and in cirrhosis with portal hypertension. Prominent superficial abdominal veins and splenomegaly suggest portal hypertension. In portal hypertension, blood flow in the veins is away from the umbilicus. Examination of the extremities may reveal edema, suggesting hypoalbuminemia secondary to chronic liver disease. Clubbing is often seen with cirrhosis. Vascular spiders are usually found in the upper extremities, in the head and neck, and above the midchest in patients with liver disease.

SUMMARY

In primary care settings, most children with GI symptoms have functional bowel disorders, almost all of which are diagnosed through the history and physical examination. With some disorders, such as GER and functional constipation, the anatomic site of dysfunction is known, and the processes reasonably well understood. For others, such as recurrent abdominal pain, non-ulcer dyspepsia, and toddler diarrhea, our knowledge of the pathophysiology is less complete. Although there is no definitive diagnostic test for many of these conditions, there are good guidelines for establishing clinical diagnoses. The clinical diagnostic criteria, such as those established for irritable bowel syndrome and physiologic jaundice of the newborn, provide reliable frameworks within which we may safely and comfortably make clinical deci-

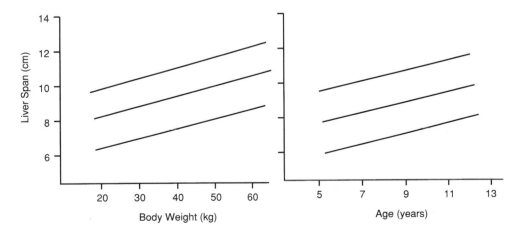

Figure 11–5 Liver span in normal children as related to body weight and age. The outer lines represent the 95% confidence limits. (Adapted from Younoszai MK, Mueller S: Clinical assessment of liver size in normal children. Clin Pediatr 4:378,1975.)

sions. This does not mean that disease cannot exist in children whose clinical presentation falls within the guidelines, only that the probability for such children to have disease is significantly lower. A finding that exceeds the boundaries of a clinical guideline, such as a newborn who goes more than 24 hours after birth without passing stool, does not identify the infant as abnormal. It simply tells us that the proba-

bility of organic disease is higher and may call for further investigation.

REFERENCE

1. Younoszai MK, Mueller S: Clinical assessement of liver size in normal children. Clin Pediatr 4:378, 1975.

chapter 12

Surgical Assessment of the Child's Abdomen

D. A. GILLIS

Often a principal objective in dealing with a child with abdominal symptoms, particularly a child whose symptoms begin acutely, is to determine the presence or absence of a visceral disease that might need surgical intervention. In acute conditions that tend to progress, such as appendicitis and intestinal obstruction, early diagnosis usually results in an improved outcome and fewer complications.

OBTAINING THE HISTORY

A detailed history is an important prerequisite for treating the whole child effectively, whether the problem of the moment happens to be medical or surgical. Especially important to the surgeon is information about preexisting disease, allergies, untoward events associated with anesthesia in the child or in family members, recent medications, familial bleeding tendencies, and recent exposure to infectious disease. Be aware that parents may have been previously unaware of the importance of these details. You might have to obtain records of neonatal events from another hospital because they may also contain important data.

APPROACH TO ABDOMINAL PAIN

Origin of Pain

Abdominal pain is the symptom that surgeons are most often asked to evaluate in children. Remember that pain is mediated by two separate neurologic pathways, visceral and somatic. *Visceral* impulses travel via the autonomic nervous system; pain from a diseased organ is experienced at a level commensurate with its innervation. Pain from small intestinal or appendiceal disease is typically felt in the periumbilical area, because the pathway is at the T10 level (Fig. 12–1). The

somatic expression of pain is mediated by locally distributed pain fibers, and the distress is felt in the area they supply. When the inflamed appendix irritates the adjacent peritoneum, the child complains of pain in the area involved, typically in the right lower quadrant.

Review the expression of visceral pain originating in various abdominal regions so that you can interpret the child's symptoms correctly. Remember, pain is often referred; for example, if fluid in the peritoneal cavity tracks beneath the diaphragm, it may irritate the immediate subdiaphragmatic peritoneum, causing pain in the lateral neck or shoulder because the diaphragmatic peritoneum is also innervated via C3, C4, and C5.

Because young children localize pain poorly, a physician's wits are challenged further. Adolescents and adults

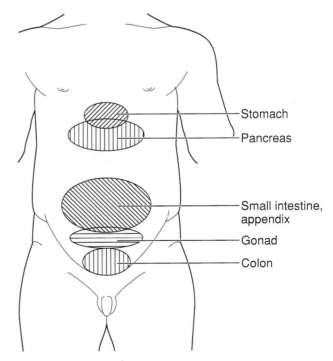

Stomach
Pancreas
Small intestine, appendix
Gonad
Colon

Figure 12–1 Visceral pain is felt over relatively wide areas.

with appendicitis typically describe their pain as starting in the periumbilical area (visceral pain), then shifting to the right lower quadrant as the parietal peritoneum becomes irritated (somatic pain). Clinicians often find it frustrating when young children (who have not read the anatomy books) fail to give them a neat description of this classic shift in location of their pain. Such children are likely to vaguely indicate the central area of the abdomen, often by passing the palm of one hand over this region. It is worth asking the young child to point, using one finger, to the area "where it hurts most," but do not be surprised if this is done inconsistently.

> **Key Point**
>
> It is quite typical for a child with acute appendicitis to point exclusively to the periumbilical area when asked where it hurts. In fact, most children point vaguely to the umbilical area whatever the cause of their pain.

EXTRA-ABDOMINAL CAUSES

Extra-abdominal sources of abdominal pain are common. In children with acute tonsillitis, abdominal pain can even dominate the clinical picture, underlining the importance of a complete and thorough physical examination. In many situations, the mechanism of referred pain remains obscure. Abdominal pain is also a common complaint in children with lower respiratory tract illness. Although this symptom is most characteristic of lower lobe pneumonias, especially of the right lower lobe, it also can occur in children with middle or upper lobe disease. In acute testicular disease, the child's initial complaint may be of severe lower abdominal discomfort, due to the innervation of the testis. Spinal or hip conditions, such as disc space disease or synovitis of the hip joint, may be confusing because the pain may be referred to the abdomen. In contrast, children with acute appendicitis often arrive at the emergency department with a distinct limp caused by protective muscle spasm. Weight bearing and movement aggravate the inflammatory process in the right lower quadrant, and the child may walk "bent over like an old man."

Finally, abdominal pain may be the principal complain in "nonsurgical" abdominal disorders, such as gastroenteritis and urinary tract infections, or in emotional disturbances, emphasizing the need for a detailed history and a truly complete physical examination in any child with abdominal pain.

THE "ACUTE ABDOMEN"

The term *acute abdomen* refers to a clinical state in which an acute intra-abdominal condition usually requires surgical intervention. For many children, the acute pain is a new experience and it may make them miserable, frightened, hostile, and uncooperative.

> **Key Point**
>
> The child's trust and cooperation must never be compromised by anything done during the clinical evaluation. Do not conceal or misrepresent an uncomfortable event, such as blood sampling or a rectal examination.

The time spent taking a history from the parents and child often helps "break the ice" and reassures the child that the physician is there to help, not to hurt.

APPROACH TO THE PHYSICAL EXAMINATION

Perform the physical examination with extreme gentleness and compassion. A famous surgeon once described a gruff colleague's bedside approach as "making a diving poke in the right lower quadrant," a method guaranteed to preclude acquiring useful information. Tell the youngster that you will try your best not to hurt, but do not promise not to cause pain; instead, say that you will "go easy," and then keep your word.

Inspecting the Abdomen

Careful hands-off observation is the essential first step. Look for distention, asymmetry, bruising, and reduced abdominal wall movement with respiration. Once you have checked the extra-abdominal areas—throat, ears, chest, and extremities—adequately, approach the abdomen gently with washed, warm hands. If the child will do so, ask him or her to "puff up" the stomach and note whether this maneuver causes pain (Fig. 12–2).

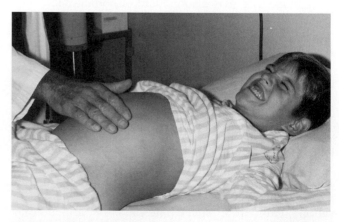

Figure 12–2 Pain is aggravated when the inflamed peritoneum is moved or stretched. "Puffing up" the abdomen causes obvious discomfort.

Hold the palm of one hand an inch or two above the umbilicus, and ask the child to push out the belly far enough to touch that hand.

If you suspect acute inflammatory disease, the diagnostic sine qua non is to identify peritoneal irritation, which may be caused by leaking fluid (blood, bile, pancreatic secretions, gastric or intestinal contents) or by pus. Tenderness produced by an acute insult to the peritoneum may be widespread, as in an intestinal perforation with spillage, or more localized, as in acute appendicitis. The physical findings should reflect the disease process accurately.

Abdominal Palpation

Always palpate gently, with a flat warmed hand, using the least amount of pressure needed to identify underlying soreness. Begin palpation in an area away from the likely site of maximal pain. Feel for muscle resistance, and watch the child's expression. With a little experience, you will find it easy to determine when to stop and move to another quadrant. Sometimes the tenderness is obvious, generalized, and marked. At other times, deep pressure can be exerted in one or two areas but much less in another quadrant. Children with acute appendicitis, for example, may tolerate a considerable amount of palpation in all quadrants except the right lower. They may help quantify tenderness if asked whether it hurts a little or a lot in each area as you assess it.

A significant clinical observation in a child with acute appendicitis is the youngster who winces as the left side of the abdomen is examined but, when asked, reports that it hurts more on the right side than where the physician pressed.

Abdominal Auscultation

Bowel sounds may be absent, but you must listen for at least 2 or 3 minutes to be sure. Bowel sounds are often hyperactive in children with "nonsurgical" inflammatory bowel problems such as acute gastroenteritis, which often causes pain and generalized tenderness. Obstructive bowel sounds are higher pitches ("tinkly"), come in rushes, and have a different auditory quality that is appreciated with experience. Bruits are heard only rarely, and most are not pathologic.

Because your stethoscope has already been used to examine the heart and lungs, youngsters will not associate this procedure with pain, yet they may be more apprehensive about the use of fingers. Therefore, while listening carefully for bowel sounds over each part of the abdomen, press the stethoscope in gently without asking whether it hurts, and simply watch the child's facial expression (Fig. 12–3). Underlying tenderness can be appreciated in this way more readily than would be possible with manual palpation. This use of the stethoscope is a valuable maneuver.

Percussion is equally important, not only to identify unusual accumulations of fluid and organ enlargement but also to recognize peritoneal irritation. Gentle percussion overcomes much of the difficulty that may be encountered with voluntary muscle resistance. Always start by percussing lightly over an area certain to be nontender, such as the iliac crest on the side away from the painful side.

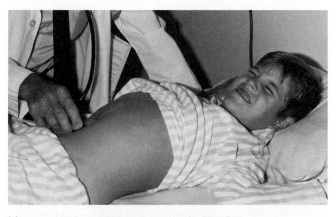

Figure 12–3 The stethoscope can be used to "feel." Gentle pressure over an area of inflamed peritoneum aggravates pain.

Rectal Examination

Rectal examination is invariably uncomfortable. Because the procedure is uncomfortable, tenderness can be difficult to ascertain or quantify, particularly in a very young child. Not infrequently, I have been told by the initial examiner, usually a junior physician, that a young child being evaluated is "tender high on the right side on rectal examination." My response? "Yes, and so are you!"

The younger the patient, the less reliable is the rectal examination in assessing localized inflammatory disease. Do not perform the examination at all if the diagnosis has already been established. If the procedure is absolutely necessary, postpone it until you have completed all other parts of the physical examination. Ideally, rectal examination should be done only once in assessing a child with an acute abdominal illness.

The examination must be preceded and accompanied by an explanation of what is being done and why. Do not tell the child it will not hurt. Lubricate the examining finger of your gloved hand well. Inserting your finger against a tightly contracted anal sphincter adds to the child's discomfort; yet if you gently apply the finger to the anus and then increase the pressure quite gradually, many children relax the sphincter considerably, making the examination easier. A rectal examination can be performed quite quickly; once your finger is in the rectum, you should complete the evaluation in less than half a minute. Rectal examination can identify the presence of a mass or significant fecal retention, and it is occasionally important in an older child in localizing an inflammatory process or similar lesion in the pelvis.

SPECIAL CONSIDERATIONS

Acute Appendicitis

> ### Key Point
>
> Despite its frequency, acute appendicitis continues to present a perplexing diagnostic challenge.

Most youngsters arriving at an emergency department with abdominal pain do not have a surgical illness, but appendicitis crops up often enough to keep us humble. In few children's diseases is bedside clinical assessment so important.

The following points about the history are important in the diagnosis of appendicitis:

1. Pain is typically the first symptom in a sequence of clinical events culminating in appendectomy.
2. Usually gradual in onset, the pain is seldom sudden and severe.
3. The pain seldom disappears completely once it begins, and it builds slowly.
4. The pain is followed, not preceded, by vomiting.
5. The child does not want to walk and is often bothered by even minor bumps when being transported by car. A child who jumps from the examining table without apparent distress probably does not have peritoneal irritation. The child with appendicitis walks cautiously. Experienced emergency department nurses often astutely observe that appendicitis seems likely after merely watching a child walk toward the examining room.
6. Many children with acute appendicitis do not vomit, but they may have nausea, and they do have anorexia, which can be identified as a significant feature by questioning the parents. Most children normally eat a good deal; parents notice a change in that pattern.
7. Diarrhea, usually mild and transient, is not uncommon and is likely to occur early in the evolution of the disease. Rarely, it may be a major symptom for as long as 2 or 3 days before diagnosis.
8. Some children complain of dysuria, particularly at a slightly later stage, if the appendix is in a pelvic location.
9. A low-grade fever is usual. Marked elevations of temperature, such as 39.5°C to 40°C usually suggest conditions other than appendicitis in children with a short history of symptoms.

> ### Key Point
>
> An underrated but important feature in the history of the child with acute appendicitis is consistent aggravation of the abdominal pain by movement.

In few children's diseases does physical examination play a more important role than in acute appendicitis. In 1889, Dr. Charles McBurney stated, "In every case, the seat of greatest pain, determined by the pressure of one finger, has been exactly between an inch and a half and two inches from the anterior spinous process of the ilium on a straight line drawn from that process to the umbilicus." More than a century later, his statement remains valid; the precise abdominal location he identified bears his name: the McBurney point.

Even with extremely careful clinical and laboratory assessment, the diagnosis may be uncertain in the early stages. Often, a period of careful observation is the most valuable diagnostic aid. This fact requires you to make a conscientious commitment to reassess the child at frequent intervals. Sometimes this approach may permit you to send a child home with the parents overnight, but only on the clear understanding that the child must return if the symptoms worsen or do not abate by early the following day. This safe approach often avoids unnecessary laparotomy without increasing the risk of complications such as perforation.

It has often been said that perforation of the appendix releases tension in an acutely distended organ, resulting in a short interval of clinical improvement followed by deterioration as peritonitis worsens. This sequence is more often talked about than seen, however, at least in children. Frank perforation is usually characterized by a longer history, greater systemic effects, and more generalized tenderness with hypoactivity or even absence of bowel sounds, indicating a paralytic ileus. Besides having more widespread and worrisome abdominal findings, children with appendiceal perforation usually demonstrate a higher fever than is seen in appendicitis without perforation; they may also show signs of clinically significant dehydration.

DIFFERENTIAL DIAGNOSIS OF APPENDICITIS

The clinical picture of acute appendicitis may be indistinguishable at times from that of a rare entity such as acute inflammation in a Meckel diverticulum or an acute inflammatory process limited to the terminal ileum (regional enteritis, or Crohn disease). It is sometimes said that a child has had "mesenteric lymphadenitis." True mesenteric lymphadenitis may occur as a result of infection with identifiable microorganisms (e.g., *Yersinia enterocolitica*), but it is greatly overrated as a diagnostic entity in children. The mesenteric lymph nodes in infants and children are typically large, particularly in the distal small bowel, and commonly react to sources of infectious stress. Thus, in children undergoing laparotomy for suspected appendicitis, the mesenteric nodes often appear large whether or not the appendix happens to be the culprit in the child's illness.

Key Point

The most important clinical feature of acute appendicitis is localized right lower quadrant tenderness.

CHRONIC APPENDICITIS

The term *chronic appendicitis* implies repeated attacks of abdominal pain that were ultimately relieved by removal of an (usually) innocuous-looking appendix.

Key Point

The idea that the appendix can be responsible for frequent or recurrent episodes of abdominal pain is difficult to sustain on the basis of objective data such as histologic findings.

Sometimes the appendix has probably become mildly inflamed because the lumen is partially obstructed (usually by a fecalith), producing transient clinical signs. In such cases, symptoms resolve only to be followed by one or two further bouts, culminating in florid acute appendicitis. Conceivably, the initial episodes in this scenario might be labeled (with the 20/20 visual acuity of hindsight) as subacute appendicitis, but this diagnosis is always retrospective. Appendectomy for recurrent bouts of right lower quadrant pain in children is ill-advised. Children who appear to be relieved of this symptom by appendectomy may simply be telling the physician that they do not want another operation. Fortunately, experience and better noninvasive diagnostic imaging techniques have largely eliminated this approach to the management of recurrent abdominal pain in children.

Key Point

For practical purposes, consider the appendix in children to be a quiescent, generally useless organ that yields a clinical picture of progressive inflammatory disease only when it is genuinely inflamed.

Acute Gynecologic Events

Ovulatory bleeding, a twisted or ruptured adnexal cyst, pelvic inflammatory disease, or ectopic pregnancy may mimic acute appendicitis. Ovulatory bleeding is by far the most common of these conditions (see Chapter 16).

Biliary Tract Disease

Biliary tract disease has been recognized in children with increasing frequency, following the widespread availability of ultrasonography. The clinical picture in children resembles that observed in adults, although a history of intolerance to fatty foods is less consistently present.

Recurrent pancreatitis, sometimes familial, may cause episodes of steady severe upper abdominal pain. This pain may be precipitated by intake of food (especially fat) and, in children, is seldom associated with demonstrable biliary tract disease, as it often is in adults. Pancreatic pain is typically epigastric and may radiate to the back. Physical findings are seldom helpful, but serum amylase values are elevated during attacks. The pain is typically severe.

Urinary Tract Problems

Although urinary infection can simulate appendicitis, remember that the child's systemic reaction is generally greater. The child is more likely to have a high fever (often with chills) and less impressive signs of peritoneal irritation. There may be a history of previous similar attacks or a family history of urinary tract infections. The diagnosis is usually confirmed by microscopic examination of a fresh urine specimen plus urine culture.

Urinary tract calculi occasionally occur in children and may be encountered, for example, on a familial basis with idiopathic hypercalciuria. Ureteral colic is one of the most severe pains that afflicts patients at any age, and it is typically colicky and excruciating.

> **Key Point**
>
> Fortunately, calculi in the urinary tract are uncommon in children, but as in adults, they cause extreme colicky (hyper-peristaltic) pain that is out of proportion to the physical findings and is more intermittent than the pain in children with acute appendicitis.

Acute Severe Abdominal Pain

The child with acute excruciating abdominal pain often presents a diagnostic dilemma. The pain is obviously severe and spasmodic, and is associated with restlessness and screaming. Curiously enough, the child with such a clinical picture seldom has a major underlying identifiable intra-abdominal disease calling for surgical intervention. In most children, the accompanying histrionics vary inversely with the gravity of the cause, which is often unidentified. The pain is usually brief and recurrent (see later). Stool retention, which may cause a transient acute distention of a portion of gut, generating colicky pain can usually be identified through the history, physical examination, or a plain radiograph of the abdomen.

Chronic Pain

The child with chronic recurrent abdominal pain can present even more of a diagnostic problem. The history is typically of recurrent bouts of short duration, usually not associated with signs of systemic illness such as fever and weight loss. Taking a careful history to try to identify a cause is fundamental. Clues may point to the presence of constipation, biliary tract disease, pancreatitis, inflammatory bowel disease, school phobia, family dysfunction, or other psychogenic causes. Often, the history is nonspecific, the attacks are self-limited, and the child's general health is good. In most children who are seen because of recurrent abdominal pain, the physical, laboratory, and imaging findings are unimpressive and helpful only in their normality. Clinical experience has supported the belief that the closer the recurrent pain is

to the umbilicus in children, the less likely it is to be of organic origin. If clinical and laboratory assessment do not reveal an identifiable disease, there is no reason to perform a laparotomy to establish a diagnosis.

Abdominal Trauma

> **Key Point**
>
> Truncal trauma is a major cause of death in children.

Most severe injuries occur in accidents involving motor vehicles, particularly when a child is struck while walking or on a bicycle. Falls are another common source of serious injury. Child abuse is recognized with distressing frequency in emergency departments. Be alert to the possibility of child abuse if there is a vague history of injury that lacks some credibility or if there are disproportionately pronounced physical findings involving areas other than the abdomen. If you suspect abuse in a child with abdominal trauma, protect the child in a hospital environment until a diagnosis is conclusively established.

Assessment of the abdomen is obviously of major significance as part of the complete evaluation of a child with multiple injuries. In every situation, the ABCs of trauma management (airway, breathing, circulatory status) are pivotal. Abdominal assessment, especially in children with multiple injuries, who frequently are obtunded, is highly significant, because the abdomen may be the site of a major visceral disruption. Identifying life-threatening hemorrhage is a high priority. In children, life-threatening hemorrhage most likely occurs from liver disruption, less frequently from major splenic or renal injuries, and on rare occasions from disrupted mesenteric or retroperitoneal vessels. The sudden escape of any body fluid (blood, bile, urine, pancreatic juice, gastrointestinal contents) into the peritoneal cavity produces signs of peritoneal irritation, as in other entities unrelated to trauma. Often the findings are diffuse, but sometimes there is a helpful localization of maximal findings in one area, such as the left upper quadrant with splenic lacerations. Free fluid may track beneath the diaphragm at an early stage and produce shoulder pain because of innervation of the subdiaphragmatic peritoneum (C3 to C5). Continued bleeding causes abdominal distention, diffuse tenderness, a "bogginess" on palpation, and evidence of cardiovascular instability related to ongoing bleeding. Appropriate imaging studies will probably be required to locate the injury and to guide definitive management. Clinical stabilization (the ABCs) must be the first priority and must not be jeopardized by a rapid trip to the diagnostic imaging department, where careful clinical monitoring can sometimes be interrupted. Abdominal paracentesis or lavage is rarely required in a pediatric patient, even if the child is obtunded.

An often neglected problem in pediatric trauma is gastric distention. Children swallow much air, especially when they are injured or apprehensive, and gastric distention may be aggravated by resuscitative measures. Injured children often present with marked abdominal distention that might suggest major visceral injury but is actually gastric distention. Judiciously passing a nasogastric tube relieves this distention promptly, and it is remarkable how often this maneuver is followed by signs of clinical improvement. It is prudent to assume that gastric emptying ceases at the time of major trauma.

Key Point

The passage of a nasogastric tube is an important adjunctive maneuver in the early assessment of the child with an injured abdomen.

Abdominal trauma does not always yield dramatic early signs. One example is injury to the pancreas, a deeply situated organ. Likewise, mesenteric injuries may yield dramatic bleeding, but these are more commonly recognized from the ischemic injury to the overlying bowel that develops within a day or two of the actual trauma. An example of this situation is a seat-belt injury.

Rupture of a Hollow Viscus

Rupture of a hollow viscus is most likely to occur in the segments of the gut that are anatomically least mobile—the retroperitoneal duodenum and the ileocecal area. Ruptures of the stomach, proximal duodenum, or colon are likely to yield physical and imaging evidence of free gas in the peritoneal cavity, whereas injuries to the small bowel often do not cause much free air; the small bowel is usually quite free of gas in normal children older than 2 years.

When interpreting abdominal physical findings and considering appropriate investigations, consider the overall status of the child with multiple injuries.

Key Point

Pay continuous attention to vital signs and the maintenance of clinical stability while diagnostic imaging and other tests are being performed.

The Newborn's Abdomen

The abdomen is a common site of major congenital anomalies, many of surgical significance. Some are suspected before birth because of hydramnios or ultrasonographic abnormalities. Most intra-abdominal anomalies requiring surgical intervention are obstructive (atresia or stenosis); the initial major symptom of those in the proximal part of the gastrointestinal tract typically is bilious vomiting.

Key Point

Assume that any newborn or young infant who vomits bile has an obstructive lesion.

The quantity of bile vomited may not be large, and the vomiting may be intermittent if the obstruction is incomplete. Physical findings are not usually helpful; therefore, it is imperative to obtain appropriate imaging studies promptly. In neonates with a high obstructive lesion such as duodenal atresia, the lower abdomen may lack its normal prominence because swallowed air cannot reached the remainder of the small bowel and colon. Remember that there is a strong association between duodenal obstructive lesions (especially duodenal atresia) and Down syndrome: About a third of newborns with duodenal atresia also have Down syndrome. Assessment of a newborn with an obstructive lesion must include careful review of other systems, because major congenital anomalies often occur in clusters (see Chapter 5).

Infants with more distal obstructive lesions, such as ileal atresia, Hirschsprung disease, and meconium ileus, are likely to present because of delayed passage of meconium. Ninety-five percent of normal full-term newborns pass meconium during the first 24 hours of life. All normal newborns pass meconium within the first 48 hours. It follows that any infant who does not pass meconium within the first 24 hours or so should be observed carefully for evidence of an underlying obstructive lesion. Very low birth weight infants are an exception. Intestinal motility in these infants is sluggish, and delayed passage of meconium is common.

Key Point

Delayed passage of meconium in newborns of normal size is analogous to bilious vomiting; it heralds the presence of an underlying obstructive lesion.

The abdomen in an infant with a distal obstruction becomes progressively more distended from continued swallowing of air, particularly after feedings begin. The newborn who did not pass meconium normally probably will not demonstrate physical findings that point to a specific lesion. Occasionally, there may be a palpable mass, such as a markedly distended loop of obstructed small bowel or meconium staining of the abdominal wall when a prenatal perforation has occurred, and sometimes loops of distended bowel are visible.

Ordinarily, the normal newborn's rectum admits your fifth finger. A gentle rectal examination plus judicious insertion of a small catheter or lubricated rectal thermometer usually excludes rare forms of low rectal atresia. In infants with Hirschsprung disease, digital rectal examination may temporarily overcome the persistently narrow and unrelaxed zone of aganglionic rectum, and withdrawal of the examining finger may be followed by a forceful passage of meconium. This sequence of events virtually ascertains Hirschsprung disease in the neonate.

Imperforate Anus

Always note the position and patency of the anal orifice. An ectopic (anteriorly placed) anal orifice, more commonly seen in girls, may be stenotic and may cause chronic constipation. When the anal orifice is absent, always inspect the perineum carefully for evidence of a fistulous connection to the rectum. In boys, a fistula may reveal itself over the first 24 hours as a streak of meconium staining along the perineal raphe, extending up toward the scrotum. Boys with imperforate anus may pass meconium in the urine because of a fistula between the rectum and bladder or urethra. From a practical viewpoint, imperforate anus in boys is a total obstruction that requires early surgical intervention, which may consist of either a primary repair if the rectum ends very close to the perineum or an initial colostomy followed by definitive repair when the infant is older. Imperforate anus is a serious malformation that is commonly associated with other major anomalies, particularly those involving the urinary tract.

Imperforate anus in girls is almost always associated with a fistulous connection to the exterior that may not be evident on first inspection. A careful examination of the area surrounding the vaginal introitus usually discloses the fistula, which is often of substantial size. This fistula is functionally important because it is large enough to allow meconium to be evacuated, making the need for surgical intervention less urgent than in boys.

Ischemic Injury to the Bowel

Newborns occasionally suffer from ischemic insults to previously healthy bowel. The two major examples of such insults are necrotizing enterocolitis and midgut volvulus. In the former, the baby, typically a low-birth-weight infant, has been stressed by prematurity, hypoxia, hypothermia, or sepsis. The infant becomes acutely ill, with intolerance to feedings, vomiting, abdominal distention, hypotension, fever, and sometimes rectal bleed-

ing. Physical findings include signs of sepsis, variable abdominal distention, and generalized abdominal tenderness. In more advanced cases, the abdominal wall may become reddened and edematous, and a palpable inflammatory mass may develop. Signs of gut perforation usually indicate the need for laparotomy. In most infants, the findings are less alarming, and much of the pathologic process seems reversible with appropriate nonoperative management, such as cessation of feedings, broad-spectrum antibiotics, and aggressive fluid resuscitation. Subsequently, obstructive signs may appear as healing progresses, and the more seriously injured segments of bowel become scarred and strictured.

Key Point

Bilious vomiting, sometimes intermittent and of relatively small volume, may be the earliest sign of a potentially lethal rotational anomaly of the midgut. Always investigate this symptom on an urgent basis.

An abnormality of intestinal rotation can set the stage for a midgut twist (volvulus) because of incomplete peritoneal attachments. The anomaly is usually referred to as *midgut malrotation*. Volvulus of the incompletely tethered bowel partially obstructs the duodenum. More important, however, it may also obstruct major mesenteric vessels in the root of the twisted mesentery. This obstruction threatens the viability of the entire midgut. Bilious vomiting may be the initial sign of this potentially devastating event, which, if identified promptly, is treatable. Vomitus-containing bile is the hallmark of an underlying obstructive process calling for urgent investigation.

Major Abdominal Wall Defects

Major abdominal wall defects may be identified antenatally on ultrasonography. The most important defects are omphalocele and gastroschisis. An *omphalocele* is the persisting presence of variable amounts of the intestinal tract, and sometimes part of the liver, outside the abdomen from which they have exited via the umbilical cord, covered only by amnion (Fig. 12–4). The underlying fascial defect may be large, and because much of the abdominal contents remain extra-abdominal during fetal life, the true abdominal cavity remains inordinately small. Omphalocele is associated with other significant congenital abnormalities in approximately 50% of affected newborns, and it may require a staged surgical repair if the true abdominal cavity is very small. In initial management, protect the intact amnion from desiccation and infection by applying moist dressings and taking appropriate measures to maintain the most sterile environment possible.

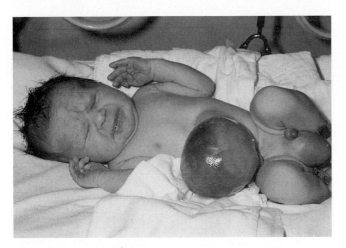

Figure 12–4 Omphalocele in newborn.

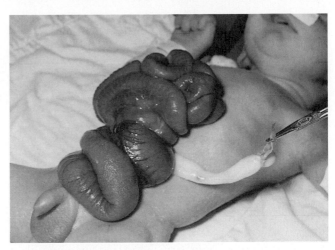

Figure 12–5 Gastroschisis in newborn.

In *gastroschisis,* there is a full-thickness defect in the abdominal wall just lateral to an intact umbilical cord, usually on its right side, allowing extrusion of bowel antenatally (Fig. 12–5). The bowel is not covered by amnion and may have been injured by prenatal exposure to amniotic fluid. The underlying fascial defect is usually small, and a primary surgical repair is generally possible. The exposed bowel requires careful handling, with emphasis on keeping it moist and as free from contamination as possible. Fortunately, the incidence of associated anomalies is low, and most babies with gastroschisis do well.

Rare and more complex abdominal wall abnormalities include gross deficiency of abdominal musculatures (the "prune belly" syndrome) and large midline defects. The large defects may involve other structures, such as the pericardium (ectopia cordis) or bladder (exstrophy), and some are incompatible with life.

Umbilical Discharge in Infants

Most often, umbilical discharge in an infant represents an exudate related to incomplete healing at the site of amputation of the umbilical cord. There is often a small polyp of moist pink granulation tissue, which is best managed by cauterization with a silver nitrate–tipped wooden applicator or by simple excision performed as an office procedure. Persistent drainage in the absence of visible granulation tissue should raise the suspicion of an underlying anomaly—either a persistently patent omphalomesenteric duct (intestinal contents) or persistent patency of the urachus (urine). Identifying these entities may require careful probing and imaging studies.

Hernias and Related Problems

Umbilical hernia is by far the most common condition seen in infants. In some parts of the world, it is found

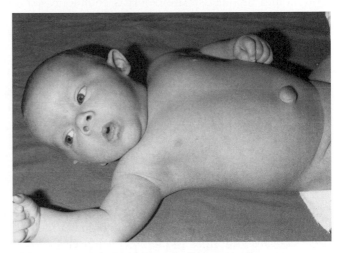

Figure 12–6 Umbilical hernia in an infant.

in most infants. Typically becoming apparent in the first few weeks of life, umbilical hernias produce a conspicuous bulge (Fig. 12–6), stretching the overlying skin. The fascial defect is usually the size of the tip of an adult's index finger, and the hernia is easily reducible when the child is not crying or straining; the size of the skin-covered bulge bears little relationship to the size of the fascial defect. As you push the contents of the hernia gently back into the abdomen, there is often a palpable and audible "squish" as the small bowel loops are returned to the abdominal cavity.

The sight and sound of an umbilical hernia bothers everybody but the baby. Because parents and other family members worry about complications and regard the somewhat unsightly bulge apprehensively, tell them that the hernia is likely to become bigger before it starts to get smaller but that it will disappear with time. Vague reassurances may fall on deaf ears. Reassure parents that (1) virtually all such hernias are self-limited, and (2) most umbilical hernias close by the child's first or second birthday, and (3) even those that persist longer may disappear spontaneously over the next couple of years. It may help to have parents feel the defect in the abdominal wall to help them realize how tiny it is.

Complications of umbilical hernia such as incarceration are vanishingly rare. Folk customs, for example, taping an object such as a coin over the fascial defect or strapping with adhesive tape, are useless, may cause skin irritation, and may delay spontaneous closure. Although surgical repair is easy enough, it is necessary only in the rare instance in which the fascial defect persists far beyond the time when it should normally close.

EPIGASTRIC HERNIA

A midline hernia, epigastric hernia occurs through a typically small defect in the linea alba between the xiphoid and umbilicus. The defect is commonly occupied by extraperitoneal fat that may not be clinically reducible. Epigastric hernias allegedly cause pain, although most are noticed incidentally by a parent or physician. These supraumbilical fascial defects do not usually undergo the typical self-obliteration that umbilical hernias do. Surgical repair can be performed at any age.

DIASTASIS RECTI

A long midline bulge extending from the umbilicus to the xiphoid is a relatively common finding, usually in infants but occasionally in older children as well. It occurs because the right and left rectus muscles are not closely approximated in the midline, and as a result, a

bulge is evident when the baby strains or cries. This bulge, caused by *diastasis recti*, can best be demonstrated if you induce the child to use the rectus muscles, as in attempting to sit up. This is not a true hernia. Diastasis recti is completely benign and will disappear gradually. No treatment is necessary.

The Inguinal Canal and Its Abnormalities

A sound approach to the management of inguinal canal abnormalities requires an understanding of the embryologic events that cause them. As a prelude to testicular descent in the male and at the same gestational stage in females, a diverticular process of peritoneum, the processus vaginalis, extends through the internal inguinal ring along the inguinal canal (Fig. 12–7). In males, this stage is followed by the normal downward migration of the testicle, which acquires a portion of its covering (*tunica vaginalis*) from the peritoneal process just described. In both sexes, the patent peritoneal process undergoes obliteration at or shortly after birth (Fig. 12–8). When this occurs, the potential for development of an indirect inguinal hernia disappears. When obliteration is incomplete, the potential for abdominal contents to enter the inguinal canal remains, constituting an indirect inguinal hernia (Fig. 12–9). The fundamental abnormality in all indirect inguinal hernias is, simply, persistent patency of the processus vaginalis, nothing more. The usual inguinal hernias in children are all of the indirect variety. Direct inguinal hernias are rare in pediatric patients.

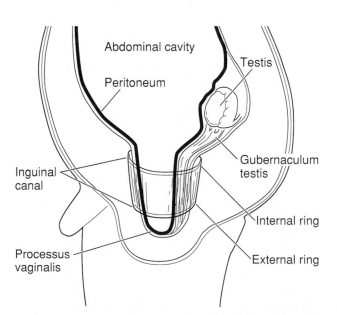

Figure 12–7 Early embryologic event in the inguinal canal. (Modified from Desjardins, J: Normal Embryological Development and Congenital Anomalies of the Inguino-Scrotal Region. Montreal, Sainte-Justine Hospital, 1982.)

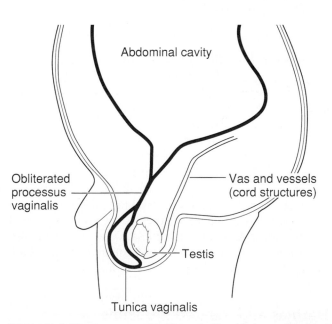

Figure 12–8 The processus vaginalis normally obliterates. (Modified from Desjardins, J: Normal Embryological Development and Congenital Anomalies of the Inguino-Scrotal Region. Montreal, Sainte-Justine Hospital, 1982.)

Hernias in children are common, and those affecting the inguinal area can cause considerable morbidity.

HYDROCELES

In the normal full-term newborn boy, expect to identify gonads in the scrotum without swelling in either inguinal canal. As the proximal processus vaginalis obliterates, it is common for some peritoneal fluid to become trapped in the tunica vaginalis of the testicle in the scrotum, constituting a hydrocele (Fig. 12–10), a common finding in newborn boys. Always regard this fluid as having been sequestered by the normal obliterative process described previously. You can confidently tell parents that the fluid will gradually be reabsorbed over the next few months. The initial appearance of a hydrocele in later infancy or childhood reflects the passage of peritoneal fluid via a patent processus (i.e., a hernial sac) into the tunica vaginalis. Consider these late-appearing hydroceles as indirect hernias because of the underlying anatomic abnormality. Parents of toddlers and young children often report that the scrotal swelling is larger in the evening and smaller in the morning, suggesting migration of hydrocele fluid back into the peritoneal cavity via the patent processus while the child is recumbent. Some authorities use the term *communicating hydrocele* to describe this finding, as opposed to the *noncommunicating hydrocele* that is so commonly seen in normal newborns. Students and physicians often comment on the fact that a hydrocele "transilluminates well."

Transillumination simply demonstrates the presence of fluid and, of itself, is seldom diagnostic.

An inguinal hernia in a child does not imply muscle weakness or attenuation, nor does it mean that there is any structural weakness in the inguinal canal floor. It is, in essence, a persistently patent processus vaginalis. Parents point to the inguinal canal area, indicating where the lump was seen, and they often say it appears intermittently, especially when the baby cries. Sometimes they describe the sudden appearance of a scrotal swelling, which may represent abdominal contents progressing down the entire length of the persistently patent processus vaginalis or peritoneal fluid that has tracked downward and accumulated in the tunica vaginalis of the testicle. In any event, the parents' description suggests patency of the peritoneal process. When this suspicion is confirmed by physical findings, an indirect hernia is the diagnosis.

Inguinal hernias in infants and children are potentially serious and can produce considerable morbidity. Unlike umbilical hernias, they do not disappear spontaneously.

Physical examination begins, as always, with inspection, which may disclose a visible swelling in the inguinal canal, scrotum, or both. Although inguinal hernias are more common on the right side than on the left, they are bilateral in 10% to 15% of patients. Sometimes the swelling is restricted to one side of the scrotum without any obvious continuity with a mass in the inguinal canal, probably because of fluid in the

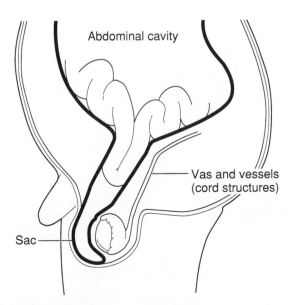

Figure 12–9 Failure of the processus vaginalis to close allows passage of abdominal contents along the inguinal canal. (Modified from Desjardins, J: Normal Embryological Development and Congenital Anomalies of the Inguino-Scrotal Region. Montreal, Sainte-Justine Hospital, 1982.)

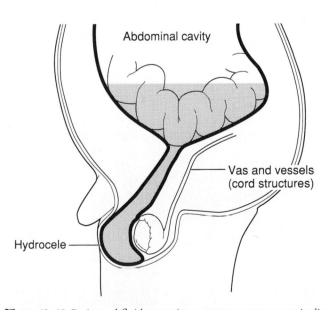

Figure 12–10 Peritoneal fluid traversing a patent processus vaginalis produces a hydrocele. (Modified from Desjardins, J: Normal Embryological Development and Congenital Anomalies of the Inguino-Scrotal Region. Montreal, Sainte-Justine Hospital, 1982.)

tunica vaginalis that occasionally imparts a bluish discoloration to the overlying stretched scrotal skin. If the swelling is continuous from the scrotum upward along the inguinal canal, fluid, bowel, omentum, or a combination of these is likely to be extending from the internal ring down to the tunica vaginalis. Sometimes, despite a clear history given by the parents, no abnormality is visible on inspection. This does not, however, exclude the presence of an underlying hernia.

Gentle palpation of an observed swelling helps determine whether it is due to bowel contained within the inguinal canal or to fluid alone. At times, the distinction is difficult. The question then is whether there is a bowel along the inguinal canal that cannot be reduced manually (*incarceration*) or simply a collection of fluid that cannot be expressed upward because of a relatively stenotic zone in the patent processus vaginalis. If the child is not irritable and the swelling has been present a considerable time and does not seem tender, chances are that the problem is not an incarcerated hernia but simply trapped peritoneal fluid (an "encysted" hydrocele). Experience usually allows a physician to make this clinical distinction confidently. It is a significant one, because incarceration of abdominal contents may damage the bowel or gonad; the latter may be damaged from pressure on the testicular vessels in the inguinal canal by the incarcerated contents. Often the hernial contents can be reduced through the inguinal ring by gentle massaging pressure. Reduction is best attempted when the child is not crying or straining. As with umbilical hernias, manual reduction may be accompanied by a palpable and audible "squish" as bowel contents return into the abdomen.

Diagnosis is relatively easy when there is a visible or palpable swelling. At times, particularly in infants, the parents clearly describe an intermittent swelling along the inguinal canal, possibly associated with transient pain, leaving little doubt that the child has an inguinal hernia (Fig. 12–11). Yet, on inspection and on initial palpation, you may find nothing. Subtler signs of a persistent patent processus vaginalis must then be sought. Because it is a tubular peritoneal structure, it adds substance or thickness to the cord structures that traverse the inguinal canal. This feature is easily appreciated on gentle palpation between the thumb and forefinger above the testicle and between it and the external inguinal ring (Fig. 12–12). The normal cord structures can be identified readily; it is usually possible to define the vas by its cordlike feel. If, besides the normal vas and vessels, there is a double-layered peritoneal sac (i.e., the patent processus vaginalis), the structures palpated are thicker than on the contralateral side.

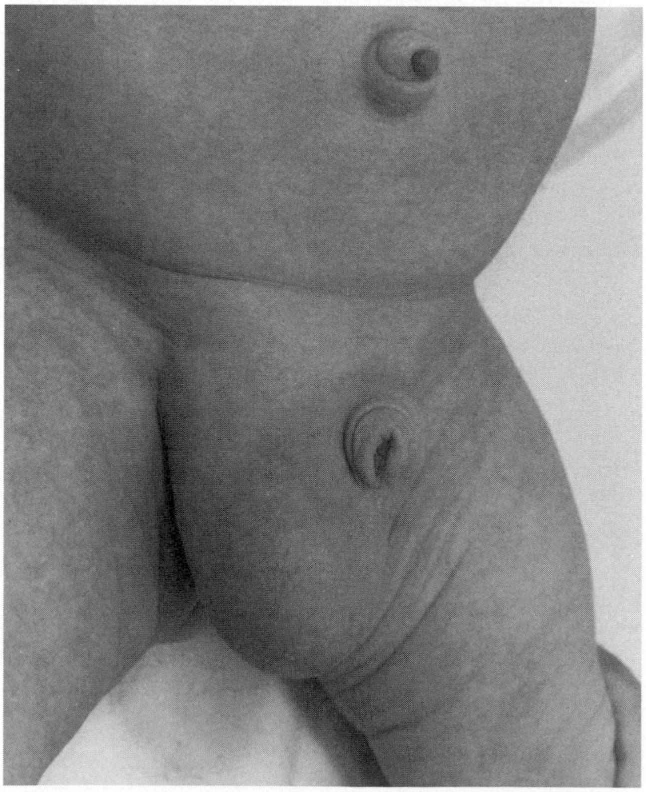

Figure 12–11 An inguinoscrotal hernia in a small infant. Note the presence also of a small polyp of granulation tissue at the umbilicus.

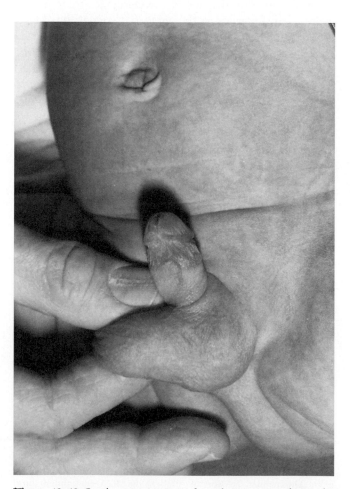

Figure 12–12 Gentle examination of cord structures above the testicle allows appreciation of the presence of an empty hernial sac.

Although less reliable, the thickness of the cord structures caused by the addition of a patent processus vaginalis may also be appreciated by putting your middle finger along the course of the inguinal canal and rubbing the underlying cord structures gently along the firm background of the canal and the pubic tubercle (Fig. 12–13). Sometimes, this gives the sensation that two surfaces (the anterior and posterior walls of the tubular processus) are rubbing against each other, described as a "silk sign" because it resembles the feel of silk surfaces rubbing against each other. The cord structures on the other side usually serve as a normal control. Appreciation of this more subtle evidence requires experience and judgment. Palpate the cord structures as part of your routine physical examination of *all* male infants. Such experience will be a great help in the identification of abnormal findings in children in whom a hernia is suspected.

In adolescents and adults, it is a common practice to invert the upper portion of the scrotal skin into the inguinal canal with the examining finger to feel for an impulse while the patient is asked to strain or cough. Never perform this technique on infants and young children; it causes the child unnecessary pain and yields no valuable information.

Inguinal hernias are far less common in girls than in boys. The clinical presentation is invariably a swelling in the inguinal canal that, as in boys, may be intermittent. On physical examination, the lump is the sine qua non for diagnosis. As in boys, you may be able to identify a sac along the inguinal canal if a lump is not present at the time of examination. The ovary is often present in the sac during the first year of life and may be identified by palpation; it is frequently not reducible. On rare occasions, the gonad presenting in the inguinal canal in an apparently normal female infant is a testicle. Surgeons recognize this structure during repair based on its gross appearance and the absence of a fallopian tube. This abnormality, *testicular feminization*, may be suspected clinically, although the external genitalia are often phenotypically female; the diagnosis is confirmed either by biopsy or by chromosomal analysis (46XY). In testicular feminization, there is a high incidence of later malignancy in the abnormal gonads; it is therefore routine practice to remove them once the diagnosis is established unequivocally. The child is raised as a female and is given hormonal replacement therapy at an appropriate age.

Abnormalities of Testicular Descent

The testicle is normally located in the abdomen until about the seventh month of gestation, when it begins to migrate downward into the scrotum, a process that takes a couple of months; it should be in a normal scrotal position at term. For reasons unknown, the right testicle descends slightly later than the left; perhaps for that reason inguinal hernias and cryptorchidism are more common on the right side.

Given the timing of normal testicular descent, it is not surprising that gonads are often not palpable in the scrotum in premature infants and may be incompletely descended in 3% to 5% of full-term babies.

Over the next several weeks after birth, testicular descent may continue, and by the end of the first year of life, it is estimated, 5% of premature infants and less than 1% of full-term infants show evidence of nondescent or incomplete descent.

The cord structures are normally enveloped by a thin extension of abdominal wall musculature known as the *cremasteric fibers*. This cremasteric musculature can contract reflexively, elevating the testicle, a normal reflex

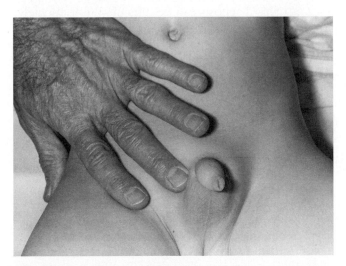

Figure 12–13 Palpation along the inguinal canal may yield findings that indicate the presence of an underlying hernial sac.

retractile phenomenon that sometimes leads to confusion between normally descended and undescended (*cryptorchid*) testes in infants and small children.

Testes should descend by the postnatal age of 3 or 4 months irrespective of the infant's gestational age at birth. It is important to distinguish between true cryptorchidism and a retractile ("yo-yo") testicle, best accomplished by careful physical examination. First, inspect the scrotum carefully. It is usually adequately developed in youngsters in whom the testicle is simply retractile, being present in the scrotum most of the time. Second, the retractile testicle can be manipulated readily on physical examination into a normal scrotal position. In some babies, it may retract rather promptly into the inguinal canal. If the gonad can be manipulated into a normal scrotal position without difficulty and without being put under tension, you can assume that a retractile testicle, and not true cryptorchidism, is present. Retractile testes almost invariably achieve a permanent scrotal position within the first few years of life without surgical or other treatment. The truly cryptorchid testicle is usually present in the inguinal canal, but it cannot be manipulated into the scrotum. In the presence of unilateral cryptorchidism, the scrotum is often underdeveloped on the affected side.

Key Point

It is important to establish the diagnosis of cryptorchidism in infancy because the optimum time for surgical repair is probably during the first 1 to 2 years of life.

Cryptorchidism is almost invariably associated with a persistently patent processus vaginalis. Thus, clinical hernias and cryptorchidism commonly coexist. Because of its tendency to produce morbid complications, the inguinal hernia is generally the dominant concern in the timing of surgical intervention. Orchidopexy is carried out at the same time as the hernia is repaired. Testicular nondescent is bilateral in 10% to 25% of cases. In rare instances, it may be impossible to identify a testicle on one or both sides, even with careful physical examination, a worrisome finding for the family that raises concerns about congenital anorchia or an important chromosomal abnormality.

Key Point

The apparent absence of *both* gonads on clinical examination calls for additional investigations.

Testes can occasionally be identified in unusual ectopic locations close to the inguinal canal or even in the perineum. It is important to be sure a testicle is present, and especially for the surgeon embarking on repair. In most cases, testes can be placed in a satisfactory scrotal position with an appropriate operation.

THE "ACUTE SCROTUM"

Acute events related to the testicle are alarming and painful. Alarm stems from the potential threat to the gonad's viability. Pain results from an insult to the sensitive gonad as the result of ischemia or inflammatory changes. Acute pain, accompanied by variable swelling that causes the child to be brought in for evaluation, may occur at any age from infancy to adolescence. The major causes are torsion of the testicle, torsion of the *appendix testis* (a vestigial remnant related to the upper pole of the gonad), and acute inflammation that is usually located primarily in the epididymis (*epididymitis*). Although the cause of epididymitis can be viral or bacterial, it is often difficult to identify.

The child with an acutely painful and swollen testicle requires immediate assessment. Occasionally physical examination reveals that the appendix testis has undergone torsion, and the tender, swollen appendix testis sometimes can be felt. It also may have a bluish discoloration because of the torsion, sometimes seen as a "blue dot" through the scrotal skin.

With torsion of the entire gonad, the organ is often relatively high and somewhat angulated in the scrotum. Pain and tenderness may make it impossible to distinguish on purely clinical grounds between an acute torsion and an acute inflammatory process. There is great urgency in making the distinction because a twisted testicle will probably survive only a few hours, so the torsion must be manually undone, usually by an open operation, which should be performed only if the diagnosis either is established or cannot be excluded. At present, the most useful diagnostic approach consists of appropriate imaging studies using techniques that can be performed rapidly, often while the operating room is being prepared in case the final diagnosis is torsion of the testicle. Torsion may also occur in an undescended testicle. When this occurs, the clinical findings are obviously most striking in the inguinal canal or upper scrotum. This diagnosis can be difficult, but fortunately, the problem occurs rarely. Remember that testicular disease can be a source of abdominal pain.

Testicular torsion may occur antenatally or in early infancy. Sometimes the earliest evidence in young infants is the presence of a discolored swollen gonad, which, when discovered, is already beyond repair. Torsion of the testicle usually occurs within the confines of the tunica vaginalis (*intravaginal*), less commonly above the attachments of the tunica vaginalis (*extravaginal*). Those that occur within the tunica vaginalis are believed to be related to an abnormal attachment of the tunica that allows greater mobility of the gonad, an anomaly that often occurs bilaterally.

An uncommon but distinct entity is so-called idiopathic scrotal edema. Usually the parents observe that their child has a red swollen scrotum with a remarkable absence of related symptoms. On examination, the erythema may extend somewhat along the inguinal canal on the same side and often downward along the median raphe between the base of the scrotum and the anus. Occasionally, the redness and swelling extend to the other side. Despite the erythema, the scrotal skin is remarkably nontender. Through the edematous skin, one can routinely palpate a normal testicle that is in good position and is nontender. The cause of acute scrotal edema is unknown, and it requires no specific treatment. Reassure the parents that it will resolve completely over a few days and that resolution may be associated with transient ecchymotic discoloration of the affected scrotal skin.

Acute scrotal pain, swelling, or both sometimes occur from trauma and occasionally may be simulated by complications related to an incarcerated or strangulated inguinal hernia. Painless enlargement of the scrotum can also be caused by a hydrocele and occasionally by a testicular neoplasm.

Acute processes affecting the scrotum or its contents are in some ways analogous to the acute abdomen, in that they require thorough history-taking and prompt, skillful physical examination.

Pyloric Stenosis

A diagnosis of pyloric stenosis, despite the advent of increasingly helpful imaging modalities, can be made in most instances by taking a thorough history and performing a careful physical examination. The gastric outlet obstruction is caused by hypertrophy of a relatively short zone of pyloric muscle that ends abruptly at the pyloroduodenal junction. The process rarely becomes clinically evident before the age of 7 to 10 days and is seldom seen beyond the age of 3 months. It is at least twice as common in boys as in girls and has a strong hereditary component. The cause is unknown.

Typically, the baby with pyloric stenosis appears normal at birth and for the first 1 to 3 weeks. Most babies vomit occasionally, and the progression of symptoms may be sufficiently subtle to escape detection until vomiting becomes persistent and the baby fails to gain or even loses weight. The infant characteristically feeds vigorously and, shortly afterward, vomits forcefully; the vomiting is typically described as *projectile*. It is just that, and in affected infants, the vomitus may clear the edge of the examining table in a trajectory of several inches or more away from the mouth. The vomitus is never bile stained, and the baby is typically described as hungry right after vomiting, unlike babies who vomit for most other reasons.

If the history suggests pyloric stenosis, proceed to the physical examination with special reference to the upper abdomen. As physicians have long been taught, first allow the baby to feed, noting the vigor with which

he or she does this. Next, with the baby supine, inspect the upper abdomen carefully, and look, under good lighting, for relative distention of the upper abdomen and visible sequential peristaltic waves moving from the left epigastric area down toward the right side of the midline as the stomach struggles against a point of distal obstruction. These waves are often dramatic and are virtually diagnostic of pyloric stenosis. Visible peristaltic waves after a feeding are often followed by early forceful vomiting; the baby then relaxes as the painful obstructive process is temporarily relieved.

Now, just after the baby has vomited, is the best time to feel for the thickened pyloric muscle, which is situated deeply in the right upper quadrant near or beneath the lateral edge of the right rectus msucle about midway between the umbilicus and xiphoid. Sit or stand on the baby's left side, use your left hand to feel for the pyloric "tumor." Gently insert the fingers of your examining hand into the right upper quadrant and beneath the area of the right rectus muscle, where the palpable, olive-like muscular lump is often found (Fig. 12–14). Gently press the thumb of your left hand just lateral to the left rectus muscle to assist in bringing the pyloric "tumor" into a palpable location. You can also feel for the mass while the baby is being fed. Feeding may relax the baby, making it easier to feel the olive. Finding the pyloric mass is so typical as to be absolutely diagnostic of the disease. Once you have felt the characteristic sensation of a pyloric "tumor," you will never forget the experience. If you have any doubt that you have felt it, then for practical purposes, you have not.

> **Key Point**
>
> In the overwhelming majority of infants with pyloric stenosis, the diagnosis can be made unequivocally on clinical grounds alone. If in doubt, ask an experienced consultant to examine the baby.

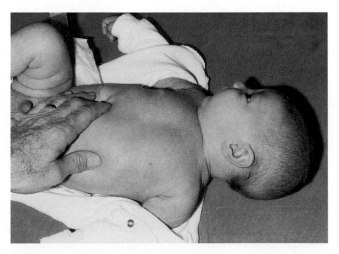

Figure 12–14 Checking for the pyloric "tumor."

If your attempts to feel the characteristic lump have been unsuccessful you may take the opportunity to do so while the baby is under general anesthesia, just before the operation (pyloromyotomy), which will make identifying the pyloric mass easier the next time you need to do so.

SUMMARY

The clinical ability to recognize pediatric abdominal conditions that call for surgical treatment is immensely important. A thorough history is a principal aid to accurate diagnosis. Understanding the neuroanatomic basis for the localization of abdominal pain is key to accurate interpretation of the child's symptoms. Astute observation should always precede palpation. When you do approach the tactile parts of the examination, gentleness and reassurance are the secrets of success. This chapter has suggested techniques for making surgical assessment of the abdomen in children more informative and less threatening. For each of the more common abdominal conditions in infants and children that requires surgery, there are important features to look for during the history-taking and special "tricks" to use during the physical examination that can make the difference between uncertainty and a reliable clinical assessment.

REFERENCE

1. Desjardins J: Normal Embryological Development and Congenital Anomalies of the Inguino-Scrotal Region. Montreal, Sainte-Justine Hospital, 1982.

chapter 13

Pediatric Neurologic Examination

JOSEPH M. DOOLEY

Many physicians feel uncomfortable when required to assess a child's neurologic status. They may be either afraid the youngster will not cooperate or uncertain of what a "normal" child should be able to do. A competent clinical evaluation, however, often precludes unnecessary investigations and prevents unwarranted psychological and financial costs for both the patient and society.

This chapter emphasizes ways to elicit cooperation from most children so that you can determine whether the findings are significant. The nervous system is an excellent model for the logical evaluation of clinical findings. Your knowledge of neurophysiology and neuroanatomy should enable you to locate the site of the problem within the nervous system or decide that the problem is caused by a more diffuse process and cannot be localized to a single lesion.

The neurologic assessment should be stimulating and enjoyable for both you and your patient. Where relevant, the description of each part of the examination is divided according to age ranges—school-aged child, preschool-aged child, and infant. At the end of the chapter, case histories are provided to show how the assessment is applied to children of different ages and to highlight some common problems in pediatric neurology.

To avoid overlooking important findings, you should approach each phase of the neurologic examination with the following categories in mind:

1. Higher cortical function or development.
2. Cranial nerves.
3. Trunk and extremities: power, tone, coordination, reflexes, and sensation.

THE LOGIC BEHIND THE APPROACH

At each phase of the assessment, try to determine the site of the lesion. Doing so makes it easier to compile a list of differential diagnoses or hypotheses. As an initial approach, divide neurologic disorders into upper motor neuron lesions (UMNLs) and lower motor neuron lesions (LMNLs). The major features of each are listed in Table 13–1. Remember that some children, such as those with leukodystrophies, may have a mixture of both UMNL and LMNL signs, and localizing the problem to a single focal lesion in such patients is not possible. In addition, children with disorders of the cerebellum or basal ganglia do not have UMNL signs.

OBTAINING THE HISTORY

When combined with hands-off observation, the history usually provides the diagnosis (see Chapter 1). The physical examination rarely reveals previously unsuspected findings.

Key Point

The history usually provides the diagnosis.

The School-Aged Child

Never intimidate the child. After introducing myself to their families, I try to establish rapport with children by asking why they think they have come to visit me and what they think is wrong. Ask youngsters their names and what they like to be called. Some children prefer to be called by a nickname.

Start the history by talking directly to the patient. This helps the youngster feel more involved in the process. Begin by talking about nonthreatening subjects, such as family members, school or teachers, television shows, music, or sports. Use open-ended questions to avoid "Yes" or "No" answers. All school-aged children deserve the opportunity to speak to the

Table 13–1   SIGNS OF UPPER AND LOWER MOTOR NEURON LESIONS

Parameters	Upper Motor Neuron Lesions: Central Nervous System Dysfunction*	Lower Motor Neuron Lesions: Peripheral Nervous System Dysfunction†
Intellect	Deficits may be found with cortical abnormalities	Normal
Cranial nerves	Abnormalities usually reflect brainstem involvement but may indicate a neuropathy	May be involved
Power	Slightly decreased, although movement more severely impaired because of altered tone	Markedly reduced; neuromuscular junction disease associated with fatigue
Tone	Increased (spasticity) with lesions affecting pyramidal pathways; rigidity seen with extrapyramidal disease	Reduced (floppy or hypotonic)
Coordination	Impaired when cerebellum or its connections are involved	May be hindered by weakness
Reflexes	Hyperactive in pyramidal dysfunction; plantar stimulation results in an extensor response (Babinski) in the great toe	Difficult to elicit
Sensation	Usually intact, but spinal cord gives a sensory level that is in a dermatomal distribution	Impaired with lesions that affect the nerve
Fasciculations		Present with anterior horn cell disease but occasionally also found with neuropathies

* Involve intracranial contents, brainstem, or spinal cord.
† Involve intracranial horn cells, nerves, neuromuscular junction, or muscles.

physician alone; it is during this part of the history that they sometimes reveal information they would otherwise withhold. The parents must be asked to leave the room for this part of the history. A child's inability to give a history may be an important observation in itself. Having gained the child's acceptance, you can now inquire about the presenting complaint.

Key Point

Every school-aged child should be given the chance to speak to the physician alone, a time when they sometimes reveal information that they would otherwise withhold. A child's inability to give a history may in itself be an important observation.

After allowing the patient to contribute as much as he or she wishes or can, ask the parents to tell you their main concerns. First, establish whether the problem is static or progressive, a distinction that will influence your differential diagnosis and subsequent inquiries. For example, a child with learning difficulties that are worsening is much more likely to have a neurodegenerative or metabolic disorder than a child whose problems are static or nonprogressive. Similarly, an intracranial lesion, such as a tumor, is much more likely if headaches are worsening than if they have been unchanged for months. Always ask details of the child's school performance, because deterioration in grades may suggest a progressive neurologic condition.

A brief but detailed history of the pregnancy is essential. Most mothers remember the pregnancy and birth in vivid detail and often have unfounded fears related to it (see Chapter 1). Reassuring a mother that the cough medicine she took during the third trimester was not the cause of her baby's meningomyelocele may relieve anxiety. Similarly, if a child has been discharged from the neonatal unit within 5 days of birth, it is extremely unlikely that significant perinatal problems occurred.

Key Point

Significant perinatal difficulties are extremely unlikely if the child was discharged from the neonatal nursery at the normal time.

The Preschool-Aged Child

Even 2-year-olds like to be involved, and a 3-year-old child may give a more accurate history than his or her distraught parent. Start the history by talking to the patient, because many children will soon become bored and distracted. The young child is most likely to cooperate if you frame requests in a gamelike fashion. The preschooler is usually happy to show a disbelieving physician that he or she can count and identify colors. Give the child the opportunity to prove you wrong. If you announce that Mickey Mouse is pink, even the most sullen child usually corrects you. The child's success and your delight with his or her performance help to improve the child's confidence in a strange environment.

To have undisturbed time during the subsequent discussions with the parents, it is essential to provide the child with age-appropriate toys. This playtime also provides an excellent opportunity to observe the child. Rarely, it may be necessary to have the child removed to another room to play.

OBSERVATION

The School-Aged Child

History-taking offers an excellent opportunity to observe the child unobtrusively. The gait of a child with a hemiparesis may be apparent as he or she walks from the waiting area to the examining room. Typically, the arm is held flexed and adducted against the chest and the leg is circumducted. The child's appearance is very important. Note the shape and size of the head (e.g., microcephaly or hydrocephalus), the shape and positioning of the eyes and ears (e.g., in Down syndrome), and any skin lesions (e.g., the facial angioma of Sturge-Weber syndrome). Asking the parents to bring in some family photographs can sometimes be useful. This allows you to compare the child's appearance with that of relatives.

Key Point

Observe the child's gait, facial appearance, use of language, and any dysmorphic features during your first encounter.

The formal neurologic examination begins during the observation phase. Strabismus or ophthalmoplegia may be apparent. The child's use of language during interaction with the parents is often more spontaneous and informative than in conversation with the physician. Dysphasia indicates dysfunction in the dominant hemisphere. Dysarthria may represent problems in the mouth, such as a cleft palate, or may be due to lesions involving cranial nerve VII, VIII, IX, X, or XII. Facial asymmetry (as in Bell's palsy) may indicate a lesion of the seventh cranial nerve (LMNL) or cerebral cortex (UMNL).

POWER

Proximal leg weakness, seen in myopathies such as muscular dystrophy, may be apparent if the child walks with a waddling gait. The Trendelenburg sign indicates weakness of the hip abductors and is reflective of proximal weakness. Normally, when the child stands on one

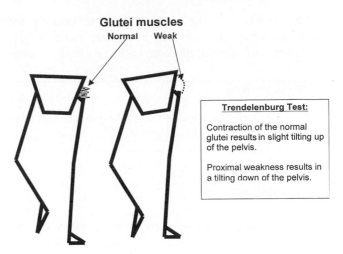

Figure 13–1 Trendelenburg test. Contraction of the normal gluteal muscles results in slight tilting up of the pelvis (*left*). Proximal weakness results in a tilting down of the pelvis (*right*).

leg, the glutei contract and the other side of the pelvis is tilted slightly upwards. When the child has proximal weakness, the glutei are not sufficiently strong, and the other hip tilts downwards. In order to maintain balance, the trunk leans over toward the side of the lesion; this is the *Trendelenburg sign* (Fig. 13–1). Weakness and wasting of the hand muscles are more likely to indicate a neuropathy. Remember that proximal weakness indicates a myopathy, and distal weakness, a neuropathy. Myotonic dystrophy, a dominantly inherited myopathy characterized by distal weakness and inability to relax the muscles, is the only major exception to this rule in childhood. During the period of observation, look for any asymmetry in limb movements.

Key Point

Proximal weakness indicates a myopathy; distal weakness indicates a neuropathy

---

Key Point

Difficulty in arising from the floor indicates weakness of the proximal leg muscles.

TONE

A limb with increased tone (spasticity, a UMNL) may be held in an unusual position. Thus, the child with a spastic arm draws with the "good" hand and keeps the spastic arm adducted against the trunk and flexed at the elbow. The spastic leg is circumducted at the hip when the child runs or walks. Always examine the wear patterns on the bottom of the child's shoes, which give invaluable information about the child's gait. When shaking hands with the child or parents, observe for myotonia, which is a difficulty in relaxing muscles. The most common cause of myotonia is myotonic dystrophy.

> **Key Point**
>
> The wear pattern on a child's shoes may give excellent clues to the origin of an abnormal gait.

COORDINATION

For older children, I use a challenging maze puzzle, which is an excellent test of coordination (Fig. 13–2). Cerebellar lesions affect the ipsilateral limb.

REFLEXES AND SENSATION

Reflexes and sensation are examined during the physical examination, described later.

ABNORMAL MOVEMENTS

The more common abnormal movements are discussed here.

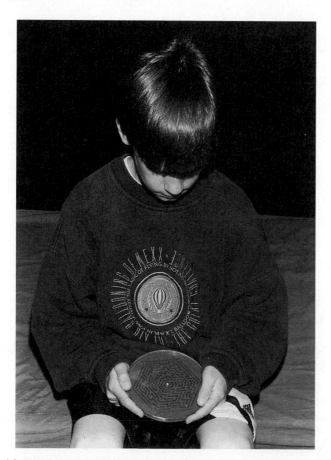

Figure 13–2 Maze puzzle.

Chorea, or *choreiform movement,* consists of quick, brief, nonrepetitive movements that vary from limb to limb and frequently involve the trunk. The child with *athetosis* has characteristic writhing movements. Both chorea and athetosis are most commonly seen in children with cerebral palsy.

Myoclonus consists of quick nonrhythmic contractions of single muscles or muscle groups.

Tremor is rhythmic and, when present during actions such as drawing, may represent benign essential or familial tremor. Intention tremor, which suggests cerebellar disease, may be seen during the finger-to-flashlight test (described below under Coordination).

Dystonic posturing, involuntarily maintained posturing of a limb in an unusual position, is seen in basal ganglia disease.

Tics are repetitive, stereotyped movements that have no purpose and usually indicate a diagnosis of Tourette syndrome. It is not unusual to meet parents who deny that they themselves have tics but who experience tics incessantly during the interview. This observation during a consultation for a child with possible Tourette syndrome is clearly of major importance.

> **Key Point**
>
> Observe both the patient and parents for abnormal movements such as tics, tremor, dystonia, athetosis, myoclonus, and choreiform movements.

The Preschool-Aged Child

In the younger child, a period of hands-off observation should always be the first part of the physical examination. I give the younger child puzzles and a pencil and paper. Giving children toys allows you to observe the youngster's manual dexterity, coordination, developmental competence, and handedness (Fig. 13–3). Observe the parent-child interaction closely. You may detect discipline problems at this stage. Drawings also reveal visual-spatial abilities, fine motor skills, and the child's level of attention. Allowing the child to play also provides important undisturbed time with the parents as you take the history.

The Infant

The period of observation of an infant is often the most revealing part of the examination. Dysmorphic features may suggest a specific syndrome. As the infant lies in the parent's arms, observe the eye movements, facial movements, and symmetry. The movements of the child might indicate weakness, as is seen in anterior horn cell (AHC) disease (Werdnig-Hoffmann disease).

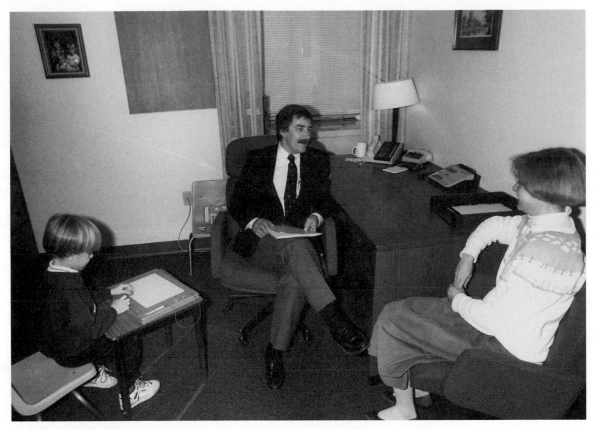

Figure 13–3 Providing drawing toys to children allows you to observe the child's hand eye coordination unobtrusively and relax the child while obtaining a history from the parent.

When tone is reduced, the infant may lie with hips and arms abducted (frog-leg position). Infants may appear to be hypotonic (floppy) from either weakness (LMNL) or central causes (UMNL). With floppiness due to an LMNL, the infant also has significant weakness and moves very little. The infant who is floppy because of a UMNL is able to move the limbs and is not weak.

THE PHYSICAL EXAMINATION

For the physical examination, the child's cooperation is necessary and is usually easy to obtain. If a child with a behavior problem refuses to cooperate, ask the parents to leave the room; this step is almost never necessary.

The School-Aged Child

I begin the physical examination of a school-aged child by playing ball with the child, thus extending the period of observation and allowing further evaluation of gait, power, and coordination as the child catches, throws, and kicks the ball.

To test proximal strength, ask the child to hop on each foot. You can also test pelvic girdle strength by asking the child to (1) arise from the supine position without using the arms, (2) do deep knee bends, and (3) "duck walk" (with hips and knees flexed). Children with mild spasticity also have difficulty performing these tasks because of their increased muscle tone.

> **Key Point**
>
> Test proximal strength by having the child arise from the floor without using the arms, do deep knee bends, and "duck walk."

Next, have the child walk on the heels and then on the toes. This request is more likely to be successful if you walk on your heels and toes at the same time. Heel walking is an excellent test, because weakness of the tibialis anterior (dorsiflexion of the foot) is an early sign of distal weakness in peripheral neuropathies. The patient with marked weakness has footdrop, which may be diagnosed from the slapping sound of the foot as the patient first walks into your office. Normally, the heel strikes the floor first, then the toes.

> **Key Point**
>
> Difficulty walking on the heels suggests distal weakness caused by a neuropathy.

Milder degrees of weakness may require additional testing. To demonstrate mild proximal weakness or spasticity, you may have to ask the child to run up and down stairs. You can easily confirm mild distal problems, however, by having the child repetitively tap each foot quickly on the ground.

Next, test cerebellar function by having the child walk a straight line in a heel-to-toe fashion (tandem gait). Other useful tests of cerebellar function are the *pirouette test*, during which the child is expected to perform three pirouettes (360-degree turns) while walking. A variant of this test is to ask the youngster to walk several times around an object (such as a chair). In both situations, the child with cerebellar disease will stumble toward the side of the cerebellar lesion. A wide-based "drunken" gait usually indicates cerebellar disease. Tapping each foot repetitively, previously described as a test for distal weakness, is also an excellent test of coordination.

Key Point

Diseases of the cerebellar hemisphere cause stumbling toward the same side as the lesion.

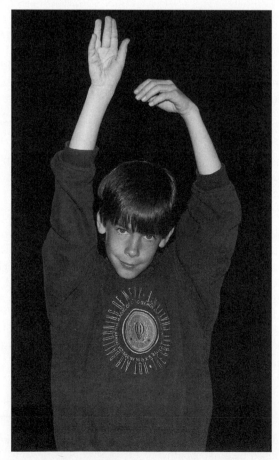

Figure 13–4 Pronator sign.

For the *Romberg test*, the child is told to keep the feet either side by side or in the "tandem" position, with one foot directly in front of the other. The child is then asked to extend the arms to the front and to close the eyes. Inability to maintain this position indicates a deficit in position sense (*proprioception*). With the eyes closed, the child is deprived of visual input and must depend on proprioception to maintain the standing position. Lesions of the cerebellum result in difficulty standing whether the eyes are open or closed. A loss of balance that occurs only when the eyes are closed is caused by a lesion in either the peripheral nerves or the posterior spinal columns.

Holding the extended and supinated arms in front of the body also tests for weakness. Children with mild weakness will be unable to maintain this position, and the arms tend to drift downward, flex at the elbow, and pronate (*pronator sign;* Fig. 13–4).

Check the spine next while the child touches his or her toes. Look for bony deformities and midline skin lesions, such as tufts of hair or sacral dimples, which may suggest underlying malformations.

Note that up to this point, you have not laid a hand on the child or used a single strange or intimidating instrument. The entire examination has been a hands-off exercise. It is now time to produce your reflex hammer and ophthalmoscope. You should, however, already have a provisional differential diagnosis in mind, which the examination will merely confirm or refute.

Key Point

At the end of the history, you should have formulated a differential diagnosis, which the examination can then confirm or refute.

If the physical examination reveals unsuspected findings, always review your history and observations to decide whether they should have led to different conclusions.

The Preschool-Aged Child

A period of ball playing is also useful for observing preschoolers. Even a child who is reluctant to leave the parent's side will usually play ball. The period of ball playing also helps establish you as an ally. You can then proceed as described for the school-aged child. Remember, however, that 4-year-olds may not successfully complete the tandem gait and that an inability to hop on one foot is not necessarily abnormal in children younger than 7 years.

You can most easily examine children younger than 6 years while they sit on a parent's lap rather than on the examining table.

Cortical Function

SCHOOL-AGED AND PRESCHOOL-AGED CHILDREN

Assess each cortical area in turn.

Frontal Lobes

The posterior frontal lobes contain the motor cortex. Deficits in a frontal lobe result in signs of upper motor neuron dysfunction on the other side of the body.

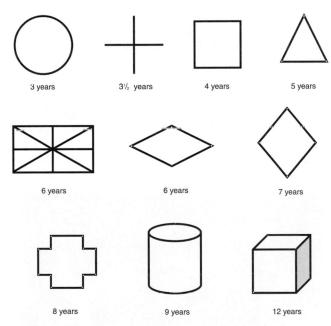

| 3 years | 3½ years | 4 years | 5 years |

| 6 years | 6 years | 7 years |

| 8 years | 9 years | 12 years |

Figure 13–5 Shapes used for testing spatial perception.

Motor aphasia appears in children older than 6 or 7 years if the Broca motor speech area in the dominant hemisphere is injured. The frontal lobes also control contralateral eye movements. An *irritative* lesion in the frontal eye fields (e.g., a seizure) causes deviation of the eyes away from the side of the lesion; in contrast, a *destructive* lesion causes deviation of the eyes toward the side of the lesion.

Disturbance of the more anterior parts of the frontal lobe may cause personality changes, irritability, and lethargy with lack of spontaneity. Sphincter incontinence may develop, and primitive reflexes, such as rooting, sucking, and grasp reflexes, may reemerge. Remember that frontal lobe lesions may be difficult to detect even if they are large.

Temporal Lobes

Temporal lobe impairment may cause personality changes similar to those seen with frontal lobe damage. Language is also represented in this lobe, and lesions of the superior and middle gyri cause *Wernicke aphasia*, characterized by impaired comprehension of word elements. Ability to read, write, and understand speech may be altered. If the nondominant temporal lobe is involved, the child has distorted perception of spatial relationships and a change in musical appreciation. Test for alterations in spatial perception by asking the child to copy geometric designs. Age-appropriate designs are shown in Figure 13–5. Bilateral involvement of the hippocampus interferes with learning. Temporal lobe injury also may produce psychotic aggressive behavior. Visual symptoms are usually represented by a homonymous superior quadrantanopia.

Memory deficits may be seen with temporal lobe dysfunction. You can test a child's immediate recall by reciting number sequences and having the child repeat them after you, either in the same order or in reverse; Table 13–2 gives examples of age-appropriate number sequences for this test.

Table 13–2   TEST FOR IMMEDIATE RECALL*

Age (yr)	"Repeat the Number After Me"			"Repeat the Number Backwards"		
2½	48	63	52	—	—	—
3	648	752	495	—	—	—
4½	4729	3852	7261	—	—	—
7	31859	48372	96183	295	816	473
9	—	—	—	8526	4937	3629
10	473859	429746	728394	—	—	—
12	72594836	47153962	41935826	81379	68582	92518
14				471952	583694	752618

*Recite each number sequence at the appropriate age level, and ask the child to either repeat it or recite it in reverse order.

Test a child's distant memory by asking the names of previous schoolteachers and locations of family vacations over the past few years; test more recent memory by asking what the child ate for supper or what television shows he or she watched the previous evening.

Parietal Lobes

Parietal lobe dysfunction produces sensory perception abnormalities. Two-point discrimination, graphesthesia, and appreciation of size, shape, and texture are all impaired. You can test these perceptions easily by asking the youngster to identify coins, a tissue, and a paper clip as you place them one at a time in one of the child's hands while the child's eyes are closed.

Children with parietal lobe deficits cannot appreciate simultaneous cutaneous stimulation on bilateral homologous body parts. Test this point by asking the child to identify (with the eyes closed) which arm you have touched; the child should be able to identify simultaneous touch of both arms.

A parietal lobe injury impairs awareness on the opposite side; cortical sensory changes are best tested during examination of sensation. Assuming that you are neurologically normal, use your own sensory perception as the normal reference.

Lesions of the parietal cortex also may cause *apraxia*, the inability to perform a series of tasks; apraxia may be present even though the patient can complete each component of the action individually. In young children with damage to the parietal lobes, growth on the affected side is usually impaired. Similarly, a smaller hand in a child with hemiparetic cerebral palsy indicates involvement of the parietal lobe. Such a child has reduced sensation in that limb and therefore has more difficulty with hand function than the child with exclusively motor dysfunction.

Occipital Lobes

Bilateral involvement causes cortical blindness. Unilateral lesions produce homonymous visual field defects.

Cranial Nerves

When testing the cranial nerves, start with the olfactory nerve (cranial nerve I) and examine each nerve sequentially until you have assessed all 12.

CRANIAL NERVE I (OLFACTORY)

The School-Aged Child

The olfactory nerve is responsible for the sense of smell. Your delight at a diagnosis of anosmia will tend to fade,

however, if the child's sense of smell returns after he or she blows his or her nose. Because children seem to have constant respiratory infections, first examine the nostrils. Then, while the child's eyes are either closed voluntarily or covered by a parent's hand, ask the child to identify the scent of common objects, such as chewing gum and chocolate, a task they should be able to perform. Never use irritants such as ammonia, detection of which involves fifth cranial nerve function.

The Preschool-Aged Child

It is seldom possible to perform an accurate assessment of the first nerve in preschool-aged children. If such assessment is clinically indicated, try to perform the technique described for the school-aged child.

CRANIAL NERVE II (OPTIC)

Always test each eye separately (see Chapter 8), and divide the examination into the following four parts.

Visual Fields

The School-Aged Child. Ask the school-aged child to point to your wiggling finger or to report how many fingers you are extending in each of the four visual quadrants while the child looks straight into your eyes.

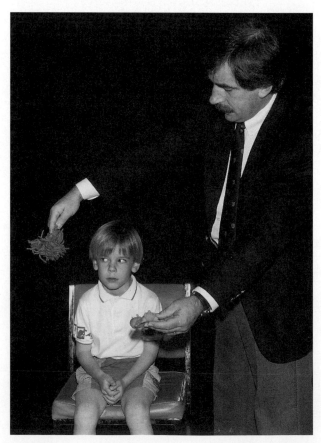

Figure 13–6 Visual field testing.

The Preschool-Aged Child. For the younger child, test the visual fields by distracting him or her with a toy in front while bringing a red toy from behind the youngster into the peripheral field of vision (Fig. 13–6). The child with normal vision should respond as soon as the toy reaches a line perpendicular to the outer canthus of the eye.

Visual Acuity

The School-Aged Child. Visual acuity can be tested as for adults, although some children with learning problems (e.g., dyslexia) should be tested with charts that contain images rather than letters (Fig. 13–7).

The Preschool-Aged Child. Use age-appropriate vision charts for the child older than 4 years. Test the younger child by offering small, interesting objects. I usually ask the parent to cover one of the child's eyes while I offer a tiny cake decoration. When the child realizes that this is "special candy," he or she readily picks it up. This is also a nice test of fine motor function. I encourage the patient to pick up the candy with each hand.

For less cooperative children, test for *opticokinetic nystagmus* (OKN) by pulling a striped cloth from one side to the other before the child's eyes. OKN consists of a slow deviation phase of the eyes in the direction the stripes are moving, followed by a rapid return (jerk) in the opposite direction. The presence of OKN indicates that the child has cortical vision. This can be a very useful test in children with hysterical blindness. Although they claim to be blind, OKN is present. If OKN is absent in one direction, suspect a hemianopia.

Key Point

Test for opticokinetic nystagmus (OKN) by pulling a striped cloth from one side to the other before the eyes. OKN consists of a slow deviation phase of the eyes in the direction the stripes are moving, followed by a rapid return (jerk) in the opposite direction.

Funduscopy

The School-Aged Child. It is difficult to distinguish papilledema from papillitis with the ophthalmoscope, but the latter is characterized by severe diminution in visual acuity.

The Preschool-Aged Child. In the preschooler, it is often reasonable to deviate from your usual order of examination by leaving funduscopy until the end of the

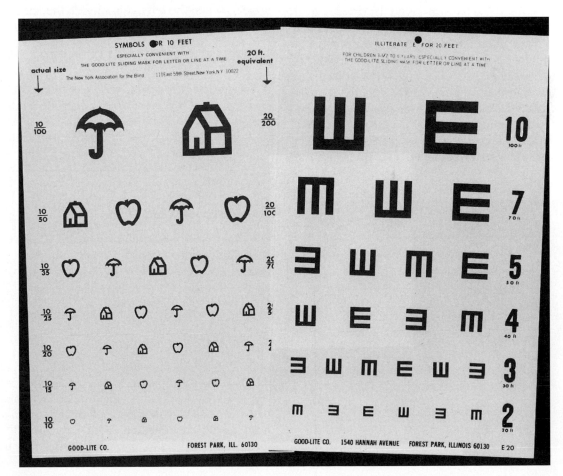

Figure 13–7 Visual chart for young children.

examination. The following technique is invariably successful:

1. Seat the child in front of you, and have the parent stand behind you; explain the procedure to the parent. Reduce the ambient light to allow pupil dilatation.
2. Ask the child to tell you whether the parent sticks his or her tongue out.
3. Not surprisingly, the child tries hard to focus on the parent, and shouts when the parent sticks out his or her tongue. Feigning anger with the parent delights the child.

With this technique, the child usually keeps the eyes still, allowing you to view the fundi. If the child cannot maintain fixation, keep the ophthalmoscope still, and view each fundus as it passes before your view while the eyes are moving.

The Infant. For infants, two techniques are valuable. Allowing an infant to suck on an object (even your finger) usually induces eye opening, and you can view the fundi without difficulty. Alternatively, have the parent hold the baby so that he or she is looking over one of the parent's shoulders. You can hold the baby's head gently but firmly while viewing the fundi (Fig. 13–8).

Pupillary Response

The pupillary response is subserved by two cranial nerves, II (afferent) and III (efferent). Test this response in children from all three age groups by moving a focused flashlight beam onto the pupil from the side; as the light is then moved to the other pupil, look for a change in the pupillary diameter. This *swinging flashlight test* compares the function of the two optic nerves. Decreased input through a dysfunctional second cranial nerve results in less constriction of both pupils when the light is shone into the affected eye. Swinging the

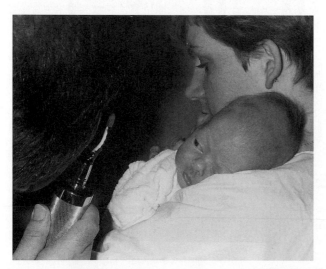

Figure 13–8 Fundus examination in an infant.

light into the normal eye then results in a greater stimulus, and the pupils constrict further.

CRANIAL NERVES III, IV, AND VI (OCULOMOTOR, TROCHLEAR, AND ABDUCENS)

The superior oblique muscle is innervated by the fourth cranial nerve, the lateral rectus by the sixth cranial nerve, and the other muscles—medial rectus, superior rectus, inferior rectus, and inferior oblique—by the third cranial nerve.

The School-Aged Child

Having the school-aged child follow a flashlight with the eyes allows you to see the light reflection, which should be centered on both pupils. If the patient has diplopia, ask him or her to report where the two images are most widely separated. Children may find it easiest to represent their diplopia by holding a pen in each hand, which they can use to demonstrate the position of each image. By having the child close each eye sequentially, establish which eye is seeing the outer (false) image. This maneuver establishes which muscle is paretic. For example, if the images are most widely separated when the child is looking horizontally to the left and the outer image disappears when the left eye is closed, the left lateral rectus muscle is responsible—signifying a left sixth nerve palsy.

Key Point

Because the sixth cranial nerve has a long course through the cranium, it is especially vulnerable to traction or pressure. Sixth nerve palsy does not help localize the site of dysfunction; it may occur with increased intracranial pressure (ICP) of any cause.

The Preschool-Aged Child

For children younger than 6 years, I place a pencil flashlight inside a plastic finger puppet. Every child readily focuses on this toy, which I move through lateral, medial, upper, and lower visual fields to observe the eye movements.

The Infant

Babies' eyes should follow an object, especially a face, that is moved from side to side at a distance of about 18 inches. In the neonate, eye movements can be tested with the *doll's eye reflex*, in which movement of the head results in deviation of the eyes in the opposite direction. This reflex remains present in coma and when fixation is prevented.

Ptosis may reflect a deficit of the third cranial nerve but also occurs in neuromuscular diseases such as myasthenia gravis. When ptosis is due to a third nerve palsy, the pupil on the affected side may be enlarged.

Key Point

Remember that in double vision, the outer image is always the false one and the images are most widely separated in the direction of action of the involved nerve and muscle.

CRANIAL NERVE V (TRIGEMINAL)

The trigeminal nerves are responsible for the muscles of mastication and for sensation to the face.

The School-Aged Child

Check the masseter muscles by asking the school-aged child to clench his or her teeth together as hard as possible. The strength of these muscles is impressive, showing why it is senseless and dangerous to try to pry open the mouth of a patient who is having a seizure. Sensation can be tested when other sensory modalities are being assessed. Test all three divisions—ophthalmic, maxillary, and mandibular.

Test the *jaw jerk reflex* by placing your thumb over the child's chin (his or her mouth should be slightly open) and then tapping on your thumb; the reflex stretches the masseter muscles, resulting in jaw closure. Both the afferent and efferent pathways are through the fifth cranial nerve. In children, the jaw closure is normally difficult to see, and brisk closure of the mouth suggests a UMNL. Do not elicit this reflex routinely; even the most trusting child will seriously question your motivation if you approach his or her face with a hammer.

Peripheral lesions of the fifth nerve are rare. Central involvement (UMNL) may occur in the cavernous sinus, where the third, fourth, and sixth cranial nerves may also be involved. Tumors at the cerebellopontine angle may involve the fifth, seventh, and eighth nerves and the cerebellar outflow tracts. Unilateral fifth nerve lesions result in deviation of the jaw to the paretic side.

The Preschool-Aged Child

In younger children, palpate the masseter muscles while the child chews.

The Infant

The masseter muscles can be palpated in infants as they suck.

CRANIAL NERVE VII (FACIAL)

School-Aged and Preschool-Aged Children

The facial nerve is responsible for the muscles of facial expression. Observing the face during the examination usually allows an excellent assessment of this nerve. Ask the youngster to forcibly close his or her eyes, wrinkle the forehead, and show his or her teeth. The facial asymmetry and weakness are not apparent during emotion-related movements, such as smiling and crying. A UMNL of the seventh nerve (above the level of pons) spares the forehead muscles. Most young children can be persuaded to imitate forced eye closure and to blow on a finger puppet or flashlight. Children with a facial palsy tend to drool from the weak side of the mouth.

All Three Age Groups

The corneal reflex depends on the fifth (afferent) and seventh (efferent) cranial nerves. Test this reflex by touching the cornea with a wisp of cotton, which is brought to the eye from the side, outside the field of vision. A substitute for this unpleasant test involves blowing gently over the cornea of one eye while your hand protects the other eye from stimulation (Fig. 13–9).

Testing taste from the anterior two thirds of the tongue (supplied by the chorda tympani) is not part of the routine neurologic examination in children.

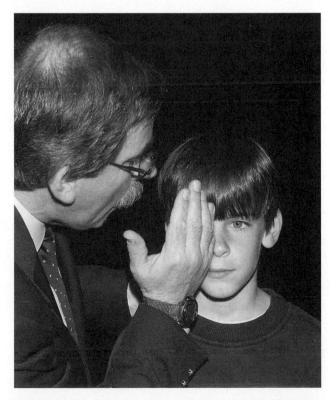

Figure 13–9 Blow gently over the cornea while your hand protects the other eye.

CRANIAL NERVE VIII (COCHLEAR AND VESTIBULAR)

The School-Aged Child

Test the acoustic nerve in a school-aged child by observing the response to rustling paper or finger rubbing. I usually test hearing by whispering numbers at a distance of 8 feet while a parent occludes one of the child's ears.

You can perform the *Rinne test* in children older than 6 years by holding a vibrating tuning fork (256 Hz) against the mastoid process (testing bone conduction). When the child can no longer hear the sound, hold the tuning fork close to the external auditory meatus (testing air conduction). Normally, air conduction is perceived for twice as long as bone conduction.

Weber's lateralizing test can also be performed in an older child. Apply the vibrating tuning fork to the midline of the forehead, and ask the child whether he or she hears sound in the center of the head or only in one ear. Normally, the sound is perceived in the midline. In ear disease, however, the sound seems louder on the affected side, because the normal environmental sounds decrease the apparent intensity of the tuning fork on the normal side. In neural deafness, the sound seems to be coming from the normal ear. If the history suggests a hearing deficit, arrange for formal audiologic evaluation.

The Preschool-Aged Child and the Infant

If the history of a preschool-aged child or infant suggests a hearing deficit, arrange for audiologic testing. Parents may report that the child wants the television volume louder than other people do or that the child is surprised when the parent "suddenly" comes into the field of vision. You can stimulate the vestibular nerve in a young child by holding him or her in your arms and rotating through 360 degrees, both clockwise and counterclockwise. Eye deviation in the direction of rotation and nystagmus in the opposite direction are normally seen. I believe this is a valuable test because it evaluates a relatively wide area of the brainstem connecting the vestibular and the oculomotor nuclei.

CRANIAL NERVES IX AND X (GLOSSOPHARYNGEAL AND VAGUS)

The School-Aged Child

Testing of the 9th and 10th cranial nerves is usually limited to observation of palatal movement. Have the school-aged child say "ah" with the mouth held widely open. Examine the gag reflex if there is any suggestion of dysfunction in the history or other aspects of the examination. Early in your career, assess the gag reflex in all patients undergoing neurologic assessment, but remember to stand to the side, because an occasional child with an excessive gag reflex will vomit.

The Preschool-Aged Child and the Infant

The younger, uncooperative child inevitably cries at some stage during the examination; take the opportunity to observe the palatal movements. As in the older child, examine the gag reflex if the history or other aspects of the examination suggest dysfunction. Children who recurrently aspirate milk or food may have an underactive reflex, whereas those with cerebral palsy may gag easily because of a hyperactive reflex. Those with defective palatal movement have difficulty making the "b," "d," and "k" sounds.

NERVE XI (SPINAL ACCESSORY)

The School-Aged Child

Assess the accessory nerve, which supplies the sternomastoid muscles, by having the school-aged child push against your hand with his or her mandible. The contracting sternomastoid on the opposite side can be palpated. Children love success, so give lots of encouragement.

The Preschool-Aged Child and the Infant

Test cranial nerve XI in the young child or infant by placing him or her in the supine position. While supporting the shoulders but not the head, push the head laterally. The child will resist the movement, and you can palpate the sternomastoid muscle.

NERVE XII (HYPOGLOSSAL)

The School-Aged Child

Assess tongue movements by asking the child to imitate you as you move your tongue from side to side. Fasciculations of the tongue while at rest indicate anterior horn cell disease.

The Preschool-Aged Child and the Infant

The examination of the 12th cranial nerve in the young patient is limited to observation when the mouth is opened.

Physical Examination of the Trunk and Extremities

The child must be asked to undress for the physical examination. It is more acceptable to undress the upper and lower halves of the body at different times. I usually examine the exposed legs first, and I ask all families to bring shorts to the consultation. The child then dresses the legs again before undressing the arms and trunk. All children, irrespective of age, deserve to have their modesty respected. Interestingly, concern about being partly undressed is most common in boys between 8 and 12 years old.

LOWER EXTREMITIES

Power

If you follow the examination procedure given in this chapter, you already tested power in the lower extremities when you had the patient hop, "duck-walk," and walk on toes and heels.

Observe the muscle bulk for wasting. In neuropathies, the wasting occurs distally and can produce pes cavus (Fig. 13–10). Diagnose pes cavus when light is seen under the arch despite pressing a hard object, such as a book, firmly against the sole of the foot. Hypertrophic appearance of the calf muscles in conjunction with proximal muscle weakness suggests muscular dystrophy (actually pseudohypertrophy, due to fatty infiltration of muscles). These pseudohypertrophic muscles feel "rubbery" to palpation. Fasciculations, due to spontaneous contractions of muscle fiber groups, are seen primarily with anterior horn cell dysfunction but also occasionally with neuropathies. They can be heard as crackling sounds when you listen over the muscle with the bell of your stethoscope.

The School-Aged Child. Undertake more formal testing with the school-aged child lying supine. Test each muscle group separately. It is useful to use a grading scale, but it is essential to document the scale you have used. I frequently find notes in charts indicating that the muscle strength in a patient's biceps was "3/6." What does this mean? One commonly used scale (from the Medical Research Council of the United Kingdom—memorandum 45[1]) is outlined in Table 13–3. As part of the routine examination, you should test (1) hip flexors, extensors, adductors, and abductors, (2) knee flexion (hamstrings) and extension (quadriceps), and (3) ankle dorsiflexion, plantar flexion, inversion, and eversion.

The Preschool-Aged Child. Place young or uncooperative preschool-aged patients on the floor. Even the most stubborn child eventually gets up. As he or she arises, assess the leg strength. Proximal weakness is characterized by the use of the arms to help the child "climb" up the legs (*Gower sign*) (see Chapter 15). Children older than 3 years should be able to stand briefly on one foot. A child who is reluctant to perform these tasks usually cooperates if you do the tasks at the same time. If this approach does not work, remember that every child rises to tiptoes to reach for an interesting toy. These maneuvers allow avoidance of the difficult question of what is acceptable strength for a child. All children should be able to support their body weight.

Key Point

All children should be able to support their body weight.

Tone

The School-Aged Child. If you are following the examination procedure given in this chapter, you have also noted muscle tone during your observation of the patient. It is difficult for students to appreciate the variations of acceptable muscle tone. The normal child younger than 12 years can passively touch his or her nose with the large toe without discomfort. In the spastic child, this maneuver is impossible, whereas the floppy (hypotonic) child can put his or her toe behind the ipsilateral ear. Normally, the ankle can be dorsiflexed 20 degrees and the hips can be abducted 60 or 70 degrees. Test clonus at the ankles by rapidly

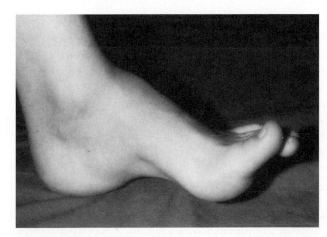

Figure 13–10 Pes cavus.

Table 13–3	SCALE FOR GRADING MUSCLE STRENGTH
0	No muscle contraction
1	Flicker of contraction
2	Movement with gravity eliminated
3	Movement against gravity
4	Movement against resistance
5	Normal power

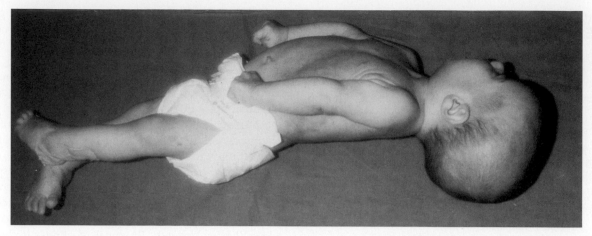

Figure 13–11 Scissoring of the legs.

dorsiflexing the foot, which is reliably done only if the ankle is relaxed. Holding the foot while talking to the child allows him or her to eventually relax. More than two or three beats of clonus is usually abnormal.

The Preschool-Aged Child and the Infant. When the young child or infant is lifted in the air, "scissoring" of the legs (Fig. 13–11) indicates increased tone (spasticity, UMNL) in the hip adductors. Because of tightness in the hip adductors, the child with increased tone also tends to sit on the floor in the "W" position, with the thighs and knees touching each other.

Key Point

"Scissoring" of the legs is an early sign of spasticity.

Coordination

The School-Aged Child. Test coordination in cooperative school-aged youngsters by having them run each heel along the shin of the other leg and then tap the knee two or three times with the heel. Repetitively tapping each foot on the ground, as noted previously, is also an excellent test of lower extremity coordination.

The Preschool-Aged Child. Most preschoolers will walk around a chair if the exercise is framed in a game format whereby the child must follow his or her parent.

Key Point

Diseases of the cerebellar hemisphere cause stumbling to the same side as the lesion.

Reflexes

School-Aged and Preschool-Aged Children. It is easy to elicit knee reflexes when you sit opposite the school-aged or preschool-aged child and rest his or her feet on

your own knees. The angle at the child's knees should be symmetrical and approximately 120 degrees. With the legs in this position, it is easy to demonstrate the reflexes by tapping just below the patella (Fig. 13–12). I discourage the use of "tomahawk" reflex hammers. Those with a "wheel" at the top work best.

You can easily obtain the ankle reflex by holding the foot at 90 degrees with your thumb on the plantar aspect and your other fingers over the dorsum. The reflex can be seen when you strike your own thumb with the hammer. If you find it difficult to elicit an ankle reflex, ask the child to kneel on the examining table or chair with the heels over the edge (Fig. 13–13), and tap over the Achilles tendon. Before concluding that a reflex is absent, try the same maneuver while you have patient clenching his or her teeth as hard as possible and trying to pull his or her interlocked fingers apart. Reflexes with a slow relaxation phase (especially ankle jerks) are seen in children with hypothyroidism.

Key Point

Areflexia is present only if reflexes cannot be elicited with reinforcement.

The *Babinski sign* was first described by Joseph Babinski in 1896. For this test, the leg should be slightly flexed and relaxed. Carefully stroke the lateral border of the sole of the foot from heel to little toe with a relatively sharp object. A positive response, indicative of corticospinal disease (UMNL), consists of dorsiflexion of the great toe and flaring of the other toes. Both my thumbnail and a car key have served me well for this test. Numerous other maneuvers that elicit the same reflex can occasionally help if interpretation of the response is hindered by either a grasp response or intolerance of the procedure. I find stimulating the dorsum of the great toe with a pin or firmly rubbing the anterior tibial region (Oppenheim reflex) is helpful.

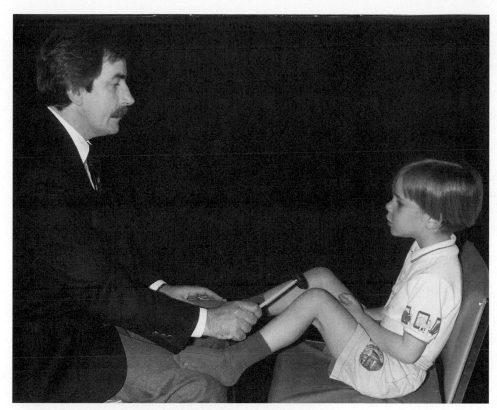

Figure 13–12 Position for testing the knee reflex.

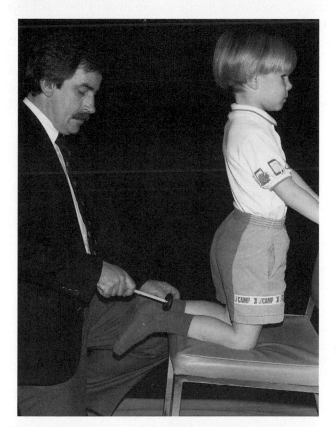

Figure 13–13 Position for testing the ankle reflex.

There has been much debate regarding the significance of the Babinski sign in children younger than 1 year. In general, it should be considered significant

only if accompanied by other evidence of a UMNL. In infants, test this reflex with the child lying supine; the head should be maintained in the midline to eliminate the asymmetric tonic neck reflex (ATNR), the knee should be extended, and the foot should be held at a 90-degree angle. If these precautions are taken, the great toe plantar flexes in the vast majority of infants, as it does in older children.

Test the abdominal reflexes, subserving thoracic segments T8 to T12, while the child lies supine on the bed or examining table. Draw a pinwheel from the lateral aspects of the abdominal quadrants toward the umbilicus, a maneuver that normally induces a movement of the umbilicus toward the stimulus. If indicated, examine the cremasteric reflex (L1, L2) by stroking the inside of the thigh with a sharp object and observing for retraction of the testis on that side. Another reflex that is sometimes valuable is the anal reflex (S3, S4, S5) or anal "wink," which is tested by scratching the skin around the anus and observing contraction of the anal ring. Absence or asymmetry of these reflexes indicates corticospinal tract involvement.

Infants. It is important to assess the primitive reflexes in all children younger than 1 year. Although there are many such reflexes, the Moro reflex and ATNR are the most helpful.

The *Moro reflex* first appears between 28 and 32 weeks' gestation and disappears between 3 and 5 months of age. Elicit this reflex by suddenly dropping the baby's head 6 to 12 inches (and catching it in your hand). The arms abduct with extension of the fingers, followed by adduction of the arms across the chest and flexion of the hips. This reflex is present in all babies during the first few months, but it normally disappears by 6 months. Look for any asymmetry between the limbs, which is also abnormal.

Obtain the *asymmetric tonic neck reflex* by turning the baby's head to one side. The arm and leg become relatively more extended on the side to which the baby looks. The limbs on the "occipital" side are flexed; this is also termed the *fencer position* (Fig. 13–14). The ATNR reflex is also seen during the first 6 months of life but is most prominent during the second and third months. It is impossible for the baby to sit if this reflex is still present, and its persistence (while the baby is awake) beyond 6 months is abnormal. Also consider the ATNR abnormal if the child cannot "break" the posture within a minute or if there is a persistent difference between the responses obtained with the head turned to either side.

The *palmar grasp reflex* is present at about 28 weeks' gestation and is replaced by voluntary grasp between 2 and 3 months of age. With frontal lobe dysfunction, this reflex may reappear.

Sensation

The School-Aged Child. Although the sensory examination often is considered the most difficult part of the pediatric neurologic examination, an easy accurate assessment is possible in most school-aged children. Using a pin, needle, Wartenberg wheel, or broken

tongue depressor for testing pain sensation in children usually causes fear and may end the examination prematurely. I use a nonthreatening pink tracing wheel, an instrument commonly used for sewing. Ask the child to close the eyes and to say "now" whenever he or she is touched and to report qualitative changes in the sensation in different parts of the limb.

If you suspect a hysterical sensory loss, ask the child to say "Yes" when you touch him or her and "No" when you do not. It amazes me how often this approach is successful. The child says "Yes" for the first few touches and replies "No" for the next few, helping persuade the parents that a more detailed review of the stresses in their child's life is warranted.

Test vibration sense using a tuning fork (128 Hz) placed over a distal phalanx. Ask the child to tell you when the vibration stops, and compare this response with your own ability to perceive vibration. To test proprioception, secure the toe or finger by holding its lateral aspects and move only the most distal phalanx. A tiny movement of 10 to 20 degrees is normally appreciated (Fig. 13–15).

The *Romberg test* also assesses proprioception. Ask the child to stand with the feet together. For a more challenging variant, ask the child to place the feet in the tandem position with one foot in front of the other in a heel-to-toe position.

The Preschool-Aged Child. Allow the child to play with the tracing wheel during the history-taking, so the tool is readily accepted at this stage of the examination. I distract the young child with a toy while I run the tracing wheel up his or her arm or leg. A child with

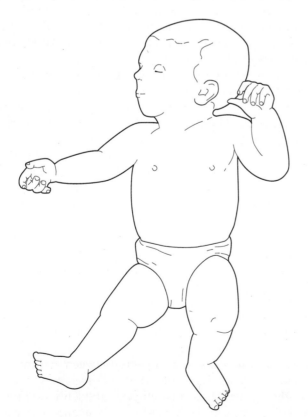

Figure 13–14 Asymmetric tonic neck reflex (ATNR).

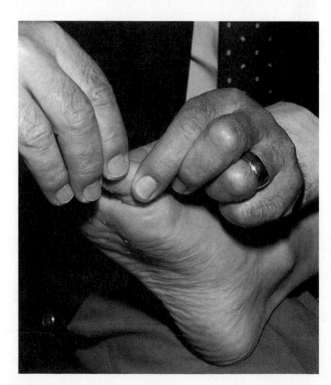

Figure 13–15 Testing proprioception.

normal sensation immediately looks at the stimulation site. If the child seems unaware of the stimulation distally but becomes more aware as the wheel is moved proximally, mark the point of apparent awareness. Repeat the test. If the findings are reproducible, further tests to diagnose a neuropathy, such as an electromyogram and nerve conduction studies, are worthwhile.

Perform sensory testing for touch with a paper tissue, being careful not to move the tissue over the skin, as this results in tickle, which is conveyed through less pure sensory pathways. Younger children can report only the presence or absence of sensation, whereas the older child can report qualitative changes.

To test vibration, place the nonvibrating tuning fork over the bony prominence of a toe or finger, repeating the procedure until the child becomes accustomed to the sensation and no longer reacts to it. Then place the vibrating tuning fork in the same position; if vibration sensation is intact, the child's response changes.

Perform the Romberg test in a preschool-aged child by having the parents cover the eyes of the child, who is told to stand with the feet together. Proprioception is not tested routinely in the young child at this stage, because the Romberg test has already been used for this aspect of the assessment.

Key Point

Respect the child's modesty, but always examine the skin thoroughly for lesions.

Before allowing the child to dress, inspect the skin thoroughly for lesions associated with "neurocutaneous" syndromes. In neurofibromatosis, there are multiple café au lait spots. In tuberous sclerosis, facial adenoma sebaceum may be mistaken for acne. Patients with this disorder also have depigmented spots (Fig. 13–16) that may have a leaf shape (ash leaf spots). The Sturge-Weber syndrome is characterized by a facial hemangioma that involves the first division of the trigeminal nerve and is associated with underlying abnormalities in the cerebral cortex on the same side. Children with this syndrome often have seizures and mental retardation in addition to other problems. Finally, check the spine for scoliosis and for cutaneous lesions. Children with a tuft of hair or apparent dermal sinus over the spine may have an underlying spinal cord lesion.

UPPER EXTREMITIES

Power

The School-Aged Child. Children with chronic hemiparesis (spasticity involving the arm and leg on the same side) usually have a smaller thumbnail on the affected side. Similarly, the nail on the large toe is smaller in even mildly hemiparetic limbs. Establish that each joint has a full range of movement. Test strength more formally by pushing against the abducted arms. Test the biceps with the child's arm somewhat flexed at the elbow and the hand held in supination. Grip the child's forearm and ask him or her to resist extension at the elbow. Test the triceps by extending the arm against resistance. Next, assess wrist extension and flexion by pushing over the dorsum and palmar aspects of the hands, respectively. Examine finger strength in the older child as in the adult. If you allow the child to "win" some of these contests of strength, he or she is encouraged to make greater effort, allowing you to assess muscle strength more accurately.

Key Point

Chronic hemiparesis is associated with a smaller thumbnail on the affected side.

The Preschool-Aged Child and the Infant. Test upper extremity strength in the younger child by staging a wheelbarrow "race" (Fig. 13–17). In this maneuver, the arms support the total body weight.

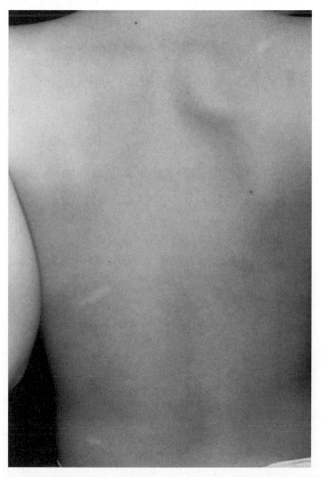

Figure 13–16 Depigmented lesions.

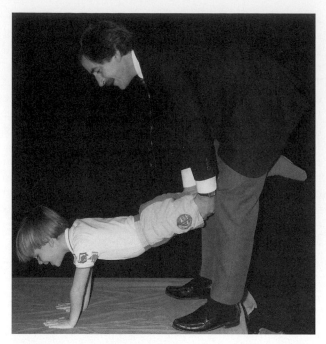

Figure 13-17 Wheelbarrow position.

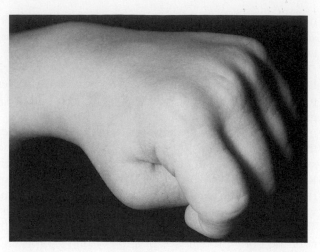

Figure 13-18 Fisting.

You can easily examine shoulder adductors by lifting the young child with your hands under the axillae. Assess distal strength by getting the child to pull a toy from you. In the child younger than 5 years, test the proximal power of the arms by holding the child under the axillae without supporting the chest. Your hands act as hooks; the child should be able to support his or her own weight.

Tone

The School-Aged Child. Test tone in the upper extremities of the school-aged child by holding the hand and alternately pronating and supinating the forearm. Increased tone in the arms is often most apparent in the hands, where the thumbs are held tucked in under the fingers in a "fisted" position (Fig. 13-18). Your confidence in distinguishing normal and abnormal tone depends on the number of children you have examined. Take every opportunity to assess muscle tone in your pediatric patients, and you will quickly appreciate the range of normal muscle tone in children.

The Preschool-Aged Child. If the preschool-aged child is uncooperative, you may assess the tone more easily by holding each forearm and then shaking it to observe wrist movements. If you accompany these movements with silly noises, the child is more likely to cooperate. This maneuver is difficult to resist and is a more reliable way to assess muscle tone in the young child.

The Infant. Hold the infant in horizontal suspension. The floppy baby hangs like an inverted U (Fig. 13-19), whereas the spastic child hyperextends the trunk. When pulled to sit, the normal neonate shows some evidence of neck flexion. The *scarf sign* is a helpful test

for upper extremity tone; to test for it, adduct the arm as far as possible. In the normal infant, the elbow can be brought to midline, touching the chin.

Coordination

The School-Aged Child. Ask the school-aged child to touch your finger and then his or her nose. Be sure to make him or her stretch to reach your finger, because tremor may be apparent only during the last few centimeters of extension.

The Preschool-Aged Child. Coordination is assessed easily and accurately in a child 18 months or older by asking him or her to press a penlight bulb with his or her index finger or great toe. I present this request as a "magic test." When the child touches the light bulb, switch off the light. The young child believes he or she has magically turned off the light and is delighted. The more mature child is pleased to inform the physician that he or she has not been fooled by so simple a trick. This test is as accurate as any performed in the adult.

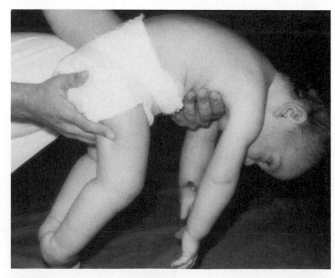

Figure 13-19 Prone floppy baby.

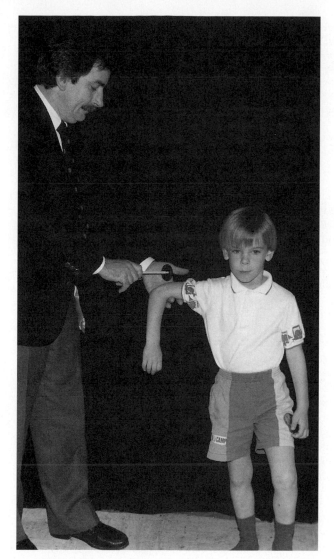

Figure 13–20 Position for testing the triceps reflex.

Test fine motor function by asking the child to screw a nut and bolt together, pile a series of blocks, and, for the older child, to sequentially approximate the thumb with each finger. Difficulty performing rapid repetitive movements (tapping the hand on the leg) and alternating movements (pronation-supination, as in screwing in a light bulb) may indicate cerebellar disease or dyspraxia. Dyspraxia, the inability to perform a series of tasks despite being able to do each segment individually, is usually due to parietal lobe disease.

Reflexes

School-Aged and Preschool-Aged Children. Examine the deep tendon reflexes in a school-aged or preschool-aged child as you would in an adult. For the biceps reflex, the child's arms should rest in his or her lap with the elbows partially flexed. I place my finger over the tendon and then hit my own finger, thus persuading the child I do not want to hurt him or her and also allowing me to feel muscle movement during the reflex. You can more easily test the triceps reflex by

abducting the arm 90 degrees with the elbow flexed to 90 degrees (perpendicular to the ground) (Fig. 13–20). In this position, the reflex can be seen easily, and it is difficult for the child to resist. Elicit the *Hoffman reflex* by holding the patient's hand in the pronated position and flicking the terminal phalanx of the middle finger down. In children with UMNL, the thumb flexes and adducts and the other fingers also flex.

Sensation

Testing sensation in the arms is as described previously for the legs.

Then, auscultate the head for bruits. As many as 60% of normal children 4 to 5 years old and 10% of children 10 years old have audible intracranial bruits that are of no clinical significance. Benign bruits are softer and less harsh than bruits associated with vascular lesions. The only way to confidently make this distinction is to listen to the cranium of every child you examine. Measure the head circumference and palpate the anterior fontanelle and cranial sutures.

Case Histories

Now that you have read over the entire procedure for neurologic assessment, try applying this approach to the following case histories.

Case 1

History. Jason, a 10-year-old fifth grader, comes to you because of headaches. What questions might you ask him? Remember that the history that you obtain from Jason will be much more valuable than that provided by his parents. Table 13–4 provides some guidelines for questions that might be valuable in this situation.

Jason reports that the headaches began 2 weeks ago and are becoming steadily more severe. In reply to your questions, he says that the pain is both sharp and throbbing, and he locates it by pointing with one finger over his right temporal region. When asked if the pain comes on at any particular time of the day, he confirms that the headache awakens him at about 6:00 AM.

The information shown in Table 13–4 should make it apparent that these findings are worrisome, suggesting raised intracranial pressure (ICP). The early-morning predominance reflects an aggravation of the slight increase in ICP that normally occurs at night.

Jason vomits with the headaches but he says he does not feel sick, a finding also suggesting raised ICP. Children who vomit with migraine typically have associated nausea.

Over the past 2 weeks, he has not gone out to play with his friends, but he has missed only 2 days of school. In response to questioning he says he has not been hit on the head.

Table 13–4   CHARACTERISTICS OF HEADACHE PAIN AND POSSIBLE MEANING

Question	What the Answer May Indicate
When did headaches begin?	Chronic headaches are less likely to be due to significant disease
Are they getting worse?	Headaches due to increased intracranial pressure often become progressively more severe
Where are they located?	Migraine headaches switch from side to side
	Tension headaches tend to occur like a band around the head
	Headaches due to increased intracranial pressure may always be located in the same position
What type is the pain?	Migraine is usually described as throbbing
	Tension headaches are typically "pressing," but tumors (increased intracranial pressure) can produce throbbing, pressing, or sharp pain
When does the pain occur?	Migraine is episodic and often occurs in the afternoon but will occasionally wake the patient
	Tension headaches may last all day but do not interfere with sleep
	Pain due to increased intracranial pressure is worse in early morning and may awaken the child
Does the headache interfere with play?	Migraine and increased intracranial pressure disrupt the child's activities
	Tension headaches are complained of but do not interrupt anything; the child may use them to avoid unpleasant tasks
Are there associated symptoms?	Tension headaches are seldom associated with other symptoms
	Migraine is usually seen with anorexia, nausea, vomiting, photophobia, phonophobia, and visual symptoms such as flashing lights
	Increased intracranial pressure results in vomiting and may cause diplopia, due to a nerve palsy
What relieves headache?	Migraine is relieved by a brief period of sleep
	Increased intracranial pressure is seldom relieved by any specific factor
	Tension headaches are helped by stress reduction
Is there a family history of headaches?	Such a history is common in migraine and stress headaches
Has the child shown any changes in personality, ability, or thinking?	Such changes are more likely to be associated with significant disease
Are the headaches triggered by any foods, activities, or events?	Migraine is often triggered by stress, specific foods, or tiredness

---

Key Point

To assess the severity of the pain, ask whether it interferes with play. Insignificant headaches may prevent school attendance but not participation in sports and other pleasurable activities.

Learning more details of a patient's school performance is often an easy way to document cognitive function. Jason is described by his teachers as an excellent student who is always at the top of his class. He has had difficulty concentrating over the past 2 weeks, probably reflecting the severity of the headache pain. Children who have difficulties in school may have other problems, such as attention deficit hyperactivity disorder or learning disabilities, which require a thorough developmental assessment (see Chapter 6).

Jason tells you that he has sometimes seen double over the past couple of weeks. The remainder of his history is unremarkable.

What Is Your Differential Diagnosis? The history indicates that Jason almost certainly has some lesion that is causing increased ICP. With the information provided, you cannot predict where such a lesion is located, but your differential diagnosis is focused on either a tumor or, possibly, hydrocephalus. Other "space-occupying lesions," such as a subdural hemorrhage and abscess, are unlikely because both of these conditions would be expected to cause more profound illness.

What Will Be of Particular Interest during the Period of Observation? As you watch Jason walk into your office, he appears to have a mild limp, suggesting weakness of his left leg. The family reports that this is a recent change in his gait. His ability to answer your questions and his conversation with you suggest that he has normal intelligence. Similarly, his speech is clear, indicating that he does not have dysfunction of the 9th, 10th, or 12th cranial nerves. Intermittently throughout the history, Jason closes one eye, which he says is because he is seeing double (diplopia). This suggests a problem with cranial nerves III, IV, or VI. He seems concerned about his headaches. By contrast, many children with stress or tension headaches report terrible headaches but appear unconcerned as they play in your office.

Has the Period of Observation Helped You Localize Jason's Problem? The presence of a recent change in gait, with left leg difficulties, suggests a problem in the right hemisphere. The diplopia is most likely secondary to a sixth nerve lesion. As noted previously, this is not a helpful "localizing" sign because the sixth cranial nerve has a long course and is especially vulnerable to traction or pressure.

How Will Your Physical Examination Help Confirm Your Suspicion of a Right Hemisphere Lesion? Jason has difficulty running because his left leg tends to turn in. As he runs, you notice that his left arm is held adducted and swings less than his right. He is unable to hop on his left leg, cannot repetitively tap his left foot, and has difficulty with fine movements involving the left hand. He throws a ball better with his right hand, even though he is left-handed. These findings suggest spasticity of the left arm and leg.

Examination of the cranial nerves reveals bilateral papilledema, which reflects increased ICP. His double vision is most marked when Jason looks to the left, and the outer image disappears when he closes his left eye, therefore indicating that the responsible nerve is the left sixth cranial nerve. His power is probably normal, although you are uncertain whether he is slightly weak on the left. His tone, however, is definitely increased in both the left arm and leg, and he has five beats of clonus at the left ankle. The reflexes are also more brisk in the left limbs, and the plantar response shows dorsiflexion of the great toe. His coordination is reduced on the left, but you think that this finding is due to the spasticity (increased tone) rather than to cerebellar dysfunction. His sensation is normal.

What Is Your Differential Diagnosis Now? All your findings confirm your initial suspicions and point to an expanding lesion of some sort that affects the right motor cortex. The findings are not specific for any particular disease or lesion.

How Will You Manage This Patient? Jason requires urgent computed tomography (CT) or magnetic resonance imaging (MRI) of his head. Scanning demonstrates a tumor in the right posterior frontal lobe. He is referred for neurosurgical consultation and undergoes successful surgery.

Case 2

History. George is a 5-year-old whose parents are concerned that he has problems keeping up with his friends in physical activities.

What Are Your First Questions to Establish a Differential Diagnosis in This Boy? You should initially ascertain whether George has a progressive or static condition and whether he has a UMNL or an LMNL.

The family thinks he has more difficulty now than a year ago, suggesting a progressive process. They also think he is weaker than the other children, indicating a probable LMNL. They believe George has most difficulty running up stairs. This may reflect proximal weakness. He has no difficulty unscrewing bottles, suggesting normal distal strength. Remember that neuropathies result in distal weakness. The family does not think George fatigues very easily, although he does not have the same stamina as his friends. Thus, he is unlikely to have myasthenia gravis, a disorder of neuromuscular transmission that is characterized by fatigue. The poor stamina is a nonspecific reflection of weakness.

The remainder of his history is unremarkable, but his mother reports that she had a brother who died at 18 years of age after many years in a wheelchair.

What Other Questions Would You Ask This Family? What Is Your Differential Diagnosis? Note that, as in most conditions, the diagnostic clues are in the history. George has progressive weakness, which is probably most marked in his proximal muscles. This suggests a progressive myopathy or disease of the anterior horn cells. He is less likely to have a neuropathy, because his distal strength seems intact, and he is unlikely to have myasthenia gravis. Childhood myopathies can most easily be divided into the muscular dystrophies, congenital myopathies, and metabolic and inflammatory myopathies.

What Do You Expect to See as You Observe George? As you walk to the examining room with this family, you notice that George has an unusual gait. His hips seem to swing from side to side (Trendelenburg gait). During the interview, he settles on the floor to play with some toys. When he moves to another area of the office, he has difficulty rising to his feet. He seems to push himself up using his hands on his legs. This, of course, represents the classical Gower maneuver, typically seen in children with proximal muscle weakness.

Despite this apparent weakness, George looks quite muscular and has particularly big calf muscles. What is the significance of this observation?

What Will Your Physical Examination Find? George's cranial nerves are normal. In particular, there is no evidence of tongue fasciculations. He cannot arise from the floor without arm assistance, and he is unable to "duck-walk" or hop on one foot. He tends to walk on his toes but has reasonably normal distal strength. His muscle bulk is increased in the deltoid and gastrocnemius muscles. Tone is reduced in the extremities, but he has passive dorsiflexion of the ankles to only 90 degrees. His reflexes are difficult to elicit, especially at the knees, but plantar responses are downgoing. His coordination and sensation are normal. Auscultation of his muscles is normal.

What Is Your Diagnosis at This Stage and How Will You Proceed? The examination has confirmed your suspicion of proximal weakness. Your differential diagnosis before the examination was of either AHC or muscle disease. The absence of tongue fasciculations, absence of abnormal muscle sounds on auscultation, and the presence of deep tendon reflexes all make AHC disease unlikely. George, therefore, is most likely to have muscle disease. The increased tone at his ankles is common in children with muscle disease. When muscles are held in a contracted position for a prolonged period, they eventually shorten, with resultant contractures. George's muscle hypertrophy in the presence of progressive weakness and the history of a maternal uncle with weakness strongly suggest a diagnosis of Duchenne muscular dystrophy. The diagnosis must be confirmed with genetic studies, muscle biopsy, or both.

Case 3

History. Three-year-old Peter is brought to see you because he frequently trips when running.

What Questions Will Help You Form a Reasonable Differential Diagnosis? First, you must establish whether Peter's problems are acute or chronic. When the parents are asked about his developmental milestones, they say that he first walked at 22 months and that he has always been clumsy. He cannot ride a tricycle, and he becomes frustrated when he cannot keep up with the other 3-year-olds at preschool. The family does not think his problem is getting worse, but it is certainly not getting better. He has not lost any skills.

At this stage, you have evidence that Peter does not have a neurodegenerative condition, but you do not know whether his problem is due to a UMNL or LMNL. Further questions about his development may help sort out whether his problems are related to weakness (LMNL) or central deficits (UMNL). His parents say that he had no difficulty speaking, but he did not crawl until he was 11 months old. His social skills have always been normal. The history, therefore, suggests a normal cerebral cortex but does not exclude damage to a restricted part of the cortex.

Because alterations in tone help to distinguish central (UMNL) from peripheral (LMNL) deficits, you ask the parents whether they have ever noticed that Peter's legs were "different." They report that they have always believed his left leg was stiffer than his right leg. This suggests spasticity—a UMNL—despite the otherwise normal language and social development.

The presence of spasticity that is not getting worse indicates a diagnosis of *cerebral palsy* (CP), which is defined as a nonprogressive disorder of movement with onset in early childhood.

Were there any problems at birth to suggest a cause? Although perinatal difficulties occasionally can give rise to cortical damage and subsequent CP, it is now clear that, at most, only 8% to 14% of cases of CP are caused by perinatal problems. Most are due to prenatal problems (before birth). Chorionitis is a possible prenatal precursor of CP and is much more common in premature babies.

Key Point

Cerebral palsy is seldom caused by perinatal problems.

Like Peter, most children with CP are the products of normal pregnancy, labor, and delivery. Peter's parents report he has always been healthy. They say he is clumsy but not weak, further evidence that he does not have an LMNL problem.

What Is Your Differential Diagnosis? Although delay in achieving motor milestones is most often caused by global developmental delay, Peter's normal speech and social skills exclude this possibility. The history does not suggest an LMNL as a cause of his tripping, and the parents report that he has not lost any skills, thus ruling out neurodegenerative diseases. One should still consider the possibility of hydrocephalus, but the differential diagnosis should focus on possible causes of CP. These can be divided into prenatal, perinatal, and postnatal problems. Prenatal difficulties may be suggested by signs of congenital malformations or anomalies. CP involving one side of the body (*hemiparesis*) may be the result of a fetal vascular insult (stroke) during pregnancy. Perinatal problems are usually excluded if the patient was discharged from the neonatal nursery at the usual time. Children who suffer an insult in the perinatal period sufficient to result in long-term neurologic impairment always have neurologic difficulties as neonates. Postnatal causes of CP include trauma and infection such as meningitis. These are easily excluded by means of a thorough history.

What Should You Observe? As you watch Peter, you notice that he tends to turn his left foot in and swing his leg from the hip (circumduct) when he runs ahead of you up the hall (Fig. 13–21). While drawing, he holds the pencil in his right hand and keeps the left arm flexed tightly across his chest, supporting your suspicion that he has a hemiparesis. He has no evidence of weakness as he rises from the floor. Your conversation with him supports his mother's claims that he is a smart little boy.

Examination of the wear patterns on the bottom of the shoes shows that the left shoe has signs of the unusual wear of the left toe, caused by scraping of the foot along the ground.

What Aspects of the Physical Examination Deserve Particular Attention? The cranial nerve

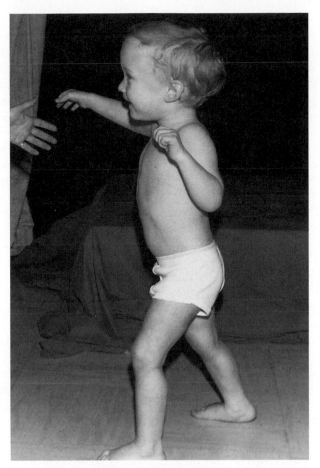

Figure 13–21 Hemiparetic gait.

examination shows a left homonymous hemianopia. This is a very important finding, because Peter's inability to see objects on his left side will influence practical aspects of his life, such as where he should be seated in school. The rest of his cranial nerves are normal.

His muscle power is normal, but the tone is increased in his left arm and leg, and he has hyperreflexia on the left. His left plantar response is upgoing. Sensation in his left hand appears to be decreased, and the nail beds of the thumb and great toe are smaller on the left than on the right. This difference in nail size suggests the chronic nature of Peter's problems and is associated with involvement of the parietal lobe.

Peter's coordination is hindered by the changes in tone, but there are no findings to suggest cerebellar disease.

What Is Your Differential Diagnosis and How Will You Manage This Patient? All the findings point to a lesion in the right hemisphere, and with the history of early onset and no progression, your diagnosis of CP is most likely correct. A computed tomography scan is worthwhile because it may indicate the origin of his CP. On clinical grounds, you predict that the right hemisphere will be found to be smaller than the left and that there may be a porencephalic cyst in the right hemisphere. The latter is a result of the prenatal insult that damaged the right

hemisphere. The CT scan confirms your clinical suspicions but does not add to your knowledge of the pathogenesis of Peter's CP. You counsel Peter's parents that his problems did not begin at the time of birth and that the parents themselves were not responsible for his CP. This is a topic that you will probably have to address again with them in the future.

Case 4

History. Four-month-old Amanda is brought to the pediatric clinic because her parents report that she has sudden "jumps" or "spasms." They have already seen a physician, who assured them that she is completely normal, but they are convinced that she is different from their older child.

The history begins with the first time they noticed these "spasms." Amanda's father reports that she appears to startle for no reason. This began at about 4 weeks of age and continues, even when she is feeding quietly. Although all babies of this age have the primitive Moro reflex, this reflex is precipitated by a stimulus; babies should not startle spontaneously.

When the parents are asked to describe and demonstrate the "spasms," they say that she suddenly draws her legs up from the waist, nods her head, and adducts her arms across the chest. This lasts only a second or two, and then she seems irritable. They do not think she loses consciousness, but it is difficult to be sure because each episode is so brief. These spells can occur at any time and interrupt her feeding if they happen while she is breast-feeding. There are no apparent abnormal eye movements or other unusual limb movements. Amanda seems normal to her parents in every other way.

The pregnancy was uncomplicated, and the delivery was at term. Amanda and her mother were discharged from the hospital on the fourth day of life. (I find that the age at discharge from the nursery is a good indicator of perinatal problems. If the infant is sent home within the first few days of life, it is unlikely that there were significant complications.)

The developmental history is more worrisome. Amanda began smiling only 2 weeks ago (at 14 weeks of age). When lying on her abdomen (prone), she does not get her head off the bed; at this age, she should be able to lift her head and chest off the bed while bearing support on her elbows.

The family history identifies an uncle who was mentally retarded and had frequent seizures. Amanda's parents are unrelated, and both report no health problems.

Does Amanda Have a Neurologic Problem? During the history, you observe Amanda as she lies in her mother's arms. She is very quiet, and the parents report that she is always like this. Many children who are developmentally delayed appear "too good"; in fact, they are better described as apathetic. While you talk to the family, Amanda has numerous small movements that are the "spasms" the parents described. The sudden jerk of her arms and legs with flexion of the neck is called *myoclonus*. Unprecipitated movements of this type are almost always seizures. When they occur in infants, they are called *infantile spasms*. The preceding description is classic for this type of seizure, which is still poorly recognized by many physicians.

The other striking observation is this child's lack of interest in her surroundings. There are no dysmorphic features in this pretty baby and no other features to suggest a diagnosis at this stage. However, the parents do interact appropriately with her.

What Will the Physical Examination Show? A complete developmental assessment is essential in this baby. You have difficulty getting her to smile in response to playing and tickling, and the parents are similarly unsuccessful.

Her cranial nerves are normal, as is her power. When pulled to a sitting position, she has very poor head control, and the tone in her trunk and extremities is also reduced. Testing coordination is impossible in Amanda, because she will not reach for a rattle, although she should at 4 months of age. She has hyperreflexia in all four extremities. Her sensation appears intact.

When you examine her skin, there is a small (1.5 × 1 cm) depigmented spot on her trunk, in the shape of a leaf. On examination under an ultraviolet (Wood) lamp, two more similar lesions are visible. These "ash leaf spots" typify tuberous sclerosis. When you ask the parents about any skin abnormalities, Amanda's father reports that he has several that are not easily seen during the winter but are obvious during the summer because they do not tan like the surrounding skin. He also has lesions that look like acne on his cheeks and reports that the physicians could never make them disappear despite intensive treatment. This, of course, is the adenoma sebaceum of tuberous sclerosis, which both father and daughter have.

What Investigations Should Be Performed to Confirm Your Diagnosis of Tuberous Sclerosis? You order a CT scan for Amanda, which shows small areas of calcification around the ventricles. Her infantile spasms are treated, but she progresses to have intellectual impairment and has other seizures when she is 2 years old. Her father has no apparent difficulties. Tuberous sclerosis is a condition with variable expression. Amanda would not have been diagnosed had you not examined her skin, and her parents would not have received appropriate genetic advice for this autosomal dominant condition.

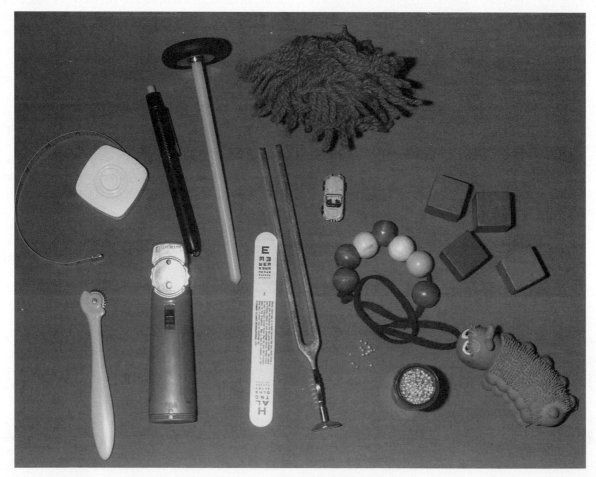

Figure 13–22 Some simple instruments that can be used in the neurologic examination.

SUMMARY

The neurologic examination can be made fun for children while allowing a thoughtful analytic approach to diagnosis. The use of simple instruments and toys (Fig. 13–22) can increase the child's enjoyment of the experience. On completing the evaluation, first hypothesize the location of any deficit in the nervous system that might account for the findings; then try to decide what disease processes could produce such a lesion. Base the need for further investigations on the differential diagnosis, always forming a specific question that each investigation should answer. The most important part of the physical examination is the period of hands-off observation.

As the case histories presented in this chapter demonstrate, the differential diagnosis is usually already formed by the time the physical examination is begun; nonetheless, you should never omit the physical examination. In Case 3 (Peter), the examination exposed a visual field defect, an important finding that will alter the approach to this little boy, because he will have difficulty seeing the left side of the blackboard in school. Consider how every presenting complaint affects the child's life. Although parents may not worry about migraine headaches after they have been assured that the child does not have a tumor, the child may be devastated at missing sleepovers because of his headaches. Similarly, you and the parents may tolerate a child's seizures that are almost completely controlled, but the child may live in terror of having a seizure in the classroom or school cafeteria. You must be sensitive to the emotional needs of your patients.

REFERENCE

1. Medical Research Council: Aids to the examination of the peripheral nervous system. London, Bailliere Tindall, 1986.

SUGGESTED READINGS

Fenichel GM: Clinical Pediatric Neurology: A Signs and Symptoms Approach, 4th ed. Philadelphia, WB Saunders, 2001.

chapter 14

Psychiatric Assessment of Children and Adolescents

HARRIET L. MACMILLAN, JAN E. FLEMING,
and ELLEN JAMIESON

Psychiatric problems, which include emotional and behavioral disorders, occur commonly among children and adolescents. Community studies indicate that approximately 1 in 5 children and adolescents suffers from some type of psychiatric disorder; at least 12% of young people have clinically important mental disorders. The physician is in a unique position to identify children and adolescents with psychiatric difficulties by means of the history-taking techniques outlined in Chapter 1 as well as through the use of the principles of assessment discussed here.

This chapter focuses on clinical skills that are useful in identifying psychiatric disturbance in childhood and adolescence. We do not tell how to diagnose or classify specific psychiatric disorders. We address interview techniques for children, adolescents, and parents and suggest ways of assessing common emotional and behavioral problems.

We hope the assessment strategies described here will help clinicians working with children and adolescents to separate symptoms that require further evaluation or treatment from those that do not.

First, we provide guidelines for the format and content of the clinical interview, including specific aspects of interviewing children and adolescents and their parents about emotional and behavioral problems. We then focus on eliciting information about some of the most common psychiatric conditions, including disruptive behavior problems, substance abuse, eating disorders, emotional disorders, and somatoform problems. Special sections summarize approaches to asking about child maltreatment, interviewing patients with mental retardation, and considering cultural issues. We discuss the importance of the physical examination and then describe the use of standardized instruments and questionnaires. For the sake of brevity, we use the word *child* to refer to patients of all ages up to 18 years, unless otherwise specified.

CLINICAL INTERVIEW

Format

The clinical interview with children and their parents is the best way to assess behavioral and emotional disturbances. It is not unusual for a child and family members to be uncomfortable about discussing mental health concerns and to be reluctant about attending the interview. Children may have received no information about the visit, and may have little understanding about the need for the assessment. Establishing a friendly atmosphere and clearly outlining the plan for assessment (e.g., explaining who will be interviewed in what order) helps reduce anxiety and facilitates the gathering of information. You should encourage family members to express their concerns and ask them why they have come to see you. Be prepared for responses such as "Because my family doctor told me to." Follow up such comments by asking the family members what they hope to accomplish by this meeting, apart from what others may have suggested. If the child is in a two-parent family, both parents should be asked to attend the first interview. If only one parent attends, emphasize the importance of a subsequent interview with the other parent.

The following guidelines are useful in planning the interview:

The child and parents should be seen together for at least part of the initial session. With a young child, you can begin the interview with the child and parents together, and then spend time with the child alone. When you are seeing an adolescent, it often helps to start by interviewing the child alone and then asking the parents to join the interview.

At some point in the first session, the child should be interviewed separately. Children may be reluctant to reveal certain information in the presence of their parents. Young children may not feel free to talk about how things are at home, and adolescents may be uncomfortable discussing topics such as sexuality and drug use in the presence of their parents.

Preschoolers, particularly those older than 2 years, should also be seen alone. Although it can be difficult to maintain a conversation with very young children, it is important to observe, even briefly, how the child behaves without the parents present. During this time, evaluate the child for the abilities to play, to relate to you, and to explore new surroundings. A child may be reluctant to separate from a caregiver, but with reassurance (for example, about the parent's close proximity), you can manage to see most children individually.

Although adolescents may attend an appointment on their own, you must at some point have contact with their parents to carry out a comprehensive assessment. Clearly explain this need to the adolescent before making any contact with the parents. With adolescents as with younger children, it is important to obtain information from multiple sources.

Parents should also be interviewed separately for part of the session. Children are very sensitive to history reported by a parent in their presence. Parents and clinicians sometimes assume that a preschool-aged child will not understand comments they make in the child's presence. Particularly when discussing sensitive issues (e.g., concern about a possible separation from a partner), ensure that the child is not present. It is your responsibility to safeguard the child against hearing potentially harmful information inappropriately. If your office does not have facilities for a young child to be supervised while the parents are interviewed alone, make a second appointment for them to return without the child.

Key Point

In assessing psychiatric problems, it is important to interview the child alone. Even very young children may be reluctant to talk about certain issues in the presence of parents.

Setting

The issue of privacy has been mentioned in Chapter 1. Although privacy in interviews with adults is often emphasized, children's need for privacy is frequently overlooked. Ensure that the child's interview is free of intrusions and cannot be overheard (as described previously).

Ideally, the room should contain small chairs and a table, suitable for preschoolers, or at least a place where you can join the child at his or her eye level. You will find that it is often helpful to get down on the floor so as to be at the same level as the child. Doing so helps engage the child and makes the situation less intimidating.

When interviewing children and youth, make sure some toys and drawing materials are available. Toys help build rapport and decrease anxiety, and they can also be used to explore the child's wishes, fears, impulses, and relationships. However, too many toys and activities can be distracting. Useful play materials are nontoxic washable markers or crayons, paper, building blocks, male and female dolls, a dollhouse with accompanying figures and furniture, and a toy telephone. Board games may help engage a child initially, but their use rarely leads to the gathering of clinically meaningful information.[1] They are typically highly structured and provide little opportunity for imaginative play.

Length

Interviews about behavioral and emotional problems often require more time than assessment of physical problems. All of the people concerned must have the opportunity to establish rapport, because exploring psychiatric issues can be stressful. We recommend that you set aside 45 minutes to 1 hour for the first encounter regarding a mental health problem. The child's age, developmental stage, and ability to be seen alone influence the proportions of time you spend with the child alone, the parents alone, and the child and parents together. It is more important to establish a positive rapport with the patient and family than to adhere to a rigid schedule for the assessment. For example, some young children can tolerate being seen alone for only very brief periods. You should structure the length of time with each person accordingly.

Key Point

When you interview children and families about emotional and behavioral problems, set aside 45 minutes to 1 hour for the first encounter.

Confidentiality

Inform both parents and children early in the interview about issues of confidentiality. You should not assure children and adolescents of absolute confidentiality of your discussions; if questions about self-harm or abuse arise, you will have to speak to parents and authorities. If you "promise" a child or adolescent you will not share anything from their interview with any other person and subsequently a problem such as abuse surfaces during the interview that you must disclose to others, the child may feel betrayed, and the therapeutic alliance may be seriously disrupted. We find it useful to inform the child in developmentally appropriate terms that what is discussed is confidential unless it involves someone's safety (e.g., people hurting themselves or being hurt by others). With young children, it is helpful to explore their understanding of the concept of safety.

Here is an example of how to discuss confidentiality:

1. Say, "I won't tell anyone what you and I talk about without you saying it's all right, unless it has to do with someone's safety."
2. Then ask, "Do you know what safety means?" Often, depending on the age, the child can provide an explanation.
3. It is still helpful to clarify what you mean by *safety*. Say, "If you or someone you know is hurting themselves or being hurt by someone else, then that's a problem with safety."

You and the child can decide together what information can be discussed with parents. Often a focus on themes, rather than specific comments, can be shared, with the child's permission. You might say, "I will be meeting with your parents, but we can decide together what is OK to talk about with them."

Parents are sometimes reluctant to have their child interviewed alone. They may be worried about what their child will say about them or their home situation. They should be reassured that obtaining the child's perspective is a routine part of your assessment.

APPROACH TO OBTAINING THE PRESENTING HISTORY

Whenever possible, the history of an emotional or behavioral problem should be obtained from multiple informants, preferably including the child, parent (both if more than one is available), and the teacher or daycare personnel.

It is well documented that there is only moderate agreement among informants describing the same child, including parent-child agreement. Reasons for these differences are as follows:

- People have different access to information; for example, children may not tell parents about feelings such as anxiety and sadness.
- People have varying perceptions of behavior; what is of great concern to one parent may not seem problematic for the other.
- Psychiatric problems may be specific to certain situations; for example, a child may be highly anxious at school but not at home, or vice versa.

Case History

Case 1

Shirley, age 7 years, and her parents are referred by their family physician because of her teacher's concerns about the child's withdrawn behavior at school

and lack of friends. According to her parents, Shirley plays well at home with her 4-year-old sister, and often helps with chores around the home. She appears happy and enjoys doing errands with her mother. Neither parent has observed any problems with Shirley. They thought that she was probably just shy at school and would become more sociable with time. Her second grade teacher has noted early in the year, however, that Shirley does not interact with her classmates and often wants to stay in the classroom during recess. Shirley appears to understand her schoolwork and completes it without difficulty; however, she resists saying anything in class and refuses to work in groups with other children. She often stays behind until everyone else has left the classroom.

When you interview her individually, Shirley initially denies having any problems. She says that her parents and her sister are her friends and that she does not need anyone else. As you probe further, however, Shirley admits to being very lonely, feeling too self-conscious to interact with peers. She acknowledges feeling so worried about meeting other children that she hates school. Together, you and Shirley talk about sharing this information with her parents. At first Shirley is hesitant, but then she agrees that it is important for her parents to know how she has been feeling.

Both parents are supportive of Shirley as she tells them, with your help, about how she has been feeling at school. They agree to meet with the teacher to discuss ways of helping Shirley with her anxiety about interacting with classmates. You refer them to a child psychiatrist for further assessment to determine whether Shirley needs additional treatment for her anxiety symptoms.

Key Point

Seek the history of emotional and behavioral disturbances from several sources, including the child, parents, and teacher or daycare worker.

The following guidelines describe an approach to obtaining the presenting history from both parents and children.

Encourage Each Person to Describe the Problem in His or Her Own Way. Open inquiry followed by more focused questions provides the most information. Examples of open versus more directive questions are given in Chapter 1. At times, a child or adolescent responds repeatedly with "I don't know." It is important to determine whether the patient genuinely does not understand or whether he or she is giving this response to avoid answering the questions. Rephrasing the question or giving examples can help with the former situation. When you suspect avoidance, you may find it helpful to ask the patient directly, but in a nonthreatening way, whether the repeated "I don't know" answers mean that he or she is having trouble comprehending or whether there are barriers to answering the question. Then explain how such responses can be confusing, and that you would prefer an alternative answer such as "I don't want to talk about that," if the child is avoiding the question.

Seek Detailed Descriptions of the Behavioral or Emotional Symptoms. Ask for specific examples of the behavior.

Avoid Leading Questions or Statements that Suggest the Answer. An example of a leading statement is "I bet that really made you angry." A better approach would be to ask "How did you feel when that happened?" Young children, in particular, may be prone to conform to an interviewer's expectations.

Ask About the Impact of the Problem. How much does the behavior affect the child's and family's functioning? For example, if the problem is oppositional behavior, you need to ask the following questions:

- How often is the behavior happening?
- What happens in response to the behavior?
- Who in the family is most affected by the child's behavior?
- Does the child feel that his or her behavior is a problem?
- When the child behaves in an oppositional way, how does it affect other family members?

Ask about the Presence of the Chief Complaint Across a Range of Activities and Situations. For example, is the child fearful only at night?

Ask About Historical Data. Inquire about data such as developmental milestones using direct questions; an open approach works best for questions about relationships and feelings.

Specific Features of the Interview with the Parent or Parents

Studies show that it is essential to interview both parents (if both are available) in the assessment of an emotional or behavioral problem. Reports by one parent about the perspective of the other are often inaccurate. Often, you can obtain details of the personal, familial, and social background only from the parents, particularly if you are assessing a younger child.

Ask parents about their own childhood. Useful questions are as follows:

- Who was in your family?
- Tell me about your family when you were growing up.
- What is your best memory of growing up?
- What is the worst (or most painful) memory of your childhood?

- What happened in your family when someone got in trouble?
- Who did you go to for help?

Inquire about relationships between the parents and grandparents. For example, prompt parents as follows:

- Tell me about the relationship between *your* parents (both then and now).
- How did you and your mom get along?
- How did you and your dad get along?

Ask about communication patterns, family alliances, and parent-child interactions, including discipline and control, with the following questions:

- How do people in the family get along?
- What do you and [child's name] do together? (ask of each parent individually)
- What happens when [child's name] gets into trouble?
- Do you have fun as a family?
- Does your family have problems with money?
- Who disciplines [child's name] in the family? (Avoid overly directive questions, such as "Do both of you discipline [child's name]?")
- How are decisions in the family made?
- How do people in the family share their feelings?
- How often has your family moved?

Explore useful screening issues as listed in Chapter 1. Some aspects of the history (e.g., family violence) are more appropriately discussed with each parent separately. However, parents sometimes learn more about their partner when they are interviewed together about past and family history.

Key Point

It is essential to interview both parents (if both are available) to gain their individual perspectives, which can sometimes vary considerably.

Specific Features of the Interview with the Child

1. Maintain a reasonable physical distance from the child to avoid intrusiveness or intimidation.
2. Ask for the child's preferred name, and make sure to introduce yourself to the child.
3. Explain clearly the purpose of the interview, and give a brief description of what topics will be covered.
4. Begin with nonthreatening general questions. Allow the child to describe the family situation, recreational activities, and interests. Examples of

such inquiries are "Tell me who's in your family" and "Tell me what you like to do after school."

5. Follow the child's lead, but do not let the interview become disorganized. Once a topic is introduced, try to maintain the focus until you obtain the necessary information.

6. Avoid note-taking as much as possible. If you must take notes, explain their purpose to the child.

7. Tailor the length of the interview to the individual child and to the nature of the problem; if the child appears tired or upset, do not hesitate to shorten the session.

Specific Features of a Family Interview with Parents and Children

Family discord and disruption are strongly linked to psychiatric problems in children. The importance of family dynamics has been highlighted in Chapter 1; it is essential to assess (even briefly) the interpersonal relationships and interactions of at least the parents and child with the presenting complaint, and preferably the child's siblings. Family interviewing is occasionally contraindicated, for example, in child abuse if the alleged perpetrator is a family member or when there is the potential for violence. Guidelines for family interviewing in the course of a psychiatric assessment are as follows:

1. Respect confidentiality; do not reveal information obtained during individual sessions unless permission is obtained.

2. Elicit information from all family members; do not allow one family member to dominate the session.

3. Do not focus solely on the problems. Ask about strengths and positive attributes of the family as well. For example, what do family members enjoy doing together?

4. Adopt a neutral stance, but always be prepared to identify and deal with any inappropriate behavior. For example, if a parent makes cruel or degrading comments to a child, address the inappropriateness in a direct but empathic manner. "I sense that you are angry, but comments such as those will not be helpful to [child's name]. Try talking about what bothers you without making critical comments to [child's name]."

5. Pay careful attention to nonverbal messages, behaviors, and expressions when you are assessing family functioning. For example, watch for the youth who rolls his or her eyes in response to a parent's statement and for the parent who casts angry glances at a partner.

Information from Collateral Sources, Including Schools and Community Agencies

Information from teachers, child-care personnel, and other community agencies can help greatly in the psychiatric assessment of children and youth. However, you should make contact with the school or outside agencies only after (1) you have obtained signed permission to do so from the parents and (2) you have informed the child that you will be doing so. Teachers can provide details about academic progress and can describe the child's relationships with peers and school personnel. School information is essential if the child is having difficulties in the school setting. Personal contact (by telephone or interview) with the teacher who knows the child best usually yields the most comprehensive data. It is also important to explore the teacher's perception of the child's difficulties and the teacher's attitudes toward the child. Contact with workers and access to reports from community agencies is particularly helpful when you are dealing with children who are in foster care or have been recently adopted.

Key Point

Contact the school to find out about the child's academic performance and relationships with peers. First obtain permission from the parents, and inform the child of your plan before acting on it.

ELICITING INFORMATION ABOUT PSYCHIATRIC DISORDERS

Child and adolescent psychiatric disorders are commonly divided into the broad categories of emotional and behavioral problems. The following sections suggest specific ways to assess symptoms in these two areas. Classification systems, such as that described in the 4th edition of the *Diagnostic and Statistical Manual of Mental Disorders* (DSM-IV), published by the American Psychiatric Association,[2] provide detailed information about the criteria used in making a specific diagnosis. The DSM is a classification system; it is not a tool for the identification of psychiatric disturbances in children and youth. For readers interested in further information, Morrison and Anders[1] provide a useful summary of DSM-IV as it applies to children. They emphasize that DSM-IV "is a snapshot in time" and that the criteria change as new information about mental disorders in childhood and adolescence becomes available.

ELICITING INFORMATION ABOUT BEHAVIORAL PROBLEMS

When determining whether a behavior problem is abnormal, you must assess its frequency, duration, and context. For example, some behaviors, such as temper tantrums, are normal when they occur at certain ages (between 18 months and 4 years) or at a low frequency. Explore the circumstances of the behavior as well as the outcome. For example, in the case of antisocial acts, who was the victim? Was it someone known to the child, or was it a stranger?

Disruptive Behavior Problems

Disruptive behavior is one of the most common problems brought to the attention of pediatricians. What distinguishes these behaviors from other psychiatric problems is the destructive, intrusive, and sometimes dangerous nature of the behavior that affects others.

Many children are inaccurate reporters of attentional or other disruptive behavioral problems. They may be unaware of their own excessive activity or may underreport aggressive behavior. Give careful attention to reports of behavioral problems by children, parents, and teachers and to the level of agreement among them.

When assessing children and youth with behavior problems, you might wish to consider the following issues:

- Has there been a recent change in the family that could affect the child?
- What are the frequency and severity of punishments? (Be alert for child maltreatment; see later)
- Are there family stresses that worsen the behavior?
- Does the child have an understanding of the symptoms?

Specific questions about disruptive behavior problems are "Have you ever been in trouble with the teacher? Some kids your age steal things—what about you? Have you been in any fights at school? Have you ever been expelled from school?" and "Do you know anyone who carries a weapon, such as a knife or a gun?" Questions you might ask about anger and aggression are "What makes you angry?" "What do you do when you get angry?" and "Do you use fighting to work out your problems with other kids your age?"

Substance Abuse

Many adolescents and some younger children experiment with drugs, whereas a smaller number of adolescents actually use drugs on a regular basis. Adolescents use alcohol and tobacco more than other classes of drugs. The true extent of child and adolescent substance abuse is difficult to determine because of such factors as difficulty differentiating casual from regular usage. Many adolescents who misuse substances have other psychiatric conditions, such as disruptive behavior problems, anxiety, and depressive disorders. You may find the following framework helpful in assessing substance abuse:

1. Ask about alcohol, smoking, and other drug use directly, including the frequency, duration, and most recent use. Ask "What experiences have you had with alcohol?" rather than "Do you drink alcohol?" As a lead-in to this area of questioning, you may want to inquire about drug and alcohol use at the child's school; for example, ask "How common is it for kids at your school to use marijuana?"
2. Ask about the desired effect of drug or alcohol use (for example, to get high, to feel less nervous, or to forget about problems).
3. Ask specifically about any problems arising from drug or alcohol use, such as parental concern, withdrawal symptoms, and legal involvement. For example, ask "Does anyone hassle you about how much you drink?" "Has anyone ever told you they think you have a drug problem?" "The day after a party, do you ever feel like you need a drink?" "Have you ever been in trouble with the police?"
4. Inquire about associated risk-taking behavior, including the use of needles and sexual practices.
5. Remember to ask about abuse of prescription or over-the-counter medications.

Key Point

When exploring risk-taking behaviors such as drug use, ask specific and direct questions. For example, "How much alcohol do you drink?"

These questions can help determine the extent and pattern of substance abuse. Although the occasional or experimental use of drugs should not be overemphasized, youth often underreport drug and alcohol use and deny associated impairment. Maintain a high index of suspicion, and ask adolescents carefully about their drug and alcohol consumption.

Eating Disorders

Eating disorders include a variety of conditions, such as anorexia nervosa and bulimia nervosa. Anorexia and bulimia can be difficult to detect, particularly in the early stages. Ask any child or adolescent presenting with a possible eating disorder about attitudes toward eating and weight. Explore the patient's impression of his or her body image (current and ideal) in detail; often, asking the youth to draw a picture of himself or herself or the family can identify disturbances of body image that may be denied or minimized during an interview.

Examples of questions to ask such patients are as follows:

- Have you ever lost so much weight that someone said you were too thin?
- Are there any parts of your body you do not like?
- Do you think you are too fat?
- Have you tried to lose weight?
- Have you ever tried to lose weight by making yourself throw up?

Patients with eating disorders are often reluctant to disclose information about their eating behaviors. It can be useful to ask adolescents about the existence of any rules they follow with regard to when, where, and what they eat.

Eliciting Information about Emotional Disorders

Determining the presence of an emotional disorder such as depression or anxiety can be difficult, because some features of the conditions are extremes of normal emotions. An emotional symptom becomes abnormal if it:

- Intrudes on the child's life (that is, the symptom is associated with significant distress).
- Is persistent rather than transient.
- Occurs in many activities; for example, a child is worried about doing well in several areas of his or her life.
- Is associated with impairment; for example, the child reports feeling sad, and school reports indicate deterioration in academic functioning.

Depression

Major depressive disorder occurs in approximately 5% of adolescents and is more common in girls than boys. Although much less common than in adolescents, serious clinical depression does occur in children, especially those with a history of depressive disorder in one or both parents. Studies have found that clinical depression in prepubertal children either occurs equally in boys and girls or is more common in boys. In assessing

depressive disorder in a young person, consider the following issues:

1. Determine whether the patient has a sad affect, such as downcast eyes, quiet voice, slowing of speech or movements, and lack of spontaneous speech.
2. Consider that in depressed children and teenagers, irritability, not sadness, can be the primary mood disturbance. Ask whether the child has been more grumpy than usual with family and friends.
3. Ask the child how much of the time he or she feels sad or "down." Occasional feelings of sadness are common, but persistent or frequent symptoms suggest depression. Younger children may have difficulty determining how long they have had feelings of sadness. It can be helpful to relate duration to meaningful events in a child's life, such as the end of the school year.
4. Listen for expressions such as feeling "empty" or "hopeless." These statements often indicate the presence of a depressive disorder. Morrison and Anders[1] suggest asking children what three wishes they would choose if given only three; such an approach can help elicit statements about hopelessness or a wish for death (see later discussion of suicidal ideation and behavior).
5. Ask about interest in friends and school as well as about energy level. Typically, depressed teenagers lose interest in some activities but may report feeling better when in the presence of their friends.
6. Inquire about changes in eating and sleeping patterns. Depressed adolescents may show either a decrease or an increase in weight and amount of sleep.
7. Ask about suicidal thoughts and behavior (see later discussion of suicidal ideation and behavior).

Anxiety

Anxiety, like depression, ranges across a continuous spectrum from normal to abnormal. As with sadness, a central question about anxiety is how severely it impairs the child's life. Does the anxiety interfere with the child's ability to participate in developmentally appropriate activities?

Other diagnostic considerations that may help determine the presence of pathologic anxiety include the following:

1. What is the level of distress experienced by the child or adolescent?
2. When the anxiety-provoking situation is not present, what is the child's level of anxiety?

3. What are the age and developmental level of the child? A 4-year-old child who experiences anxiety upon separation from a parent presents a different clinical picture from that of a 13-year-old child with the same symptoms.

In determining whether emotional symptoms are abnormal, consider the intrusiveness and impact of the problem in the child's life. For example, how much is anxiety interfering with daily activities?

Although older children and adolescents generally understand the concept of anxiety, younger children should be asked about things that frighten or worry them. Children may manifest anxiety through physical symptoms; headaches and stomachaches are particularly common. Although parents are often aware of these common physical symptoms, children and adolescents may not mention other symptoms, such as sweating, palpitations, dizziness, trouble breathing, and fear of dying.

One anxiety condition that was thought to be rare in children and adolescents is obsessive-compulsive disorder. Recent studies, however, have made it clear that this condition often begins in childhood and may affect as many as 1% to 2% of adolescents. Young persons may keep their obsessive thoughts and compulsive behaviors secret. It is important to ask whether children experience an urge to check things repeatedly or have a specific order in which they have to do certain tasks.

Case History

Case 2
Robert, age 13 years, has always been an excellent student and well liked by his peers. In eighth grade, his marks began to slip and his mother has noticed that he is tired and subdued much of the time. She and Robert's father separated 2 years ago, but Robert is able to spend time with both parents and appeared to adapt to the situation reasonably well. When Robert's mother meets with the teacher this year, she is informed that Robert has not been completing his assignments. Robert's mother expresses confusion, because her son typically spends 3 hours a night in his room on homework.

Robert is referred to the school guidance counselor, who develops a rapport with him. He confides to the counselor that he has trouble completing his work because of the tasks he has to do before starting his assignment. At first the counselor thinks Robert means chores, but on further questioning, she realizes that he is referring to certain rituals. Robert explains that he has to count things in his room (such as the books on the shelf) and the number of words on the pages of his assignment before he can do his homework. If he loses count, he must start over, and frequently he becomes so tired that he

does not finish his assignment. According to Robert, he must follow these rituals to ward off bad events, such as the illness of his mother or father. Robert admits that this "sounds crazy" but says he cannot stop himself from counting.

There is often considerable overlap among symptoms of anxiety and depressive disorders in both childhood and adolescence.

Suicidal Ideation and Behavior

Suicidal behavior is uncommon in childhood and early adolescence but increases significantly in older adolescence. Many people falsely assume that young children do not experience suicidal thoughts and are not at risk for attempting suicide. Research suggests that about 10% of teens between 14 and 16 years of age experience thoughts of suicide. Ask the child or adolescent directly about thoughts of suicide. Such questions should usually be asked without the parent present. You can ask questions such as "Have you ever thought that life is not worth living?" and "Have you ever thought about taking your own life or not being alive anymore?"

For an adolescent who admits to experiencing suicidal ideation or attempting suicide, your next step is to assess intent by asking about the events and precipitants leading up to the episode or associated with the thoughts of suicide. Children vary in their level of comprehension about death, depending on their age and developmental stage. In evaluating suicidal ideation or behavior, you should explore the child's or adolescent's concept of what would happen. Examples of possible questions are "What did you think would happen if you tried to kill yourself? Did you think you would die?" and "What happens when people die?"

Key Point

Ask routinely about suicidal thoughts and behavior. Children and adolescents rarely volunteer such information.

When asking about possible precipitants or stressors, avoid minimizing problems. Although the breakup of a relationship or embarrassment among peers may not seem like major stressors to some people, such experiences can be extremely demoralizing and associated with feelings of hopelessness among adolescents.

The risk that a child with suicidal ideation will complete suicide increases with the following associated features:

- Clear intent
- Planned suicidal act with a lethal method
- Presence of a psychiatric disorder, particularly depression, delinquency, or substance abuse

- Hopelessness about change in the future
- Male gender
- Poor family supports
- Previous attempt
- Recent loss or other negative life event

Somatoform Disorders

Somatoform disorders are psychiatric disturbances that are characterized by physical symptoms that may resemble those of other medical conditions but have no identifiable anatomic or physiologic cause. Examples are somatization disorder (a pattern of recurring somatic complaints), conversion disorder, and hypochondriasis. Assessment calls for a careful history about the onset of the symptoms as well as about precipitating, aggravating, and relieving factors associated with them. It sometimes helps to consider the patient's affect during the description of the physical complaints (for example, the adolescent who appears disinterested while describing serious symptoms). Nevertheless, it is essential to remain alert for the presence of medical illness and to remember that a patient can have an underlying physical illness and psychiatric symptoms in association with it.

Psychosis

Children and adolescents can show the same symptoms of psychotic illness as adults, although such symptoms are uncommon in childhood. The two main features of psychotic disorders are hallucinations and delusions. You should differentiate these potentially serious symptoms from other, more common and benign phenomena, such as imaginary companions and fantasies.

HALLUCINATIONS

Inquiry about hallucinations should include both auditory and visual experiences. You can incorporate the questions into the systems review focusing on eyes and ears, asking, for example, "Do you have any problems with your eyes?" and "Do you ever see things that other kids do not see?" Ask similar questions about auditory hallucinations. Remember that hallucinations that occur only while a person is falling asleep or waking up generally are normal phenomena. When asking about hallucinations, explore the source, location, number, identity, and content as well as the effect of these experiences on the adolescent. If the child does have hallucinations, consider drug intoxication, seizure disorder, infection, and metabolic disorder in addition to a primary psychiatric disorder.

DELUSIONS

A *delusion* is a false belief that cannot be changed by logical argument or evidence against it. Such beliefs often involve bizarre or unusual thinking. Few studies have carefully assessed delusions in childhood; they are rare before late adolescence. Among psychotic adolescents, delusions are often paranoid or persecutory. For example, a teenager may complain of being followed or poisoned. Sometimes delusions have religious themes. A useful question is "Have you ever believed something that other people thought was odd or strange?"

Key Point

Although children may have erroneous views about people or events, actual delusions are rare in childhood.

Inquiring about Child Maltreatment

Children and adolescents are often victims of some type of maltreatment, such as physical abuse, sexual abuse, neglect, emotional abuse, or exposure to domestic violence. According to a recent Canadian community survey,[3] between 1 in 3 and 1 in 4 adults reported experiencing either physical or sexual abuse during childhood. Much less is known about the prevalence of other types of maltreatment. In most regions, it is the responsibility of child protection agencies to carry out investigative interviews when child maltreatment is suspected. Nevertheless, you should include questions about child maltreatment in any general assessment.

Examples of questions to elicit concerns about child maltreatment are as follows:

- What things do you worry about?
- What happens in your family when someone gets in trouble?
- Has anyone ever touched you in a way that made you feel uncomfortable or upset?
- Has anyone ever made you do something sexually you did not want to do?

This clinical area is an exception to the earlier comments about note-taking during assessment. If a child or adolescent discloses information about any type of maltreatment, attempt to document the statements verbatim. It is helpful to record the wording of the questions you ask as well as the child's response. It is generally not advisable to ask detailed questions about a disclosure of maltreatment, because in many jurisdictions, a child protection agency worker must obtain the disclosure. Similarly, the use of anatomically correct dolls should be reserved for specialized interviews requested by the child protection agency and performed by a clinician trained in their use. Children should not be subjected to multiple interviews by clinicians without specialized training in this area.

Although videotaping offers a complete record of an interview, it has associated problems. Videotapes may be used inappropriately; for example, details about how the child was interviewed may take precedence over the child's verbal statements. At this time, there is insufficient advantage for videotaping of psychiatric interviews to recommend its use, even if abuse is suspected.

Interviewing Patients with Mental Retardation

As in any clinical encounter, you should adapt the duration, format, and questions of a psychiatric assessment to what the child and family can tolerate. In addition to cognitive impairment, patients with mental retardation may have other behavioral and emotional problems, such as aggression, self-injury, hyperactivity, depression, and anxiety. Sometimes the psychiatric assessment of children and adolescents with mental retardation is neglected, particularly when their verbal skills are impaired. There is evidence that emotional disorders are present to a greater extent in patients with mental retardation than in those without, but often such problems are not recognized. Following are some important considerations for interviewing a pediatric patient with mental retardation:

1. Before meeting the child, learn about his or her life situation, living arrangements, and school experience.
2. Be clear about the reason for the visit, and explain carefully what will be done.
3. Ensure that you see the patient alone, even if you have difficulty communicating with him or her.
4. As the interview progresses, check to ensure that the patient understands your questions.
5. Be flexible about the pace and duration of the interview.

Morrison and Anders[1] declare that one of the major challenges in interviewing mentally retarded children and adolescents is to "pitch the questions at just the right level—neither so complex as to confuse nor so simple as to insult." They recommend paying close attention to the patient's response to the first open-ended question as a way of gauging how to conduct the remainder of the interview.

Cultural Considerations

Each culture has unique developmental pathways and varied expressions of emotional dysfunction. The way in which a child or youth with psychiatric disturbance presents can be strongly influenced by cultural factors. You should adhere to the following principles when assessing cultural determinants:

1. Ask the youth or parents for help in understanding their specific culture.
2. When seeing a patient from a culture with which you are unfamiliar, learn from the literature about specific cultural factors.
3. Consult with colleagues. Sometimes a patient or family may appreciate the opportunity to see a clinician who has an in-depth understanding of their culture. For example, some clinicians have spent considerable time learning about Aboriginal health and may be able to provide important insights about emotional and behavioral problems of someone who is Aboriginal. (For further information on cross-cultural pediatric care, see Chapter 2).

PHYSICAL EXAMINATION

The physical examination has been discussed in detail in other chapters of this book. It is an important part of any psychiatric assessment because (1) behavioral and emotional problems can have physical causes, (2) various conditions (e.g., anorexia nervosa) may cause growth impairment and malnutrition, and (3) certain psychiatric symptoms and conditions may be missed if you do not perform a physical examination. For example, psychosis can occur as a side effect of certain medications, and eating disorders can lead to significant electrolyte disturbance and dehydration.

Key Point

The physical examination is an important part of any psychiatric assessment. Various psychiatric conditions have physical causes or sequelae.

STANDARDIZED INTERVIEWS AND QUESTIONNAIRES

Structured psychiatric interviews and rating scales for both children and parents have been developed to improve the validity and reliability of observations and information about emotional and behavioral problems. Generally, these tools are most useful for research purposes; however, a few measures may be helpful to the clinician.

Structured interviews are comprehensive and reduce the chance that an area will be forgotten. They were developed originally to improve the quality of information collected during mental health assessments. However, they are typically time-consuming and may interfere with building rapport.

Questionnaires or rating scales that ask about behavior can be useful for obtaining information from multiple sources. Generally, these scales are focused on behaviors and do not ask in-depth or detailed questions. Such scales can be particularly helpful when you are seeking information from schools. The following teacher questionnaires have satisfactory reliability and validity:

Conners Teacher Rating Scale (helps in assessing attention deficit and hyperactivity symptoms)[4]
Child Behavior Checklist (CBCL) (asks about emotions/behaviors)[5]
Revised Behavior Problem Checklist (asks about emotions/behaviors)[6]

Each of these instruments has parallel versions for completion by parents, so that systematic information can be obtained about a list of behaviors. These are screening instruments, however, and should not be used for making specific diagnoses.

Key Point

Questionnaires such as the Conners Teacher Rating Scale can be useful in collecting information about behaviors but should not be used for making specific diagnoses.

SUMMARY

A thorough history from multiple informants is the most important part of any psychiatric assessment. The approaches described in this chapter are closely linked with other skills in pediatrics and can help you understand behavioral and emotional problems in childhood. It is important to seek detailed descriptions of the psychiatric symptoms from the child and parents and to gather information about family history and parent-child interactions. Ask about positive attributes of the family; do not focus solely on problems. Contact with schools and community agencies can be extremely helpful and is often an essential part of understanding a child's emotional or behavioral disturbances.

Several conditions, such as depression, anxiety disorders, disruptive behavioral problems, substance abuse, and eating disorders, are common in young persons. If you do not inquire specifically about these problems, they will be missed. Psychiatric disturbances are underrecognized and hence, undertreated; as a pediatric clinician, with your knowledge about development and child health, you are in a uniquely qualified position to carry out psychiatric assessments.

REFERENCES

1. Morrison J, Anders TF: Interviewing Children and Adolescents: Skills and Strategies for Effective DSM-IV Diagnosis. New York, Guilford Press, 1999.
2. Diagnostic and Statistical Manual of Mental Disorders, 4th ed. Washington, DC, American Psychiatric Association, 1994.
3. MacMillan HE, Fleming JE, Trocmé N, et al: Prevalence of child physical and sexual abuse in the community: Results from the Ontario Health Supplement. JAMA 278:131–135, 1997.
4. Conners CK: Conners' Teacher Rating Scale—Revised. North Towanda, New York, Multi-Health Systems, 1997.
5. Achenbach TM: Manual for the Child Behaviour Checklist 4–18 and 1991 Profile. Burlington, Vermont, University of Vermont Department of Psychiatry, 1991.
6. Quay HC, Peterson DR: Manual for the Revised Behavior Problem Checklist. Coral Gables, Florida, University of Miami, 1987.

SUGGESTED READINGS

Hughes JN, Baker DB: The Clinical Child Interview, 2nd ed. New York, Guilford Press, 1990.
Lewis M (ed): Child and Adolescent Psychiatry: A Comprehensive Textbook, 2nd ed. Baltimore, Williams & Wilkins, 1996.
Morrison J, Anders TF: Interviewing Children and Adolescents: Skills and Strategies for Effective DSM-IV Diagnosis. New York, Guilford Press, 1999.
Rutter M, Taylor E, Hersov L (eds): Child and Adolescent Psychiatry: Modern Approaches, 3rd ed. Oxford, Blackwell Scientific, 1994.
Saywitz K, Camparo L: Interviewing child witnesses: A developmental perspective. Child Abuse Negl 22:825–843, 1998.

chapter 15

Pediatric Musculoskeletal Examination

BIANCA A. LANG

The 6-year-old boy who presents with a limp and no other complaints or the 18-month-old girl who has one swollen knee can pose a diagnostic dilemma. Although most children with musculoskeletal pains do not have a serious underlying problem, some do have a potentially life-threatening or debilitating disease that requires urgent recognition and treatment. The first step toward distinguishing between a condition that requires treatment and one that calls for studious neglect is to understand normal variants and their spontaneous evolution. This understanding avoids unnecessarily meddlesome and expensive treatments and soothes parents enormously. Common musculoskeletal concerns include the child with feet (one or both) that turn in or out, legs that appear bowed, flat feet, a peculiar gait, and occasional stumbling. Most are self-correcting variants of normal skeletal growth, sometimes traceable to intrauterine position or familial characteristics. They are not deformities and should not be labeled as such when you talk to parents.

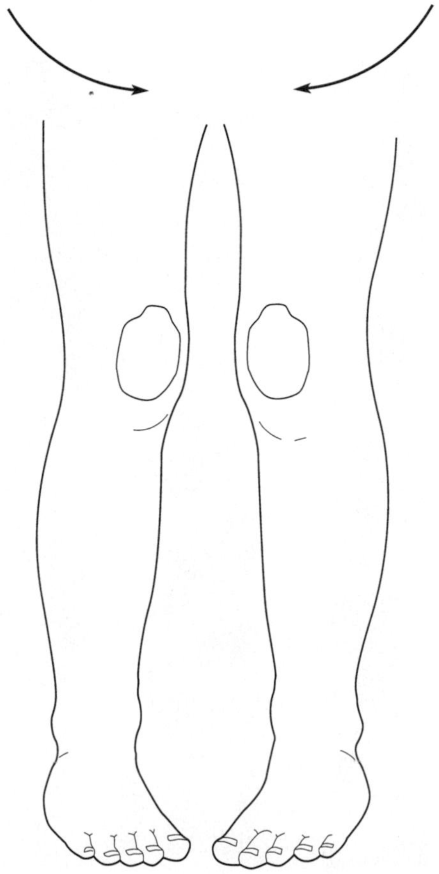

NORMAL MUSCULOSKELETAL VARIANTS

Torsional Phenomena

Torsional phenomena occur in at least half the infant and toddler population, varying considerably in degree. In a child whose feet turn inward, you must first decide whether it is the feet, femora, or tibias that are responsible. Does the torsion originate above or below the knee?

Internal Femoral Torsion (Femoral Anteversion)

When children have internal femoral torsion, the patellas show "internal strabismus" (Fig. 15–1). Gently rotate the knees so that the patellas face forward. If internal femoral torsion is the problem, the feet suddenly and miraculously point directly forward.

Once you understand the "in-toeing" mechanism, it becomes obvious that special "orthopedic" shoes, mistakenly prescribed as "corrective," usually exaggerate the in-toeing because of their sheer weight.

Figure 15–1 Internal femoral torsion: "internal strabismus" of the patellae.

Perfectly normal shoes almost invariably exaggerate in-toeing as well. It usually helps to demonstrate this phenomenon to the parents by having the child walk with and without shoes, after which they frequently realize that the problem is really not as bad as it seems.

Key Point

Special shoes are rarely indicated for treating children's leg and foot problems, whether real or perceived. Internal femoral torsion, a normal developmental phenomenon, is the most common cause of in-toeing in children between 3 and 12 years of age.

Internal Tibial Torsion

Internal tibial torsion is a normal phenomenon seen in children 6 to 18 months old. It is noticed especially when they begin to walk and can vary greatly in degree. If the patellas point directly forward and the feet appear normal in a child with in-toeing, the likely cause is tibial torsion. As with femoral anteversion, the "deformity" typically appears worse when the youngster puts on shoes and may cause the child to stumble a bit more than average. Reassure the parents that this phenomenon disappears in most children by age 2.

Bowleg (Genu Varum) and Knock Knees (Genu Valgum)

Mild lower extremity bowing is the norm in infants and young children (Fig. 15–2). Internal tibial torsion often accompanies physiologic bowing and accentuates the bowed appearance. No treatment is necessary. By age 2 years, physiologic bowing spontaneously corrects itself in most children. Many healthy children, including those who have had physiologic bowing as toddlers, gradually "convert" to develop some degree of genu valgum after 2 years of age (Fig. 15–3), which usually disappears spontaneously by 8 years of age.

In a few children, physiologic bowing or knock knee may be quite marked, raising concerns about possible underlying disease. If bowing increases after the child begins to walk, you should rule out pathologic causes, such as Blount disease, rickets, and metaphyseal dysplasia. Genu valgum may also develop in extremely obese children, the result of bearing excessive weight. It may also occur in pathologic conditions such as metabolic bone disease (rickets or renal osteodystrophy).

Toeing-Out

Toeing-out, sometimes quite marked, is noted when some perfectly healthy youngsters begin to walk. This

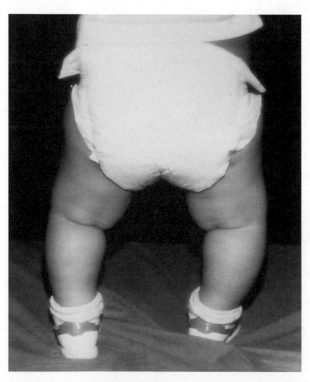

Figure 15–2 Genu varum (nonrachitic bowing of the legs), a transient normal variant requiring no treatment.

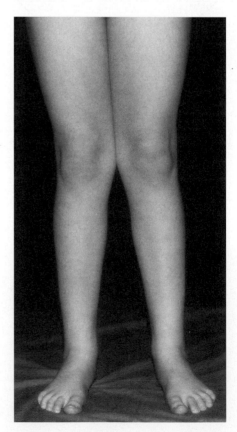

Figure 15–3 Physiologic knock knee, a self-correcting condition that requires no treatment.

eversion of the legs, not the feet, may look peculiar but does not interfere with walking and generally corrects spontaneously 6 to 12 months later. It is usually due to external rotation of the hips or to external tibial torsion. When it is due to external rotation of the hips, rotating the hips to a normal position during the examination corrects the "abnormality" and helps the parents understand its nature. No treatment is necessary.

Metatarsus Varus (Forefoot Adduction)

In metatarsus varus, the forefoot turns inward in relation to the long axis of the heel (Fig. 15–4). The critical clinical issue is to determine whether the foot deformity is fixed or flexible. Mild to moderate flexible metatarsus varus usually corrects itself, because it is the result of intrauterine position or "packing." A severe or fixed metatarsus varus may require serial casting or an orthotic device. If you are in doubt about the severity of this condition in a child, consult a pediatric orthopedist.

Flat Feet

Flat feet are the norm in children younger than 2 to 3 years of age and in older children who show greater than average joint mobility. Usually asymptomatic, this normal variant is often simply part of generalized hypermobility. In such children, the normal body weight is sufficient to cause flattening of the feet. When the youngster sits on a table, the longitudinal arch miraculously reappears as the feet are suspended in space.

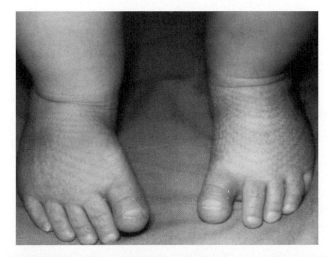

Figure 15–4 Metatarsus varus. The key clinical issue is the extent of flexibility of the deformity.

Key Point

Often, at least one parent has similar generalized ligamentous laxity and joint hypermobility. Checking both parents for joint hypermobility helps them understand the child's "problem."

Toe-Walking

The most common condition that causes pathologic Achilles tendon tightening and gastrocnemius spasm is spastic cerebral palsy, but toe-walking can also be seen occasionally in perfectly normal children who favor their toes in the early months of walking before they develop a mature heel-toe gait. Toe-walking in normal children tends to be intermittent, and they tend to rest with their feet flat on the floor when they stop walking. By contrast, children with cerebral palsy have persistent toe-walking and often circumduct their legs while walking as well; they also have increased muscle tone, hyperreflexia, and tight heel cords. Although congenitally short Achilles tendon does occur, it is rare. Proximal muscle weakness, as in muscular dystrophy, and a tethered spinal cord also must be excluded in the child with toe-walking.

IMPORTANT LOCAL CAUSES OF MUSCULOSKELETAL PAIN

Musculoskeletal pain may be caused by local or generalized conditions. Local causes of hip, knee, foot, and back pain in children include many common orthopedic conditions, which are summarized here.

Hip Pain

TRANSIENT SYNOVITIS

Transient synovitis is an acute transient disorder of unknown etiology that frequently causes isolated hip pain in children younger than 10 years. Typically, the child awakens with intense groin pain that causes him or her to limp or refuse to walk. The leg is often held in a flexed and externally rotated position. Although the range of motion in one hip is limited, physical examination is otherwise normal. The most important differential diagnosis is septic arthritis, which is suggested by fever, other signs of systemic illness, marked pain, reduction in hip movement, and an elevated erythrocyte sedimentation rate.

LEGG-CALVÉ-PERTHES DISEASE

Legg-Calvé-Perthes disease is the name used for idiopathic avascular necrosis of the femoral head, usually seen in children between 4 and 10 years of age. It manifests as either acute or insidious onset of hip pain with associated limp and decreased range of motion, particularly in internal rotation.

SLIPPED CAPITAL FEMORAL EPIPHYSIS

Slipped capital femoral epiphysis occurs in adolescents. Presenting symptoms are (1) hip pain that radiates to the groin, medial thigh, and knee, (2) an externally rotated gait, (3) decreased hip internal rotation, and (4) a limp. Short obese children with delayed puberty and children who have undergone a recent, rapid growth spurt are at particular risk for chronic slipped capital femoral epiphysis. An acute slip can occur after trauma.

Knee Pain

> ### Key Point
>
> Never forget that knee pain may not originate in the knee. It may be referred pain originating in a diseased hip.

Knee pain in children is often due to one of the following causes.

PATELLOFEMORAL MALALIGNMENT

Patellofemoral pain often occurs in adolescents, particularly girls, as a result of chronic injury to cartilage secondary to subclinical instability related to malalignment. Typically, knee pain occurs with activity and is exacerbated by climbing or descending stairs, walking down hills, squatting, or jumping. The term *chondromalacia patella* is a pathologic diagnosis made when there is evidence of fragmentation of the articular cartilage on the posterior surface of the patella.

RECURRENT PATELLAR SUBLUXATION OR DISLOCATION

Recurrent patellar subluxation or dislocation is suggested when a child's knee periodically gives way in association with severe, sudden pain and inability to straighten the knee. Treatment consists of referral for physiotherapy.

SYNOVIAL PLICAE

Synovial plicae are persistent remnants of folds of synovial membrane that divide the knee joint into three compartments during fetal development. A thickened

synovial fold that runs over the medial femoral condyle typically results in medial knee pain.

OSTEOCHONDRITIS DISSECANS

Osteochondritis dissecans is a defect in the subchondral region of an epiphysis with partial or complete fragmentation of bone. The condition commonly affects the distal femur, causing acute or insidious knee pain in teenaged boys, with or without an intra-articular loose body. Complaints about a knee that aches, gives way, locks, and swells characterize osteochondritis dissecans, although teenagers often complain of a knee that gives way or aches without any evidence of disease.

OSGOOD-SCHLATTER DISEASE

Osgood-Schlatter disease is a common cause of knee pain that is localized to the tibial tuberosity in athletic teenagers. Tenderness and swelling occur at the tibial tubercle and patellar tendon insertion, which result from a microavulsion fracture due to repetitive injury.

Foot Pain

Poorly fitting footwear is a common cause of foot pain in children. Other causes are *tarsal coalition* (a coalition between the tarsal bones characterized by a rigid flat foot), *Köhler disease* (avascular necrosis of the navicular bone), and *Freiberg disease* (avascular necrosis of the second metatarsal head).

Back Pain

> ### Key Point
>
> Always take back pain in a child seriously, because an organic cause is commonly found, particularly in younger children.

Consider osteomyelitis of a vertebral body, diskitis, or tumor in all children who present with back pain. Other causes are discussed here.

Spondylolysis is a stress fracture, usually unilateral, through the pars interarticularis (usually affecting L5). Spondylolisthesis occurs in the setting of bilateral spondylolysis when one vertebral body slips forward on the one beneath (such as L5 on S1). Both conditions may cause back pain in a child older than 5 years.

Scheuermann disease (idiopathic adolescent kyphosis), a disorder of unknown etiology, is characterized by increased thoracic spine kyphosis with abnormal wedging of at least three vertebral bodies at the apex of the kyphotic curve with the presence of Schmorl nodes.

GENERALIZED CAUSES OF MUSCULOSKELETAL PAIN

Besides the orthopedic disorders that cause pain in specific bones or joints, certain conditions may cause musculoskeletal pain in any location and must be considered in any child presenting with musculoskeletal pain. The pain may be localized to one or a few sites or may be generalized.

Trauma

Whether accidental or inflicted, trauma can cause localized pain wherever it occurs. Always determine whether the child's complaints and physical findings are compatible with the extent of injury reported.

Infection

Bacterial infections such as septic arthritis and osteomyelitis usually affect a single joint or bone, particularly the knee or hip; however, multiple sites are occasionally involved. If a child is febrile and has marked pain with movement of a joint or marked bony tenderness, you should suspect infection. Redness overlying the tender area should heighten your suspicion of bacterial infection. Specific infections and postinfectious illnesses may give rise to particular patterns of joint involvement as described here.

Acute rheumatic fever produces a postinfectious migratory arthritis affecting any single joint for approximately 1 week or less. Lyme disease (a tick-borne infection) causes arthritis that usually affects a few joints, particularly the knee, shoulder, and elbow. Viral infections may be associated with acute pain in joints, muscles, or both that usually resolves rapidly with symptomatic treatment.

Tumors

Osteoid osteoma is a relatively common benign tumor causing localized bone pain, usually in the proximal femur or tibia, that worsens at night and is classically relieved by salicylates or other nonsteroidal anti-inflammatory drugs (NSAIDs).

Leukemia is the most common malignancy causing musculoskeletal pain in children. Leg pain and fatigue on exertion may be among the earliest complaints of affected children. The pain is typically localized to the metaphysis of long bones, and the severity of pain is often out of proportion to other objective findings. The child may have associated swelling of a joint, most commonly the knee, which must be differentiated from pauciarticular juvenile rheumatoid arthritis (JRA). Neuroblastoma is another important cause of bone pain in young children, the pain being due to bony metastases.

Primary bone tumors often manifest as localized musculoskeletal pain. Osteosarcoma, the most common primary malignant bone tumor in children, typically occurs in the metaphysis of the distal femur, proximal tibia, or proximal humerus in adolescents. Ewing sarcoma is the second most common malignant bone tumor in children and also usually occurs in adolescents. It is often found in the diaphysis of the femur, humerus, or tibia but may occur in any bone, including those of the axial skeleton.

Juvenile Rheumatoid Arthritis

> **Key Point**
>
> Juvenile rheumatoid arthritis (JRA) is diagnosed if a child younger than 16 years exhibits persistent arthritis for more than 6 weeks with no underlying cause

Arthritis is defined by the American College of Rheumatology as the presence of joint swelling or two or more of the following findings: (1) tenderness or pain on motion, (2) limitation of motion, and (3) increased heat. Although any joint may be affected, certain types of JRA involve specific joints predominantly, providing essential diagnostic clues.

Pauciarticular JRA typically involves four or fewer joints, most commonly the knees, ankles, or elbows but not the hip joint. It primarily affects young girls 1 to 3 years old and is frequently associated with asymptomatic uveitis and a positive antinuclear antibody test result. In a 2-year-old girl who has hip pain, other causes should be sought, such as septic arthritis and leukemia.

Polyarticular JRA involves five or more joints, most often the knees, wrists, elbows, and ankles. The cervical spine and temporomandibular joints are also often involved. Symmetric small-joint disease of the hands is particularly common in the subgroup of children with rheumatoid factor–positive polyarticular JRA.

Systemic-onset JRA is characterized by high spiking fevers, an evanescent rash, variable internal organ involvement, including hepatosplenomegaly, lymphadenopathy, pericarditis, and other serositis, and chronic arthritis. Either a pauciarticular or polyarticular pattern of arthritis may be seen. You must always exclude infection and malignancy before making a diagnosis of systemic-onset JRA.

Other Rheumatic Diseases

The spondyloarthropathies, including juvenile ankylosing spondylitis, commonly affect the large joints below the waist, particularly the knees, ankles, and hips. Boys older than 8 years who carry the genetic marker HLA-B27 are most likely to be affected. Buttock pain due to sacroiliitis and back pain also occur but usually appear later in the course of disease. Enthesitis resulting in pain in the heels, over the tibial tuberosities at the knees, and under the feet is also characteristic of the spondyloarthropathies. Similar patterns of joint involvement are seen in patients with psoriasis, inflammatory bowel disease, Reiter syndrome, and reactive arthritis.

The connective tissue diseases, including systemic lupus erythematosus, juvenile dermatomyositis, mixed connective tissue disease, and scleroderma, may manifest as arthritis, arthralgia, myositis, myalgias, or tenosynovitis that causes musculoskeletal pain. The various forms of systemic vasculitis may also manifest as arthritis, causing joint pain.

"Growing Pains"

So-called growing pains have no connection with growth (aside from the fact that they occur in growing children!). The term *growing pains* is used to describe limb pains that follow a characteristic pattern and are found by careful physical examination not to be associated with any detectable disease. They most commonly occur in children between 2 and 6 years old. The limb pains occur mainly at night, often after intensive physical activity, and can cause severe leg pain. Typically, affected children are asymptomatic during the day, and their gait is normal.

Many children who experience growing pains go to bed without complaint but wake up 1 to 3 hours later complaining of leg pain that is often severe enough to make them cry. Most complain of bilateral calf, shin, or thigh pain, or, more vaguely, of pain in the entire leg. The trunk and upper extremities are rarely affected. Commonly, a parent of such a child experienced similar pains in childhood. Affected children often find relief from a single dose of acetaminophen or from massage, in contrast to children with an underlying pathologic cause of pain, who almost never ask their parents to rub their legs. A hot bath immediately before bed seems to help prevent pains in some children. If the history is atypical or if the child has a limp, joint swelling, or bone tenderness, do not label the problem as growing pains.

Benign Hypermobility

Benign hypermobility syndrome is a common cause of joint pain, particularly in the knees, ankles, and fingers.

Table 15–1 FINDINGS IN JOINT HYPERMOBILITY*

Passive opposition of thumb to flexor aspect of the forearm
Passive hyperextension of fifth finger parallel to extensor aspect of forearm
Hyperextension of elbows to >10 degrees
Hyperextension of knees to >10 degrees
Ability to touch floor with flat of hands without bending knees

*The diagnosis of joint hypermobility requires the presence of three of these findings.

Occasionally, the affected joints appear swollen for brief periods, but the swelling resolves spontaneously. The symptoms are episodic and may be exacerbated by exercise. The clinical findings that allow you to make a diagnosis of hypermobility are listed in Table 15–1.

Diffuse Idiopathic Musculoskeletal Pain

Diffuse idiopathic musculoskeletal pain is a poorly understood condition characterized by chronic widespread musculoskeletal aching and stiffness that occurs predominantly in healthy teenaged girls. Patients often complain of fatigue, poor sleep, and awakening unrefreshed. They may have associated chronic headaches or irritable bowel syndrome. In some patients, physical examination reveals exquisite tenderness at characteristic soft tissue sites, meeting the criteria for fibromyalgia. The cause of fibromyalgia is unknown. Fibromyalgia may be primary or secondary, superimposed on a recognizable painful condition or underlying disease. The diagnosis, which is suggested by the history and the finding of specific tender points on physical examination, requires exclusion of other causes of widespread aches and pains, including hypothyroidism and depression.

Localized Idiopathic Musculoskeletal Pain

Localized idiopathic musculoskeletal pain is typically constant, severe pain that can involve any part of the body. The leg is more commonly affected than the arm, and distal involvement is more common than proximal. The pain often significantly interferes with normal functioning and is frequently accompanied by *allodynia* (pain generated by stimuli that are not normally painful). The pain may or may not be associated with symptoms and signs of autonomic dysfunction, including cool temperature, mottled purple discoloration, increased sweating or marked dryness, and diffuse swelling of the painful area. Minor injury not infre-

Table 15-2 COMMON CAUSES OF A LIMP IN A CHILD

Cause	Underlying Conditions
Local causes	
Hip	Congenital hip dislocation, Legg-Calvé-Perthes disease, septic arthritis; toxic synovitis, slipped capital femoral epiphysis
Knee	Osgood-Schlatter disease, osteochondritis dissecans, tumors
Tibia	Toddler's fracture, stress fracture, fracture through a bone cyst
Foot	Tarsal coalition, Köhler disease, tight shoes
Back	Spondylolisthesis, osteomyelitis, Scheuermann disease
Short leg	
Generalized disorders	
Bone diseases	Rickets, infections, leukemia, primary tumors
Muscle diseases	Inflammatory, congenital, metabolic myopathies
Joint diseases	Juvenile arthritis, septic arthritis
Neurologic diseases	Cerebral palsy
Psychiatric diseases	Conversion disorder

quently precedes the onset of pain, but progressive disability follows that is not consistent with the inciting event. The disorders reflex sympathetic dystrophy and chronic regional pain syndrome types 1 and 2 are encompassed in the category *localized idiopathic pain*. As in the child with diffuse idiopathic pain, other diseases that could reasonably explain the symptoms must be excluded before this diagnosis is made.

THE CHILD WITH A LIMP

> **Key Point**
>
> A limp in a child must be taken seriously; usually, a cause is found. Observation of the gait often tells a great deal about the site and nature of the problem.

Causes of an abnormal gait may be divided into the following categories:

Painful causes: injury, mechanical stress, inflammation, or a destructive process

Painless causes: leg-length discrepancy, in-toeing or out-toeing

Neuromuscular causes: weakness, spasticity, or coordination problems

A limp is frequently accompanied by pain in a child, although discomfort may not be the chief complaint

(Table 15-2). Recent pain accompanied by worsening symptoms suggests trauma, infection, slipped capital femoral epiphysis, or transient synovitis. The more prolonged the symptoms, the more likely that an abnormality will be detected on imaging studies. A limp that is worse in the morning and improves as the day progresses may be due to inflammatory disease. Limping without pain occurs in conditions such as congenital hip dislocation, leg-length discrepancy, and neurologic disorders.

THE CHILD WITH A SINGLE SWOLLEN JOINT

Six broad categories of monoarthritis are listed in Table 15-3. As with musculoskeletal pain, the location provides a diagnostic clue, particularly in rheumatic or orthopedic conditions.

Trauma is the most common cause of a single swollen joint in a child. Ask about a precipitating injury.

Infections such as septic arthritis or osteomyelitis must be considered. If the child has had a fever or recent documented infection and has recently received antibiotics, you should suspect infectious arthritis, especially if marked pain, redness, and increased heat are noted in a single joint.

Consider malignancy in a child who presents with fever, weight loss, and malaise. Leukemia, lymphoma, and neuroblastoma are by far the most common possibilities.

THE CHILD WITH MULTIPLE SWOLLEN JOINTS

The broad etiologic categories listed in Table 15-3 for a single swollen joint apply to determining the cause of

Table 15-3 CAUSES OF MONOARTHRITIS IN A CHILD

Trauma
Infection
Malignancy
Rheumatic
  Juvenile rheumatoid arthritis
  Juvenile ankylosing spondylitis
  Arthritis associated with other conditions
    Psoriasis
    Inflammatory bowel disease
    Reactive arthritis
    Reiter syndrome
    Sarcoidosis
Hematologic (hemophilia, hemangioma)
Mechanical and "orthopedic conditions"

multiple swollen joints in children, although mechanical and orthopedic conditions are less likely. Septic arthritis is also less likely, although not impossible, if multiple joints are affected. Certain infections usually affect more than one joint, including hepatitis B, Epstein-Barr virus, adenovirus, rubella, *Mycoplasma*, and Lyme disease. *Salmonella, Shigella,* and *Yersinia* may cause postinfectious arthritis of multiple joints.

In a child with acute onset of polyarthritis, you should also consider Henoch-Schönlein purpura, Kawasaki disease, serum sickness, systemic lupus erythematosus, and subacute bacterial endocarditis. Chronic polyarthritis may occur in these diseases and with mixed connective tissue disease, juvenile dermatomyositis, polyarteritis nodosa, or scleroderma. Consider also the possibility of hematologic disorders and of underlying conditions such as cystic fibrosis and immunodeficiencies.

SIGNIFICANT COMMON SKELETAL DEFORMITIES

Scoliosis is a lateral spinal curvature. A structural scoliosis is associated with a rotation deformity of the vertebrae and ribs. Idiopathic scoliosis, which accounts for 80% of cases, varies in severity and shows a sex-linked inheritance pattern.

Neurofibromatosis is commonly associated with scoliosis. Also, an underlying neuromuscular disorder such as cerebral palsy, prior vertebral trauma, irradiation to the spine, Marfan syndrome, dwarfism, or congenital heart disease may be associated with scoliosis. Elicit details about when the scoliosis was first observed and how it has progressed.

When torticollis (wryneck) is first noted between 6 and 12 weeks of age, it is a "congenital muscular torticollis" caused by contracture of the sternocleidomastoid muscle, usually on the right side. The contracture tilts the head toward the involved side and rotates the chin toward the other shoulder. The knowledge that a palpable mass, a fibroma of the sternocleidomastoid muscle, was noted in the affected muscle during those weeks confirms this diagnosis.

By contrast, a history of torticollis noted shortly after birth suggests a congenital abnormality of the cervical spine (e.g., hemivertebra). Older children may demonstrate acute torticollis after an acute pharyngitis with cervical adenitis or after trauma. Associated symptoms may also suggest the etiology. Gastroesophageal reflux is occasionally associated with an intermittent torticollis, known as *Sandifer syndrome*. Ocular causes include a fourth cranial nerve palsy and, uncommonly, congenital nystagmus (see Chapter 8). Other uncommon causes are spinal cord or posterior fossa tumors, cervical spine infections, and JRA.

Key Point

Torticollis (wryneck) should prompt the physician to ask one important question: What was the age at onset? If torticollis was present from birth, a radiograph is needed to exclude a congenital anomaly of the cervical spine.

OBTAINING THE HISTORY

Even before beginning the detailed history, ask the child's age, because age and sex yield important clues to the cause of the musculoskeletal pain (Table 15–4). Establish the purpose of the visit and determine whether the parents (1) are troubled because the child's pain is worsening, (2) were pressured by a worried grandparent into making an appointment, or (3) are simply seeking reassurance that their child is normal.

While taking the history, observe the child for signs of definite organic disease, such as a limp or difficulty using an arm.

Stress

Ask about stress. Psychosocial stresses trigger not only benign abdominal pain or tension headaches but also benign musculoskeletal pain, particularly in teenagers with diffuse or localized idiopathic pain syndromes. Stress may not be immediately obvious, but observation and questioning may reveal a highly motivated "overachiever" who is under considerable family pressure, other recent stresses at home or at school, or an abnormally symbiotic parent-child relationship. Sexual abuse may be a hidden cause of unexplained musculoskeletal pain, and you should suspect physical abuse if the child has extensive bruising or multiple fractures.

Timing of Symptoms

Find out when the symptoms began, and determine their course. Musculoskeletal pain that has been unchanged for many years is unlikely to be due to significant disease. A notable exception is osteoid osteoma, which may cause persistent mild and inconstant symptoms for several years before medical attention is sought. Malignant bone tumors have a much more fulminant course but may cause pain with few other symptoms for weeks or months before diagnosis.

Locating Pain Sites and Establishing Severity

Asking a child "Show me with one finger where it hurts" and asking the parents to describe where the

Table 15–4 AGE RANGE AND SEX PREDOMINANCE FOR COMMON MUSCULOSKELETAL DISORDERS IN CHILDHOOD

Musculoskeletal Disorder	Peak Age Range (yr)	Sex Predominance
Trauma	Any age	Female and male
Infection	Any age*	Female and male
Malignancy		
Osteoid osteoma	Any age (most 10–20)	Male > female
Primary malignant bone tumor	≥10	Female and male
Secondary bone tumor	Any age	Female and male
Juvenile rheumatoid arthritis		
Pauciarticular		
Type I	1–3	Female >> male
Type II	>8	Male > female
Polyarticular		
RF-negative	2–5	Female > male
RF-positive	>10	Female >> male
Systemic-onset	Any age	Female and male
Juvenile ankylosing spondylitis	>8	Male >> female
Transient synovitis	4–8	Male > female
Legg-Calvé-Perthes disease	4–9	Male > female
Slipped capital femoral epiphysis	8–16	Male > female
Osteochondritis dissecans	>10	Male > female
Growing pains	4–13	Female and male
Fibromyalgia	>10	Female >> male
Reflex sympathetic dystrophy	>10	Female >> male

Abbreviation: RF, rheumatoid factor; >, greater than; >>, much greater than.
* Septic arthritis is most common in children 3 years or younger.

child usually complains of pain may help locate the cause of musculoskeletal pain in children.

Although children find it difficult to describe their discomfort, they give fairly consistent descriptions in several disorders. For example, they describe growing pains as heavy, deep aching, or cramping that, unlike most other musculoskeletal pains, is relieved by massage. Children with diffuse idiopathic pain syndromes often describe their pain as ill-defined, diffuse aching pain with stiffness; in some localized idiopathic pain syndromes, the pain may be described as burning pain.

Having the child or parent describe the severity of the pain does not help distinguish an organic from a nonorganic cause, because significant disease may cause only moderate pain, whereas a child with a benign condition may complain of severe pain. Knowing whether the pain interferes with function and how it affects the child and family helps you evaluate its severity. Musculoskeletal pain with no obvious organic basis may produce weeks of school absence in the child with diffuse or localized idiopathic pain, whereas many children with JRA and obvious organic joint disease rarely miss school and manage to keep up with their peers.

Key Point

Always take seriously any pain severe enough to limit a child's play, because an important underlying physical or emotional cause is usually found for such pain.

Aggravating and Relieving Factors

Discovering what alleviates the pain or worsens it is a diagnostic aid. Increased activity aggravates musculoskeletal pain from mechanical causes, such as patellofemoral malalignment, which is aggravated by climbing stairs, deep knee bends, and prolonged periods of knee flexion. Other mechanical causes of pain, such as plica syndrome, Osgood-Schlatter disease, joint hypermobility, and stress fracture, are all aggravated by exercise.

Pain from a mechanical cause is usually less severe in the morning and worsens with activity during the day. By contrast, pain that is worse in the morning and gradually improves with increased daytime activity characterizes inflammatory disease and suggests arthritis. Growing pains occur at night and disappear the next morning, only to recur on subsequent nights. Pain from an osteoid osteoma worsens at night but is usually unilateral if the lesion arises in an extremity. By contrast, growing pains are almost always bilateral. Although pain from a malignant bone tumor may intensify at night, it usually remains constant throughout the day. Often, pain from infection is fixed, day and night. Pain due to diffuse and localized idiopathic pain syndromes is frequently unremitting during the day but does not awaken the child at night.

Preceding Trauma

Always ask about possible trauma, because subtle injuries, even a minor penetrating wound to the foot or a rose thorn prick to a finger, can give important clues to the child's problem. Not infrequently, a minor fall brings attention to a previously unrecognized swollen joint secondary to JRA or another underlying abnormality. Occasionally, minor trauma can cause a pathologic fracture in the presence of an underlying abnormality such as a bone cyst. If the child has a bleeding disorder, a minor injury may lead to significant bleeding in a joint.

Repetitive minor trauma can result in an "overuse syndrome," so ask about a child's participation in sports, which might cause little leaguer's shoulder, little leaguer's elbow, or tennis elbow. Also, recent vigorous physical activity after a prolonged period of inactivity increases the risk of a stress fracture.

Previous Infection

Elicit details of any previous infections. A sore throat due to β-hemolytic streptococcal infection or scarlet fever preceding migratory joint symptoms by a latent period of 2 to 5 weeks suggests acute rheumatic fever. A gastrointestinal or genitourinary infection 2 to 4 weeks before the onset of joint pain suggests a reactive arthritis. Always ask about recent treatment with antibiotics or other medication. Antibiotic use for any reason can result in a partially treated septic arthritis or osteomyelitis, obscuring the typical clinical manifestations; some medications can produce drug reactions or serum sickness. Certain viral infections, especially influenza A and B, may be followed by sudden onset of acute muscle pain and tenderness, usually affecting the calf muscles. The calf pain is often so severe that the child refuses to walk but will crawl around on hands and knees. This acute myositis usually resolves spontaneously in a few days.

A history of a tick bite, visit to a tick-infested area, or a rash suggestive of erythema migrans raises the possibility of Lyme disease, named after the town of Old Lyme, Connecticut, where it was first recognized.

Associated Symptoms and Signs

Key Point

The critical question that helps determine the underlying cause of musculoskeletal pain in a child is "Are there associated symptoms or signs?"

Joint pain associated with early-morning stiffness suggests inflammatory joint disease. The mother may report that the child moves slowly on awakening and refuses to climb stairs or "walks like a little old man." The morning stiffness may last from 5 or 10 minutes to several hours. Recurrent stiffness after an afternoon nap or a long car ride, known as the "gelling phenomenon," also characterizes inflammatory disease. Swelling, redness, and warmth over one or more joints also suggest inflammatory disease. A history of limping always indicates a significant problem, even if other symptoms are minimal.

If you suspect an underlying connective tissue disorder, take a detailed history, including a complete functional inquiry, because these illnesses frequently affect multiple organ systems. Has the child experienced fever, weight loss, anorexia, or fatigue? A few specific questions about the head and neck provide a clue in children whose multisystem complaints suggest an underlying connective tissue disorder. They include questions about alopecia, recurrent mouth ulcers, sicca symptoms (dry eyes, dry mouth), facial swelling, and dysphagia.

Constitutional symptoms such as fever, fatigue, anorexia, and weight loss may also occur with infection, systemic-onset JRA, or malignancy, particularly leukemia or neuroblastoma. Abdominal pain, diarrhea, and fever should raise the suspicion of inflammatory bowel disease or bowel infection such as *Yersinia* infection with joint involvement. A detailed history may also uncover symptoms suggesting fibromyalgia, such as constant fatigue, generalized stiffness, recurrent headaches, abdominal pain, and symptoms of anxiety or depression.

Asking about previous musculoskeletal complaints is important. The presence of an underlying illness such as hemophilia, hypothyroidism, inflammatory bowel disease, or cystic fibrosis may also establish the etiology of the musculoskeletal complaint. Immunodeficiency states, in a child with a history of recurrent infections, may manifest as arthritis that is clinically indistinguishable from JRA. Recent immunization, particularly with rubella vaccine in older children, can occasionally cause an arthritis that may persist for weeks.

Because adult rheumatoid arthritis is common, a family history of this disease has little diagnostic value. Certain forms of arthritis, particularly those associated with the genetic marker HLA-B27, do have a genetic predisposition, so ask about a family history of ankylosing spondylitis, psoriasis, inflammatory bowel disease, Reiter syndrome, and other collagen vascular disorders. A positive family history may also be seen with Legg-Calvé-Perthes disease and osteochondritis dissecans.

APPROACH TO THE PHYSICAL EXAMINATION

Observation

Watch the child closely. Observe for any obvious abnormalities while the child is walking or playing. If the youngster is old enough, begin the examination with nonthreatening activities that will help establish the extent of physical limitation. To detect subtle abnormalities in one limb, ask the child to hop on one foot at a time while you hold one of his or her hands. Note whether the child grasps your hand more firmly when supported on the affected leg (Fig. 15–5). Ask the

youngster to walk on the heels and toes to determine whether there is impairment due to muscle weakness or due to local pain or tenderness. A simple screening technique to assess either strength or lower extremity joint disease is to ask the child to squat and walk across the room "like a duck" (Fig. 15–6). A normal "duck-walk" makes significant joint disease in the knees and hips extremely unlikely.

> **Key Point**
>
> Rule out a primary muscle disorder such as dermatomyositis or muscular dystrophy by testing pelvic girdle muscle strength.

To test pelvic girdle muscle strength, ask the child to sit on the floor and then stand up; often, with proximal muscle weakness, the child cannot rise from the floor without assistance or without either using a chair or table or "climbing up the legs"—placing the hands on the thighs to assist, a phenomenon (Fig. 15–7) known as the Gower maneuver.

With the child sufficiently undressed to give you a good view of the legs and pelvis, observe the gait during walking and running over a good distance. Check the mechanics of walking, including heel strike, follow-through, and push-off. Be sure that flexion and

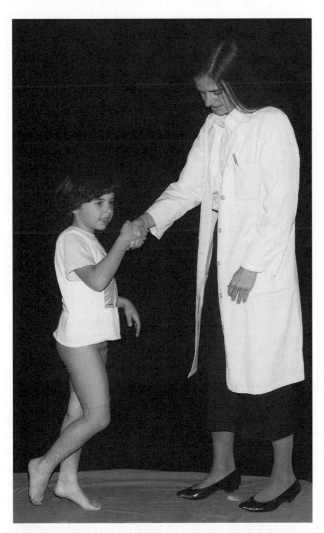

Figure 15–5 When there is pain or weakness in one leg, the child may grasp the physician's hand for added support when hopping on the affected leg.

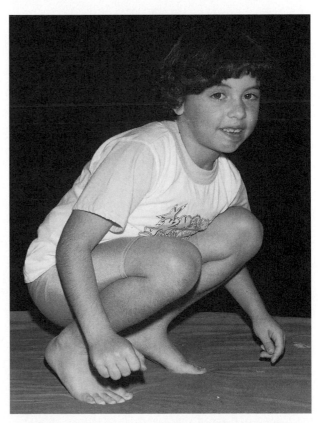

Figure 15–6 Squatting like a duck, a good screening test for weakness or other lower limb problems.

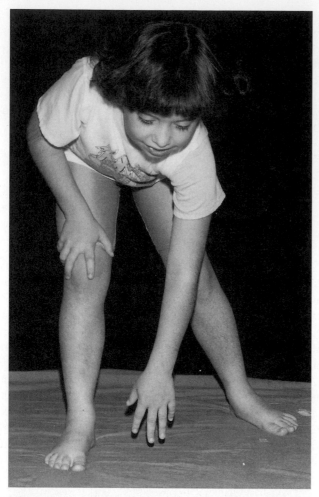

Figure 15–7 The Gower sign. A child with weak proximal leg muscles "climbs up her legs" when getting from the floor to a standing position.

extension of the ankles, knees, and hips are normal. Examine the gait with the child's shoes on, then with the child barefoot. Ill-fitting shoes can cause foot pain at any age.

When a child spends a shorter time bearing weight on the painful leg than on his or her normal one, the gait is described as *antalgic*. The following characteristic gait patterns help localize the problem:

- Push-off is avoided in a painful forefoot or in pain at the Achilles tendon insertion.
- Heel strike is avoided in a painful heel.
- Persistent flexion of the knee is seen when the joint is swollen and painful.
- A Trendelenburg gait results from hip disease or hip girdle weakness; it is characterized by shifting of the head and trunk to the side of the affected hip when the child bears weight on the affected leg.
- The common gait abnormalities, in-toeing and out-toeing, may be caused by any of the rotational deformities discussed earlier along with normal variants.

Back Examination

Look at the child from behind while the youngster stands upright. If the spinal dimples are level, there is no significant leg-length discrepancy (Fig. 15–8). Inspect the lower back for the presence of a tuft of hair, midline nevi, angioma, lipoma, or a central dimple, suggesting an underlying vertebral and spinal cord abnormality. If the spinal cord is tethered by a bony spicule or fibrous band (*diastematomyelia*), the child may present with back or lower extremity pain or may be asymptomatic for years.

Next, with the child still standing, examine the back for scoliosis. Observed from behind, the shoulders should be level. Note any scapular prominence. With nonstructural scoliosis, a lateral curve is present that is flexible and is corrected with side bending to the convex side; with structural scoliosis, the curve is not corrected with side bending. A structural thoracic scoliosis leads to deformity of the rib cage, with the ribs on the convex side of the curve protruding on forward bending to produce a "rib prominence" on that side (Fig. 15–9). Ask the child to bend forward at the waist, keeping the knees straight and allowing the arms to hang down freely. This position accentuates even a slight rib or lumbar asymmetry. Inspect the back for compensatory secondary curves above and below the major curve. These secondary curves help keep the head aligned over the pelvis. If the child has a leg-length discrepancy, correct it before checking for scoliosis.

Key Point

When assessing a child with scoliosis, search for café au lait spots that suggest neurofibromatosis. Conduct a thorough neurologic examination, including abdominal reflexes, to exclude a neuromuscular cause, and evaluate the child's height and secondary sexual characteristics to help predict future growth patterns.

Scoliosis must be severe to produce back pain in a child; mild scoliosis cannot explain a child's back pain and suggests some other underlying pathologic process, such as osteoid osteoma, spinal cord tumor, infection, or spondylolisthesis. If you detect significant scoliosis in a child, screen all of his or her siblings.

Examine the youngster's back for evidence of decreased or excessive thoracic kyphosis or lumbar lordosis. Excessive thoracic kyphosis appears as "round shoulders" or a "rounded back" and, in the adolescent, may be caused by poor posture or by Scheuermann disease. In Scheuermann disease, unlike poor posture, the kyphosis persists when the child lies prone and is emphasized by forward bending. With the child bending forward, observe how the lumbar spine forms a smooth curve from the thorax to the

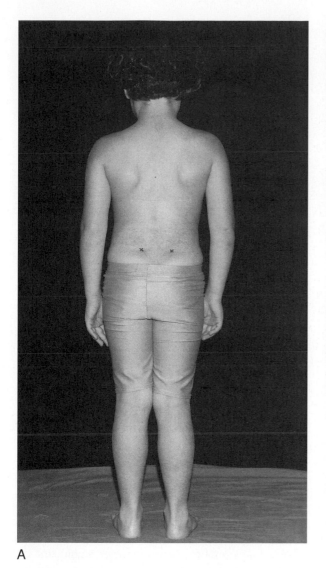
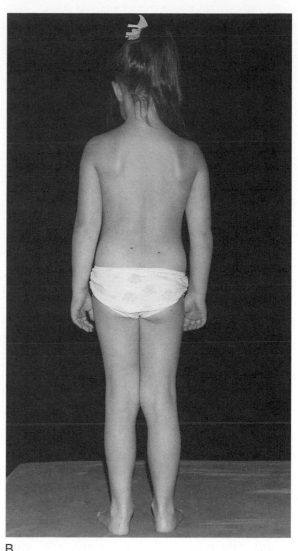

A   B

Figure 15–8 Spinal dimples should be level when there is no leg length discrepancy. *A,* normal. *B,* Child with mild overgrowth of the left leg secondary to juvenile rheumatoid arthritis involving the left knee.

sacrum. Back flattening in the lumbar area suggests disease ranging from chronically limited movement secondary to juvenile ankylosing spondylitis to acute limitation from vertebral osteomyelitis or even a spinal tumor.

Teenagers often have tight hamstring muscles that prevent full hip flexion and may appear to limit lumbar flexion; slightly bending the knees can increase the range. Hamstring tightness and marked restriction of forward hip flexion are common in patients with symptomatic spondylolisthesis with or without associated tenderness on palpation of the lower back. Perform a straight leg raising test to assess hamstring tightness further.

Be sure to differentiate hamstring tightness from a nerve root problem. With the patient supine, flex the hip while keeping the leg straight. Normally, flexion to 80 to 90 degrees is possible. In the presence of a normal hip, limitation of flexion with pain occurring

below the knee as well as in the hamstring area suggests nerve root disease. To help confirm nerve root irritation, flex the knee to allow further flexion of the hip, and then straighten the knee to see whether doing so induces pain (Lasègue test); then ease knee flexion to a tolerable degree and dorsiflex the ankle (Bragard test); pain with this maneuver confirms a nerve root problem.

Have the child lie in a prone position, and palpate the spine, the paravertebral muscles, and the sacroiliac joints. Test back movement in older children thoroughly. Check lateral flexion by asking the child to tilt sideways without bending forward and to touch the tips of the fingers to just below the sides of the knees. Normally, the fingertips can touch the head of the fibula (Fig. 15–10). To test rotation, first have the patient straddle a chair to stabilize the pelvis and cross the arms across the chest to stabilize the shoulder girdle; then ask the patient to rotate the trunk (Fig. 15–11).

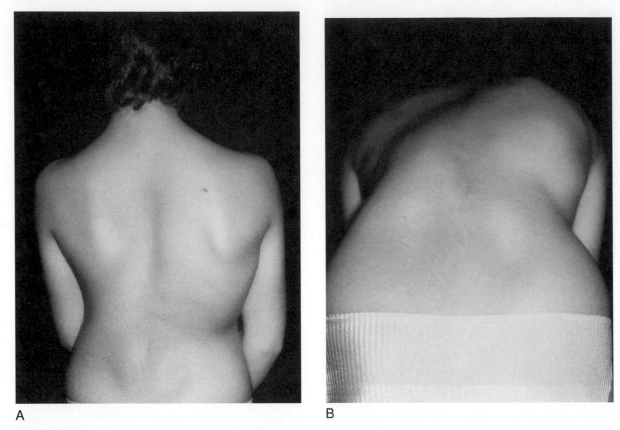

A   B

Figure 15–9 Scoliosis. Mild degrees of scoliosis *(A)* become more obvious when the child is asked to bend forward *(B)* and is inspected from the rear.

Cervical Spine Examination

Facing the child, inspect the child's neck for evidence of torticollis. In infants, palpate for a firm nontender mass in the body of the sternocleidomastoid muscle, which would suggest congenital muscular torticollis; the mass may resolve spontaneously by 4 to 6 weeks of age. Palpate for tightness or contracture of the sternocleidomastoid muscle. Measure the infant's skull, and look for secondary facial and skull asymmetry. Facial flattening on the side of the abnormal sternocleidomastoid muscle can occur with untreated torticollis.

Key Point

In a child diagnosed with congenital muscular torticollis, remember to examine the hips, because 20% of children with congenital torticollis also have congenital hip dislocation.

Next, observe the cervical spine from the side, noting the presence or absence of the normal cervical lordosis. Palpate the paravertebral muscles and the spinous processes to detect tenderness or masses. Test the range of motion—extension, flexion, rotation, and lateral flexion. Normally, the cervical spine extends so that the child's occiput touches the upper back, and the young-

ster looks directly at the ceiling (Fig. 15–12*A*). Loss of extension is often the most sensitive test for early cervical spine involvement in JRA (see Fig. 15–12*B*), whereas flexion may remain normal despite significant cervical disease. To test rotation, ask the child to look toward each shoulder; the normal range is 80 to 90 degrees. Ask the child to touch each ear to the shoulder to test lateral flexion; the normal range is 45 degrees.

Temporomandibular Joint Examination

Inspect the temporomandibular (TM) joint for overlying swelling just anterior to the tragus of the ear. Do not confuse this swelling with parotid gland swelling, which extends over the angle of the jaw behind and below the ear. Look for micrognathia. Mandibular growth may be impaired by arthritis affecting the TM joints in childhood (Fig. 15–13), and facial asymmetry may develop if one TM joint is more severely affected than the other.

Test jaw movement when the child opens the mouth widely. Because the jaw is smaller on the side of the more severely affected TM joint, the jaw shifts slightly toward the affected TM joint when the child opens the mouth wide. The interdental distance—the distance between the upper and lower central incisor teeth when

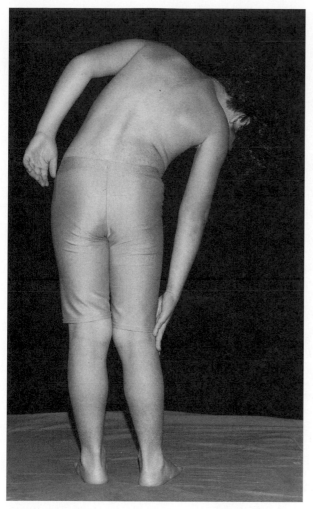

Figure 15–10 Testing lateral flexion of the spine. The child can normally touch the head of the fibula with the fingertips. Make sure that the child does not "cheat" by bending forward to reach the lower leg.

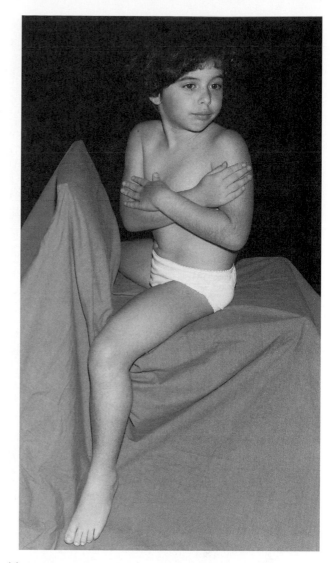

Figure 15–11 Testing spinal rotation. Straddling the chair stabilizes the pelvis, and crossing the arms stabilizes the shoulder girdle. The child is then asked to turn as far as possible to each side.

the child opens the mouth maximally—is at least 3 cm in a normal child (Fig. 15–14). Palpate the mandibular condyles for tenderness, and try to appreciate their normal rounded contour, which may be lost with persistent arthritis. Crepitus may be present if the cartilage separating the condyle from the temporal bone is eroded.

Peripheral Joint Examination

Examining the peripheral joints helps document the presence or absence of arthritis. Have older children sit on the edge of the examining table; infants and younger children can sit on the parent's lap.

The examination of each joint consists of (1) inspection for swelling, redness, and deformity, (2) palpation for tenderness, synovial thickening, and effusion, and (3) assessment of active and passive ranges of movement.

It is also essential to examine the bones proximal and distal to the joints. Examine the child scrupulously for bone tenderness. A useful technique to pinpoint

bone tenderness uses the eraser on the end of a pencil. The periosteum is extremely sensitive to pain, and bone tenderness may result from trauma, osteomyelitis, or subperiosteal leukemic infiltrates.

Approach to the Examination of Specific Joints

HAND EXAMINATION

It is least threatening for a child if you begin the peripheral joint examination by inspecting the hands. Check the fingers for psoriatic nail pitting (Fig. 15–15), clubbing, periungual erythema, nail fold vasculitic infarcts (Fig. 15–16), loss of the distal finger pulp, ulcerated fingertips, and sclerodactyly. Note any swelling, redness, deformity, or asymmetry between the two hands (Fig. 15–17).

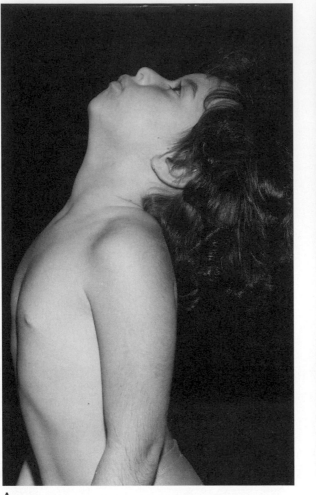
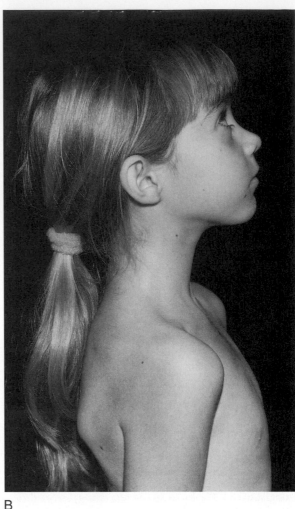

A   B

Figure 15–12 *A,* Normal degree of cervical spine extension. *B,* Marked limitation of extension (in juvenile rheumatoid arthritis) accompanied by typical upward gaze.

Palpate the individual distal interphalangeal (DIP), proximal interphalangeal (PIP), and metacarpophalangeal (MCP) joints, searching for evidence of tenderness, increased warmth, synovial thickening, or effusion. Bimanual palpation using the thumbs and index fingers of both hands detects effusions of the MCP joints. MCP joints are located 1 cm distal to the knuckles, and swollen MCP joints cause the depressions between the knuckles, normally visible when a child makes a fist, to disappear. To assess active flexion of the small joints of the hand, ask the child to make a fist. Evaluate the passive range of motion, noting the presence or absence of "stress pain," which occurs at the extreme ranges of joint movement.

Key Point

The MCP joints normally flex to 90 degrees and extend to 30 degrees; the PIP joints flex to 120 degrees and extend to 0 degrees; and the DIP joints flex to 80 to 90 degrees and extend to 0 to 10 degrees.

Pain, swelling, and limited finger movement may also result from *tenosynovitis,* an inflammation of the tendon sheaths. Palpate each tenosynovial sheath for swelling, tenderness, or crepitus. Sometimes, discrete nodules, palpable in the individual tendons, may obstruct normal finger flexion and extension, causing *triggering,* an involuntary hesitation in flexion or extension caused by sticking of a flexor tendon within its sheath. Before concluding the hand examination, inspect the bony and soft tissue structures; cool temperature, hyperesthesia, blue mottled discoloration, increased sweating, and bizarre posturing suggest reflex sympathetic dystrophy.

WRIST EXAMINATION

Inspect the wrist for deformity or malalignment. In JRA, ulnar posturing (deviation) of the wrist is not uncommon, and volar subluxation may occur with longstanding or severe disease. Examine the wrist for evidence of swelling along the joint line, which would

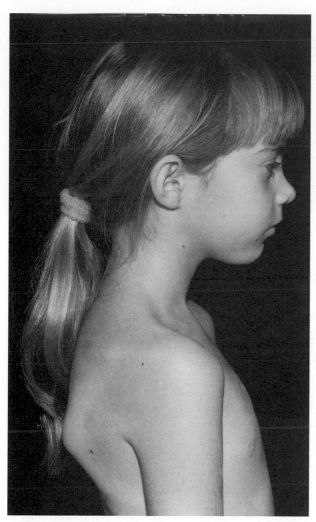

Figure 15–13 Early micrognathia associated with juvenile rheumatoid arthritis. In some affected children, this sign can be much more pronounced.

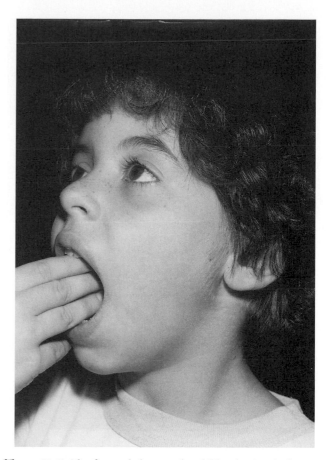

Figure 15–14 The fingers belong to the child, who is asked to put them in her mouth as a quick screening test for loss of interdental distance. The mouth should admit at least three fingers in the position shown.

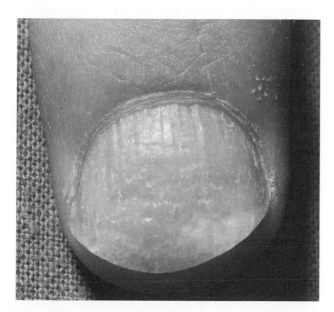

Figure 15–15 Typical nail pitting associated with psoriasis.

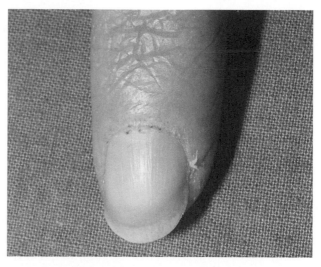

Figure 15–16 The dark spots on the nail bed represent small vasculitic infarcts, seen typically in connective tissue diseases.

indicate an effusion. Swelling may also be seen over the dorsum of the hand distal to the wrist joint (Fig. 15–18); its presence suggests tenosynovitis of the extensor tendon sheaths, which is confirmed if the swelling moves as the child opens and closes the fist. When the fingers are actively extended, the distal margin of the

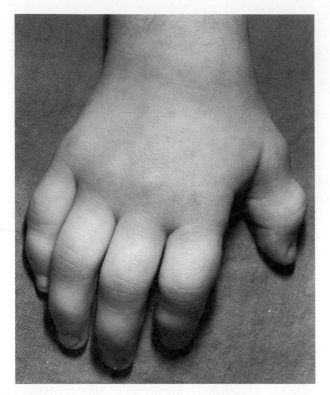

Figure 15–17 Marked swelling of the interphalangeal joints with flexion contractures in juvenile rheumatoid arthritis.

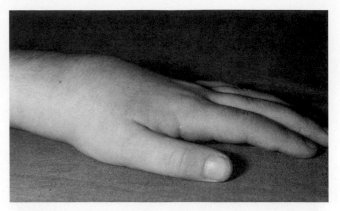

Figure 15–18 Swelling over the wrist and dorsum of the hand in juvenile rheumatoid arthritis.

swelling moves proximally and appears to "tuck in"; hence, this phenomenon has been called the *tuck sign* (Fig. 15–19). Observe the range of motion at the wrist; in most children, flexion and extension to 80 to 90 degrees are possible.

Forearm supination and pronation occur at the distal and proximal radioulnar joints. Test these movements with the child's arm held at the side, the elbow flexed to 90 degrees, and the hand held in the neutral position with the thumbs up. Supination is normally possible to 90 degrees (palms up), and pronation to 85 degrees (palms down).

ELBOW EXAMINATION

Examine the elbow for swelling, tenderness, increased warmth, and range of motion. The elbow normally flexes to at least 145 to 150 degrees and extends to at least neutral (complete extension) and, frequently, to 10 degrees of hyperextension, especially in girls. Carefully palpate the elbow for swelling; you can most easily detect an effusion by moving the elbow from flexion into extension, reducing the intra-articular space. Simultaneously palpate the joint over the lateral or medial aspects to feel the fluid bulge. Examine the posterior surface of the proximal ulna for rheumatoid nodules, which may occur in the small subgroup of children with rheumatoid factor–positive polyarticular JRA.

SHOULDER EXAMINATION

The shoulder mechanism consists of the glenohumeral joint and the shoulder girdle. The deltoid muscle produces the normal rounded contour of the shoulder, a contour that is lost with anterior shoulder dislocation or with significant muscle atrophy from primary muscle or joint disease (Fig. 15–20). Inspect the shoulder for normal contour and for an effusion, which results in an anterior prominence just lateral to the coracoid process.

Test mobility at the shoulder joint by asking the child to perform the following active movements:

1. Reach the hands and arms as high above the head as possible. Typically, the child with JRA that restricts movement at one shoulder tilts the head toward the abnormal side to minimize the obvious limitation of shoulder motion (Fig. 15–21).
2. Clasp the hands behind the neck, to test external rotation, and then scratch the middle upper portion of the back with both hands, to check internal rotation.

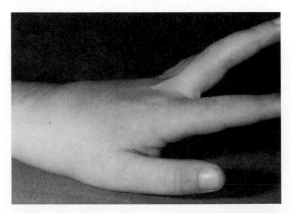

Figure 15–19 The tuck sign. When the child extends the fingers, the swollen extensor tendon sheath moves proximally and produces a bulge on the dorsum of the hand.

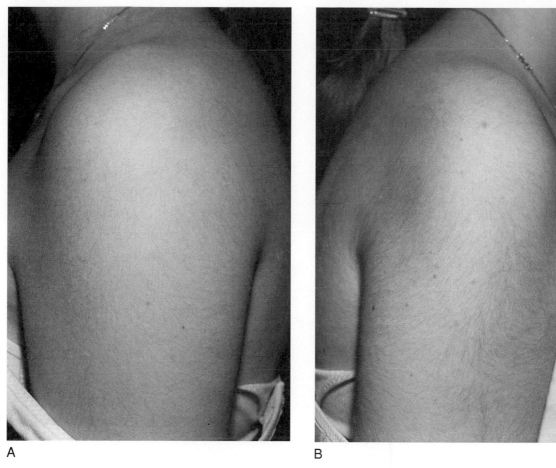

A   B

Figure 15–20 A 14-year-old girl with juvenile rheumatoid arthritis. *A*, Her left shoulder appears normal. *B*, On inspection, her right shoulder shows marked atrophy of the shoulder girdle, visible anteriorly and posteriorly.

If a child's active movements are restricted, test passive movements individually with the shoulder abducted to 90 degrees and the elbow bent to 90 degrees. Rotate the shoulder externally (up) and internally (down). The normal range for both external and internal rotation is 90 degrees.

| **Key Point** |

Although the shoulder is an uncommon site of involvement in JRA, limited external rotation is commonly the first sign of shoulder joint disease.

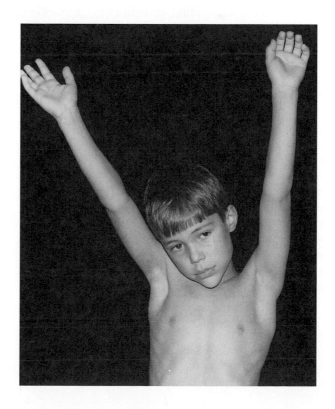

Figure 15–21 Testing range of motion of the shoulder. The child is asked to raise the hands above the head with palms facing each other. This boy has limited abduction of the right shoulder. Typically, he tilts his head toward the affected side when asked to perform this maneuver.

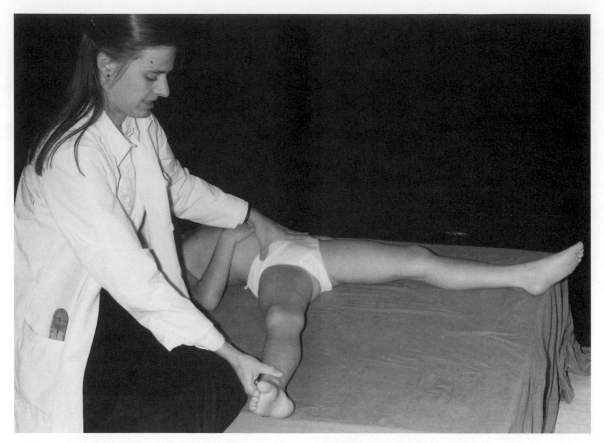

Figure 15-22 How to test hip abduction. Use one hand to stabilize the pelvis. Normal range is 40 to 50 degrees.

HIP EXAMINATION

Ask the child to lie supine on the examining table, or reposition the younger child or infant in a recumbent position on the parent's lap. Observing the child's posture and position is critical in examination of the hips, because these joints are too deep to inspect directly. Suspect significant hip disease in the child who holds the hip in flexion and external rotation.

A screening test for hip disease in addition to the "duck-walking" test is the *log roll*, a painless test to detect muscle spasm secondary to hip joint irritability. With the child lying supine, place your hand on the thigh, and gently roll the hip into internal and external rotation, noting any resistance, which would suggest hip disease. To assess the range of hip movement accurately, you must place your other hand on the child's pelvis to stabilize it (Fig. 15–22). When the pelvis moves, the end of hip movement has been reached. Normal hip mobility varies significantly with age and is generally greater in infants than in older children.

Test hip flexion by asking the child to bring the knees to the chest (normal range, 120 degrees). Move the leg laterally and medially to test abduction (normal range, 40 to 50 degrees) and adduction (normal range, 25 degrees). Test abduction in each leg individually; if you test the legs together, compensatory spinal curving will create a false impression of normal leg abduction even if one hip has limited abduction.

It is best to examine hip rotation with the child lying prone and to symmetrically move the legs into external and internal rotation with the knees flexed, so that you can more easily appreciate pelvic movement, especially if you are an inexperienced examiner (Fig. 15–23). Flex the knee to 90 degrees, move the foot outward to test internal rotation (normal range, 40 to 45 degrees), and swing the foot inward to test external rotation (normal, 30 to 40 degrees). Loss of internal rotation is often the first sign of hip involvement in children with joint inflammation. A valuable sign of hip disease is external rotation of the hip as it is flexed from the extended position. Diminished abduction and internal rotation of the hip may be the earliest and sometimes the only abnormalities detected in the child with Legg-Calvé-Perthes disease or slipped capital femoral epiphysis.

Measure leg length from the anterior superior iliac spine to the medial malleolus, preferably with a steel tape (Fig. 15–24). It is important to position the patient supine with the legs fully extended and parallel and with the pelvis level.

A fixed flexion deformity of the hip may not be obvious on your initial observation of a child. Clues to a flexion contracture include accentuated lumbar lordosis and a tendency to stand with one knee slightly

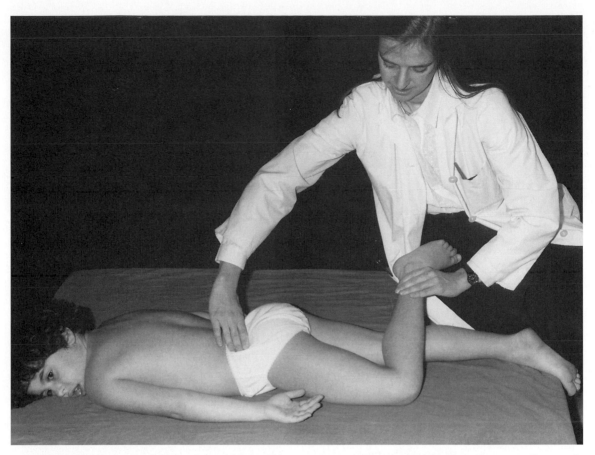

Figure 15–23 Testing external rotation of the hip. The child should be prone. Use one hand to stabilize the pelvis. Normal external rotation is 30 to 40 degrees.

bent despite the absence of knee disease. Perform the *Thomas test*, to detect a fixed flexion deformity, as follows (Fig. 15–25): (1) bring the child's knees up to the chest so that the lumbar lordosis becomes flat, and then (2) lower each leg in turn to the limit of extension with the spine still flat on the examining table.

Keep one hand under the child's lumbar spine as the hip extends, because the lumbar spine can move into lordosis and mask a fixed flexion deformity even with the other knee held to the chest. Inability to rest the leg on the table with the lumbar spine flat indicates a fixed flexion deformity. Measure the remaining angle.

Use the *Trendelenburg test* to evaluate a painful hip or to gauge hip girdle weakness in the older child who will cooperate. Ask the child to stand on one leg; normally, the pelvis rises slightly on the side opposite to the leg one stands on, because the hip abductors contract on the weight-bearing leg. When hip abductor muscles are weak, the pelvis drops downward on the side opposite to the weight-bearing (affected) leg (Fig. 15–26).

The Ortolani test is used specifically to detect the "click" or "clunk" of congenital hip dislocation in the newborn (see Chapter 4). In an older infant or a child with untreated congenital hip dislocation, the result is always negative, because the dislocated femoral head can no longer be reduced into the acetabulum. Late diagnostic signs of congenital hip dislocation are a

painless limp, asymmetric posterior skin folds on the thighs, a shortened thigh (because the femoral head no longer remains in the acetabulum), and tightened muscles around the hip joint, which restrict hip movement, particularly abduction.

KNEE EXAMINATION

Inspect the knee for obvious swelling, redness, or evidence of injury. The first sign of a knee effusion is loss of the normal concavity along the medial side of the patella. Check for the characteristic swelling over the tibial tuberosity seen in Osgood-Schlatter disease. Inspect the quadriceps muscle for wasting. Note any knee deformity. The most common knee deformity seen in children with JRA is a flexion contracture, which should be measured with a goniometer (Fig. 15–27). Bony overgrowth at the knee may occur with JRA because of epiphyseal overgrowth in the affected knee and may contribute to a leg-length discrepancy. Posterior subluxation of the tibia is demonstrable when the knee is bent to 90 degrees and the proximal tibia sags posteriorly. This condition is an uncommon complication of JRA. Some children, including those with generalized ligamentous laxity, may have genu recurvatum (hyperextensible knees).

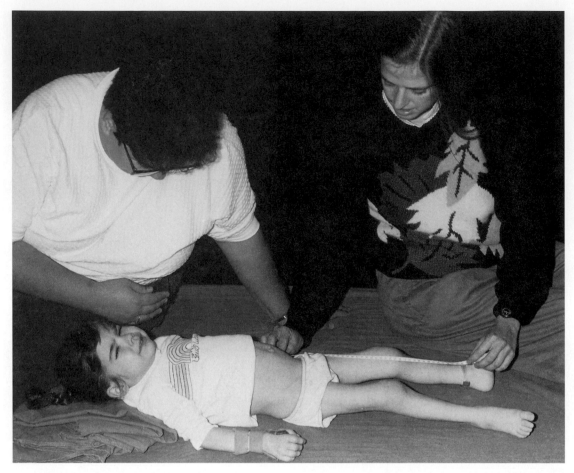

Figure 15–24 Technique for measuring true leg length, from the anterosuperior spine of the iliac crest to the inferior edge of the medial malleolus.

A high patella that faces outward suggests greater risk of recurrent patellar dislocation.

Inspect the knee for angulation, which is often seen in growing children. A line drawn from the midpoint of the inguinal ligament to the midpoint of the ankle should cross the center of the patella. Genu varus (bowleg or nonrachitic leg bowing) is physiologic in infancy, when the tibiofemoral angle is less than 15 degrees varus and the deformity is symmetric. At roughly 18 months, the child's legs appear straight, and by 2 to 4 years, the tibiofemoral angle changes to valgus. With increasing age, the valgus gradually reduces to the slight valgus of the normal adult.

Ignore knock knees in a child younger than 7 years, unless the valgus is greater than 15 degrees or there is evidence of asymmetry. Asymmetric angular deformity or evidence of knee instability with a lateral thrust (bowleg) or medial thrust (knock knee) that occurs immediately on weight-bearing is not seen in physiologic bowleg or knock knee. Such a finding indicates an underlying pathologic condition, such as Blount disease, rickets, or a growth plate injury.

After inspecting the knee, palpate for a joint effusion using several techniques. Elicit the *bulge sign* to detect a small to moderate effusion by milking fluid out of the medial recess into the suprapatellar pouch and then stroking the lateral recess in a downward direction to move the fluid back into the medial recess; the latter maneuver creates a "fluid bulge" in the knee's medial aspect between the patella and femur.

To demonstrate a large knee effusion, use the *patellar tap*, as follows: Empty fluid from the suprapatellar pouch by pressing firmly on the suprapatellar pouch with one hand; then use the other hand to tap the patella against the femur. The presence of a palpable tap indicates a large effusion. This is a less sensitive maneuver than the bulge sign and is not always specific. Occasionally, a child with a knee effusion may also have a popliteal cyst (Baker cyst), best detected when the patient lies prone or stands upright. Most Baker cysts disappear spontaneously. They require no treatment when asymptomatic but may rupture spontaneously, causing acute calf pain and swelling that may be confused with a deep vein thrombosis.

Palpate the knee for joint line tenderness with the knee flexed to 90 degrees. Tenderness along the entire joint line suggests synovitis and may be associated with thickened synovium that obscures the normal bony

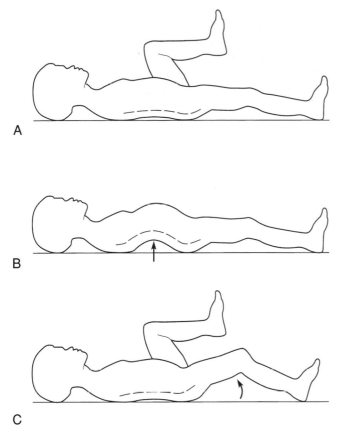

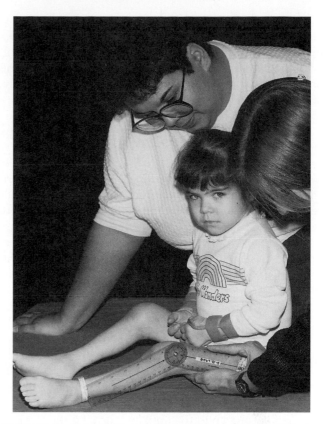

Figure 15–27 A child with juvenile rheumatoid arthritis and flexion contractures of the knees. The degree of contracture should be measured at each visit with the goniometer.

Figure 15–25 Thomas test. *A,* Normal. *B,* Increased lumbar lordosis masking a hip flexion deformity. *C,* Hip flexion deformity unmasked by flexion of the other hip. Estimate the angle between the table and the patient's leg to measure the flexion contracture.

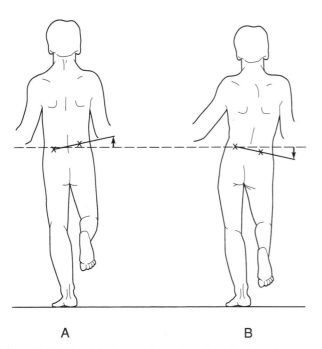

Figure 15–26 Trendelenburg test. *A,* when the patient stands on one leg, contraction of the gluteus medius muscle on the supported side should elevate the pelvis on the unsupported side. *B,* With a positive Trendelenburg test result, which occurs with weakness of the hip abductors, the pelvis on the unsupported side descends. (*X* indicates a dimple overlying the posterosuperior iliac spines.)

landmarks. Tenderness localized to the medial or lateral aspects of the joint line may suggest a meniscal tear in an older child. Perform a *McMurray test* by holding the child's heel in one hand while holding your other hand over the patient's flexed knee. Rotate the tibia externally and internally over the femur while slowly extending the child's knee; a palpable or audible clunk or click, sometimes associated with pain, may be detected with a meniscal tear.

Palpate the insertion of the patellar tendon into the tibial tuberosity for evidence of tenderness, warmth, or swelling. Such findings in only one tibial tuberosity suggest Osgood-Schlatter disease. If both are affected, particularly if there is tenderness at the sites of insertion of other tendons or ligaments, suspect *enthesitis,* an inflammation at the point of insertion of a tendon, ligament, or capsule into bone, commonly seen in children with juvenile ankylosing spondylitis.

A child should be able to flex the knee enough for the heel to touch the buttock, an angle of 130 to 150 degrees. An older child's flexion may be limited by the calf muscle bulk and by the hamstrings. When the knee is extended, the child should be able to achieve a straight leg; often children have 5 to 10 degrees of hyperextension. Note any crepitation during knee flexion and extension. Crepitation may occur with osteochondritis dissecans, which may be accompanied by tenderness of the affected femoral condyle, or with patellofemoral problems with patellar tenderness.

Test the medial and lateral collateral ligaments by stressing them both with the knee extended and flexed approximately 20 degrees. The ligaments are tight when the knee is in full extension, and no movement should be possible. Slight movement occurs normally when the knee is flexed to 20 degrees, but such movement is painless and limited.

Assess the cruciate ligaments, which normally prevent anterior and posterior instability of the knee and limit medial rotation, as follows: With the knee flexed to 90 degrees, pull the upper tibia forward to test the anterior cruciate ligament; pull the upper tibia backward to test the posterior cruciate ligament. Contracted hamstring muscles can prevent the tibia from moving forward even if there is a complete disruption of the anterior cruciate ligament; therefore, first ensure that the hamstring muscles are relaxed. Normally, there is little movement with this maneuver.

Evaluate patellar pain with additional tests:

Apprehension test: Try to move the child's patella laterally; resistance or anxiety suggests a tendency to recurrent subluxation.

Test for inflammation associated with patellofemoral malalignment: Press downward on the patella, asking the child to simultaneously lift the extended leg against gravity. This contracts the quadriceps muscle and moves the patella upward, resulting in pain and crepitus in patellofemoral malalignment. There is associated tenderness on palpation along the inferomedial edge of the patella.

Assessment for medial patellar plica syndrome: Palpate for tenderness over the superomedial border of the femoral condyle, with locking or snapping during knee joint movement.

ANKLE AND FOOT EXAMINATION

Inspect the ankle and foot for swelling, redness, trauma including the presence of a foreign body, and evidence of deformity, such as a clubfoot, pes cavus (high arch), or pes planus (flatfoot). If you find a pes cavus deformity, you must exclude underlying neurologic conditions such as spinal dysraphism, Charcot-Marie-Tooth disease, and Friedreich ataxia. In pes planus, or flatfoot, the feet characteristically have a flattened longitudinal arch, valgus hindfoot, and abduction of the midfoot and forefoot (see earlier discussion).

Palpate the foot and ankle to localize areas of tenderness or swelling that may occur secondary to injury. Ankle injuries are common, but only 12% to 15% result in fractures. The Ottawa Ankle Rules[1] may help you determine the likelihood of a fracture and the need for radiographs. According to these rules, if the child cannot bear weight or has tenderness at the posterior edge or tip of the malleolus, a fracture is likely, and a radiograph should be obtained. Localized tenderness and swelling of the foot may also occur with stress fractures (particularly at the second metatarsal) or an ingrown toenail. Pain, tenderness, and swelling over the navicular with a limp and a tendency to walk on the lateral edge of the foot suggest Kohler disease (avascular necrosis of the navicular).

After palpating the joints and bony structures of the feet, palpate the Achilles tendon for tenderness, because tendonitis may occur from overuse. Tenderness at the points of attachment of the Achilles tendon and of the plantar fascia to the calcaneus also occurs with enthesitis.

Test the range of movement at the three major joints of the foot and ankle. These movements are dorsiflexion (normal range, 15 to 20 degrees), plantar flexion (normal range, 40 to 50 degrees) at the true ankle joint, inversion (normal range, 20 degrees), and eversion (normal range, 20 degrees) at the subtalar joint, and pronation and supination at the midtarsal joints. Limited movement at the ankle or foot may be caused not only by joint inflammation but also by tarsal coalition, a bony or cartilaginous bridge between tarsal bones that typically causes a rigid flat foot with limited painful motion at the subtalar joint; confirm this diagnosis with an oblique radiograph of the foot.

Lateral compression of the metatarsals is a good screening test for inflammation of the metatarsophalangeal (MTP) joints. Perform this maneuver extremely gently, because it can cause intense pain if one or more MTP joints are inflamed (Fig. 15–28). If the child complains of pain on compression, examine the MTP joints individually to identify the affected joint. Examine the toes for swelling or deformity. Diffuse swelling of a toe that gives it a sausage-like appearance, termed *dactylitis*, may occur with infection, psoriasis, and Reiter syndrome. Common toe deformities include hallux valgus, syndactyly (webbing deformity), polydactyly, and overlapping fifth toe.

Muscle Assessment

Muscle assessment includes inspection of muscle bulk for wasting. Synovitis results in reflex inhibition of muscles acting across a joint, leading to wasting, which may be noticed as early as within one week. Widespread wasting of muscles around a joint tends to occur with arthritis, whereas localized muscle wasting is more characteristic of a local mechanical or peripheral nerve problem.

Muscle power is very important to assess. If you have followed the examination procedure described in this chapter, you have already screened muscle power when observing the child's gait and with a number of maneuvers described in the observation section of the physical examination—hopping, toe- and heel-walking,

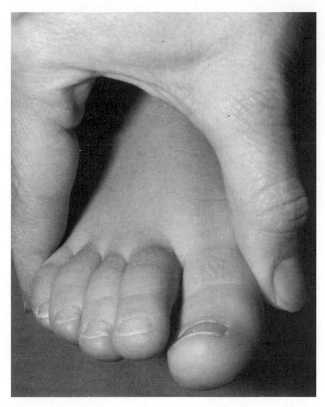

Table 15–5 SCALE FOR GRADING MUSCLE STRENGTH

Grade	Percentage of Function	Activity Level
0—None	0	No evidence of muscle contractility
1—Trace	15	Evidence of slight contractility; no effective joint motion
2—Poor	25	Full range of motion without gravity
3—Fair	50	Full range of motion against gravity
4—Good	75	Complete range of motion against gravity with some resistance
5—Normal	100	Complete range of motion against gravity with full resistance

From Cassidy JT, Petty RE: Textbook of Pediatric Rheumatology, 4th ed. Philadelphia, W.B. Saunders, 2001.

Figure 15–28 Screening for inflammation of the metatarsophalangeal joints with the metatarsal compression test. The response "Ouch" constitutes a positive result.

and checking for Gower sign. To assess trunk and neck flexor strength in a child old enough to cooperate, ask him or her to perform five sit-ups and then, while lying supine, to hold his or her head above the pillow for 60 seconds.

You can make a more formal assessment of power performed by using a simple grading scale, shown in Table 15–5. Keep in mind, however, that there is considerable individual variability among both patients and examiners, and strength assessments that use this scale are estimations. Further description of the assessment of muscle power can be found in Chapter 13.

General Medical Examination

A complete physical examination is very important in the assessment of a child with musculoskeletal complaints and may yield valuable diagnostic clues. Determining the child's growth percentiles may show evidence of failure to thrive, and the presence of hepatosplenomegaly or lymphadenopathy may suggest an underlying systemic disease.

Subcutaneous rheumatoid nodules are seen in the 5% to 10% of children with JRA who have rheumatoid factor–positive polyarticular disease. These nodules are firm, nontender, and usually mobile. They are most commonly seen below the olecranon but also occur over other pressure points, joints, tendon sheaths including the Achilles tendon, and the occiput. They must be distinguished from benign rheumatoid nodules, which may be single or multiple and tend to occur over bony prominences such as the tibia, scalp, and dorsum of the foot; these nodules occur in healthy children and usually regress spontaneously, although they may recur.

Children with a history of a scaly rash, "eczema," or psoriasis may have psoriatic arthritis. Frequently, children must be examined completely undressed, because an intermittent evanescent rash may be discovered whose appearance can be almost pathognomonic of systemic onset JRA, even when the child shows absolutely no joint involvement. The rash, which is salmon pink and morbilliform or maculopapular, often includes characteristic small (1 to 2 mm) circular or semicircular pink lesions with paler centers. It may be extremely transient, present in the evening and gone 2 hours later. Because no single laboratory test can diagnose JRA, this telltale rash may be the one feature that helps diagnose the disease in a child with fever of unknown origin. The more often you inspect children with systemic-onset JRA, the more often you will find the rash and clinch the diagnosis.

Eye findings also may provide a diagnostic clue in the child with joint problems. Redness, photophobia, pain, or impaired vision may occur when acute iritis is associated with the seronegative forms of arthritis, including Reiter syndrome. An irregular pupil in a child with arthritis suggests untreated chronic uveitis associated with JRA.

Pauciarticular juvenile rheumatoid arthritis in young girls is often associated with chronic asymptomatic iritis, which is commonly detectable only by slit-lamp examination before visual loss occurs.

SUMMARY

Musculoskeletal complaints are common in children. Therefore, it is essential to be comfortable and skilled in their assessment. This chapter has outlined the common normal musculoskeletal variants that frequently arouse concern in parents but, in most cases, require no investigation or intervention. The differentiation of uncommon but serious causes of musculoskeletal problems, such as rheumatic diseases and malignancy, from more common causes, such as injuries, infections, and orthopedic conditions, has been reviewed. At times, additional laboratory tests and imaging studies are necessary to complete a patient's evaluation, but such investigations rarely establish the diagnosis on their own. Whether a child presents with a painful extremity, a limp, or a swollen joint, a detailed history followed by a skilled physical examination and a period of observation are the three most valuable diagnostic aids available in establishing the correct diagnosis and answering parents' concerns.

REFERENCE

1. Stiell IG, Greenberg GH, McKnight RD, et al: Decision rules for the use of radiography in acute ankle injuries: Refinement and prospective validation. JAMA 269:1127–1132, 1993.

SUGGESTED READINGS

Cassidy JT, Petty RE: Textbook of Pediatric Rheumatology, 4th ed. Philadelphia, WB Saunders, 2001.
Morrissy RT: Lovell and Winter's Pediatric Orthopedics, 5th ed. Philadelphia, Lippincott Williams & Wilkins, 2001.

chapter 16

Clinical Endocrine Evaluation of the Child

SONIA R. SALISBURY AND ELIZABETH A. CUMMINGS

Pediatric endocrinology has special appeal because most childhood endocrine disorders are treatable. A specific diagnosis is usually possible on clinical grounds alone. Do not be intimidated by the myriad of hormone assays and endocrine tests that are needed to evaluate excesses or deficiencies. We have neatly arranged them all in an interrelated hormone map, which shows the feedback control of hormone action (Fig. 16–1). A good practice is to draw such a picture as you are explaining the details of hormone action to the family. Doing so slows down your explanation and makes you translate the medical lingo while still providing the correct names for hormones.

Probably the most common endocrine complaints parents express concern a child who is too small, too fat, too thin, or too tall or whose sexual development is premature or delayed. On first hearing such complaints, listen; do not be judgmental. Even if there is no serious disease, the family or child needs a careful assessment and a clear explanation. Be prepared to spend time helping individuals understand and accept the variations of normal development, and talk directly to the child about his or her self-perception and future prospects for growth and development.

CHIEF CHARACTERISTICS OF THE CHILD WITH GROWTH HORMONE DEFICIENCY

Most short children do not have growth hormone deficiency (GHD), but because GHD is so highly treatable, it must be carefully considered and excluded. In children, GHD may be organic (tumor, cranial irradiation, or congenital malformation) or idiopathic. Hypothalamic-pituitary failure of growth hormone (GH) secretion can occur alone or in combination with deficiencies of one or several pituitary hormones.

Certain midline defects are often associated with GHD, including cleft palate, choanal atresia, a single upper central incisor, and optic nerve hypoplasia (with or without an absence of the septum pellucidum, which is revealed by computed tomography or magnetic resonance imaging). Recent advances in molecular biology have shown that many cases of GHD with or without midline defects that were previously thought to be sporadic actually have a specific genetic basis.

Key Point

In examining children who are unusually short, always ask about a history of symptoms that may suggest hypoglycemia in infancy and early childhood. Because growth hormone is a major counterregulatory hormone to insulin, deficiency of this hormone makes some children susceptible to hypoglycemia, particularly during fasting periods or during mild illness when food intake is marginal.

When asked about symptoms of hypoglycemia, parents of a child with GHD may describe episodes in which the youngster was found limp, glassy-eyed, stuporous, and possibly unresponsive to verbal commands. Most parents have successfully tried the natural cure, fruit juice or its equivalent. If the child is left untreated, convulsions may result, bringing the child to immediate medical attention. Unlike febrile seizures or epilepsy, a hypoglycemia episode rarely ends in spontaneous recovery without administration of sugar.

Parents of a child with idiopathic or early childhood GHD usually report that the child has always been smaller than others but that the difference became more noticeable when he or she started school. Often, no height record is available, so always ask how frequently the child's shoe and clothing sizes have changed.

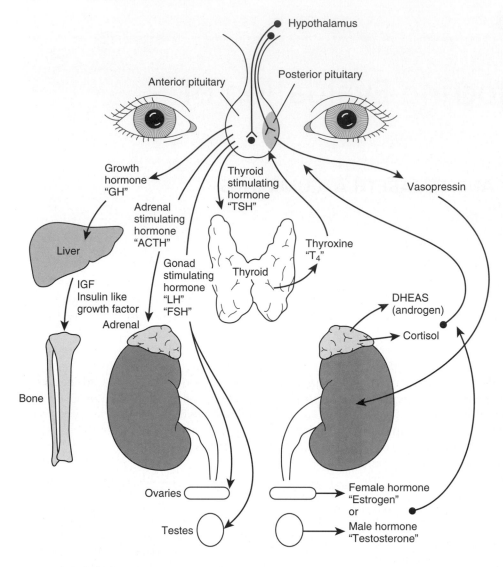

Figure 16–1 A map of the endocrine system. Draw the appropriate portion of the map as you sit with the family and the child. It is a way to explain hormone deficiencies or excesses. Tell the family that they are at the same stage as a first-year medical student, getting their first lecture in endocrinology. Tailor the drawing to the specific disorder, however, to avoid giving them the whole lecture.

New-onset growth failure with GHD in an older child is more likely due to a destructive lesion, such as a tumor or previous cranial irradiation. Assessment of a child with short stature at any age must include careful questions about headaches.

Headaches due to tumor often occur without a precipitating cause, at night or in the early morning, and may or may not be accompanied by vomiting. It is rare for children or adolescents in whom physical examination detects optic atrophy or a visual field defect to have recognized a visual problem themselves. Ask whether they have felt an increase in thirst and urination, which may suggest diabetes insipidus.

Case History

Case 1

Terry, age 12 months, whose parents say he has had an uncontrollable thirst and a constantly wet diaper from early infancy, is placed on the floor in the examining room. There are four bottles of water in his toy bag. Before removing his toys, he first takes all the bottles out of the bag and positions them in the corners of the room.

Diabetes insipidus is generally classified as central (destruction or maldevelopment of the hypothalamic-pituitary vasopressin axis) or nephrogenic (one example of which is the congenital X-linked variety illustrated in the case history). Terry had a family history of excessive water drinking in his male relatives, making the diagnosis nephrogenic, not pituitary, diabetes insipidus.

APPROACH TO THE PHYSICAL EXAMINATION OF A CHILD WITH POSSIBLE GROWTH HORMONE DEFICIENCY

Children with GHD are described as "cherubic" (Figs. 16–2 through 16–4). They appear younger than their

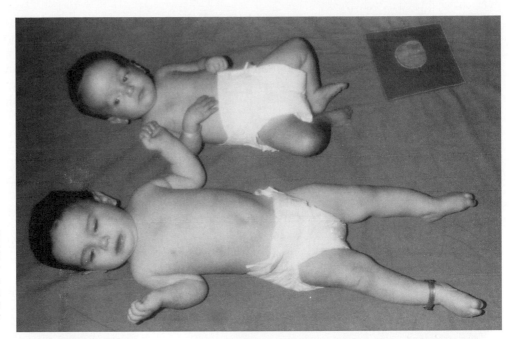

Figure 16–2 Hypoglycemia in infancy. The larger infant had hyperinsulinism in the neonatal period, which was treated by pancreatectomy. She is shown here at age 12 months beside a very small infant of the same age who has hypoglycemia secondary to growth hormone deficiency.

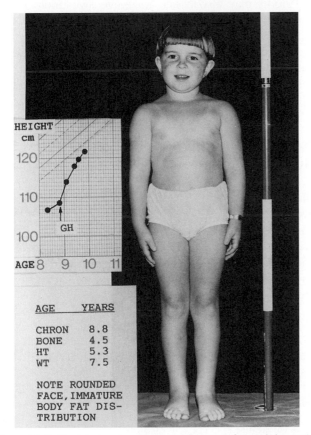

HEIGHT cm

120

110

GH

100

AGE 8 9 10 11

AGE	YEARS
CHRON	8.8
BONE	4.5
HT	5.3
WT	7.5

NOTE ROUNDED FACE, IMMATURE BODY FAT DISTRIBUTION

Figure 16–3 Crystal, showing the typical features of growth hormone deficiency before treatment. Inset is the growth curve after treatment with growth hormone.

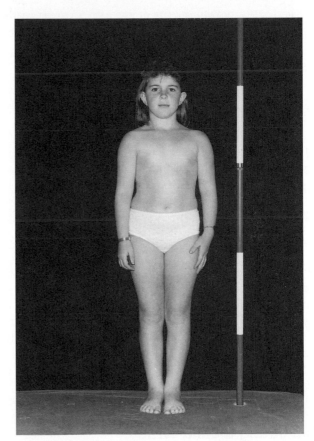

Figure 16–4 Crystal, 2 years later, after treatment with growth hormone.

chronologic age, having a rounded face, chubby limbs, and "puddling" (or dimpling) of the anterior abdominal fat. Because of these children's infantile appearance, which is further enhanced by a high-pitched reedy voice, adults may baby them or classmates may carry them around like pets.

Height and weight percentiles (see Fig. 3–4) are usually discrepant in GHD, with a high weight-to-height ratio. This is a major clue to the need for detailed endocrine investigation. Chronic disease, especially inflammatory bowel disease, may be quite silent and manifest as short stature but, by contrast, a low weight-to-height ratio.

You can see the poorly developed muscle bulk of a child with GHD on inspection and appreciate it by running your hands over the limbs. The hair is fine and wispy, and tooth eruption is delayed. In boys, the penis may be quite small (less than 2.5 cm); remember to push the suprapubic fat pad as flat as possible, in case a normal-sized penis is merely buried in a thick fat pad.

Examination must include careful funduscopic and visual field assessment.

Investigate a growth velocity of less than 5 cm per year in children aged 5 years to puberty; a growth velocity of less than 4 cm per year is pathologic (see Chapter 3).

You cannot assess short stature or analyze growth velocity without examining the breasts and genitalia to determine the child's pubertal stage (see Fig. 3–9).

CHIEF CHARACTERISTICS OF THYROID DISORDERS IN CHILDREN

Structure, Function, Signs, and Symptoms

Typically, the history is the most important diagnostic aid in evaluating thyroid disorders, although the physical findings serve to bolster your suspicions. Thyroid size does not reflect thyroid function. First sort out the functional state: hypothyroid, hyperthyroid, or euthyroid (normal function). Then examine the thyroid to see whether it is too big or contains any lumps and to search for associated lymphadenopathy.

Evaluating a Child with Hyperthyroidism

Symptoms of hyperthyroidism are the same in children as in adults, but it is the parents or teachers who usually complain about the child's restlessness and irritability. The child often does not complain, although the symptoms are obvious to everyone else. The following questions will elicit the essentials:

Has the child's behavior changed?

In the office setting, is the child fidgeting but trying to be attentive? This is the biggest difference in behavior between hyperthyroidism and attention deficit–hyperactivity disorder (see Chapter 6).

Have learning difficulties been detected recently at school?

Has the child's handwriting deteriorated? Tremor and involuntary muscle contractions affect the neatness of writing.

Does the child laugh or cry more readily than before or suddenly vacillate between laughing and crying? Emotional lability is often striking in hyperthyroidism.

Does the child throw the bedclothes off, have difficulty falling asleep, or awaken during the night?

Is the child, particularly an older child, extremely fatigued? Restlessness and hyperactivity at the onset of hyperthyroidism may be followed by extreme fatigue.

Parents may also notice excessive sweatiness in the child, who may ask to wear only light clothing. Although loose bowel movements are often listed among the manifestations, the characteristic change is greater frequency and softer stool consistency. If tachycardia is present, the child is rarely aware of it. Larger appetite, with either failure to gain weight or loss of weight, is also typical.

Evaluating a Child with Hypothyroidism

Like children with hyperthyroidism, children with hypothyroidism rarely complain of symptoms (Table 16–1), perhaps because the changes develop so insidiously that neither child nor parent notices the difference. When symptoms go unrecognized for years, linear growth is profoundly impaired and may be the presenting feature.

Table 16–1 PHYSICAL FINDINGS THAT MAY BE SEEN IN HYPOTHYROIDISM

Short stature
Decreased height-to-weight ratio
Slow thickened speech; low croaking voice
Slow pulse
Cool, dry scaling skin with decreased body hair
Dry lifeless hair
Pale puffy face
Periorbital puffiness
Palpable stool in descending colon (constipation)
Enlarged calf muscles
Delay in relaxation phase of deep tendon reflexes

Case 2

Shauna, age 15 years says, "I was the tallest in my class in fifth grade, but I have not grown since then, and my periods haven't started" (Fig. 16–5).

Your physical examination reveals all the physical findings for hypothyroidism that are listed in Table 16–1. You particularly note the characteristic puffiness around Shauna's upper face and eyes. In this case, because of profound hypothyroidism, there is also a more generalized swelling including the neck.

With treatment for hypothyroidism, Shauna's menses start almost immediately. She grows an inch and loses 4 kg (9 lb) during 4 months of therapy.

Causes of Childhood Hypothyroidism

The most common cause of hypothyroidism in childhood is autoimmune thyroiditis (Hashimoto disease, or lymphocytic thyroiditis). Lymphocytic infiltration causes firm diffuse enlargement of the thyroid and a pebbled surface. The anterior pituitary, sensing the lack of thyroid hormone (loss of feedback inhibition), increases secretion of thyroid-stimulating hormone (TSH), causing the thyroid to enlarge further. Although the gland can grow in response to TSH, it cannot necessarily keep up in terms of thyroxine (T_4) production. Because the autoimmune process is destructive, some patients have a small or undetectable thyroid gland at presentation. A child with hypothyroidism secondary to hypothalamic-pituitary disease does not have thyroid enlargement (a goiter).

Congenital hypothyroidism is usually due to either absence of the thyroid or a hypoplastic thyroid that may be ectopic (located anywhere along the line of descent from the back of the tongue to the anterior neck.) In a few infants, hypothyroidism is caused by a congenital enzyme defect in thyroid hormonogenesis. In such instances, a goiter is present. In many countries, congenital hypothyroidism is now detected in the presymptomatic stage, before any significant intellectual deficit occurs, through blood spot screening between the second and fifth days of life. If congenital hypothyroidism is left untreated, the clinical manifestations may not become fully apparent until around the third month of life.

Thyroid hormone is essential for adequate development of brain cell function and interneuronal connections. With absence of the hormone over the first few months of life, the infant suffers marked and irreversible developmental delay, the intellectual deficit progressing with each passing week. Universal newborn screening for hypothyroidism is therefore essential.

The infant with untreated congenital hypothyroidism has a low core body temperature, slow pulse rate, prolonged neonatal jaundice (because of poor hepatic conjugation of bilirubin), dry skin and hair, a large posterior fontanel (greater than 0.5 cm), poor head control, poor muscle tone, an enlarged tongue, a characteristically puffy face, and a hoarse cry (Fig. 16–6). The parents may report poor feeding and constipation. If acquired

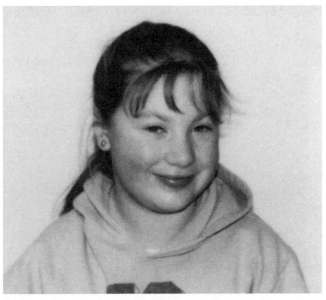

A

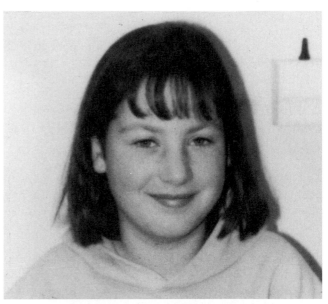

B

Figure 16–5 A, Shauna, showing the typical facial features of profound hypothyroidism. Note the puffy face and neck and the coarse, dry hair. B, Shauna after 4 months of treatment with thyroid hormone.

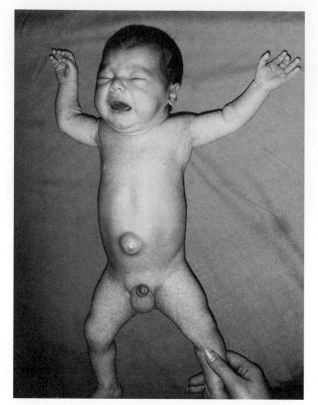

Figure 16–6 Typical appearance of congenital hypothyroidism in a 3-month-old baby.

hypothyroidism develops after the age of 2 or 3 years, no permanent intellectual deficit is thought to occur.

Acquired hypothyroidism must be ruled out in any child with unexplained growth retardation. The child's appetite is generally diminished, yet there is a modest weight gain, leading to a disproportionate height-to-weight ratio. Such children are not massively obese; by contrast, prepubertal obese children generally grow well in height. Constipation is a common feature. In children with type 1 diabetes mellitus, you must always rule out the coexistence of autoimmune thyroid disease, usually lymphocytic thyroiditis.

APPROACH TO THE PHYSICAL EXAMINATION OF THE CHILD WITH A THYROID DISORDER

As with other pediatric examinations, always begin with the hands-off approach. Children are often ticklish, and touching the neck may elicit giggles and squirming, making it difficult to see the thyroid. Sit the child on a chair or examining table, with good light and in a relaxed atmosphere. If the child is old enough and cooperative, ask him or her to take a sip of water, first hold the water in the mouth without swallowing, and then swallow. Observe the area just above the sternal notch to see whether the small thyroid gland moves up and down during swallowing (Fig. 16–7). Next, ask the

child to hyperextend the neck. This maneuver makes thyroid enlargement more obvious, and sometimes, it is the only way to see the gland easily.

Examining Newborns and Young Infants

In a newborn or young infant, use a different technique to examine the thyroid. Place your hand under the child, between the scapulae, and raise the baby's shoulders, allowing the head to fall back gently until it rests on the examining table or a parent's lap. If the thyroid is enlarged, this maneuver will expose it, allowing you to palpate with the second and third fingers of your other hand (Fig. 16–8).

Key Point

In a normal newborn, the thyroid cannot be felt. A newborn baby's thyroid that can be felt is probably enlarged.

Examining Young Children and Adolescents

In the young child or adolescent, first observe the gland, Then, after gaining the child's cooperation, palpate it. We generally examine from the front, as follows: Rest both thumbs gently over the lobes of the thyroid, and ask the child to swallow. While the child swallows, move your thumbs with the child's skin, up and down over the thyroid to outline its size. Note any nodules or irregularities you feel. You can also examine thyroid in the traditional way, from behind the child: Place the second and third fingers of your examining hand over the gland to estimate its size, and ask the child to swallow. We often joke with older children who "hate" to have their necks touched that we have never choked anyone and are not allowed to!

Always measure and record the gland size so that any significant changes between visits are documented. With a measuring tape, measure from upper to lower pole and the greatest vertical dimension of the isthmus. Record the results in diagrammatic form, indicating any nodules or other irregularities.

The normal thyroid weight in grams corresponds approximately to the child's age in years; a normal adult gland weighs 20 to 25 g and is the size of your thumb from the distal interphalangeal joint to the tip. The thyroid can be palpated in most older children. Because its normal consistency is soft, the contours can barely be seen, and the gland is rather flat when the child hyperextends the neck. Once the thyroid gland becomes firm, as in autoimmune thyroiditis (Hashimoto disease), or hard, as in carcinoma, you should recog-

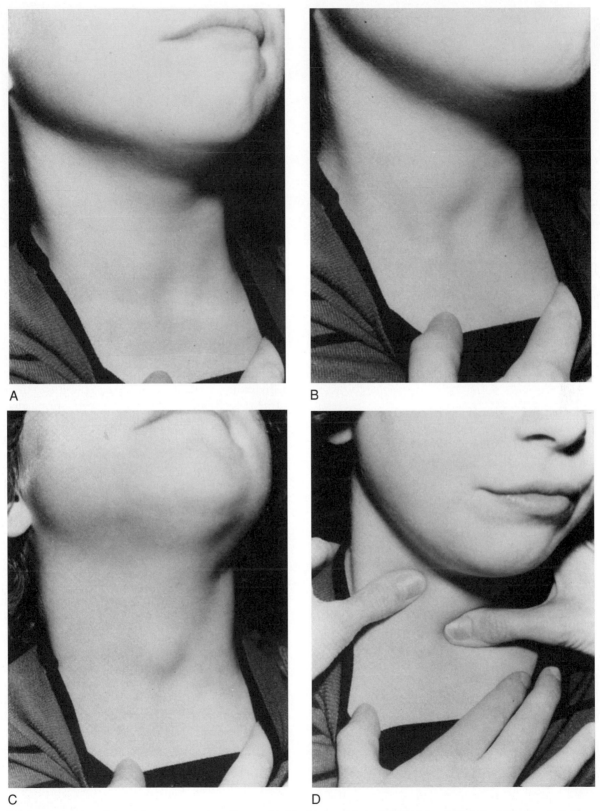

A

B

C

D

Figure 16–7 Demonstration of thyroid enlargement in a 12-year-old girl with a nodule in the right lobe. A, Little is visible at rest. B, The enlarged right lobe moves upward and becomes more obvious with swallowing. C, With neck extension, it is readily visible. D, Palpation of the nodule from the front.

nize the difference in consistency, even though enlargement may not be striking. Some carcinomas may not be hard to the touch.

Most midline neck masses are thyroid glands or thyroid remnants. A central rounded midline mass between the thyroid and the chin is almost certain to be

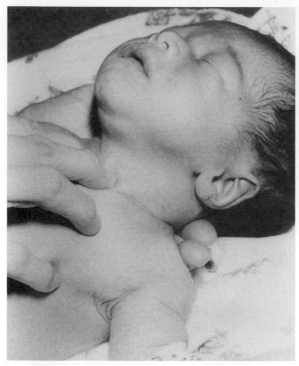

Figure 16–8 Palpation of the thyroid gland in an infant.

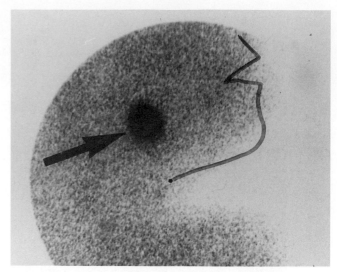

Figure 16–10 Thyroid scan in an infant demonstrating uptake of the radionuclide at the base of the tongue in a lingual thyroid, (arrow).

a thyroglossal duct cyst (Fig. 16–9), derived from a remnant of the thyroglossal duct, which runs from the foramen cecum of the tongue downward to the cricoid cartilage during fetal development. When the child sticks out the tongue, the mass moves upward. The child may present initially with an infected thyroglossal duct cyst. Sometimes, the gland fails entirely to migrate downward from the foramen cecum and manifests clin-

ically as an oval or rounded midline mass at the base of the tongue (Fig. 16–10). This lingual thyroid usually represents *all* the thyroid that the child has. Most lingual thyroids are treated with daily therapy using L-thyroxine, which suppresses pituitary thyrotropin (TSH) secretion, causing the lump to shrink markedly.

The thyroid may be absent, small, ectopic, or enlarged. If both lobes are enlarged fairly symmetrically, it is described as diffusely enlarged. The normal gland may have slight undulations on palpation, but if you find one or more distinct lumps, the child has a solitary nodule or a multinodular goiter, respectively.

Key Point

The uninformative term *goiter* denotes any thyroid enlargement but reveals nothing about the functional or anatomic diagnosis. A diffuse or nodular enlargement gives the child a sensation of difficulty swallowing but rarely causes true dysphagia. Press your finger gently over your own trachea just above the sternal notch to understand the sensation that children feel with even slight thyroid swelling. Enlargements may be painful and tender to touch. A change in the voice may occur if the enlargement damages the recurrent laryngeal nerve or if the vocal cords become myxedematous in severe hypothyroidism.

A diffusely enlarged, nontender gland that is soft to somewhat firm in consistency is compatible with Graves disease. By contrast, a tender, diffusely swollen gland in a child who withdraws when the gland is touched is likely to represent subacute thyroiditis attributed to a viral cause. Thyroid-stimulating antibodies interact with the TSH receptor on the thyroid cell, producing the constant stimulation of Graves disease. In subacute thyroiditis, disrupted cells produce a sudden thyroid hormone discharge, causing a transient hyper-

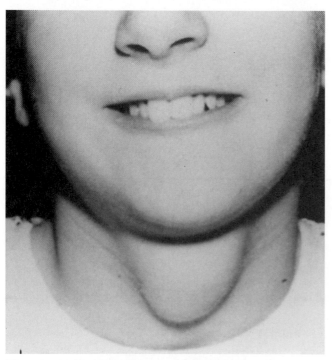

Figure 16–9 Thyroglossal duct cyst, a midline neck mass.

thyroid period, which is often followed by a longer hypothyroid state and then by euthyroidism within 3 to 6 months. A similar sequence is seen in a condition called *silent thyroiditis,* so called because it is not painful. Silent thyroiditis is most common in the postpartum period but does occur at all ages and in both sexes; it has an autoimmune etiology.

If one or more nodules are found in a child with hyperthyroidism, the cause is probably a benign adenoma, called *toxic nodular goiter,* that is overproducing thyroid hormone. This condition is seen more commonly in adults. The discrete smooth oval or round nodules are firmer than the surrounding gland but not rock-hard. When the child swallows, they move up and down and are not fixed to extrathyroidal tissues. Rare TSH-secreting pituitary adenomas can cause diffuse thyroid enlargement and systemic signs of hyperthyroidism but without the eye findings characteristic of autoimmune (Graves) disease.

Eye examination yields important clues for diagnosis and management of thyroid disease. In hyperthyroidism, the palpebral fissures are widened and blinking is diminished, giving the child a staring appearance. In autoimmune Graves disease, the eye muscles swell to several times their normal size, and the retro-orbital fat pad enlarges, causing the eye to bulge out of the orbit (*proptosis*), often with injection (prominent small surface vessels) and edema of the bulbar conjunctiva (*chemosis*). Because individuals with proptosis have difficulty closing their lids, corneal ulceration may occur, causing red, sore eyes, particularly in the morning. Ask the parent whether the child closes the eyes when sleeping. Without adequate tears and closed lids, the cornea becomes dry and vulnerable to ulceration. Enlarged ocular muscles produce an imbalance of extraocular muscle function, sometimes sufficient to cause diplopia, which may be unrecognized by affected patients until they are asked to look upward and outward, the direction of gaze in which diplopia can first be elicited. Usually, there is some loss of convergence, and the child cannot cross the eyes to the usual extent when trying to follow the physician's finger as it is moved toward the nose.

Thyroid bruits are characteristic of Graves disease, but this sign is not very useful in children. The problem with auscultating the neck in children is that if you press hard enough with the stethoscope, you can make anything whistle.

Infants may be born with neonatal hyperthyroidism from transplacental passage of thyroid-stimulating immunoglobulin, an antibody produced in a mother who has active or treated Graves disease with persistent circulating antibody. Although these babies have the same signs as older children, they are more likely to have hyperthermia and cardiac arrhythmias and to develop congestive heart failure.

> **Key Point**
>
> Neonatal hyperthyroidism must be treated, but it is a self-limited condition. It subsides when maternal IgG disappears from the infant's circulation.

Euthyroid States

Someone who has had hyperthyroidism may continue to have a palpably enlarged thyroid gland, even though the disease has disappeared spontaneously or has been treated. Not all patients with autoimmune (Hashimoto) thyroiditis become hypothyroid; some remain euthyroid for years and may never have hypothyroidism.

Ruling Out Thyroid Carcinoma

Children who have single or multiple nodules are usually euthyroid. When a nodule is found, the parents are understandably concerned about cancer. It is not always possible to rule out thyroid cancer on clinical grounds alone, but some characteristics can influence your suspicions. Carcinoma in children may go undetected for many years and is generally asymptomatic; the swelling may be more readily recognized by someone who does not see the child every day. Thyroid carcinoma (usually the papillary type) is typically hard, not merely firm. It may be smooth and oval, but if it has extended beyond its capsule, it may feel irregular. More than one nodule decreases the likelihood of carcinoma but does not exclude it completely. Benign adenomas or simple colloid cysts also may present as single or multiple nodules.

> **Key Point**
>
> Assessment of the thyroid gland should always include palpation of the cervical lymph nodes. Even in the absence of a palpable thyroid mass, a hard, enlarged cervical lymph node raises the possibility of thyroid carcinoma.

Because external irradiation to the head and neck is associated with an increased incidence of both benign and malignant thyroid lesions, patients who have been exposed to therapeutic irradiation should be examined annually.

> **Key Point**
>
> Whenever you detect a thyroid nodule, question the family carefully about prior radiation exposure.

Medullary carcinoma, the best-recognized familial thyroid tumor, has an autosomal dominant pattern of inheritance and often appears in childhood. The tumor originates in the parafollicular or C cells that produce calcitonin. It is essential to screen children with a positive family history of medullary carcinoma.

CLINICAL CHARACTERISTICS OF DISORDERS OF CALCIUM METABOLISM IN CHILDREN

Hypercalcemic States

Hypercalcemia causes constipation, polyuria, and thirst. Other complaints are mood changes and "epigastric distress." Belly pain in an infant usually manifests as vomiting, and mood changes manifest as fussiness and crying.

CAUSES OF HYPERCALCEMIA

Always consider the possibility that excessive amounts of vitamin D (or A) may have been ingested by a hypercalcemic child.

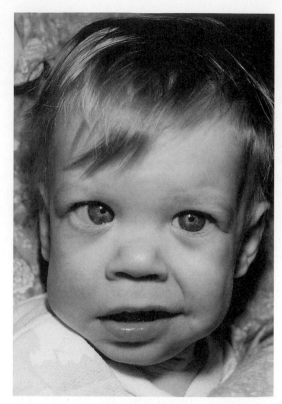

Figure 16–11 The facial appearance of a toddler with Williams syndrome.

Hypocalcemic States

Maternal hyperparathyroidism can result in transient symptomatic low serum calcium levels in the newborn, a fact that emphasizes the need to take a good history of the mother's health for every baby you examine.

APPROACH TO THE PHYSICAL EXAMINATION OF A HYPOCALCEMIC CHILD

The following case history illustrates the approach to the physical examination of a child with hypocalcemia.

Case History

Case 3
Two sisters with hypoparathyroidism, Susan and Betty, have had well-regulated levels of serum calcium while receiving the usual therapeutic doses of vitamin D and supplementary calcium. Now, within a month of changing foster homes, they demonstrate extreme lethargy, marked constipation, and bedwetting. You order serum calcium measurements, and calcium levels are found to be high for both girls. You sit with the new foster parents and go over their routine for administering calcium and vitamins to the babies. You discover that the foster parents have been giving Susan and Betty 10 times the recommended dose. After this error is corrected, the serum calcium levels in both babies normalize over several weeks.

Some infants with idiopathic infantile hypercalcemia have a characteristic facial appearance (Williams syndrome), consisting of full cheeks, a wide mouth, and a stellate iris, typically associated with supravalvular aortic stenosis or other cardiovascular lesions (Fig. 16–11). An asymptomatic condition known as *familial hypocalciuric hypercalcemia* is generally discovered incidentally or during family screening studies. The etiology is an autosomal dominant defect in the calcium-sensing receptor. The volume of urine does not increase (and so neither does the thirst) because the urine calcium level is low, partly explaining the paucity of symptoms. Because the condition is caused by a calcium-sensing defect, the serum parathyroid hormone level is usually in the normal range, not suppressed as it would be in a normal individual.

Case History

Case 4
Amanda, age 7 years, began to have seizures due to hypocalcemia when she was 3 years old. During these short-lived episodes, her eyes roll upward, her hands twitch, and her legs stiffen. The seizures are heralded by a choking sound coming from her room that the parents can hear. Incorrectly diagnosed with epilepsy, she has remained seizure-free on anticonvulsant medication but has persistent cramps in her hands and feet, which the parents relieve by rubbing them or by placing her in a hot bath. Amanda also has intermittent "funny feelings"

(paresthesias) in the ends of her fingers. The cramps and the paresthesias are secondary to the hypocalcemia. Although her developmental milestones have been normal, she has repeated kindergarten and is distractible and talkative, all findings that are at least partly related to the chronic hypocalcemia.

Your physical examination reveals that Amanda's height and weight are on the third percentile; her blood pressure and pulse are normal. She appears anxious and chronically ill. Her skin and hair are dry and without luster, and she has bilateral clouding of the lenses, demonstrated by a decreased red reflex (this finding later proves to have been caused by bilateral cataracts, a complication of long-standing hypocalcemia).

Although her tooth development is delayed, Amanda has no enamel abnormality. Less than 30 seconds after you inflate the blood pressure cuff around her upper arm above her systolic pressure, her fingers become hyperextended with partial flexion at the metacarpophalangeal joints (carpal spasm, or *Trousseau sign*; to demonstrate this sign in suspected hypocalcemia, leave the cuff on for up to 3 minutes.) Tapping in the area just anterior to her earlobe, below the zygomatic arch, at the top of the parotid gland where branches of the facial nerve exit, causes her to purse her lips. (Known as *Chvostek sign*, this response can be elicited in many otherwise normal children, but in individual children with hypocalcemia who are examined repeatedly, the presence and intensity of the sign serve as a useful marker for the presence and severity of hypocalcemia.) You also elicit a positive peroneal sign by tapping with a reflex hammer over the lateral peroneal nerve where it runs around the fibula's upper end, about 2 cm below the fibular head. The increased neuromuscular excitability secondary to low ionized calcium causes her foot to jerk quickly upward and outward.

The remainder of the physical examination is unremarkable. Specifically, you detect no abnormality of facial features or congenital heart disease, which would suggest DiGeorge syndrome, and no shortening of the fourth or fifth metacarpal, as seen in pseudohypoparathyroidism.

You finally attribute Amanda's hypocalcemia to hypoparathyroidism. Despite the absence of any family history, you judge the etiology to be autoimmune, caused by antibodies to parathyroid tissue. Treatment with vitamin D and calcium replacement is successful.

Hypocalcemia may occur secondary to hypoparathyroidism or *pseudohypoparathyroidism* (an abnormality of the parathyroid hormone receptor) or in association with vitamin D deficiency. The most common causes of hypoparathyroidism (aside from surgical removal of the gland) are autoimmune destruction and absence or maldevelopment of the parathyroid glands. This condition may also be associated with aortic arch abnormalities and absence or diminished function of the thymus (*DiGeorge syndrome*). Children with pseudohypoparathyroidism typically show moderate obesity, with ovoid facies, mild to moderate intellectual deficit, and short fourth or fifth metacarpals (see Fig. 16–29). When the child makes a fist, the fourth and fifth knuckles are short, a sign also seen in girls with Turner (karyotype XO) syndrome.

Vitamin D deficiency and vitamin D receptor abnormalities are associated with hypocalcemia and rickets. Affected children present in infancy when they begin to bear weight on their legs. Signs and symptoms include bony metaphyseal flaring, bowing of the legs, palpable beading at costochondral junctions (*rachitic rosary*), and bony pain, which may manifest as weakness, gait disturbance, and regression of motor skills. Infants with hypocalcemia and rickets are often irritable and do not like to be handled. Sometimes, fad diets are the cause of vitamin D deficiency. *Hypophosphatemic rickets*, a genetic abnormality of renal handling of phosphate, manifests as rickets without hypocalcemia.

CHIEF CHARACTERISTICS OF ADRENAL DISORDERS IN CHILDREN

Key Point

Recognizing adrenal disorders in infants and young children can be lifesaving; the endocrinologist is unlikely to be first on the scene.

The Endocrine Basis of Signs and Symptoms

Cortisol and aldosterone are essential for survival, whereas adrenal androgens are responsible for initiating the growth of pubic and axillary hair and the oiliness of skin and hair and for changing the child's body build in the immediate preadolescent years (the physiologic anabolic steroid effect). Subsequently, the testes and, to a lesser extent, the ovaries play an essential role in completing this process of *adrenarche*. Endocrinologists are probably the only physicians who care about the presence of pubic and axillary hair, but we recommend that you take an interest as well.

Overproduction of adrenal cortical hormones may change a child's appearance dramatically. Antenatal exposure of a female fetus to excess androgens causes sexual ambiguity; postnatal exposure results in partial sexual precocity in males and virilization in females.

Aldosterone excess causes hypertension, a rare primary adrenal abnormality in childhood; cortisol excess produces Cushing syndrome.

Pheochromocytoma, a tumor of the adrenal medulla or extra-adrenal chromaffin neural crest tissue, causes sustained or paroxysmal hypertension because of excessive secretion of catecholamines (epinephrine and norepinephrine). Headaches and flushing are among the cardinal symptoms.

Evaluating Cushing Syndrome

The overwhelming majority of obese children do *not* have Cushing syndrome, but the few who do may be difficult to identify. Cushing syndrome most commonly occurs as a result of exogenous administration of glucocorticoids. Whether cortisol excess is of exogenous or endogenous origin, the degree of excess determines the severity of the clinical features. Most prepubertal obese children are tall for their ages and have a significant family history of obesity, but the child with Cushing syndrome displays a recent weight gain, poor statural growth, and fatigue or mood changes.

Observe the child from all sides to assess body fat distribution. In adults with Cushing syndrome, the adiposity is clearly central; they have slim limbs, thin hands, and a rounded face. Young children with Cushing syndrome have more generally distributed body fat that is still maximal in the face, trunk, and cervical region (the "buffalo hump"), but the adiposity is chunkier and more solid in the very young, almost seeming to bury their small features (Fig. 16–12). We never tell patients that they have a "buffalo hump," preferring the term "increased cervical fat pad" because it sounds less derogatory.

Striae (stretch marks) are unusual before the teen years. In Cushing syndrome, these marks are violaceous rather than the pink to silver color seen in obesity or during rapid growth in normal adolescents. Check the scalp hairline. Fine lanugo hair growing down from the scalp to the forehead, from the occipital region to the nape of the neck, and sweeping down the lateral cheek suggests excess cortisol exposure. A small amount of fine hair may be distributed over the entire body, including the pubic region. Cortisol excess increases red cell production, giving the child a ruddy, plethoric complexion. It also inhibits protein synthesis, resulting in muscle atrophy, decreased strength, thin fragile skin and vasculature, and susceptibility to bruising. Osteoporosis, a significant sequela, may be manifested by back pain due to vertebral compression fractures. This condition is particularly evident in children who receive high-dose glucocorticoid therapy for long periods to control a primary disease (see Fig. 16–13).

When both glucocorticoid and adrenal androgen are in excess, secondary sexual hair may appear in an oth-

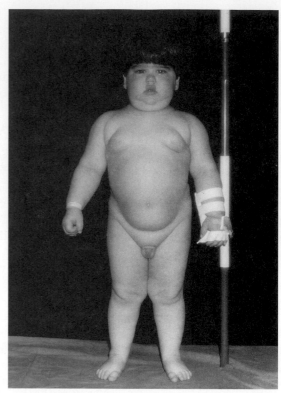

Figure 16–12 Clinical features of Cushing syndrome in a 4-year-old boy.

erwise prepubertal child. In a boy, this finding is not accompanied by an increase in testicular size, because the androgen is adrenal rather than testicular in origin.

Cortisol enhances norepinephrine's action on the vasculature and has some intrinsic mineralocorticoid effect, increasing sodium retention; therefore, the blood pressure may be elevated or at the upper limit of normal.

Once you suspect Cushing syndrome, how can you localize its cause? Increased pigmentation suggests a pituitary etiology, such as an adenoma with increased adrenocorticotropic hormone (ACTH) secretion, although the pigmentary change is far less dramatic than in Addison disease. Always note the parents' complexion so as not to be misled by familial pigmentary characteristics. Pituitary tumors can press on the optic chiasm, causing visual field defects—classically, bitemporal hemianopsia with optic atrophy (see Chapter 8). On clinical grounds alone, it can be extremely difficult to differentiate Cushing syndrome with a central etiology from that caused by an adrenal tumor. Sophisticated imaging and laboratory investigations are usually required to make the distinction.

Androgen Excess

CHIEF PHYSICAL CHARACTERISTICS

The physical changes induced by androgen excess depend on the child's age and sex. It is crucial to deter-

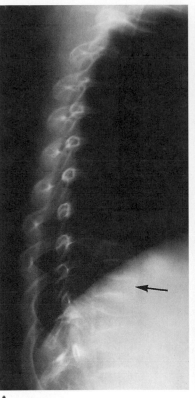
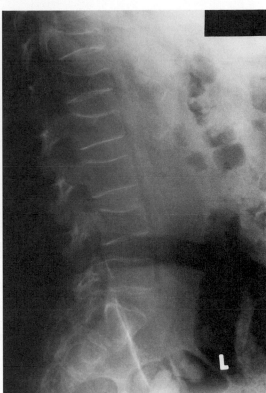

Figure 16-13 A, Spinal radiograph of a 10-year-old boy with Duchenne muscular dystrophy who experienced severe osteoporosis after receiving high doses of glucocorticoid for 3 years to improve muscle function. Note the marked wedging of the anterior vertebral bodies, which caused the patient so much pain that he was unable to continue to crawl and was no longer able to assist with transfers from bed to wheelchair. B, After treatment for 2 years, the vertebral bodies show improved density. The patient's pain disappeared, and his mobility was restored to the previous level.

A   B

mine whether the child has true virilization and whether the onset was antenatal or postnatal (Table 16–2).

BENIGN PRECOCIOUS ADRENARCHE

Adrenarche is the normal physiologic increase in adrenal androgen production that initiates pubic and axillary hair growth, increased oiliness of the skin and hair, and mild acne. In benign precocious adrenarche, pubic hair, axillary hair, or both, appear prematurely—before age 9 in boys or age 8 in girls—and may antecede true puberty by several years.

The absence of penile enlargement in boys or of clitoral enlargement in girls distinguishes benign precocious adrenarche from pathologic virilization. If a female fetus was exposed to excessive androgen in utero, the clitoris enlarges, and the labia may fuse posteriorly (Figs. 16–14 through 16–17).

CONGENITAL ADRENAL HYPERPLASIA

Congenital adrenal hyperplasia (CAH) is the most important cause of antenatal virilization of a male or female fetus. The most common cause is a deficiency of the 21-hydroxylase enzyme, which blocks the production of cortisol. Precursors are shunted toward the normal androgen pathways stimulated by high levels of ACTH. Be alert to this possibility in any female

Table 16–2 ADRENAL OR GONADAL EXCESS ANDROGEN STATES

Physiologic variation from normal
   Precocious adrenarche (benign)
      Excess adrenal androgen, only for age
Virilization of female and enhanced virilization of male
   Congenital adrenal hyperplasia
      21-hydroxylase enzyme deficiency
         Salt-losing
         Non–salt-losing
      11-hydroxylase enzyme deficiency
   Adrenal/gonadal tumors
      Benign
      Malignant
   Male limited precocious puberty
      Testotoxicosis (Leydig cell hyperplasia)
Mild virilization or hirsutism
   Late-onset congenital adrenal hyperplasia (female)
   Polycystic ovary syndrome (Stein-Leventhal syndrome)
   Idiopathic
   Exogenous source (precocity of male if given in
     prepubertal years)

newborn in whom the external genitalia are ambiguous and prevent instant sex assignment. Explain to the parents that all males and females start embryonic life looking the same. Call the genital organ a phallus, not a penis or clitoris. Refer to the patient as "your child" or "the baby," instead of "he" or "she" until sex assignment can be made. CAH is a much more difficult

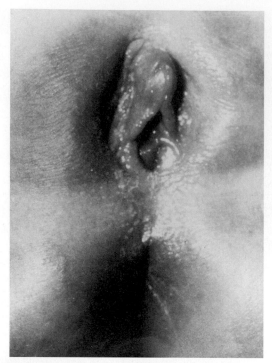

Figure 16–14 Normal external genitalia in a female infant.

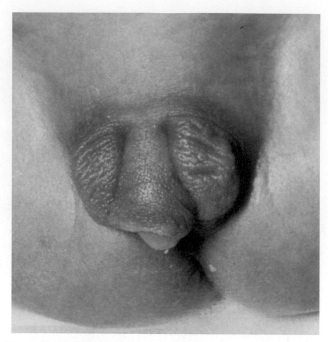

Figure 16–16 More pronounced clitoral enlargement in a female infant with congenital adrenal hyperplasia. The urethra and vagina share a common small opening on the perineum.

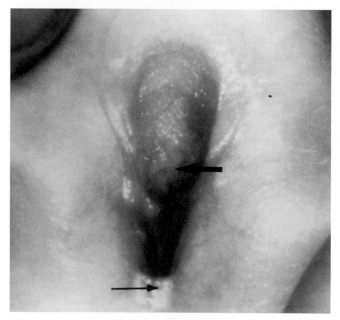

Figure 16–15 Enlarged clitoris *(thick arrow)* and partial posterior labial fusion *(thin* arrow) in a female infant with congenital adrenal hyperplasia due to 21-hydroxylase deficiency.

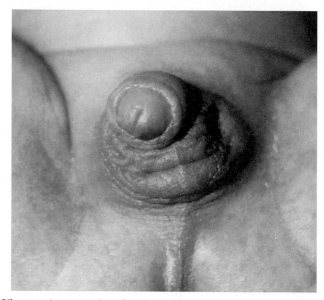

Figure 16–17 In this female infant with congenital adrenal hyperplasia, the clitoral enlargement is so extreme that the phallus resembles a penis with a male urethral meatus. This girl even underwent a circumcision before diagnosis at age 10 days.

diagnosis in the male infant or the wrongly classified female, who becomes symptomatic toward the end of the first week of life or soon afterward. In affected boys, the penis does not look very different from normal. The systemic manifestations are lethargy, weak cry, difficulty feeding, vomiting, and, on examination, evidence of increased pigmentation.

The clinical presentation of classic salt-losing virilizing CAH is dramatic, and early recognition and treat-ment are lifesaving. The infant with this condition may present in shock and is profoundly dehydrated, limp, and pale, with little response to painful stimuli (Fig. 16–18). The clinical tip-off may be that the extent of collapse and shock far exceeds the reported level of gastrointestinal loss from diarrhea and vomiting.

Simple (non–salt-losing) virilizing CAH, if not recog-nized in infancy, may be detected as the child becomes older because of an unusual growth spurt and hyper-

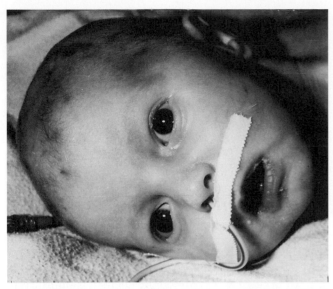

Figure 16–18 This 20-day-old, full-term baby with untreated adrenal insufficiency shows the sunken eyes, dry mucous membranes, mottled skin, and anxious look of impending cardiovascular collapse.

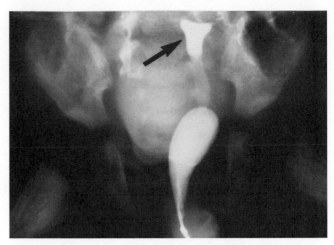

Figure 16–19 Genitogram of the patient shown in Figure 16–18. The radiograph demonstrates the bladder, uterus *(arrow)*, and vagina.

androgenism. Such a child has compensated adrenal (cortical) insufficiency, with an excessively stimulated intact androgen pathway.

A defect in the 11-hydroxylase enzyme causes cortisol deficiency and virilization, as in 21-hydroxylase deficiency, but the affected infant is also hypertensive (because of excess accumulation of 21-deoxycortisol acetate), a feature that stresses the necessity for accurate blood pressure recording, even in newborns. The less common deficiency of 3β-hydroxysteroid dehydrogenase results in ambiguous genitalia in both male and female infants. (See Chapter 5 for a detailed discussion of the clinical approach to the child with ambiguous genitalia.)

Approach to the Physical Examination of a Child with Congenital Adrenal Hyperplasia

High ACTH levels cause increased nipple and labial or scrotal pigmentation, yet in normal neonates, some darkening is expected because of exposure to maternal estrogen. Measure the phallus length, and check the terminal urethral position. Examine the labial or scrotal area for testicles. If they are not palpable, check the groin areas for undescended testicle, which occurs in about 3% of full-term newborns; undescended testicle may be unilateral or bilateral, but most commonly the testicles are partially descended. By 1 year of age, less than 1% of testes remain undescended.

Key Point

When the external genitalia appear ambiguous and testicles are palpable, the differential diagnosis is narrowed, and 21-hydroxylase or 11-hydroxylase deficiencies are excluded.

The female child with hyperandrogenism due to CAH has an enlarged clitoris and normal internal female sexual organs (Fig. 16–19). In a newborn, the enlarged clitoris may resemble a male phallus so closely as to be indistinguishable. The child whose genitalia are shown in Figure 16–17 actually underwent a circumcision 10 days before the signs of acute adrenal insufficiency appeared.

In the female infant or small child, the uterus is felt as a small midline lump in front of the anterior rectal wall on digital rectal examination. It feels slightly larger than the tip of your little finger. Look carefully to see whether there is a urethral orifice separate from and anterior to the hymenal ring. When the lower end of the vagina has not formed, as occurs in some females with CAH, there is a fistula from vagina to urethra, with a common external opening. A milder anatomic abnormality may be clitoral hypertrophy with partial fusion of the posterior labia; in this abnormality, the joining skin is thickened, not grayish and transparent as in benign labial agglutination (see Fig. 16–7), a common phenomenon in female infants.

Boys with the common forms of CAH have an enlarged penis. If the condition is diagnosed after the infancy period, such children will mature rapidly and develop increased muscle bulk because of the excessive testosterone secretion.

The term used to describe a urethral opening on the perineal surface in boys is *perineal hypospadias*. Take care to determine genetic sex by karyotyping to avoid assigning male gender to a female child with CAH. At the other extreme is the child with a normal XY karyotype who has ambiguous genitalia because of an androgen receptor abnormality (Fig. 16–20).

The genetic male with complete androgen resistance (also called *testicular feminization*) has normal female external genitalia and breast development but little or no pubic or axillary hair. The condition may not be recognized until the patient comes to medical attention

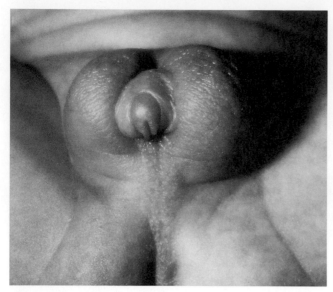

Figure 16–20 Ambiguous genitalia in a male infant with androgen resistance. Note testicles that are present in the scrotum.

because of primary amenorrhea, which is due to absence of the uterus and the upper two thirds of the vagina. Palpating the groin and labia reveals testicular swellings in the patient, which were missed in early childhood but are now larger because of puberty.

HIRSUTISM

Excessive facial or body hair in adolescent girls is most distressing, but you should explain that it is usually simply a variation of normal. Hair growth increases in the androgen-dependent areas: on the upper lip, chin,

and cheeks, between the breasts, across the chest, shoulders, and back (including the sacral area), up the linea alba, across the abdomen, down the inner thigh, and on the limbs and digits. Generally beginning at puberty, hirsutism becomes more troublesome with age. Pay attention to hirsutism that develops at puberty so you can offer investigation and treatment before the hair growth becomes well established and impossible to reverse (Fig. 16–21).

The etiology of hirsutism may be nonclassic CAH, in which the enzyme block is only partial. Affected patients have no evidence of adrenal insufficiency but, because of 21-hydroxylase enzyme deficiency, may experience precocious adrenarche and, at puberty, hirsutism. Another cause is polycystic ovary syndrome (PCOS), in which the hair follicles are excessively sensitive to androgen. This is a common female metabolic and reproductive disorder (prevalence roughly 5%), characterized by irregular menstrual cycles, relative infertility, hyperinsulinism, and usually central obesity. Originally called the Stein-Leventhal syndrome, PCOS is typified by multiple nontumorous ovarian cysts, anovulatory cycles, and hirsutism and begins around the time of puberty. In some cases, precocious adrenarche is the forerunner. There is a strong familial incidence, although the genetics have not been clearly defined; therefore, always ask about hirsutism in female relatives. Associated high insulin levels, a risk factor for type 2 diabetes mellitus, are also characteristic. In every case, look for *acanthosis nigricans*. This thickened, raised, velvety brown appearance to the skin folds in the neck, axillae, or groin, between the breasts, or over pressure points like the elbow or knuckle is the hallmark of hyperinsulinism (Fig. 16–22). Usually, affected

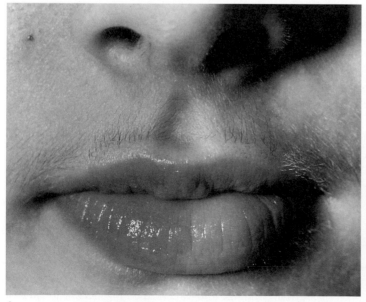

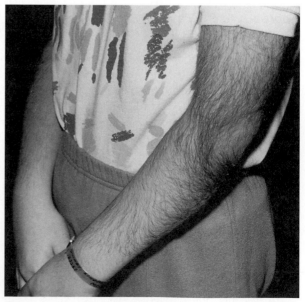

A   B

Figure 16–21 Hirsutism in an 11-year-old young girl: A, facial hair; B, arms.

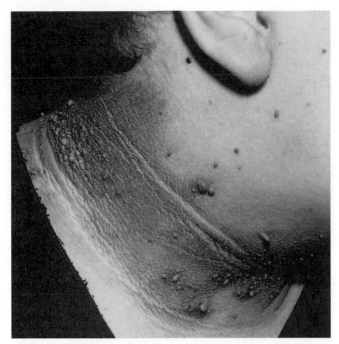

Figure 16–22 Acanthosis nigricans of the neck in a teenager with type 2 diabetes mellitus. This is a severe case, with extensive pigmentation and skin thickening and pseudopolyps called *acrochordons.*

children have been accused of not washing their necks, but no amount of scrubbing helps.

Key Point

All adolescent girls with increased body hair with or without irregular menses should be screened both for polycystic ovary syndrome and type 2 diabetes mellitus.

Adrenal Insufficiency

Adrenal insufficiency may be primary, due to adrenal failure, or secondary, caused by pituitary failure and inadequate secretion of ACTH. An important acquired cause of secondary adrenal failure is discontinuation of glucocorticoid medication before the suppressed hypothalamic-pituitary-adrenal axis has had a chance to recover. When taking the medical history of a child who has recently been receiving glucocorticoid medication, inquire about the type of medication, the dose, mode of adminisration, and whether the dose has been increased or tapered recently.

The clinical presentation is early and acute in hereditary disorders of adrenal steroid hormone synthesis. In patients with an autoimmune destructive process, however, symptoms rarely develop until after the toddler stage and are so gradual that family or physicians recognize the changes only in retrospect. Symptoms include fatigue, nonfading summer tan, list-lessness, decreased muscle strength, dizziness, faintness on standing quickly, decreased appetite for food but increased craving for salt, and weight loss. The mother of one of our patients with this disorder commented that her son liked so much salt on his hamburger, even the dog would not eat it. Small children lick salt shakers because their craving is so great.

If the diagnosis goes unrecognized, an adrenal crisis eventually occurs, with nausea, vomiting, high fever, diarrhea, extreme listlessness, and shock. These symptoms of adrenal crisis also occur with secondary adrenal insufficiency. Mild illnesses such as the common cold may precipitate the symptoms and are often more protracted and severe in the child with adrenal insufficiency than in other family members.

APPROACH TO THE PHYSICAL EXAMINATION OF A CHILD WITH ADRENAL INSUFFICIENCY

The child in an acute adrenal crisis is dehydrated and extremely lethargic. Recumbent blood pressure may be normal but falls precipitously upon standing or sitting. In primary adrenal failure, there is increased pigmentation over pressure or friction points (such as elbows [Fig. 16–23] or knees) and on buccal surfaces, gingival margins, nail bases, palmar creases, and scars that develop after the disorder begins. Even pigmented nevi darken. This darkening is due to increased ACTH production, which stimulates melanocytes. (The first 13 amino acids in the ACTH sequence are identical to those in melanocyte-stimulating hormone.)

In adolescent girls with primary adrenal failure, pubic and axillary hair either fails to appear or is scanty. In affected adolescent boys, by contrast, testicular testosterone ensures normal secondary sexual hair development. In both adolescent boys and girls with secondary adrenal failure, because the pituitary gland fails to secrete ACTH and gonadotropins, secondary sexual hair does not appear and skin pigmentation is unchanged.

If adrenal insufficiency is long-standing, particularly in primary Addison disease, the intravascular volume is contracted, and the heart small; the heart looks like a teardrop on a radiograph. Aldosterone, even in physiologic amounts, in the absence of cortisol is not sufficient to maintain normal homeostatic control of blood pressure. An adrenal crisis with cortisol deficiency is severe and life-threatening whether of adrenal or pituitary origin. The only difference is that in the adrenal crisis due to primary adrenal failure, the salt deficit is exceedingly large, the blood volume reduced, and serum potassium level high, a combination of manifestations that may cause cardiac arrhythmias.

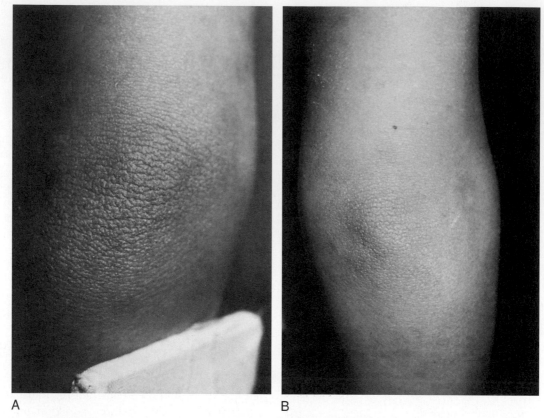

A   B

Figure 16-23 Pigmentation of the elbow in Addison disease before (A) and after (B) treatment.

CHIEF CHARACTERISTICS OF PUBERTAL DEVELOPMENT: PRECOCIOUS, DELAYED, AND NORMAL VARIANTS

General Definitions

The occurrence of pubertal changes before the age of 8 years in girls or 9 years in boys and the delay of pubertal changes beyond age 14 years in girls or 16 years in boys should be evaluated. Puberty depends on secretion of luteinizing hormone (gonadotropin) releasing hormone (LHRH) through increased activity of the LHRH "pulse generator."

Central precocious puberty is idiopathic in about 70% of cases. Identifiable causes include hypothalamic tumors and *hamartomas* (normal tissue in a tumorous collection). Noncentral precocious puberty does not originate in the hypothalamic-pituitary axis; it results from increased sex hormone secretion from the adrenal glands or gonads. CAH is one example. See Table 16-3 for a list of the causes of precocious puberty.

Obtaining the History

Although establishing when secondary sexual changes began is helpful in a child with precocious puberty, the

Table 16-3 CAUSES OF PRECOCIOUS PUBERTY

Type of Precocious Puberty	Underlying Cause
Central	Idiopathic
	Hypothalamic hamartoma
	Germinoma (pinealoma)
	Other cerebral tumors or malformations
	Hypothyroidism secondary to cranial irradiation
Gonadal	Precocious thelarche (? central)
	Ovarian cysts, benign
	McCune-Albright syndrome (polyostotic fibrous dysplasia of bone, ovarian cysts, large irregular café-au-lait spots)
	Leydig cell hyperplasia (familial testotoxicosis)
	Gonadal tumors (male and female)
	Premature menses (? Central)
Adrenal	Precocious adrenarche
	Congenital adrenal hyperplasia
	Adrenal tumors
Iatrogenic	Exogenous sources

reported sequence may be approximate because of the gradual nature of puberty. An exception is the time of the first menstrual period, which most girls remember. Vaginal bleeding may occasionally be a first sign of puberty; remember the possibility of sexual abuse or self-insertion of foreign objects.

For a child whose pubertal development is abnormal, you must evaluate the psychosocial impact. Is excessive masturbation a problem? How do the parents deal with the problem? Do they hug and cuddle this 4-year-old who looks and sounds like a small man but acts like a small child (Fig. 16–24)?

A family history of similar delay can reassure the teenager, often a boy, who shows slow pubertal maturation. In girls, excessive physical activity—gymnastics, ballet, or running—can delay secondary sexual development and menarche. Similarly, eating disorders inhibit sexual maturation and may cause secondary amenorrhea.

Cerebral insults, such as birth asphyxia, hydrocephalus, and cranial irradiation, can be associated with premature or delayed puberty. Because the hypothalamus, pituitary, and optic chiasm are in close anatomic proximity, expanding masses may produce a combination of decreased vision, GHD, and either precocious or delayed puberty.

Approach to Physical Examination of Children with Precocious Puberty

Take height measurements 6 months to 1 year apart so you can calculate the child's growth velocity (see Chapter 3), which is accelerated. Chronic or acute increases in intracranial pressure, secondary to a central tumor, cause optic atrophy or papilledema. Carefully document the visual acuity, visual fields, and extraocular movements. Occasionally, children with hypothyroidism experience precocious puberty, but they are short, with decreased growth velocity for age. Look for *café au lait spots*, brown macular pigmented areas on the skin with either a smooth border, consistent with neurofibromatosis, or an irregular outline, consistent with McCune-Albright syndrome (polyostotic fibrous dysplasia) (Fig. 16–25). Both conditions can be associated with precocious puberty, the former with central precocious puberty. In McCune-Albright syndrome, the precocious puberty is not central, and the child may have multiple ovarian cysts and completely suppressed pituitary gonadotropins, but menses often begin before the age of 4 years.

Acne is an early pubescent sign, and oily hair and adult-type body sweat odor are manifestations of both adrenal and gonadal activity. Tell the parents that it is appropriate for the child to use deodorant and to shave the axillary hair to avoid teasing.

To examine a child's breasts, observe the contour and record the breast diameter. Is the nipple pale, thin, and transparent (Fig. 16–26), as in isolated breast enlargement (*precocious thelarche*)? This common reversible condition seen in toddlers does not usually progress to true precocious puberty. Alternatively, is

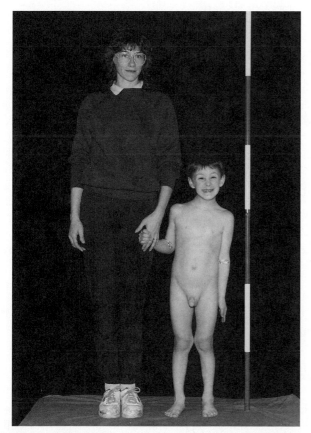

Figure 16–24 Precocious puberty in a 4-year-old boy due to Leydig cell hyperplasia (activation of the LH [luteinizing hormone] receptor). Note the increased size of the phallus, maturity of the scrotum, and muscular body habitus.

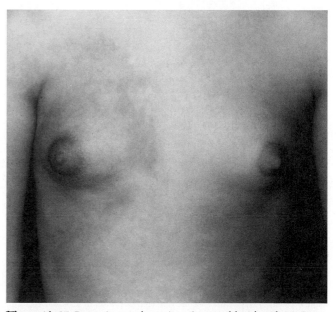

Figure 16–25 Precocious puberty in a 3-year-old girl with McCune-Albright syndrome. Note how mature the breasts and nipples appear. A large café au lait spot covers most of the right breast.

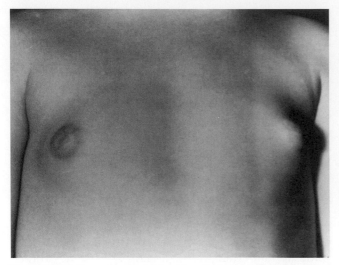

Figure 16-26 Precocious thelarche. Note the immature appearance of the nipples in this self-limited breast enlargement of toddlers.

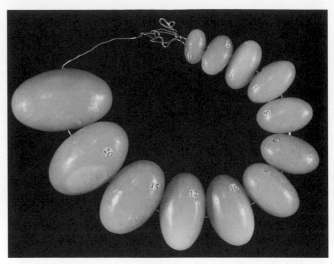

Figure 16-28 An orchidometer. Note the numerical volumes in milliliters printed on the beads. Prepubertal testicles are 1 to 3 mL.

the areola dark, indicating high circulating estrogen levels, with a prominent nipple mound, as seen in the 3-year-old girl with McCune-Albright syndrome shown in Figure 16–25? This child demonstrated precocious puberty with menses at age 18 months. Note also the irregular contours of the café au lait spot over the right breast—a clue to the etiology of the precocity.

When there is a significant postnatal increase in circulating estrogen, regardless of its source, the labia minora become enlarged and thickened (Fig. 16–27), vaginal secretions (leukorrhea and/or menses) begin, and breast buds appear.

Male breast enlargement, known as *gynecomastia*, is caused by a temporary increase in the estrogen-to-testosterone ratio. This is usually a benign, spontaneously regressing manifestation of puberty, occurring in most teenage boys. It can nevertheless be very distressing to an adolescent, especially if pronounced. In rare instances, the enlargement can be so extreme and psychologically distressing as to require pharmacologic treatment or surgery.

TESTICULAR EXAMINATION

The main differentiating feature between adrenal and central (hypothalamic) causes of sexual precocity is that when the testosterone is adrenal in origin, the testicles remain small.

Estimate testicular volume with the use of an orchidometer (Fig. 16–28). A volume of 4 mL is equivalent to 2.5 cm long and corresponds with Tanner stage 2 (see Fig. 3–9). Enlargement suggests a testicular origin for androgen production. If you only have a tape measure, you can derive the testicular volume from measurements of width and length, using the following formula:

$$\text{Volume} = \text{width} \times \text{length}^2 \times 0.71$$

At Tanner stage 3, testicular volume is between 10 and 12 mL.

Physical Findings in Delayed Puberty

Although the most common cause by far of delayed puberty is physiologic (constitutional) delay, usually associated with delayed growth, the history and physical examination help exclude pathologic causes. A classification dividing the causes into central (hypothal-

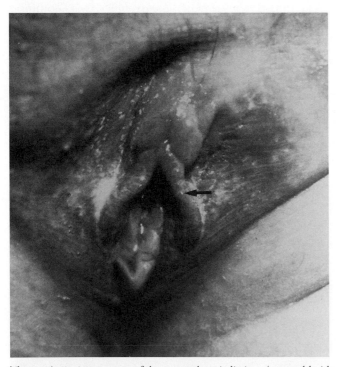

Figure 16-27 Appearance of the external genitalia in a 4-year-old girl with central precocious puberty. The enlarged labia minora are indicated by the *arrow*. Compare with the normal prepubertal appearance shown in Figure 16–14.

Table 16–4 CAUSE OF DELAYED PUBERTY

Type of Delayed Puberty	Causes
Central	Physiologic delay
	Malnutrition (including anorexia nervosa)
	Intensive physical training
	Chronic illness
	Hypothalamic and/or pituitary
	Developmental/genetic
	Destructive
	Surgical
	Radiotherapy
	Tumor
	Drugs (e.g., cyproterone acetate, luteinizing hormone agonists)
	Other endocrine (including hypothyroidism and hyperprolactinemia)
Gonadal	Developmental
	"Vanishing testes" caused by antenatal testicular torsion
	Anatomic abnormalities of female genital tract
	Chromosomal
	XXY Klinefelter syndrome
	XO Turner syndrome
	Immunologic
	Autoimmune endocrinopathy (oophoritis)
	Destructive
	Surgical removal of gonads
	Radiotherapy/chemotherapy

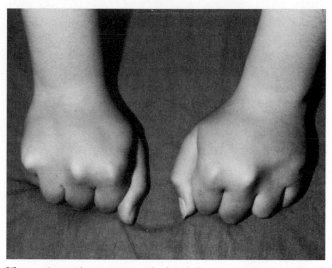

Figure 16–29 The patient's right hand demonstrates a short fourth metacarpal, and the left hand, short fourth and fifth metacarpals. To elicit this sign, tell the patient to make a fist with each hand. Then place a pen or your finger across the third, fourth, and fifth knuckles to see whether they all line up.

amic and/or pituitary) and gonadal is given in Table 16–4. Although the list is not exhaustive, it provides an orderly approach to the evaluation of teenagers who are worried about their sexual development. Their stature may be normal or shorter than normal, and their growth velocity is below normal for their chronologic age. The exceptions are boys with Klinefelter syndrome (karyotype XXY gonadal dysgenesis), who are tall with disproportionately long arms and legs, normal adrenarche, and small testes, which may be cryptorchid. These children are often overweight and may show delayed social and intellectual development.

In girls, the most common causes of pubertal delay are physiologic (familial or constitutional), poor food intake (as in anorexia nervosa), intensive competitive physical training (as in ballet or gymnastics), and chronic illness.

When pubertal delay is combined with short stature in girls, always consider Turner syndrome (karyotype XO), the physical characteristics of which include a short, wide-based neck, low anterior and posterior hairline, shield-shaped chest, absence of breast development, increased elbow-carrying angle, a short fourth metacarpal (Fig. 16–29), and spoon-shaped nails with lateral margins buried deeply in the pericuticular skin. In some girls, the signs of Turner syndrome are very subtle, especially if the karyotype demonstrates mosaicism, and the presence of breast development does not preclude the diagnosis. Children with Turner syndrome undergo normal adrenarche, so pubic hair and axillary hair are expected at the appropriate age.

In girls with otherwise normal sexual maturation but delayed onset of menarche or secondary amenorrhea, galactorrhea suggests prolactinoma. Although such a tumor is more common in adults, it may begin in adolescence. Boys with prolactinomas can have similar failure of pubertal progression.

Inability to smell (*anosmia*) or an impaired sense of smell (*hyposmia*) may accompany hypothalamic hypogonadism, an association that can be explained because the neurons producing LHRH share their origin with the olfactory nerve. Test the sense of smell (see Chapter 13) in any child with small (and often undescended) testicles and a small penis (less than 2.5 or 3 cm in length and circumference). Remember that it is the intrauterine fetal testosterone level that is responsible for the development of the normal penis size at birth.

CLINICAL CHARACTERISTICS OF DIABETES MELLITUS IN CHILDREN

Type 2 Diabetes Mellitus

Strong predictors of type 2 diabetes mellitus (DM) in overweight children are first- or second-degree relatives with diabetes and the presence of acanthosis nigricans (see Fig. 16–22). Not all children who are obese have diabetes. The increase in rate of type 2 DM in young people is related to rising rates of obesity in the general population. Obesity in a child older than 6 years, especially when accompanied by parental obesity, correlates with adult obesity, a risk factor for type 2 DM, and is also an independent risk factor for cardiovascular disease. Careful documentation of the family history should alert you to a genetic predisposition to obesity and a possible diagnosis and prevention. Because of concerns about self-esteem, calling attention to personal characteristics of an individual is frowned upon. We often ask parents whether they have any concerns about the child's growth or weight. Gently questioning the child about lifestyle habits may elicit associated poor eating and exercise habits. However, population-based remedies are needed to promote change on a large scale, because individual counseling is often unsuccessful.

The presentation of type 2 DM is generally insidious, with few symptoms at first, much as in adults. With time, however, polyuria and polydipsia develop once the blood glucose level is sufficiently high. Many children have ketonuria, and diabetic ketoacidosis can even occur. With improved public and health professional awareness, children with type 1 DM progress less frequently to ketoacidosis than in the past. However, most are ketotic (have acetone breath and ketones in the urine) and are thin. Children with type 2 DM are overweight, but as our population becomes progressively more obese, we are seeing more overweight children, even among patients with onset of type 1 DM, making this differentiating feature not entirely reliable. In certain racial groups such as African Americans or Native North Americans, it is *more likely* that the diagnosis will be type 2 DM rather than type 1 DM, but not invariably so. Similarly, in white teens, type 1 DM is most common, but type 2 DM is increasing in this population as well. The presence of acanthosis nigricans strongly points to type 2 DM as the cause of the diabetes (see Fig. 16–22).

Acute Presentation of Type 1 Diabetes Mellitus or Acute Decompensation in a Child Previously Diagnosed

The diagnosis of diabetes mellitus is generally based on a history of polyuria, polydipsia, and recent weight loss. Symptoms such as abdominal pain and vomiting suggesting a flulike illness are quite common, especially as the metabolic state deteriorates. An accumulation of ketone bodies (β-hydroxybutyrate and acetoacetate), which results from insulin deficiency and glucagon excess, causes ketoacidosis. The likelihood that a child will present with acute decompensated diabetic ketoacidosis is higher both in children younger than 5 years and in children and adolescents with previously diagnosed type 1 DM in whom poor adherence to recommended treatment schedules (such as insulin omission), severe intercurrent illness, or both, are superimposed. Although obtunded, they usually recognize person, place, and time and are seldom truly comatose. The history is typically short, a few days to several weeks, with a progressive increase in severity of the symptoms. There may be a family history of diabetes, thyroid disease, or both.

The physical signs reflect acidosis, ketosis, and dehydration. Respiratory compensation for the acidosis results in characteristic rapid but deep sighing (Kussmaul) respirations. The breath has the sweet odor of acetone; it smells like nail polish remover. Look for signs of dehydration, such as dry mucous membranes, lack of tears, decreased tissue turgor (tested by picking up a pinch of anterior abdominal wall skin, then releasing it to see whether it springs back quickly or remains tented), and low blood pressure. Low circulating volume in states of dehydration may be best appreciated from the rapidity of the heart rate rather than the measurement of the blood pressure, which may be low only when measured in the upright position, a dangerous maneuver in the patient with acute presentation or decompensation of diabetes.

A high blood glucose level, estimated at the bedside, usually eliminates other conditions from the differential diagnosis. In relatively rare instances, transient stress hyperglycemia and glycosuria can develop in association with severe infections or in acute asthma treated with β-agonists. Affected individuals do not appear to be susceptible to development of diabetes at a later date. Refer to standard pediatric texts for a full discussion of childhood diabetes.

Table 16–5 contains a useful checklist for significant issues in the history and physical examination of the child with known diabetes who returns for assessment of diabetes control (Figs. 16–30 and 16–31).

SUMMARY

Most pediatric endocrine disorders are diagnosed in the first instance on the basis of the history and physical findings. In each disorder, signs and symptoms can be explained logically, on the basis of an understanding of the normal hormonal pathways, physiologic effects, and feedback mechanisms. Such an approach makes the clinical findings in childhood endocrinopathies predictable, removing much of the mystery and pointing the way to appropriate management.

Table 16–5 CHECKLIST OF SIGNIFICANT ISSUES IN HISTORY AND PHYSICAL EXAMINATION FOR ASSESSMENT OF DIABETES CONTROL

History	Meal plan and compliance; mealtime problems
	Insulin
	Dose, frequency
	Timing
	Sites
	Adjustment for blood glucose
	Self-monitoring of blood glucose
	Frequency
	Results in book/device memory
	Device/calibrated?
	Hypoglycemia
	Day/night
	Warning/no warning
	Mild/moderate
	Severe (definition: cannot help self)/seizure
	Usual treatment
	Exercise
	Ask what sports
	Intercurrent illnesses
	History of gastric discomfort or frequent loose stools may suggest celiac disease (gluten-sensitive enteropathy), as common an associated disease as Hashimoto thyroiditis; poor control of diabetes despite following guidelines may be a useful clue
	Dental care (silent dental infection is a common cause of poor control)
	Emotional or psychosocial problems
	Family functioning/coping
	School progress
	Smoking/drinking
	Safe sex
	Driving
	Test blood sugar before driving?
	Carry sugar to treat "lows"?
	Wearing a medical alert bracelet or medallion?
Physical findings	Growth and pubertal development
	Blood pressure
	Funduscopy for microangiopathy (microaneurysms, exudates)
	Dental examination
	Goiter or evidence of hypothyroidism (up to 10% of diabetic children experience Hashimoto thyroiditis)
	Acanthosis nigricans (see Fig. 16–22) (a sign of hyperinsulinism, present in children with, or at risk for, type 2 diabetes mellitus
	Hepatomegaly (fatty infiltration associated with poor control)
	Monilial vaginitis in girls/balanitis in boys
	Insulin injection sites (hypertrophy [Fig. 16–30], lipoatrophy)
	Neuropathy (ankle jerks, vibration sense)
	Mobility of finger joints (reduced by increased glycosylation of tissue proteins when blood glucose is chronically high)
	Necrobiosis lipoidica diabeticorum (Fig. 16–31) (a rare but characteristic dermopathy of diabetes; a yellowish or salmon colored, circular, raised lesion with a central area of atrophic fragile skin; generally located over the shins)

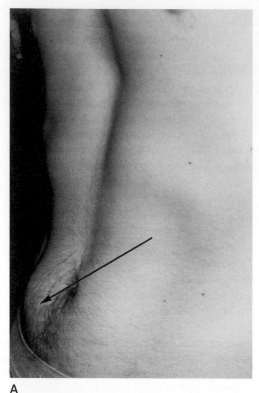

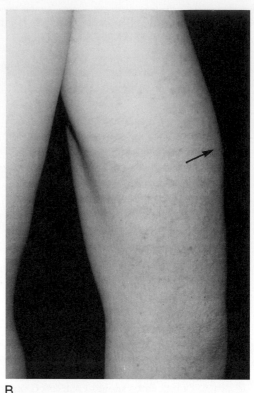

A

B

Figure 16–30 Lipohypertrophy in a teenager with type 1 diabetes mellitus who administered most insulin injections into a favorite spot: A, lower abdomen; B, upper arm.

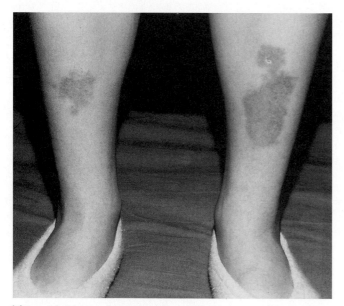

Figure 16–31 Necrobiosis lipoidica diabeticorum, a skin condition associated with diabetes, is found most commonly on the shins.

SUGGESTED READINGS

Becker KL, Bilezikian JP, Brenmer WJ, et al: Principles and Practice of Endocrinology and Metabolism, 3rd ed. Hagerstown, MD, Lippincott Williams & Wilkins, 2001.

Hall JG, Froster-Iskenius UG, Allanson JE: Handbook of Normal Physical Measurements. Toronto, Oxford University Press, 1989.

Mahoney CP (ed): Current Issues in Pediatric and Adolescent Endocrinology. Pediatr Clin North Am 37:1255–1523, 1990.

Sperling MA: Pediatric Endocrinology, 2nd ed. Philadelphia, WB Saunders, 2002.

Styne DM (ed): Pediatric Endocrinology. Pediatr Clin North Am 44:269–529, 1997.

Wilson JD, Foster DW, Kronenberg HM, Larsen PR (eds): Williams Textbook of Endocrinology, 9th ed. Philadelphia, WB Saunders, 1998.

chapter 17

The Sports Preparticipation Physical Examination

PAUL G. DYMENT

Better known as the "sports physical," the sports preparticipation physical examination was for many years more of a time-honored ritual than a useful technique to prevent either sports injury or a medical catastrophe on the playing field, such as sudden cardiac death. When conducting these examinations, most primary care physicians performed the traditional medically oriented clinical examination, emphasizing auscultation of the heart and chest and checking for inguinal hernia in boys.

Unfortunately, such examinations detect abnormalities that require further evaluation or disqualify the athlete from sports participation in some sport in only about 1% of participants. Any suspicious finding of such examinations was generally a condition of little consequence, such as an innocent heart murmur, transient proteinuria, or mild or transient hypertension, none of which would raise the athlete's risk from participation in athletics. With such a low "return," it is not surprising that physicians may have considered such examinations to be so infrequently productive that their performance became cursory, reducing even further the likelihood of detecting a true abnormality.

At least one study, however, has shown that when a brief but systematic examination of the musculoskeletal system is performed in addition to the medical examination, abnormalities are detected in more than 10% of high school athletes, most of which are persisting signs of previous injuries.[1] It is believed that *most sports injuries are re-injuries*. The musculoskeletal component of the sports preparticipation examination is performed principally to detect the residua of incompletely healed or incompletely rehabilitated injuries, such as the patellofemoral syndrome, ankle and knee ligament instabilities, and long-standing abnormalities such as tight hamstring muscles, any of which can contribute to the production of athletic injuries.

The sports preparticipation examination should be performed at least 6 weeks before the start of the sport season, so that if rehabilitative exercises are indicated, they can be prescribed with reasonable hope that the athlete will perform them for long enough to reduce the likelihood of injury when he or she begins more vigorous play. Obviously, sports preparticipation examinations that are performed just before the fall football season and have "cleared" students to play football should not be considered approval for them also to play ice hockey later in the school year. Some of these students could well have sustained a play-limiting injury during the football season. Schools and other organizations responsible for the well-being of athletes must develop systems by which all potential players, before *every* sport season, complete questionnaires concerning recent injuries, to identify athletes who require another preparticipation assessment by a physician.

Ideally, as a student's primary care physician, you should perform the "sports physical" in your office. You should "convert" this clinic visit into a health maintenance examination, consisting of (1) a thorough medical examination, (2) a screening musculoskeletal examination, and (3) a review of the psychosocial issues of importance in this age group. This visit is usually the only opportunity you will have during that year to offer your patient general anticipatory guidance.

The scope and techniques of the medical examination are thoroughly presented in other chapters in this book. Also, a useful sports-oriented medical history is described in detail in a consensus statement published by a group of professional medical societies concerned with the health care of young athletes.[2] The most important question in the medical history concerns musculoskeletal complaints and previous injuries, which, if present, should prompt performance of an additional joint-specific examination.

All athletes undergoing a preparticipation examination should receive the general musculoskeletal

Table 17–1   THE TWO-MINUTE ORTHOPEDIC EXAMINATION

Figure	Instructions	Observations
17–1	Stand facing examiner	Acromioclavicular joints, general habitus
17–2	Look at ceiling, floor, over both shoulders; touch ears to shoulders	Cervical spine motion
17–3	Shrug shoulders (examiner resists)	Trapezius strength
17–4	Abduct shoulders 90° (examiner resists at 90°)	Deltoid strength
17–5	Full external rotation of arms	Shoulder motion
17–6	Flex and extend elbows	Elbow motion
17–7	Arms at sides, elbows 90° flexed; pronate and supinate wrists	Elbow and wrist motion
17–8	Spread fingers; make fist	Hand or finger motion and deformities
	Tighten (contract) quadriceps; relax quadriceps	Symmetry and knee effusion; ankle effusion
17–9	"Duck walk" four steps (away from examiner with buttocks on heels)	Hip, knee, and ankle motion
17–10	Back to examiner	Shoulder symmetry, scoliosis
17–11	Knees straight, touch toes	Scoliosis, hip motion, hamstring, tightness
17–12	Raise up on toes, raise heels	Calf symmetry, leg strength

Adapted from Sports Medicine: Health Care of the Young Athlete, 2nd ed. Elk Grove Village, IL, American Academy of Pediatrics, 1991.

screening examination described here, which can generally be completed in 2 minutes. A systematic approach ensures that no component is forgotten. To facilitate thoroughness, you can photocopy Table 17–1 and refer to it during an examination.

THE TWO-MINUTE ORTHOPEDIC EXAMINATION

While facing the athlete, give him or her each of the instructions listed in Table 17–1, and observe how they are carried out (Figs. 17–1 through 17–12). You should demonstrate most of the maneuvers yourself in addition to explaining them.

If you detect an abnormality during the screening musculoskeletal evaluation, such as an incompletely rehabilitated ankle sprain, you can usually allow the athlete to play, advising him or her to undergo several weeks of rehabilitative exercises first to decrease the risk of re-injuring the ankle. Only rarely will you detect a condition during either the medical or the orthopedic component of the preparticipation evaluation that would prevent an athlete from playing a sport; fortunately, you can now consult at least two consensus guidelines to help make this sometimes tough decision.[2, 3]

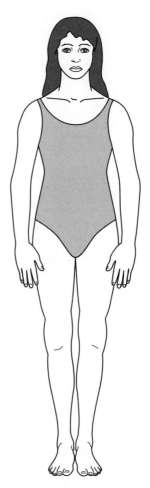

Figure 17–1 *Instructions:* Athlete stands straight with arms at the sides, facing the physician. *Normal findings:* Symmetry of upper and lower extremities and trunk. *Common abnormalities:* Enlarged acromioclavicular joint, enlarged sternoclavicular joint, asymmetric waist (leg length difference), swollen knee or ankle. (Used with permission of Ross Products Division, Abbott Laboratories Inc., Columbus, OH 43215. From For the Practitioner: Orthopedic Screening Examination for Participation in Sports, Ross Products Division, Abbott Laboratories Inc., 1978.)

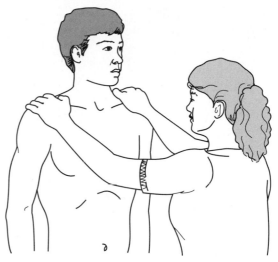

Figure 17–3 *Instructions:* Athlete shrugs the shoulders while the examiner holds the shoulders down. *Normal findings.* Trapezius muscles appear equal, and left and right sides have equal strength. *Common abnormalities:* Loss of strength or loss of muscle bulk may indicate shoulder or neck muscle injury. (From For the Practitioner: Orthopedic Screening Examination for Participation in Sports. Columbus, OH, Ross Products Division, Abbott Laboratories Inc, 1987.)

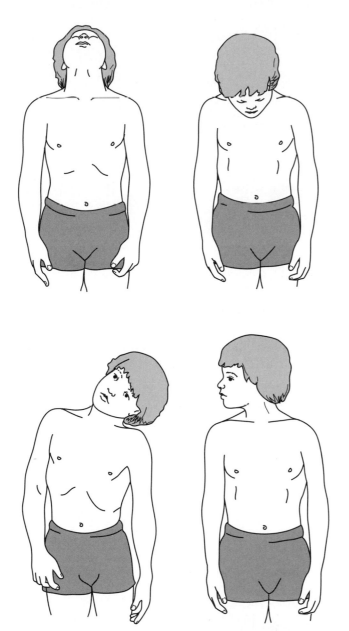

Figure 17–2 *Instructions:* Athlete looks at the ceiling and at the floor, touches the right (left) ear to the shoulder, and looks over the right and left shoulders. *Normal findings:* Athlete should be able to touch the chin to the chest and the ears to the shoulders, and look equally over the shoulders. *Common abnormalities:* Loss of flexion, loss of lateral bending, and loss of rotation, all of which may indicate a previous neck injury. (From For the Practitioner: Orthopedic Screening Examination for Participation in Sports. Columbus, OH, Ross Products Division, Abbott Laboratories Inc, 1987.)

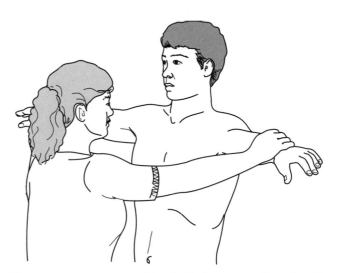

Figure 17–4 *Instructions:* Athlete holds the arms out from the sides horizontally and lifts them while the examiner holds the arms down. *Normal findings:* Strength of the two arms should be equal, and the deltoid muscles equal in size. *Common abnormalities:* Loss of strength and wasting of the deltoid. (From For the Practitioner: Orthopedic Screening Examination for Participation in Sports. Columbus, OH, Ross Products Division, Abbott Laboratories Inc, 1987.)

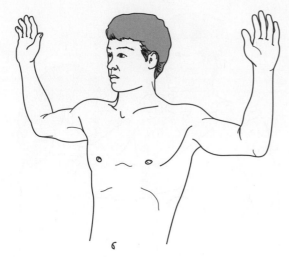

Figure 17–5   *Instructions:* Athlete holds the arms out from the sides with the elbows bent downwards about 90 degrees. Then athlete rotates the arms anteriorly until the hands are in the vertical position shown in the illustration. *Normal findings:* Hands go back equally to at least the vertical position. *Common abnormalities:* Loss of external rotation may indicate a shoulder problem or a previous dislocation. (From For the Practitioner: Orthopedic Screening Examination for Participation in Sports. Columbus, OH, Ross Products Division, Abbott Laboratories Inc, 1987.)

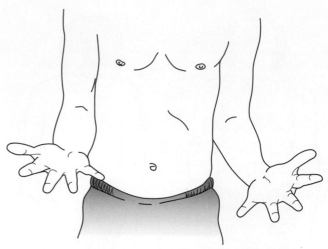

Figure 17–7   *Instructions:* Athlete holds the arms down at the sides with elbows bent 90 degrees, then supinates and pronates the palms. *Normal:* Palms should go from facing the ceiling to facing the floor. *Common abnormalities:* Lack of full supination or pronation may indicate previous elbow, forearm, or wrist injury. (From For the Practitioner: Orthopedic Screening Examination for Participation in Sports. Columbus, OH, Ross Products Division, Abbott Laboratories Inc, 1987.)

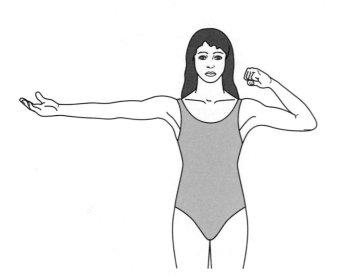

Figure 17–6   *Instructions:* Athlete holds the arms out from the sides, palms up, and then completely extends and then flexes the elbows. *Normal findings:* Equal motions left and right. *Common abnormalities:* Loss of extension or flexion may indicate an old elbow injury. (From For the Practitioner: Orthopedic Screening Examination for Participation in Sports. Columbus, OH, Ross Products Division, Abbott Laboratories Inc, 1987.)

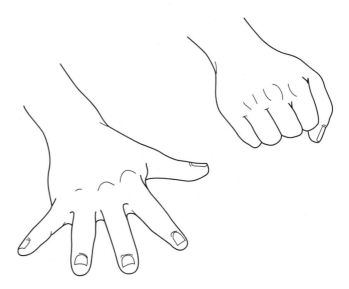

Figure 17–8   *Instructions:* Athlete makes fists, opens the hands, and spreads the fingers. *Normal findings:* Fists should be tight and fingers straight when spread. *Common abnormalities:* Protruding knuckle or a swollen or crooked finger may indicate an old finger fracture or sprain. (From For the Practitioner: Orthopedic Screening Examination for Participation in Sports. Columbus, OH, Ross Products Division, Abbott Laboratories Inc, 1987.)

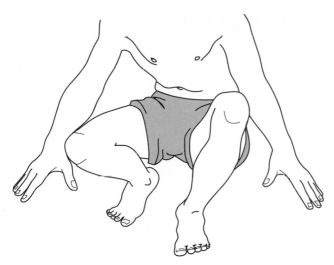

Figure 17–9 *Instructions:* Athlete squats on the heels, then duck-walks four steps and stands up. *Normal findings:* The maneuver is painless, the heel-to-buttock distances are the same on the left and right, and knee flexion is equal during the walk. *Common abnormalities:* One heel kept closer to the ground suggests an old ankle sprain on that side. (From For the Practitioner: Orthopedic Screening Examination for Participation in Sports. Columbus, OH, Ross Products Division, Abbott Laboratories Inc, 1987.)

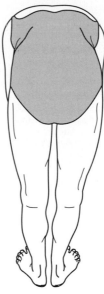

Figure 17–11 *Instructions:* Athlete bends forward slowly with the knees straight to touch the toes. *Normal findings:* Athlete can bend to almost touch the toes without discomfort. *Common abnormalities:* An inability to flex the spine very far suggests low back pain or tight hamstrings. (From For the Practitioner: Orthopedic Screening Examination for Participation in Sports. Columbus, OH, Ross Products Division, Abbott Laboratories Inc, 1987.)

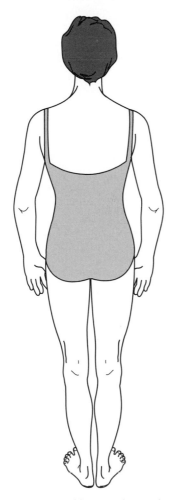

Figure 17–10 *Instructions:* Athlete stands straight with the back to the examiner. *Normal findings:* Symmetry of shoulders, waist, thighs, and calves. *Common abnormalities:* Scoliosis, trapezius muscle loss, or a high hip or asymmetric waist suggests a leg length difference or scoliosis, and a small calf or thigh suggests weakness from an old injury. (From For the Practitioner: Orthopedic Screening Examination for Participation in Sports. Columbus, OH, Ross Products Division, Abbott Laboratories Inc, 1987.)

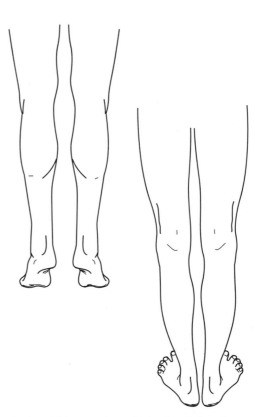

Figure 17–12 Athlete stands on the heels and then the toes. *Normal findings:* Equal elevation left and right, and symmetry of the calf muscles. *Common abnormalities:* Wasting of calf muscles suggests an old ankle or Achilles tendon injury. (From For the Practitioner: Orthopedic Screening Examination for Participation in Sports. Columbus, OH, Ross Products Division, Abbott Laboratories Inc, 1987.)

REFERENCES

1. Thompson TR, Andrish JT, Bergfeld JA: A prospective study of preparticipation sports examinations of 2,670 young athletes: Method and results. Cleveland Clin Q 49:225–233, 1982.
2. American Academy of Family Physicians, American Academy of Pediatrics, et al: Preparticipation Physical Evaluation, 2nd ed. Minneapolis, Physician and Sports Medicine (McGraw-Hill), 1997.
3. American Academy of Pediatrics, Committee on Sports Medicine and Fitness: Medical conditions affecting sports participation. Pediatrics 107:1205–1209, 2001.

SUGGESTED READING

American Academy of Orthopedic Surgeons and American Academy of Pediatrics: Care of the Young Athlete. Elk Grove Village, IL, American Academy of Pediatrics, 2000.

chapter 18

Pediatric Gynecologic Assessment

JOAN B. WENNING

The most frequently neglected or poorly performed part of the physical examination of children is the examination of the genitalia. Explanations for this fact include the examiner's personal inhibitions and inexperience, reluctance to cause anxiety or embarrassment to the child, and the parents' inhibitions. This is unfortunate, because examination of the genitalia may reveal unsuspected abnormalities requiring treatment or provide information that helps establish a diagnosis.

When an examination of the genitalia in young or adolescent girls is carried out tactfully and skillfully, it is remarkable how little anxiety is produced and how quickly any anxiety can be diffused. Making a genital examination a routine part of a girl's physical examination from an early age may help to promote lifelong compliance with regular gynecologic assessments.

Anxiety and tension are highly communicable "disorders." If a physician is apprehensive about performing a gynecologic assessment, the apprehension is quickly communicated to the patient. Using a soft reassuring voice, showing respect for the child's privacy and modesty, and chatting about unrelated issues important to the child, such as school, family, and hobbies, help most children undergo a gynecologic assessment in a reasonably relaxed way.

APPROACH TO THE PHYSICAL EXAMINATION

An infant or very young child can be examined most easily while she is semirecumbent on her mother's lap with her hips flexed and abducted. Put lateral and downward pressure on the labia majora so you can visualize the introitus, hymen, and lower third of the vagina (Fig. 18–1). An alternative, equally effective technique is to grasp the labia majora gently between your thumbs and forefingers and gently draw them forward (Figs. 18–2 and 18–3).

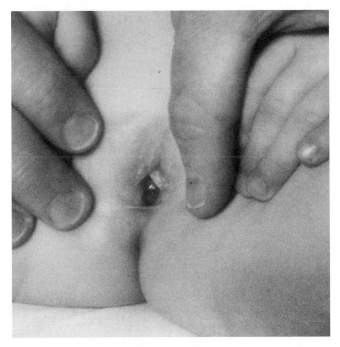

Figure 18–1 Lateral retraction of the labia majora while a prepubertal girl lies in a frog-legged position.

A child who is 2 years or older also can be examined in the knee-chest position. The child holds her bottom in the air with her knees 10 to 15 cm (about 4 to 6 inches) apart, allowing her stomach to sag against her thighs. Have an assistant or parent gently retract the labia majora on one side laterally and upward while you do likewise on the other side. This positioning facilitates inspection of the external genitalia and causes the pubococcygeus muscle to relax, allowing the vagina to fall open. You can visualize the entire length of the vagina and frequently identify the cervix. Use the otoscope (without a speculum) to provide magnification and good illumination along the length of the vagina. Do not allow the otoscope to touch the external genitalia or enter the vagina.

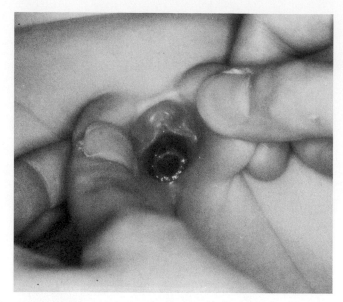

Figure 18–2 Forward retraction of the labia majora facilitates inspection of the hymenal area in this prepubertal child. An annular hymen is easily seen.

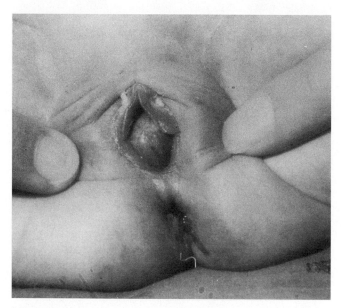

Figure 18–3 A mucocolpos, easily seen with lateral retraction of the labia majora.

Key Point

The technique for the examination of the genitalia must be tailored to the child's age.

Examination of External Genitalia

Examination of the external genitalia should consist of a systematic inspection of the clitoris, urethra, labia majora, labia minora, perihymenal tissues, hymen, posterior fourchette, and perineal body. Document the hymenal configuration and confirm its patency.

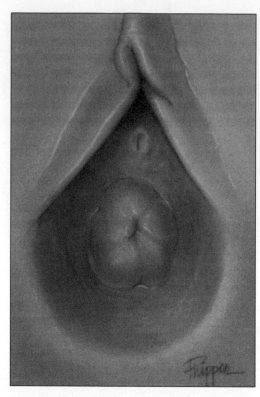

Figure 18–4 Posterior rim hymen. (From Pokorny S: Physical examination of the reproductive systems of female children and adolescents. Curr Probl Obstet Gynecol Fertil 8:202, 1990.)

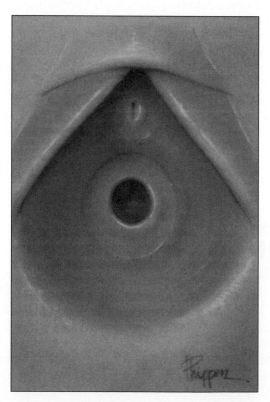

Figure 18–5 Circumferential hymen. (From Pokorny S: Physical examination of the reproductive systems of female children and adolescents. Curr Probl Obstet Gynecol Fertil 8:202, 1990.)

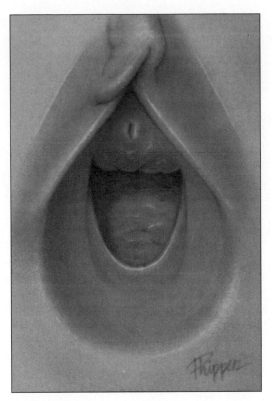

Figure 18–6 Fimbriated hymen. (From Pokorny S: Physical examination of the reproductive systems of female children and adolescents. Curr Probl Obstet Gynecol Fertil 8:202, 1990.)

Variations in normal hymenal configuration have been well described (Figs. 18–4 to 18–6). Fimbriated hymens are characterized by redundant folds of hymenal tissue with scalloped rims that circumscribe the vaginal introitus. Annular or circumferential hymens are smooth uniform skirts of hymenal tissue that completely surround the vaginal introitus. Posterior rim or crescentic hymens appear as smooth folds of tissue arranged from 2 o'clock through 11 o'clock around the introitus, with minimal or no hymenal tissue present inferiorly under the urethra.

The hymenal orifice at the introitus varies in size and placement, the variations being directly influenced by the configuration of the hymenal tissue. You should be able to identify microperforate hymen, imperforate hymen, and cribriform hymen. The orifice of a microperforate hymen can be difficult to identify, but gentle probing directly beneath the urethra with a small moist swab helps locate the opening. Transverse hymenal bands and tags have been reported to be present in 3% to 4% of newborn females.

The transverse diameter of the hymenal opening is most commonly measured with the child in the semirecumbent position previously described. The knee-chest position consistently produces larger measurements. Therefore, always record the position the child was in when the measurement was made. The diameter of the vaginal opening varies with the child's level of relaxation during the examination, age, and stage of pubertal development. The transverse diameter of the hymenal opening also varies with its configuration.

There is overlap in diameters recorded for varying age groups. Between the ages of 5 and 10 years, however, the upper normal limit of the transverse diameter of the hymenal orifice (in millimeters) should not exceed the child's age in years. In a child in whom the transverse diameter is larger than expected for age, suspect a prior penetrating injury of the vagina.

Periurethral bands are observed in approximately 50% of prepubertal girls. These bands are bilateral in 91%, creating false pockets on either side of the urethral meatus.

The appearance of the labia and perihymenal tissues may suggest that the child has been exposed to endogenous (or possibly exogenous) estrogen. The labia and perihymenal tissues of an unestrogenized prepubertal girl are poorly developed and appear red. Labial agglutination (Fig. 18–7) and chronic skin changes such as increased pigmentation may suggest a chronic inflammatory process. Document the presence of a purulent discharge, smegma, or leukorrhea. A thicker, lesser fusion of the posterior aspect of the labia minora may suggest excessive androgen stimulation due to congenital adrenal hyperplasia, especially if the labial fusion is associated with clitoral enlargement. If it appears that clitoromegaly is present, measure the clitoris glans in both its transverse and longitudinal diameters. Normal values for clitoral size at various ages and stages of sexual development are available in pediatric gynecologic references.

Indications for Vaginoscopy

Instrumentation of the vagina is rarely required in the evaluation of prepubertal girls. Indications for vaginos-

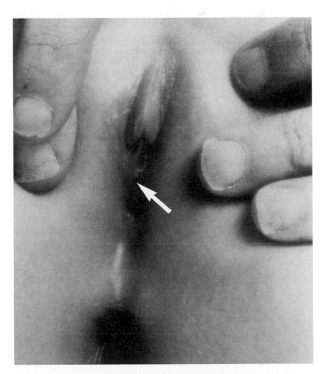

Figure 18–7 Labial agglutination. *Arrow* points to the line of fusion between the labia minora.

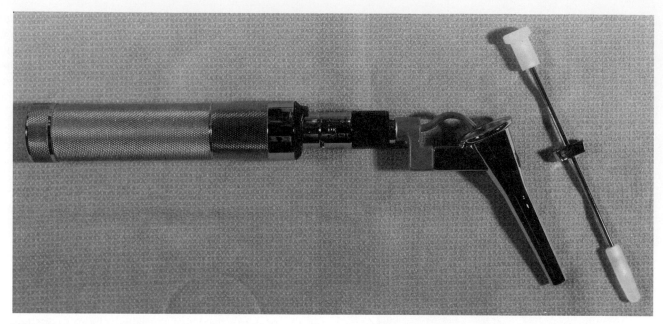

Figure 18-8   Welch Allyn pediatric anoscope may be used as a vaginoscope.

copy include undiagnosed vaginal bleeding, refractory vaginal discharge, and suspicion of intravaginal foreign body. Before beginning vaginoscopy, show the child all the instruments, and let her touch them (Fig. 18–8). If you intend to obtain cytologic and bacteriologic specimens during vaginoscopy, use only water as a lubricant.

Office vaginoscopy can be successfully carried out when the child understands what is to be done and trusts you. Because the vagina of a prepubertal girl is a short (4 to 5 cm), nonpliant cylinder that can be traumatized easily, gently place any instrument. The hymenal membrane is particularly sensitive; applying 2% lidocaine jelly to the introitus may help make the examination less uncomfortable. If the child is tense and the hymenal opening does not relax, postpone vaginoscopy until the child is less anxious and better able to cooperate. A child should never be forcibly restrained in the course of such an examination. On rare occasions, the gynecologic examination of a very young or very anxious child may best be carried out with the use of anesthesia or conscious sedation.

Bacteriologic Cultures

Obtain bacteriologic cultures from the prepubertal child's vagina instead of endocervical cultures because (1) bacterial infections such as *Neisseria gonorrhoeae*, group A *Streptococcus*, and group B *Streptococcus* cause vaginitis as well as cervicitis and (2) it is technically difficult to obtain endocervical cultures from a prepubertal girl in an office setting.

Key Point

Even the seemingly simple task of obtaining a culture specimen from the vagina can be difficult because the prepubertal vaginal mucosa, being hypoestrogenic, is easily abraded.

It is important to premoisten culture swabs with nonbacteriostatic saline solution or sterile water. Use appropriately sized swabs for culturing. The Calgiswab (available from Spectrum Laboratories Inc., Houston, TX) is particularly useful for obtaining gonorrheal and routine cultures from the vagina (Fig. 18–9). Swabs taken must be placed immediately in the transport medium and plated without undue delay. The small calcium alginate swab cannot be used for *Chlamydia* testing, unless batch tested, because calcium alginate is toxic to some strains of this organism. Always choose the smallest swab available for sampling, but confirm with your microbiology laboratory that the swabs chosen are appropriate.

Vaginal cultures may be obtained while the child is either in the knee-chest position or in the supine position, whichever effects the greatest relaxation of the hymenal orifice, allowing the swab to be passed into the vagina without touching the sensitive hymenal membrane. Some clinicians report success with the use of vaginal irrigation specimens for culture. A malleable plastic sterile eyedropper or butterfly catheter tubing, encased in a red rubber catheter and with the needle removed, has been used to flush the vagina with sterile nonbacteriostatic saline solution or sterile water.

Bimanual rectoabdominal examination is indicated in any prepubertal girl who presents with undiagnosed

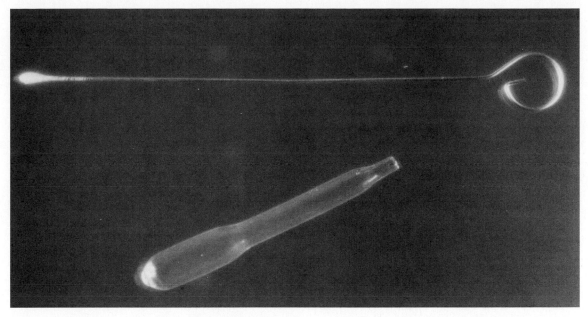

Figure 18–9   A Calgiswab (*top*) or a plastic eyedropper (*bottom*) can be used to obtain bacteriologic specimens from the prepubertal vagina.

vaginal bleeding or in whom an intravaginal foreign body or a pelvic mass is suspected. As mentioned previously, the vagina in prepubertal girls is short, non-pliant, and easily abraded. You can obtain more information if you perform a rectoabdominal examination with the child in a supine, frog-legged position. Bimanual examination should enable you to identify the small uterus as a midline structure. Ovaries are abdominal organs in prepubertal girls; therefore, they should not normally be palpable on bimanual examination.

Examining Adolescent Girls

The gynecologic examination of an adolescent girl begins with the interview. If a young girl is uncomfortable being interviewed alone and requests her parent's presence, you must make sure to phrase the questions so that the girl is aware that she, and not her parent, is the patient and is the person controlling the interview. If it is difficult to separate parent from child, defer confidential personal questioning to another visit, when the youngster may be more relaxed. Some physicians establish "ground rules" with the teenager and her parents, telling them that at a predetermined age, such as 12 years, you will spend some time talking with the young girl alone. It is very important, when dealing with adolescents, that you convey to them a sense of self and reassure them that everything they tell you is confidential and will not be directly conveyed to their parents without their consent. You also must establish with a young patient that if she is pursuing life-threatening behaviors, you will be compelled to involve other health care providers and her parents, even without her consent.

OBTAINING THE HISTORY

A complete gynecologic history can provide an indication of whether gynecologic disease is present. Document the age of menarche and the age and progress of pubertal change (thelarche, adrenarche; see Chapter 16). The mother's age at menarche is often a good predictor of when her daughter will experience her first menstrual period. Menarche commonly occurs 2 years after thelarche, when breast development reaches Tanner stage 4.

Menses can be characterized in terms of duration of flow, amount of flow, and interval between menses (Fig. 18–10). The normal duration of flow varies from 3 to 7 days. Persistence of menses for longer than 10 days warrants intervention. When asking about the cycle interval, make sure that the days of menstrual flow are included in the estimate. Day 1 of the menstrual cycle is the first day of the menstrual flow. A range of 25 to 35 days should be accepted as falling within the range of normal; shorter or longer intervals may require evaluation and treatment. Cycles may remain anovulatory for 2 to 4 years after menarche. Therefore, early cycle irregularity may reflect immaturity of the hypothalamic-pituitary-ovarian axis rather than gynecologic disease.

It is often difficult to obtain a reliable impression of the amount of flow. The reported number of menstrual pads or tampons used per day is unreliable because a fastidious girl may change pads or tampons when they are only slightly soiled. Asking about symptoms such as low energy, fatigue, and dizziness may help to identify the girl who is anemic secondary to menorrhagia.

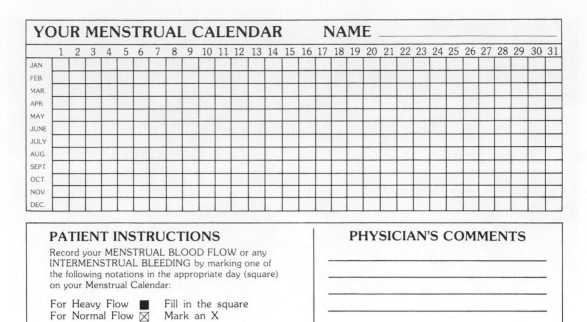

Figure 18–10 The menstrual calendar is a useful tool for prospectively recording menses. (Courtesy of Dr. JEH Spence, Ottawa Civic Hospital, Ottawa, Ontario, Canada.)

Key Point

Occasionally, determinations of hemoglobin and hematocrit levels may be the most reliable way to tell whether a patient's menstrual flow is truly heavier than normal.

Normally, the physiologic discharge varies in consistency and amount throughout the menstrual cycle, in response to cyclic production of both estrogen and progestin. Before both menarche and the establishment of ovulatory cycles, the mucoid discharge may be copious as a result of unopposed estrogen stimulation, and this excessive production of mucus may in turn cause vulvar irritation. Taking the time to talk about the discharge and explaining that the secretions come from the endocervical glands in response to normal cyclic ovarian hormone production may help allay unspoken anxieties in both the girl and her parents. Frequently, patients and parents may mistakenly perceive such physiologic discharge as indicating infection or pelvic inflammatory disease.

You must ask any adolescent girl questions about sexual practices because (1) many adolescents are sexually active at an early age and (2) issues of sexual orientation can arise in this age group. Be sure to frame the questions in an open and specific manner. You may simply ask, "Some of my patients of your age are in a relationship. Are you?" If the patient's answer is affirmative, ask, "Is your partner a male or female?" If the patient is sexually active, ask (1) whether she notes bleeding after or pain with intercourse, (2) whether she enjoys intercourse, and (3) what she is using for birth control. It is also important to establish that she is using her contraceptive method correctly and consistently. You can form an impression about her susceptibility to risk-taking behavior by asking how many boyfriends she has had over the past year and with how many of them she has had sexual intercourse. These questions will set the stage for a frank discussion about substance abuse, interpersonal violence, sexually transmitted diseases, safe sex, homosexuality, and the patient's own sexual experiences. She may want to discuss these issues with you but may be uncomfortable about initiating the discussion. It is important to delve into issues that may also make you a little uncomfortable. Information pamphlets on human sexuality, sexually transmitted diseases, and contraception should also be available in any clinical setting where adolescent patients are treated.

Many young girls are shy and nervous about an impending pelvic examination. Unfortunately, in "preparing" her daughter for the visit, a mother who is herself uncomfortable about pelvic examinations may have conveyed these anxieties to her daughter.

Key Point

Before asking an adolescent girl to undress, sit and explain, with the aid of pictures and instruments, exactly what will happen in the course of the examination.

Give the patient privacy to disrobe, provide her with a gown, and be sure she is appropriately draped throughout the examination.

APPROACH TO THE PELVIC EXAMINATION

Always precede a pelvic examination with a general physical examination. This more familiar examination gives your patient time to become comfortable with you and helps relieve some anxiety. Appraise and stage the secondary sexual characteristics, and look for evidence of an underlying endocrinopathy. Breast and pubic hair development can be staged according to the Tanner classification (see Chapter 3). Note the presence of axillary hair or of adult sweat odor. Thyroid gland enlargement, galactorrhea, and signs of androgen excess such as acne, oiliness of the skin, and hirsutism are all important findings. In the course of the general physical examination, you can give the patient much useful information about the changes she may be noticing in her body.

Tailor the pelvic examination to the presenting complaint and the stage of pubertal development. Inspection of the genitalia alone offers much information. Systematically examine the clitoris, labia majora, labia minora, perihymenal tissues, hymen, posterior fourchette, and perineal body. While looking at the labia, assess whether the mucosal appearance and secretions are in keeping with exposure to estrogen. Thickening of the perihymenal tissues and increased development of the mons, labia majora, and labia minora both suggest an estrogen effect. The configuration and patency of the hymen can be documented by inspection alone. Note the presence of leukorrhea or of secretions at the introitus. The presence of obvious secretions at the introitus provides indirect evidence that a normal cervix is present and that there is no obstruction between the cervix and perineum.

When first examining a young girl who is not sexually active, it is best not to attempt instrumentation of the vagina. As noted earlier, evaluation with the child in the knee-chest position allows visualization of the entire length of the vagina and inspection of the cervix. Culturing the vagina is much easier in adolescents, because the estrogenized mucosa is thick and less easily traumatized. Swabbing, therefore, does not produce the same abrasive discomfort as in a nonestrogenized prepubertal girl.

Bimanual examination of the pelvis in the adolescent girl who is not sexually active is best carried out by rectoabdominal examination with the girl in the supine frog-legged position. Rectoabdominal examination is generally perceived as less threatening by young girls who are not sexually active. A single-finger vaginal examination can produce enough patient anxiety and discomfort to preclude obtaining any useful information about the internal genitalia.

Pelvic examination of the sexually active adolescent requires instrumentation of the vagina. A complete gynecologic assessment includes both a Papanicolaou

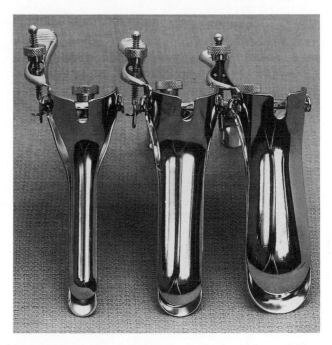

Figure 18–11 A variety of vaginal specula should be available so that the appropriate-sized instrument is always used. *Left to right*: Huffman, Pederson, and Graves specula.

(Pap) smear and culture of the endocervical canal for sexually transmitted diseases.

Various specula are available to facilitate the examination (Fig. 18–11). The Pederson and Huffman specula are best in pediatric practice because they are much narrower than the Graves speculum, the standard instrument used in adult gynecologic practice. Before performing a speculum examination, show the patient the instrument and explain how you will use it. It is easiest to examine adolescent girls when they are placed in the lithotomy position and properly positioned at the end of the examination table. Take the time to encourage the patient to breathe quietly and deeply during the examination and to relax the abdomen and buttocks. The patient should allow her knees to fall loosely open, effecting a further relaxation of the perineal muscles. Warm the speculum under warm (not hot) water; use only water for lubrication to facilitate insertion of the speculum into the vagina. Before inserting the speculum, gently retract the labia laterally with a gloved hand, bringing the hymenal opening into view and preventing inadvertent pinching of the labia when you insert the speculum.

As you insert the speculum, exert gentle pressure posteriorly, because any anterior pressure compresses the sensitive urethra. Next, open the blades of the speculum to bring the cervix into view. Gently swab away the mucus covering the exocervix, and inspect the cervix for any plaques, areas of whiteness, ulcers, or polyps. Nabothian cysts are not abnormal findings (Fig. 18–12). Note the transitional zone at the junction of the columnar and squamous epithelia (Fig. 18–13). It

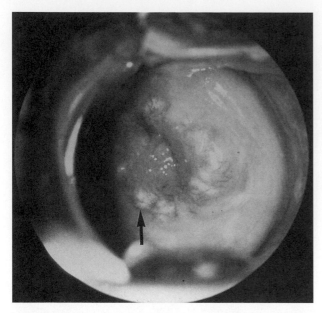

Figure 18–12 Cervix visualized with the aid of a speculum. *Arrow* points to a benign nabothian cyst.

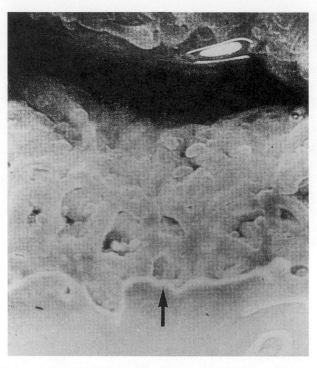

Figure 18–13 Photomicrograph of the cervix showing the cervical os and columnar epithelium (*top*), the transitional zone (*arrow*), and squamous epithelium (*bottom*).

is the transitional zone that must be sampled when you obtain a Papanicolaou smear. In adolescents, it is not uncommon to see red-looking columnar epithelium on the exocervix. Do not mistake this finding as an indication of cervicitis.

Always obtain specimens in the following sequence:

1. Take two samples of vaginal secretions with a balsa-wood stick or a cotton-tipped swab. Suspend one specimen in a drop of sodium chloride, and the other in a drop of a 10% potassium hydroxide solution placed on regular microscope slides. These slides can be examined later under the microscope for the presence of *Trichomonas*, clue cells, or hyphae.

2. Obtain the Papanicolaou smear specimen before other cervical specimens (Fig. 18–14).

3. Use a wooden Ayre spatula to sample exfoliated cells on the exocervix at the squamocolumnar junction. Place the longest tine of the spatula within the endocervical canal, and rotate the spatula 360 degrees in each direction.

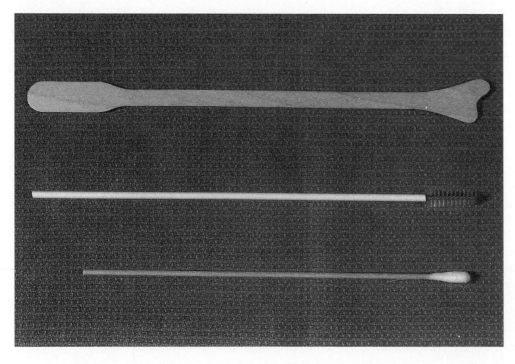

Figure 18–14 Equipment required to obtain a Papanicolaou smear consists of the Ayre spatula (*top*) and either a cytology brush or a cotton-tipped swab (*bottom*) for sampling of the endocervical canal.

4. Next use a saline-moistened cotton-tipped swab or a cytology brush (Cytobrush, available from Precision Dynamics Corp., San Francisco, CA) to sample the endocervical canal.

5. Thinly smear the collected specimens on glass slides and immediately fix them with 95% ethyl alcohol.

Key Point

Air-drying slides before fixation produces artifacts that make the slide specimens impossible to interpret; therefore, slide specimens must be fixed immediately.

When you collect culture specimens for sexually transmitted diseases, it is always important to sample the endocervical canal; use firm swabbing to ensure an adequate cell sample. Culture specimens are taken first for gonorrhea and either plated immediately on Thayer-Martin agar plates or placed in Stuart charcoal transport medium. Also, submit a smear of endocervical canal secretions for Gram stain. The last swab collected should always be for detection of *Chlamydia*. Rapid detection techniques, such as the enzyme immunoassay (Chlamydia Swab Collection Pack, Beckman Coulter, Inc., Fullerton, CA) or the fluorescein-conjugated monoclonal antibody slide test (MicroTrak, Syva Co., Palo Alto, CA), require purposeful endovaginal swabbing. In many laboratories, polymerase chain reaction (PCR) technology is replacing enzyme immunoassay methods.

When all necessary cytologic and bacteriologic specimens have been obtained, withdraw the speculum slowly, gently rotating the blades so you can visualize the mucosa along the entire length of the vagina. Once you have completed inspection of the vagina, perform a bimanual examination, using a standard lubricant jelly. In an adolescent girl, discretion should dictate whether you should perform a one- or two-finger vaginal examination. Examine the anterior, posterior, and lateral vaginal fornices. During this examination, you can delineate the position and size of the uterus and identify any adnexal fullness. Normally, moving the cervix in any direction should not produce discomfort. If the patient is uncomfortable with cervical motion, adnexal disease may be present.

After palpation of the vaginal fornices and side walls, use one hand on the lower abdomen to gently palpate and outline the uterus and adnexa. To palpate the uterus, use the fingers inserted into the vagina (vaginal fingers) to lift the uterus upward to the hand on the abdomen (abdominal hand), which is placed suprapubically. When palpating the uterus, assess its size, shape, position within the pelvis, and mobility. A nulliparous uterus is normally the size of a golf ball. When palpating the adnexa, place the vaginal fingers into the lateral vaginal fornix, and gently sweep them along the posterior pelvic

wall, sacrum, and side wall. Place the abdominal hand laterally, just above the iliac crest. Gently bring the vaginal and abdominal hands together, allowing the adnexa to slip through your fingers. A normal ovary is about the size of an almond. The ovary is normally tender to pressure, producing some mild visceral pain. When palpating the ovary, characterize its size, shape, consistency, location, mobility, and degree of tenderness.

After completing the abdominovaginal examination, perform a rectovaginal examination, with your index finger in the vagina and your middle finger in the rectum. This step allows you to assess the rectovaginal septum for thickening or nodularity.

During the pelvic examination, you may use a hand mirror to give the patient an anatomy lesson and to review the physiology of puberty and menstruation with her. You can discuss many anticipated developmental changes and common menstrual problems, giving her an opportunity to express concerns that she might not otherwise mention. Once the physical and pelvic assessments are complete and the patient has dressed, sit with her and review all the findings. Most girls need to be reassured that they are normal healthy young women.

APPROACH TO ASSESSMENT FOR SEXUAL ABUSE

Obtaining the History

Unfortunately, increasing numbers of prepubertal girls are presenting to their physicians for a gynecologic assessment because of allegations of sexual abuse. Despite whatever interviews may have been obtained before this examination, you should obtain sufficient history to reach an unbiased understanding of what actually happened. This interview allows the child to become comfortable with you and enables you to learn the child's familiar terms for her body parts. Also review the child's past medical history, because this knowledge may be important in the interpretation of physical signs.

Some young girls need to have their mother or another supportive person present during the interview. Others may be more comfortable talking to you alone. Therefore, always give the child the choice of who will or will not be present during the interview. Do not assume, however, that the child's mother is always the best person to have present during the interview. The child (1) may be angry with her mother if she believes that her mother has recognized the abuse and failed to protect her or (2) thinks that her mother does not believe what she has disclosed.

At times, a female nurse wearing a uniform, which indicates she is a caring health care professional, is the best person to have present during the interview. The interview does not have to delve deeply into family dynamics, but it should provide a clear understanding of what went on, allowing for appropriate interpretation of findings. Remember that the disclosure may be incomplete because of the child's inability to talk freely about what happened. Never shorten the physical evaluation on the basis of the history alone. (For further information about interviewing in cases of suspected abuse, see Chapter 14.)

Approach to the Physical Examination

It is your responsibility to document accurately the presence or absence of physical findings that have legal significance. Use sketches or color photographs, and carefully record any abnormalities seen. Approximately two thirds of young girls who have been sexually abused have no physical findings that would help to substantiate their allegations; therefore, never assume that the absence of abnormal physical findings signifies a lack of abuse. As with any young child, begin with a general physical examination. This familiar procedure decreases the child's anxiety and gives her time to become more comfortable with you. It also allows you to look for clinical signs that may suggest coexisting physical abuse or neglect.

The examination of the genitalia is no different from that previously described. The systematic examination of the external genitalia should include a search for evidence of trauma, such as scarring, erythema, abrasions, fingernail lacerations, bites, and ecchymosis. With the aid of magnification and a good light, carefully inspect the hymen and perihymenal tissues for evidence of microtrauma. You can use an otoscope, a hand-held magnifying glass with a good examining lamp, or a colposcope (Fig. 18–15) to facilitate this evaluation. Interestingly, the colposcope does not seem to intimidate children, perhaps because the instrument keeps the examiner at a distance. Significant physical findings are transections of the hymen, intravaginal synechiae, and abrasions of the posterior fourchette.

Three-site screening (throat, vagina, and anal specimens) for sexually transmitted diseases is now recommended only if specific risk factors are identified. These risk factors are (1) assault by multiple perpetrators, (2) the presence of a genital injury, (3) the presence of perianal discharge, and (4) past history of a sexually transmitted disease either in the patient or in the perpetrator if the perpetrator is known. If such screening is deemed appropriate, obtain culture specimens from the throat, vagina, and anus for testing for gonorrhea and *Chlamydia*. Vaginal secretions should be suspended in saline solution and checked for *Trichomonas* and clue cells.

Instrumentation of the vagina in the prepubertal girl is almost never required as part of a sexual abuse assessment. If the upper vagina requires exploration because of bleeding or concerns about a penetrating injury, examination under anesthesia may be the best way to proceed in a previously traumatized child.

Always include an evaluation of the perianal area in your abuse assessment. Document the presence of perianal skin tags, scars, and pigmentation changes. Perianal soft tissue variants have been described in nonabused children, but findings that suggest abuse are anal dilatation greater than 20 mm without stool in the

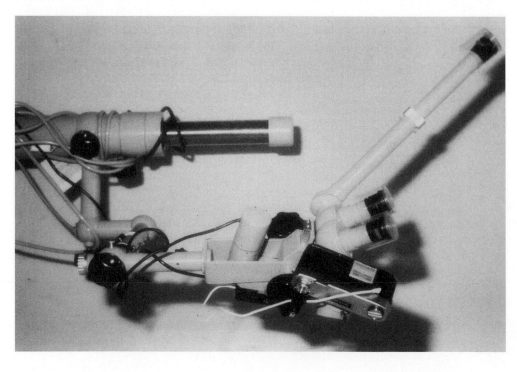

Figure 18–15   Colposcope.

rectal ampulla, irregularity of a dilated anal orifice, and persistence of a prominent anal verge.

Be cautious about offering an opinion as to whether sexual abuse has occurred on the basis of physical findings alone. The significance of many anatomic observations has not yet been established unequivocally. Currently, studies are under way to collect normative data describing the many variations of genital anatomy in nonabused prepubertal children.

Blood specimens for syphilis and hepatitis B serologic testing should be collected from all children with suspected abuse. Clear-cut guidelines have yet to be formulated for human immunodeficiency virus (HIV) testing. At this time, it is prudent, after discussion with the family, to test a child who has been assaulted by a stranger or by an individual known to have exhibited high-risk behavior (i.e., homosexuals, intravenous drug abusers). Repeat testing should also be offered for syphilis, hepatitis B, and HIV 3 to 6 months after the initial test.

ADOLESCENT CONTRACEPTION

Pregnancy is a leading cause of hospital admission among teenage women. By the end of high school, 50% of students have had sexual intercourse. Only 50% of teenagers use a contraceptive at first intercourse. Most adolescent pregnancies are unplanned and follow unprotected intercourse or ineffective use of a contraceptive method rather than failure of contraceptive method. Women who first give birth at an early age have subsequent children more rapidly, have more unwanted and out of wedlock births, and experience greater marital instability and lower educational attainment than women who have their first children later in their lives. Babies born of teenage mothers are more likely to be small for dates, to be born prematurely, and to have low Apgar scores at birth, factors associated with greater perinatal mortality. The chances of growing up in poverty, having school difficulties, trouble with the law, and child abuse are recognizably higher in children of teenage mothers.

Teens who use drugs, alcohol, or tobacco are more likely to be sexually active. Some report that they participated in intercourse as a result of excessive alcohol intake and later regretted such activities.

The personal cost to the young woman having an unintended pregnancy is considerable. In Canada, one in five teenage mothers uses services for abused women, and one in six has been treated for alcohol or drug addiction. The rate of a second pregnancy within 3 to 6 months of the first delivery is as high as 40% among adolescent mothers. At 2 years postpartum, the percentage of second pregnancies increases to 50%. It is estimated that 80% to 90% of repeat pregnancies in teenagers are unplanned and unwanted. Innovative

postpartum programs are needed for these teenagers; the programs must furnish infant and well-child care as well as support, enhance the parenting skills of, and provide contraception and lifestyle advice to the mother. More frequent and earlier visits should be scheduled, as 50% of teenagers fail to abstain from intercourse before their 6-week postpartum visit. Teenage mothers are at increased risk for depression and suicide, and many experience isolation and parenting difficulties.

The younger the adolescent girl, the less likely she is to request birth control from her physician. Therefore, it is important to talk openly and nonjudgmentally with adolescent patients and offer them information concerning sexuality and contraception. During such discussions, you can present abstinence as a positive choice; however, if abstinence is not the adolescent's choice, you must offer appropriate contraceptive options.

It is useful, when discussing various contraceptive methods, to have both concise information pamphlets and samples of the methods available for scrutiny—oral contraceptive pills (OCPs), intrauterine contraceptive devices, spermicidal creams, condoms, and diaphragms (Fig. 18–16).

Key Point

Fertility awareness methods of contraception are of little value in adolescent patients because of their inherent noncompliance and because their cycle intervals are frequently irregular.

Female barrier methods are not an acceptable contraceptive choice for most adolescents. The diaphragm is a dome-shaped rubber cup with a flexible rim that is inserted together with a spermicide into the vagina before intercourse. Many adolescents feel uncomfortable with the internal manipulation this barrier method requires. The most common cause of diaphragm failure in adolescents is nonuse. Reported first-year failure rates for diaphragms range from 2.1 to 18.6 pregnancies per 100 woman-years of use.

Another option is the contraceptive sponge, made of collagen impregnated with the spermicide nonoxynol 9. Individual fitting is not required, as it is for diaphragms, because the sponge is available in one size only; however, it still requires insertion into the vagina. As with the diaphragm, this manipulation makes its use unacceptable to many adolescents. The pregnancy rate in users of the contraceptive sponge is 13 to 15 per 100 woman-years of use; thus, a better option is the condom plus the contraceptive sponge or another spermicide.

Spermicides (foam, gel, films) are available without a prescription, but 26% of women become pregnant

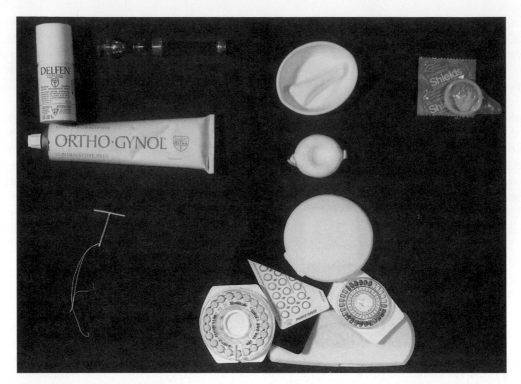

Figure 18–16   Counseling about contraceptive choices is facilitated by a complete kit of available devices.

within the first year of typical use of these products. Nonoxynol 9 is in many spermicide products, but there are now concerns that it may increase the risk of HIV transmission because it frequently induces vaginal irritation, which disrupts the integrity of the vaginal mucosa.

The condom is a barrier method that is actually more effective than the diaphragm in preventing pregnancy. Unfortunately, it is often very difficult for a girl to ask her partner to use a condom, underscoring the importance of discussing contraception with both male and female patients. The lubricated latex condom without spermicide is effective in protecting against both sexually transmitted diseases and pregnancy. First-year failure rate among typical users averages about 12%. It is necessary to give unsolicited detailed instructions to the adolescent, who may be too shy or embarrassed to ask just how a condom is used properly.

The female vaginal condom is available but should be deemed a method of protection against sexually transmitted diseases rather than a contraceptive method. The failure rate for the female condom is 21% in the first year of typical use.

The intrauterine contraceptive device (IUCD) is not commonly used in the young adolescent patient. The IUCD is frequently poorly tolerated by nulliparous patients because of associated menorrhagia and increased dysmenorrhea, but this issue may become less problematic with the progestin-containing systems now available. Perhaps more important than these adverse effects is that a young patient may have multiple sexual partners and therefore be at great risk for

contracting pelvic inflammatory disease with its long-term sequelae of chronic pelvic pain, infertility, and ectopic pregnancy. Because of an adolescent's potential greater risk for these complications, the use of an IUCD should be discouraged.

The low-dose OCP is the most effective means of preventing an unintended pregnancy. The lowest expected first-year failure rate is 0.1%. Frank discussion of the risk and benefits of OCPs often helps allay patients' concerns about its use. Healthy adolescents who are not overweight, are normotensive, and do not smoke have a low risk of developing life-threatening complications. The pill's contraceptive effect is secondary to inhibiting ovulation, thinning of the endometrial lining, changes in the cervical mucus that render it impermeable to sperm, and interference with fallopian tube motility.

Key Point

The OCP is directly or indirectly protective against pelvic inflammatory disease, ectopic pregnancy, iron deficiency anemia, ovarian neoplasms, fibrocystic breast disease, and endometrial cancer. Common adverse effects of the pill are nausea, depression, exacerbation of migraine headaches, and breast tenderness. Most of these effects can be avoided by selecting the appropriate preparation.

Because the adolescent girl is frequently an erratic, inconsistent user of the pill, "breakthrough bleeding" can be a problem. You can enhance compliance with the use of the pill by discussing breakthrough bleeding with the patient and instructing her on how to avoid it. Unfortunately, if breakthrough bleeding becomes a problem, it often makes the patient discontinue using the pill altogether, underscoring the necessity of close follow-up of adolescent patients through the first few cycles of pill use.

Advise the young patient that if she encounters problems with pill use, she should contact you or a well-trained nurse directly. Promoting such communication makes patients' use of the OCP more consistent and enables most problems to be addressed easily. With each return visit, talk to the patient about what she is doing to prevent pregnancy, so that you can identify and correct improper and inconsistent contraceptive use. If she uses a contraceptive erratically, talking about unintended pregnancy and its impact on her life may help to enhance her compliance.

All patients should be made aware of the existence of emergency postcoital contraception. First coital experiences are frequently unprotected. A condom may break or a diaphragm become displaced during intercourse; thus, postcoital methods have a place in the contraceptive armamentarium. Formerly the most commonly used regimen involved the use of a combination 50-µg pill, such as norgestrel–ethinyl estradiol (Ovral). Two tablets are given immediately to a patient who has had inadequately protected intercourse within the preceding 72 hours; the dose is repeated 12 hours later. This regimen frequently produces quite marked nausea, despite routine premedication with an antiemetic. Approximately 50% of women have difficulties with vomiting. If vomiting occurs within 2 hours of pill administration, the dose should be repeated. Emergency contraceptives containing levonorgestrel are now available (Plan B) and are reportedly associated with less nausea. More than 98% of women treated with these agents do not become pregnant as a result of that single exposure. Withdrawal bleeding, an indicator of treatment success, can be expected to occur within 21 days in 98% of women treated. Shortening of the cycle is seen in 20% of women. Women who do not have a spontaneous episode of bleeding 21 days after treatment should undergo serum pregnancy testing.

Long-acting injections of progestins such as medroxyprogesterone acetate (Depo-Provera) have been recognized as being an effective alternative means of providing contraception to women. The standard recommended dose is 150 mg every 90 days, given as a deep intramuscular injection. Ovulation is inhibited for 3 months after injection. This medication also produces atrophy of the endometrium and alters cervical mucus so it does not facilitate sperm transport. Complications related to this method of contraception include menstrual cycle disturbance varying from unpredictable breakthrough bleeding to amenorrhea, weight gain, and increased frequency of headaches. Studies of medroxyprogesterone have demonstrated a failure rate of 0.3 pregnancies per 100 woman-years.

A system in which polymeric silicone capsules of levonorgestrel (Norplant) are inserted under the skin of the upper arm is available. Levonorgestrel is a synthetic progestin that exhibits no significant estrogenic activity. The levonorgestrel slowly diffuses from its capsules, and the device is effective for up to 5 years of use. The mechanism of action is similar to that of medroxyprogesterone. The agent inhibits ovulation, thickens cervical mucus so as to make it impermeable to sperm, and produces an atrophic endometrium. The failure rate of this method is 0.4% over a 1-year period. Side effects include headache, mastodynia, acne, and weight gain. Menstrual abnormalities ranging from amenorrhea to intermenstrual bleeding are also seen. The cost of the implantable capsule makes its use prohibitive for most adolescent patients.

SUMMARY

The inclusion of gynecologic evaluation in every girl's physical examination increases familiarity and comfort with this assessment for both you and the child. Performing the assessment on many children enables you to discriminate between normal anatomic variants and pathologic changes. As a young girl approaches puberty, this examination gives you an excellent opportunity to offer information about developmental changes and sexuality in a casual, nonthreatening manner. Describing the concerns about sexuality expressed to you by other children often induces a shy girl to reveal her own concerns or misconceptions. The gynecologic examination is not difficult. It should be carried out in an organized fashion with appropriately proportioned instruments and diagnostic tools readily at hand. The confidence and thoughtfulness with which you approach the assessment is apparent to both child and parent.

SUGGESTED READINGS

Bays J, Chadwick D: Medical diagnosis of the sexually abused child. Child Abuse Negl 17:91, 1993. (Excellent illustrations.)
Berenson A, Heger A, Andrews S: Appearance of the hymen in newborns. Pediatrics 87:458, 1991. (Excellent illustrations.)
Berenson A, Heger A, Hayes J, et al: Appearance of the hymen in prepubertal girls. Pediatrics 89:387, 1992. (Excellent illustrations.)
Committee on Child Abuse and Neglect, American Academy of Pediatrics: Guidelines for the evaluation of sexual abuse of children: Subject review. Pediatrics 103:186, 1999.
Atabaki S, Paradise J: The medical evaluation of the sexually abused child: Lessons from a decade of research. Pediatrics 104:178, 1999.
Hatcher R, Trussell J, Stewart F, et al: Contraceptive Technology, 17th ed. New York, Irvington Publishers, 1998.
Huffman J, Dewhurst C, Capraro V: The Gynecology of Childhood and Adolescence, 2nd ed. Toronto, WB Saunders, 1981.

Pokorny S: Physical examination of the reproductive systems of female children and adolescents. Curr Probl Obstet Gynecol Fertil 8:202, 1990.

Pokorny S, Kozinetz C: Configuration and other anatomic details of the prepubertal hymen. Adolesc Pediatr Gynecol 1:97, 1988. (Excellent illustrations.)

Blythe M, Rosenthal S: Female adolescent sexuality. Obstet Gynecol Clin North Am 27:125, 2000.

The rights of the adolescent: The mature minor. J SOGC 23:343, 2001.

Pokorny S: Configuration of the prepubertal hymen. Am J Obstet Gynecol 157:950, 1987.

chapter 19

Clinical Assessment of the Skin in Children

LAURA A. FINLAYSON

Problems of the skin or its appendages are common in children, and it is therefore important to assess the skin in a logical and organized manner. In fact, a skin condition is the chief complaint for approximately 15% of patients in a family doctor's or pediatrician's office and is a secondary concern for other patients. A number of cutaneous conditions occur almost exclusively in infants and children, and most *dermatoses* (skin conditions) that are seen in adults are also seen in youngsters. There are many hereditary and congenital skin conditions (*genodermatoses*). Most common infectious diseases of childhood have cutaneous manifestations, and cutaneous involvement is a major feature of several multisystem disorders.

A child's skin is more reactive than that of an adult. It is more likely to blister and is more susceptible to warts and certain other infections. When children are ill, they are more likely than adults to have multisystem manifestations of illness. For example, they may demonstrate a complex of symptoms that could include rash, fever, anorexia, lethargy, and diarrhea. Paradoxically, physicians often regard skin diseases as relatively trivial in the vast scope of medicine—"the least of the patient's problems"—but the patient may be more concerned about cutaneous problems than about a more serious internal problem that is not visible to others. For example, a teenager with both psoriasis and cystic fibrosis may consider the psoriasis the more difficult of the two to accept.

Some physicians consider skin diseases difficult to diagnose for a variety of reasons. Because skin has a limited repertoire of reaction patterns, several disease processes may cause similar rashes. In addition, there are many variations in the appearance, location, and severity of both common and rare diseases of the skin, so a condition may look quite different in different patients. Finally, many skin conditions have one or more unhelpful protracted Latin names that are difficult to remember.

Despite these factors, it is possible to develop a simple, practical approach to most dermatologic problems. If you can assign a skin condition to a broad mor-phologic group on the basis of its appearance, you can learn or refer to lists of the conditions within the group. After a time, you will find it easier to recognize the primary lesions that identify the morphologic groups and the variations in common skin conditions in each group. Table 19–1 lists the most common skin problems seen in children and classifies them by morphologic appearance.

This chapter reviews the history and physical examination of the skin and illustrates the approach to diagnosis through case history examples. Color plates illustrate

Table 19–1 MORPHOLOGIC CLASSIFICATION OF COMMON PEDIATRIC SKIN CONDITIONS

Skin Lesion	Examples
Macules	Freckles, junctional nevi, tinea versicolor
Patches	Café au lait spots port-wine stains, vitiligo
Maculopapular rashes	Viral exanthems, drug eruptions
Papules	Warts, molluscum contagiosum, insect bites, compound nevi
Papules with burrows	Scabies
Papules with comedones	Acne
Plaques (nonscaly)	Mastocytomas, sebaceous nevus
Papulosquamous eruptions	Psoriasis, pityriasis rosea, lichen planus, fungal infections
Vesiculobullous eruptions	Friction blisters, acute contact dermatitis, herpes infections, bullous impetigo, staphylococcal scalded skin syndrome
Eczematous eruptions	Atopic dermatitis, seborrheic dermatitis, contact dermatitis, diaper dermatitis
Nodules or tumors	Epidermoid or pilar cysts, neurofibromas, lipomas
Alopecia	Alopecia areata, trichotillomania, tinea capitis

many of the problems discussed as well as some nevi commonly seen by pediatricians. Details and photographs of most pediatric dermatologic conditions can be found in the works cited in the Suggested Readings.

Key Point

Classifying a child's skin disease into one of several broad groups (e.g., maculopapular, papulosquamous, vesiculobullous) on the basis of the history and physical examination is a good start, even if a specific diagnostic label cannot be applied.

OBTAINING THE HISTORY

As always, a detailed history is fundamental in assessing each child's problem. Clues from casual inspection may direct your line of questioning and make the interview more efficient; but even if the diagnosis is obvious from a single glance, take the time to obtain a thorough history.

When children are too young to give a history firsthand, you can generally rely on the parents' interpretations. A baby who scratches constantly is almost certainly experiencing pruritus, although some itchy infants are irritable and sleep poorly but scratch very little. Children are suggestible; a 7-year-old who is asked, "Does your rash itch?" will almost certainly answer, "Yes." Instead, ask the child whether the rash bothers him or her in any way, and ask the parent whether the child sleeps well at night or is scratching frequently. Pruritus from any cause is always worse at night, because (1) there are fewer external distracting stimuli and (2) the warmth of the bedclothes causes vasodilation in the skin, which exacerbates itching. Some skin conditions, such as poison ivy dermatitis and lichen planus, are intensely itchy, and relieving the pruritus may be more important than improving the rash.

Initially, you are seeing the child's skin problem at a particular moment in its evolution. The parents' description of its appearance at the onset and careful documentation of its evolution are therefore very important. Acute skin eruptions are usually dynamic, and the distribution or morphology may change rapidly. By contrast, chronic eruptions are more likely to have a stable appearance.

Key Point

Acute skin eruptions can change rapidly. A rash that is undiagnosable one day may be quite obviously diagnosable the next day.

Table 19–2 EXAMPLES OF TERMINOLOGY MOST PARENTS UNDERSTAND

Medical Term	Lay Term
Macule	Dot
Papule	Little bump
Nodule	Big bump
Plaque	Raised or thickened area
Vesicle	Little blister
Bulla	Big blister
Pustule	Pus pocket, pimple
Desquamation	Scaling, flaking
Crusts	Scabs
Excoriations	Scratch marks
Comedones	Blackheads, whiteheads

Some patients and parents are incredibly observant when it comes to skin, and others notice no details at all. Let both patient and parents give their descriptions, then ask for clarification. Use terms they will understand, such as those suggested in Table 19–2.

Some words used to describe skin eruptions are nonspecific and are often used improperly by patients or physicians. An example of such nonspecificity is the word *blister*. If a child presents with a vesiculobullous eruption, ask the following questions (in words they can understand):

- How long ago did they start?
- How long does each blister last?
- Did all the blisters start at once?
- Are the blisters localized or generalized?
- Do they arise on an erythematous (red) base or on normal skin?
- What color is the fluid within them—serous (clear), purulent (cloudy), seropurulent, hemorrhagic (bloody), or serohemorrhagic (pink)?
- Are the blisters tense or flaccid?
- Do they break easily?
- Is there associated tenderness or itching?
- Has the child had any contact with infectious disease?
- Have there been any blisters in the mouth or in the genital area (mucocutaneous lesions) or on the scalp?
- Has the child had any systemic symptoms?
- What has been put on the skin before or after the blistering started?

Answers to such questions will narrow the differential diagnosis.

For a rash, ask what the child and parents think caused it. Their suspicions may turn out to be correct, or they may have an unfounded fear (e.g., skin cancer) that can be put to rest.

Ask for details of exacerbating or relieving factors and of seasonal influences on the course of the skin problem. Some types of dermatitis become worse in the winter because of the lower humidity. The influence of sun exposure is an important factor. Conditions such as lupus erythematosus are exacerbated by sun exposure, whereas psoriasis usually improves significantly with sun exposure.

Sometimes you need to find out what routine care is given to the skin and the clothing that is in contact with it. For instance, in eczematous eruptions, you must learn how often the child is bathed, what kind of soap and detergent are used, and what moisture creams or other preparations have been applied to the skin.

Key Point

Frequently, several topical agents have been applied before the child visits a physician, and it is important to find out what has been used both before and after the problem began.

Some proprietary medications may be bland and soothing and provide symptomatic relief. Others may contain active ingredients that are inappropriate for the child's problem or are in the wrong concentration. Some may contain ingredients that are common topical sensitizers and may aggravate the skin problem. Ask about any prescribed topical medications used before the current assessment of the child. Often, parents may not remember the names of topical preparations. If necessary, call the pharmacist to find out what was prescribed.

Obtain a detailed history of all prescribed or over-the-counter oral medications, including doses and duration of administration. Ask specifically about non-prescription medications, such as acetylsalicylic acid, acetaminophen, and cold remedies. Drugs can cause rashes of all descriptions, although the most common are maculopapular eruptions, urticaria, and erythema multiforme. Ask about any previous reactions to medications, and document the type and severity of each.

Request details of any previous skin problems; these may or may not be related to the presenting problem. Some conditions, such as atopic dermatitis, can resolve only to flare up years later under certain circumstances.

Ask about any associated systemic symptoms, such as fever, malaise, cough, sore throat, anorexia, diarrhea, and joint pains.

Obtaining a family history is important, because numerous skin conditions are genetically determined, and many chronic dermatoses are considered hereditary, although they may be polygenic or exhibit incomplete penetrance. Sometimes an environmental trigger may unmask a disease in an individual who is genetically predisposed. For example, a sore throat commonly precedes the development of guttate psoriasis.

A patient presenting with a genodermatosis or a neurocutaneous syndrome may or may not have a known family history of the disorder. Absence of a family history may be due to the following factors:

- A high mutation rate (50% for neurofibromatosis)
- Recessive inheritance or incomplete penetrance causing the condition to skip generations
- An extended family history that may be unknown

Many skin conditions occur on clothed skin and are not considered a proper topic of conversation between generations. False-positive family histories are also occasionally obtained when past diagnoses have been wrong or are misunderstood.

At times, the family history is not as important for diagnosis as for prognosis. For example, a teenager with multiple large and irregular nevi who has a family history of malignant melanoma is at significant risk for development of a melanoma; therefore, advise him or her about sun protection, regular self-examinations, and periodic professional examination to prevent melanoma or detect it in an early, curable stage. The positive family history is a significant risk factor in this case.

Key Point

Ask about recent travel outside the country to properly diagnose nonendemic infections or to find out about environmental conditions such as high heat and humidity, which can induce or exacerbate a skin condition.

APPROACH TO THE PHYSICAL EXAMINATION

When you begin the physical examination of the child's skin, you should have in mind a general differential diagnosis based on the details of the history. Sometimes, after examining the skin, you will find that additional history is required. For example, if the history suggests an exacerbation of atopic dermatitis and you find multiple crusted vesicles on examination, you need to ask about the patient's contact with people who have cold sores, because eczema herpeticum is a likely cause of this flare-up.

Good light is essential to adequate examination of the skin. Its importance is often overlooked. Natural light is best, and it may help to move the patient near a window. However, natural light is not always available in clinics and hospital rooms, and fluorescent light may distort colors and minimize subtle skin changes. For examination of localized lesions, using a spotlight can help. Also, a magnifying glass helps you to appreciate details.

Examine the Entire Skin Surface

Always look at the entire skin surface, even if the history suggests a localized problem. The dermatologic examination includes the entire skin, the visible mucous membranes, and the skin appendages (hair, nails, and sweat glands), for the following reasons:

1. There may be involvement of other skin sites that no one had recognized, such as a small raised scaly plaque on the scalp or nail pitting in a child with possible psoriasis.
2. Other cutaneous manifestations may be found that relate to the presenting complaint, such as reticulate white plaques on the buccal mucosa of a child with possible lichen planus. These findings can help to confirm or rule out a diagnosis.
3. Other unrelated but important skin problems may be discovered. For example, the presenting complaint may be warts on the hands, but a complete skin examination may reveal a malignant melanoma on the back.

The extent, distribution, and severity of a skin problem are best appreciated by undressing the child and viewing most of the skin at once. You can, however, perform this step after the youngster is more comfortable with the examination procedure. Older children feel more self-conscious about being unclothed for a skin examination than they are by the same extent of undress for a chest or neurologic examination. Give the child a gown, and leave the room while he or she changes into it. It is acceptable to uncover and examine one area at a time in a gowned patient, but do not try to peek under tight clothing. For children younger than 2 years, a gown is unnecessary. The toddler's sense of modesty is relatively undeveloped, and it is much easier to examine the child properly when he or she is wearing nothing more than a diaper or underpants.

Wear examining gloves if the child has eroded or oozing lesions and when you examine the mucous membranes. Generally, however, gloves are not necessary and tend to make the youngster feel uncomfortable.

Key Point

You can learn much if you simply start the examination by assessing the distribution and extent of the skin problem and the presence or absence of symmetry. Is the condition generalized or localized? Are the scalp, face, and neck involved? Is the eruption predominantly proximal or distal, and are the palms and soles involved? Are there any mucous membrane lesions?

Primary Lesions

A lesion is referred to as *primary* if it is the first change to occur in the skin because of the disease. *Secondary* lesions can be caused by external factors, such as scratching and secondary infection, or may evolve from the primary lesion. Proper assessment of the type of primary lesions present is essential. The patient may have just one type of primary lesion or a variety of primary and secondary lesions.

MACULES AND PATCHES

A *macule* is a small (less than 1 cm), circumscribed, flat area of change in skin color. Describe subtle changes, and think about what can cause such a color change (see later discussion of color changes) while continuing to examine the child. Freckles are examples of hyperpigmented macules. Alternatively, macules may be hypopigmented. Tinea versicolor, a common superficial fungal infection, may show either hypopigmented or hyperpigmented macules.

Larger, flat areas of color change are called *patches*. A good example of a patch is a port-wine stain. Often, macules and papules may coalesce. Drug eruptions and viral exanthems are typically *maculopapular*, an overused term that should be applied strictly as defined—combined macules and papules.

PAPULES

A *papule* is a small (less than 1 cm) elevated lesion that is palpable above the skin surface. Note the distribution and color. If papules are multiple, are they discrete, or do they coalesce? Comment on the shape in all dimensions (e.g., the papules are polygonal and flat-topped in lichen planus, and they are round and dome-topped with umbilication in molluscum contagiosum; Plate 19–1). Describe any change on the surface, such as scaling or crusting. Palpate the lesion to determine whether it is soft or firm, and try to distinguish which layer of skin it arises in—epidermis or dermis.

PLAQUES

A *plaque* is a raised lesion in which the surface area is greater than the elevation. Plaques can arise directly from the skin or can develop from a coalescence of papules. They can vary in size from 1 cm to huge plaques covering most of the body. Note whether the surface is smooth or scaly. Comment on any subtle changes, such as plugging of hair follicles within the plaque (seen commonly in discoid lupus erythematosus). If scaling is present, describe it in detail (see later discussion of scaling). Some eruptions show a combination of scaly papules and plaques; they are termed *papulosquamous* eruptions. The most common papulosquamous eruptions seen in the pediatric age group are psoriasis (Plate 19–2), pityriasis rosea (Plate 19–3), and fungal infections.

NODULES AND TUMORS

Nodules and tumors are circumscribed and elevated lesions that are larger than papules. Nodules tend to arise from deeper structures, therefore displaying depth as well as elevation (Plate 19–4). Tumors can arise from deep structures, the dermis, or the epidermis. As with papules, describe the shape, outline, elevation, depth, surface characteristics, and firmness of a nodule or tumor as well as its mobility on palpation.

VESICLES AND BULLAE

A *vesicle* is a small (less than 1 cm) raised cavity containing fluid. A *bulla* is a larger lesion (more than 1 cm). Both are called "blisters" by lay persons. Look at the distribution and arrangement, which may be important for diagnostic purposes. The blisters in poison ivy contact dermatitis are commonly linear in arrangement (Plate 19–5), whereas those of herpes simplex are clustered closely together. Note whether the blisters arise on erythematous skin, such as in a blistering contact dermatitis, or on apparently normal skin, such as with friction blisters. Describe the color of fluid within the lesions—serous, hemorrhagic, or a combination.

Noting whether the vesicles and bullae are tense or flaccid provides clues to the layers of skin in which they arise. Blisters that are more superficial, such as those of bullous impetigo, are more flaccid because fewer layers of cells make up the roof of the lesion, whereas those arising from deeper layers tend to be tense. The pathologic process is also likely to be more superficial if there are multiple erosions present, because these blisters rupture easily and the roof of the lesion is no longer present. Often, a small peripheral rim of epidermis is still adherent around the periphery of an erosion, indicating that this eruption is vesiculobullous (see later) even though no blisters remain intact.

Check for the *Nikolsky sign* in vesiculobullous conditions. The Nikolsky sign exists if the layers of skin can be easily separated with a gentle rubbing or shearing force (Plate 19–6). This phenomenon is seen in staphylococcal scalded skin syndrome, toxic epidermal necrolysis, pemphigus, and some forms of epidermolysis bullosa.

Search for any vesicles or erosions on the visible mucosa. It is unusual to see blisters in the intact state in the mouth because there is so much friction and trauma from eating and talking.

The group of disorders in which blisters are the primary lesions is called *vesiculobullous* eruptions. There are many causes of vesiculobullous eruptions in children. Some are rare hereditary blistering disorders, such as epidermolysis bullosa. Common infectious diseases, such as varicella (Plate 19–7), bullous impetigo, and herpes simplex, produce vesiculobullous eruptions. Skin conditions due to exogenous factors such as friction and sunburn frequently cause blistering. A vesicular reaction may be caused by various types of contact dermatitis, either irritant or allergic in origin. (A prime example of allergic contact dermatitis is that caused by poison ivy, shown in Plate 19–5.) Vascular reactions such as erythema multiforme and some forms of vasculitis may cause vesicles.

> **Key Point**
>
> Many drugs can cause various patterns of blistering on the skin. Drug eruptions are most commonly maculopapular or urticarial, but almost every pattern of skin eruption can be caused by drugs.

Finally, there is a rare group of primary vesiculobullous disorders in children, including chronic bullous dermatosis of childhood, pemphigus, bullous pemphigoid, and dermatitis herpetiformis.

PUSTULES

Pustules are similar to vesicles, but the fluid within them is a purulent exudate. Try to determine whether a pustule is associated with a hair follicle (folliculitis). Pustules frequently represent skin infections, which can be either primary (e.g., bullous impetigo) or secondary infection of another skin condition (e.g., infected atopic dermatitis). Pustules are formed by an abnormal accumulation of leukocytes with or without microorganisms and cellular debris. Not all pustules, therefore, represent infection. For example, the pustules of pustular psoriasis are sterile if the fluid is cultured, and they arise from chemotaxis of neutrophils into the epidermis.

WHEALS OR URTICARIA

A *wheal* is a transient raised lesion caused by edema within the skin. The lay term for *urticaria* is "hives," which are usually erythematous and vary greatly in size, shape, and number. They are caused by an extravasation of fluid from the cutaneous blood vessels and vasodilation. The extravasation is usually secondary to local release of histamine and other chemical mediators. The individual lesions usually resolve within 24 hours, but they may continue to evolve at different sites. The course of an urticarial eruption may therefore be arbitrarily defined as *acute* (lasting less than 6 weeks) or *chronic* (longer than 6 weeks).

Angioedema is a similar process that occurs deeper in the skin, giving a less well-demarcated localized swelling, which often is tender rather than pruritic. Patients prone to urticaria often have *dermatographism*, in which the wheals form in lines wherever pressure is exerted on the skin, such as under tight clothing. It can be demonstrated by firmly stroking the letter X on the patient's back; if dermatographism is present, an urticarial wheal will form within a few minutes (Plate 19–8).

COMEDONES

A *comedone* is a plug in a hair follicle. Usually occurring in areas with many sebaceous glands, comedones are a primary lesion in acne. The plug consists of clumped keratin and sebum. Comedones can be either closed (whiteheads) or open (blackheads). The black color of open comedones is due to oxidation of the plugged material when it is exposed to air.

BURROWS

Burrows are faint linear tunnels in the layers of the superficial epidermis, usually 2 to 7 mm long (Fig. 19–1). They are the primary lesions in scabies and are most easily found between the fingers and around the wrists and ankles. The female scabies mite (*Sarcoptes scabiei*) and some of her eggs may be visible only as a tiny black dot at the blind end of the burrow.

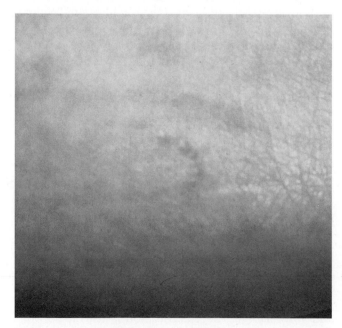

Figure 19–1 Scabies with typical burrows.

Patients with scabies usually have numerous excoriated inflammatory papules with some burrows among them. The morphology of scabies may vary with age. In an infant, there may be lesions over the entire body, including the face and scalp, whereas in older children and adults, the head area is spared. Infants may present with pustules on the palms and soles, a pattern less common in older individuals. Chronic scabies that has gone undiagnosed for months may appear as crusted nodules rather than the more typical papules and burrows (Plate 19–9).

TELANGIECTASIA

Telangiectasia represents permanently dilated superficial blood vessels in the skin. On *diascopy* (viewing through a microscope slide pressed firmly against the skin), they blanch almost completely but fill again as soon as the pressure is released. Primary telangiectasia can be hereditary, idiopathic, or a manifestation of one of several rare syndromes. Secondary telangiectasia may be related to localized inflammation, collagen vascular diseases, sun damage, liver disease, or pregnancy.

Secondary Lesions

Secondary lesions can evolve from primary lesions or can arise from external factors, such as scratching.

SCALING

Scaling, which results from the accumulation of desquamating skin cells, can be primary or secondary. It is commonly seen in disorders of keratinization. Normally, cells that are fully keratinized *desquamate* (flake off) invisibly on the skin surface. Scaling occurs if there is hyperproliferation of the epidermis, as in psoriasis, or if there is an abnormality in cohesion of keratinocytes that causes them to clump together abnormally, as in some types of ichthyosis. Describe the type of scaling as accurately as possible—coarse, fine, white, yellow, silvery, greasy, peripheral, or adherent.

CRUSTS

Crusting results from accumulation of dried exudates or transudates on the skin (Plate 19–10). A crust from dried serous fluid is honey colored and easily dislodged, a crust from purulent material is dark brown and tightly adherent, and a crust from sanguineous or bloody fluid is red-brown to black and tightly adherent. Crusts are seen on any oozing eruption, such as infected eczema or a vesiculobullous eruption.

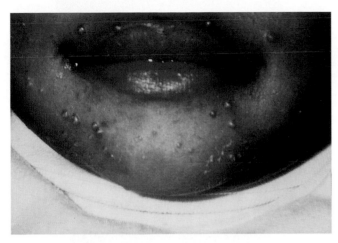

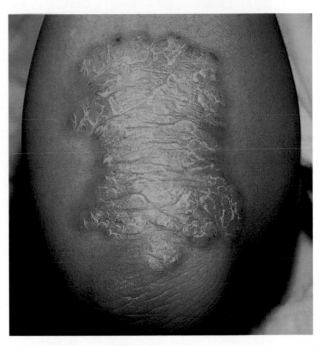

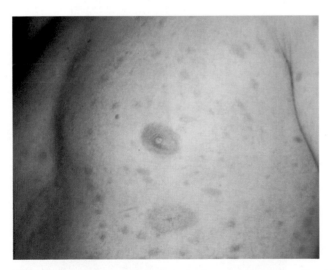

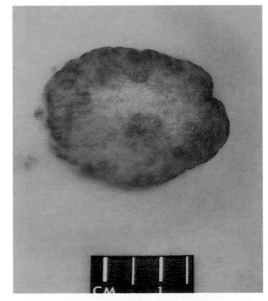

Plate 19–1 Molluscum contagiosum. Numerous dome-topped umbilicated papules. Note the small central plugs, which consist microscopically of denatured cells and viral particles (molluscum bodies).

Plate 19–2 A well demarcated, irregularly shaped plaque of psoriasis with silvery scales on the elbow.

Plate 19–3 Pityriasis rosea. Note the larger scale plaque (herald plaque) that preceded the truncal eruption of small, oval, salmon-pink plaques.

Plate 19–4 Capillary hemangioma. Strawberry-colored vascular nodule. This lesion is in the involuting stage, and the flesh-colored tissue at the center will gradually replace the vascular component as it resolves.

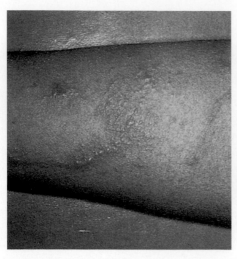

Plate 19–5 Poison ivy contact dermatitis. Note the linear distribution of vesicles resulting from brushing against the plant.

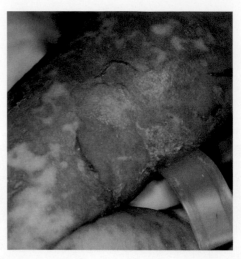

Plate 19–6 Toxic epidermal necrolysis. A diffuse erythematous vesiculobullous eruption resulting from a drug reaction. The epidermis is easily peeled away from the dermis—a finding known as the Nikolsky sign.

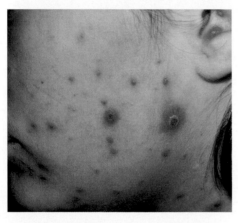

Plate 19–7 Varicella (chickenpox). Small vesicles on an erythematous base, pustules, and seropurulent crusts.

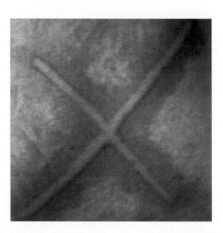

Plate 19–8 Dermatographism. A urticarial response elicited by firm stroking of the skin.

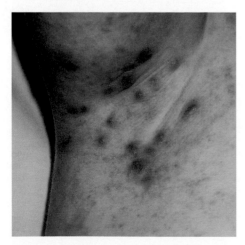

Plate 19–9 Nodular scabies. Erythematous papules and nodules in the axilla. This variant of scabies may be seen in children younger than 2 years.

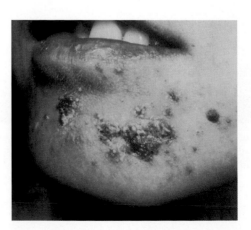

Plate 19–10 Impetigo. Grouped erythematous papules and pustules with honey-colored crusts.

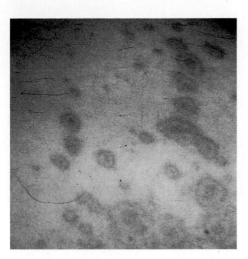

Plate 19–11 Erythema multiforme—typical target lesions.

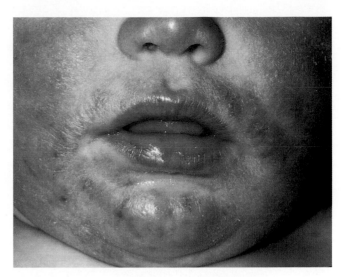

Plate 19–12 Atopic dermatitis—facial rash. Eczematous eruption on cheeks and chin with sparing and pallor around the mouth and nose.

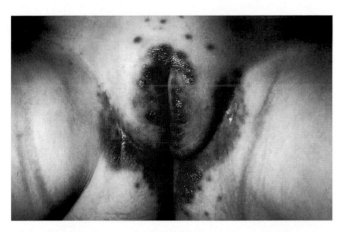

Plate 19–13 Diaper rash—candidiasis. Bright red erythematous plaques involving the deep folds of the diaper area with satellite papules and pustules.

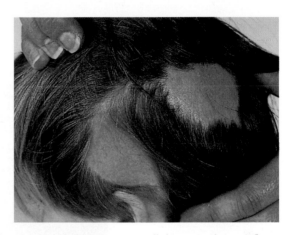

Plate 19–14 Alopecia areata. Well-demarcated, noninflammatory, hairless patches.

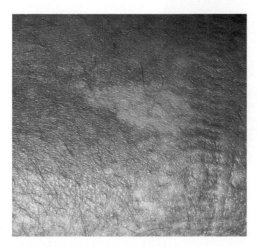

Plate 19–15 Ash leaf spot. A 2-cm, elliptical, hypopigmented patch on a limb with smaller hypopigmented macules around it—a specific skin lesion of tuberous sclerosis.

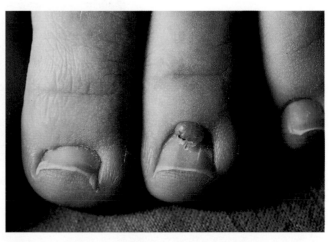

Plate 19–16 Periungual fibroma. Pink fibrous papule at proximal nail fold—a specific skin lesion of tuberous sclerosis.

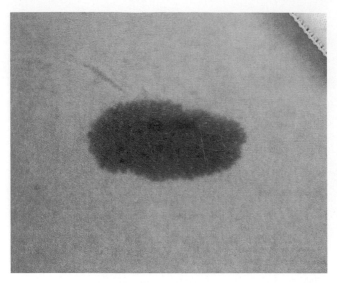

Plate 19–17 Congenital nevus. A 3.5-cm, well-demarcated, medium brown pigmented lesion with a slightly irregular border and some darker macules within it.

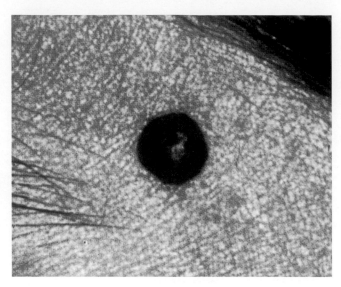

Plate 19–18 Compound nevus. An acquired 5-mm, dome-topped, dark brown pigmented papule with uniform pigmentation and regular borders.

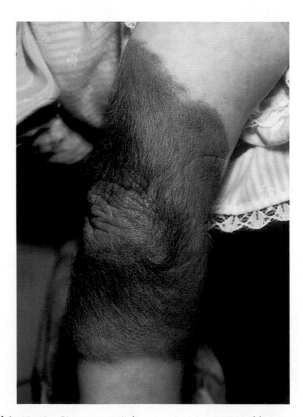

Plate 19–19 Giant congenital nevus. A giant congenital hairy nevus on the arm.

EXCORIATIONS

Excoriations are defined as linear breaks in the skin at various depths caused by scratching.

> **Key Point**
>
> Excoriations may alter the appearance of an eruption to the point that describing the original morphology properly is difficult.

In extremely pruritic conditions such as scabies, it may be necessary to look carefully to find an identifiable primary lesion (a burrow) remaining among the excoriations.

FISSURE

A *fissure* is a linear crack in the skin. Fissures are usually seen on the hands and feet, where pressure and movement may induce fissures to form on inflamed or thickened skin.

EROSIONS AND ULCERS

An *erosion* is a circumscribed loss of the epidermal layer, whereas an *ulcer* is a deeper area of loss of tissue that extends into the dermis, to subcutaneous tissue, or even deeper. When describing an ulcer, comment on the shape, size, and depth, and describe the edges—rolled, translucent, violaceous, indurated, undermined, or jagged. Note also the condition of the surrounding skin and of the base of the ulcer and the presence or absence of eschar, fibrinous debris, crusts, or granulation tissue.

ATROPHY

Atrophy results from a thinning of one or more of the layers of skin. Atrophy may be confined to the epidermis, in which very fine wrinkling is evident on the surface (referred to as "cigarette paper wrinkling"). This condition is best appreciated with tangential lighting and by gentle stretching of the skin with the fingers. Dermal atrophy causes an indentation or depression in the skin that often can be appreciated on palpation as well as on inspection.

SCAR

A *scar* results from fibrous tissue repair of skin that has been damaged below the level of the epidermis. Scars can be either *atrophic* (level with the skin) or *hypertrophic* (raised). The severity of scarring that develops after trauma varies in individuals. A *keloid* is a very hypertrophic scarring reaction that extends beyond the original area of injury and shows no sign of flattening with time. Some areas of the body, such as the upper chest and back, show much more prominent scarring than other sites because the dermis is very thick on these areas.

Special Patterns

Some morphologic terms referring to special patterns require further definition. *Annular* lesions are circular or ringlike with central clearing. *Discoid* or *nummular* lesions are round or coin-shaped without a tendency to central clearing. *Arciform* lesions form arcs or partial circles. *Polycyclic* lesions are usually multiple annular lesions that often coalesce. A *target* or *iris* lesion shows alternating circular bands of pink and darker red, resembling a target; the target lesion is the hallmark of erythema multiforme and is diagnostic if present but is not always seen in the condition (Plate 19–11).

Eczema and Dermatitis

Dermatitis simply means inflammation of the skin. The term is often used interchangeably with the term *eczema*.

> **Key Point**
>
> Lay persons usually use the word *eczema* to mean *atopic dermatitis*, but *eczema* merely denotes a morphologic appearance in which there is erythema, usually poorly demarcated, with superficial scaling and fissuring, with or without vesicles and crusting.

Eczematous disorders are often pruritic and therefore secondarily excoriated as well. They look quite different depending on the stage of the condition. Acute eczemas consist of small vesicles, oozing, crusting, and bright erythema. Subacute eczemas manifest as pink scaly patches or plaques (Plate 19–12). More chronic eczematous disorders frequently show *lichenification* (thickening of the skin with accentuation of surface markings).

Eczema is not a diagnosis but a descriptive term. Depending on the history, distribution, and clinical appearance, the term must be qualified to refer to atopic dermatitis, seborrheic dermatitis, irritant or allergic contact dermatitis, or stasis dermatitis.

Color Changes

Normal skin color is mostly determined by a combination of the individual's constitutional level of melanization (determined by hereditary or racial background) and the blood vessels underneath. Note the color of the child's uninvolved skin, and compare it with the color of the skin problem. Many skin eruptions are erythematous, and the erythema can be from inflammation, vasodilation of blood vessels, or blood that has extravasated out of the vessels (*purpura*). Diascopy may be helpful. Erythema due to vasodilation blanches when the vessels are compressed; purpura, by contrast, does not blanch.

> **Key Point**
>
> Describing the subtle hue of erythema often suggests a certain diagnosis. Erythema is violaceous in lichen planus, salmon-pink in pityriasis rosea, and beefy red in candidiasis (Plate 19–13).

In dark-skinned races, it is more difficult to assess color changes in the skin. Erythema may be difficult to detect, especially for the inexperienced examiner. Hypopigmentation, however, is more prominent in a darker-skinned patient because of the greater contrast with the normal skin color.

Secondary changes, such as scaling or crusting, may significantly alter the underlying color of an eruption, such as when the erythema of a psoriatic plaque is obscured by thick silver scales.

Increased brown color of the skin is usually due to higher amounts of melanin. Hemosiderin deposits caused by chronic extravasation of blood from blood vessels also produces a brown color, but the shade is usually more tan or yellowish.

White discoloration can result from (1) a decrease in the amount of melanin pigment, (2) a change in melanin distribution and packaging within the skin, or (3) a constriction of the cutaneous blood vessels. A variety of disease processes can cause this appearance. Both hypopigmentation and hyperpigmentation commonly occur after an inflammatory process, and these post-inflammatory pigmentary changes will gradually fade.

> **Key Point**
>
> It is important to explain to parents that postinflammatory pigmentary changes will fade, because parents often believe that the changes represent permanent scars.

Examination of the skin with a Wood lamp is useful in pigmentary abnormalities. The emitted light from this lamp is in the ultraviolet A (UVA) range, with a narrow spectrum around 366 nm, because the other wavelengths are filtered out by a special filter. The Wood lamp allows much clearer visualization of hypopigmented conditions. Because there is less pigment to absorb the light, more light is reflected back. Completely depigmented conditions, such as vitiligo, show stark contrast and appear bright white under Wood lamp examination. The lamp is also useful for detecting certain types of fungal infection, because some fungi elaborate a pigment that fluoresces when exposed to the lamp's wavelength of light.

A blue-gray color is usually caused by the presence of elongated melanocytes deep within the dermis, as in mongolian spots on the lower back of dark-skinned infants. More of the blue wavelength of light is reflected back from the surface, thus giving this color. Occasionally, a gray color develops from deposition of a drug-pigment complex or from ingestion of metallic substances such as silver compounds.

Yellowish discoloration of the skin can be due to lipid deposition, to pigments such as carotene or bilirubin, or to pigments from degenerating red blood cells, as seen in the resolving stages of purpura.

APPROACH TO THE EXAMINATION OF MUCOSA AND SKIN APPENDAGES

Buccal Mucosa

> **Key Point**
>
> Always examine the child's mouth at the end of the physical examination and after you have gained the youngster's confidence.

Many children open their mouths amazingly wide when requested to do so and do not require a tongue depressor. Comment on the state of the tongue, palate, gingiva, buccal mucosa, pharynx, and teeth. At times, examination of this area yields the diagnosis. For example, Koplik spots are visible in early measles, and reticulate white plaques on the buccal mucosa may be seen in lichen planus.

Nails

Examine the fingernails and toenails, noting the color of the nail beds and nail plates as well as the condition of the surrounding skin. Search for any thickening or subungual debris of the nail plate, which are seen in such diverse disorders as psoriasis and *onychomycosis* (fungal infection of the nail). Note changes in the nail plate, such as ridging or pitting. Pitting is seen very commonly in psoriasis.

Look for *onycholysis* (separation of the nail plate from the nail bed), which is seen most commonly in psoriasis but also in trauma and in some thyroid disorders, and is secondary to certain drug reactions.

Scalp and Hair

Many cutaneous disorders have scalp or hair manifestations that are easily overlooked. Check the scalp for areas of inflammation, scaling, and hair loss. If inflammation is present, be specific as to the morphology of the lesions: Are they erythematosus plaques with silvery scales, as in psoriasis, or scaly plaques with follicular keratotic plugging, scarring, and hair loss, as in discoid lupus erythematosus?

If alopecia is the presenting problem, decide whether it is diffuse or patchy, inflammatory or noninflammatory, and scarring or nonscarring. Assignment of the alopecia to one of these broad groups simplifies the differential diagnosis. For example, if an alopecia is patchy, nonscarring, and noninflammatory, it is probably either alopecia areata (Plate 19–14) or *trichotillomania* (hair pulling). The bald patch is smooth in alopecia areata, but broken-off hairs are seen in trichotillomania. In alopecia areata, look for so-called exclamation mark hairs, which are 1 to 2 mm in length, tapered at the attached end, and seen around the periphery of developing bald patches (Fig. 19–2).

With a hand lens, examine the character of the hair shafts and the presence or absence of a telogen (*resting phase*) bulb at the end of easily pulled hairs. Telogen hairs, which have a small hypopigmented bulb at the root end, are the hairs that come out daily with normal brushing and washing. In *telogen effluvium*, which can

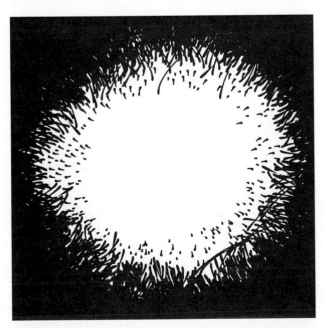

Figure 19–2 "Exclamation mark" hairs in alopecia areata.

be precipitated by pregnancy, fever, or surgery, a higher percentage of hairs are in the telogen phase, and the patient experiences a temporary diffuse loss of hair.

Several types of hair shaft defect may lead to alopecia or breakage of hairs. To detect structural abnormalities, it is necessary to examine several hairs with a light microscope or electron microscope.

Wood light examination (see earlier) has been used traditionally as a screening examination for tinea capitis. Some types of fungal infection of the scalp fluoresce under this UVA light, particularly those caused by the *Microsporum* genus. Fluorescence under Wood light examination confirms the diagnosis. Absence of fluorescent under Wood light examination does not, however, exclude the possibility of tinea capitis, because several cutaneous fungal infections do not fluoresce.

Case Histories

Case 1

Robert, age 15 years, comes to your office with the complaint of a relatively sudden onset of an extensive scaly skin eruption.

What questions are important to establish a differential diagnosis? You obtain the following pertinent history: The rash began 3 weeks ago with the appearance of a solitary raised scaly plaque, which is oval and about 3 cm wide, on his left upper chest. Over the next week, numerous smaller scaly thin plaques developed, mostly on the trunk. The rash has not changed much since then. It is not symptomatic. There has been no involvement of the scalp or mucous membranes.

Functional inquiry is normal, except that Robert had a sore throat a few weeks ago. He has been taking no prescribed or over-the-counter medications. He showers daily with a mild soap and does not apply any other preparations to his skin. He has never been sexually active and has no past history of skin problems. There is no family history of psoriasis or other skin diseases. At this point, you suspect that Robert has pityriasis rosea, on the basis of the history of the larger lesion (the herald patch) that preceded the more extensive asymptomatic eruption. With this background information, you have also considered guttate psoriasis, nummular or contact dermatitis, drug eruption, and secondary syphilis (which, although rare, must be considered in an adolescent with this history), and you have asked specific questions to help rule out or further consider those disorders.

What do you expect the physical examination to show? Robert has an extensive papulosquamous eruption most prominent on the trunk, with slight involvement of the proximal limbs and neck. There is sparing of the scalp, face, mucous membranes, palms, and soles. Oval, salmon-pink plaques are arranged parallel to the lines of skin cleavage on his trunk (*Christmas tree distribution*). The individual plaques are thin and just palpable above the skin surface; most measure about 1 cm, except for a 3-cm-diameter plaque on the left side of his chest (see Plate 19–3). There is scaling around the periphery of most of the plaques, with the free edge of the scale facing toward the center of the lesion (a "toeing-in" or "collarette" scale). His fingernails are normal.

What is your conclusion? It is now obvious that Robert has both the classic history and typical clinical appearance of pityriasis rosea. You therefore reassure him that he has a self-limited condition that will resolve without treatment in about 6 weeks.

Robert's story illustrates how knowledge of the classic features of common skin problems can make the diagnosis easy.

Key Point

Many skin conditions have characteristic historical features and physical findings. For example, the typical features of pityriasis rosea include the herald patch (actually a plaque in most cases), which precedes the more generalized eruption, Christmas tree distribution, collarette scale, and spontaneous resolution.

Case 2

Joanne, who is 8 years old, is brought in from a rural area with a preliminary diagnosis of early-onset acne. A few small red bumps were noticed around her nose when she was 4 years old. More of these lesions have developed gradually, and the original papules are still present. They have never had pus within them, and Joanne does not have "blackheads" or "whiteheads." Joanne's parents have been applying an acne gel containing 5% benzoyl peroxide for 6 months, with no improvement.

What is your line of thinking at this point? Several factors in the history so far make you question the presumptive diagnosis of acne. Age 4 years is very young for the development of acne. Joanne has had no pustules or comedones, both of which are hallmarks of acne, and there has been no improvement with treatment. You decide that a detailed history is needed.

Joanne's past medical history reveals that she had a brief seizure 2 months ago, which was never investigated because it did not recur and it is difficult for the family to travel to the city. Joanne is not taking any medications. Functional inquiry reveals that she has failed two grades in school and is much slower to learn than her sibling. She has a few light-colored birthmarks. Her mother has a few red papules around the nose and gets large "hangnails" around her fingernails and toenails.

During the interview, Joanne does not contribute to her history when asked questions; she is restless and behaves like a younger child.

What physical signs are you specifically looking for on the physical examination? Examination of Joanne's skin reveals approximately two dozen erythematous papules on her face, mostly around the nasolabial folds. These are 2 to 3 mm, bright red, firm, and smooth on top. Not all of these papules are associated with a hair follicle, as one would expect in acne, and there are no comedones or pustules.

At this point, your presumptive diagnosis is that these papules represent angiofibromas (otherwise known as adenoma sebaceum), a hallmark of tuberous sclerosis. The history of a seizure and mental slowness is also in keeping with this disorder. You continue the examination, looking particularly for other cutaneous manifestations of this syndrome. There are five faint hypopigmented patches on the trunk and limbs (the "birthmarks"), so you shine a Wood light on the skin, which makes them more obvious. Each is 2 to 3 cm in diameter, oval, and not raised or scaly (Plate 19–15). These patches are called *ash leaf macules* or patches because of their shape. Joanne also has two firm pink polypoid papules along the lateral aspects of her toenails (*periungual fibromas*; Plate 19–16). There is a localized leathery-looking plaque on her lower back, a *shagreen plaque* that represents a fibrous hamartoma.

These skin findings are pathognomonic of tuberous sclerosis and confirm the diagnosis. You now proceed to a full physical examination, because many organ systems can be involved in this disease. It is also important to ask further focused questions about the family history, asking specifically whether family members have had the neurologic, cutaneous, or renal manifestations of tuberous sclerosis. Joanne requires more specific neurologic, developmental, renal, and cardiac investigation, and the parents should undergo genetic counseling.

Key Point

Take a complete history and examine the patient's entire skin surface, even if the presenting problem is apparently localized; some skin conditions indicate the possibility of a multisystem disorder.

Case 3

Six-month-old David's parents are concerned about a very itchy rash that he has had for a month. Because there is a family history of atopic dermatitis, they have assumed that David has this form of eczema. They are frustrated by the fact that David is scratching his skin day and night, and a nonprescription-strength topical corticosteroid cream has not helped at all.

What important questions do you have for David's parents? You ask further questions appropriate for a diagnosis of atopic dermatitis, such as the onset and progression of the rash, what seems to exacerbate or relieve it, what his skin comes in contact with, and whether his skin is generally dry. However, when you ask about contact with others who may be itchy, you learn that David's uncle, who was visiting 6 weeks ago, had a rash on his trunk and limbs, and David's mother noted a few itchy bumps around her wrists just yesterday.

What specific clinical signs are you now looking for? You suspect that David has contracted a scabies infestation. On examination, you find several small pustules on the palms and soles (a common sign of scabies in an infant). David has an extensive eruption of excoriated papules on his trunk and limbs, and a few on his neck. On careful examination, you find a few 3- to 5-mm linear burrows around his wrists and ankles (see Fig. 19–1). David does not have the background dry skin of atopic dermatitis.

How do you make the definitive diagnosis of scabies? At the end of one burrow, there is a tiny black dot. With a hand lens, you are able to lift the dot out with a needle tip without hurting the child. Microscopic examination clearly shows a mite (*Sarcoptes scabiei*). You can now reassure his parents that David does not have eczema but does have scabies, a common and readily treatable condition. You give them exact written and verbal instructions on how to treat scabies topically with permethrin and how to prevent re-infestation by washing personal clothing and linens. You also emphasize that household contacts must also be treated, even if they are asymptomatic.

Key Point

Try to extract the scabies mite from a burrow with a needle, or by gently scraping with a scalpel blade. Examine the tissue with a microscope; if you can identify a mite, the diagnosis is unequivocal.

Case 4

Two-year-old Maria is brought to the emergency department by her parents in the late evening. She has been perfectly well until 24 hours earlier, when erythema developed in the diaper area and around her mouth. She became febrile (39.5°C), and oral acetaminophen relieved the fever for only a few hours. Gradually, Maria became irritable and anorexic, and she cried frequently, even when she was picked up. Her skin had become generally red, and her parents noted the development of some blis-

tering and crusting on her buttocks, lower back, and face. They have given her no medications other than acetaminophen.

What clinical signs are you likely to note on examination? Maria is irritable and cries when handled, even by her mother. Her core temperature is 39.5°C. A generalized, bright red, blanching erythema of the skin is most noticeable around the lower trunk. There is superficial radial fissuring and crusting around her mouth and under her eyes. Some erosions are present on her buttocks, perianal area, and back, and there are several intact flaccid vesicles containing serous fluid arising on erythematous skin over pressure points. You apply a gentle lateral shearing or slow rubbing force on the erythematous skin, which results in detachment of the epidermal layer, leaving an erosion—the Nikolsky sign.

Can you now make a clinical diagnosis? Maria has the typical manifestations of staphylococcal scalded skin syndrome, caused by a localized infection with *Staphylococcus aureus* phage type 71. This organism elaborates a systemic epidermolytic toxin that separates the layers of the epidermis and produces an acute, generalized superficial bullous disorder. People older than 8 years are able to neutralize the toxin and therefore rarely manifest the disease. Although the condition is self-limited, the affected child may experience significant secondary fluid and electrolyte abnormalities because of loss of the skin barrier. You therefore admit Maria to the hospital and begin treatment with intravenous anti-staphylococcal antibiotics and fluid replacement. She recovers quickly and completely, with no residual scarring.

Key Point

Recognition of an acute infectious disease affecting the skin leads to early initiation of appropriate treatment and prevention of complications.

SUMMARY

Dermatology, unlike beauty, is more than skin deep. Clinical assessment of the child with a dermatologic complaint requires a thorough history, the purposes of which are (1) to define precisely the evolution of the skin lesions and their relationship to environmental and other influences and (2) to detect possible relationships between the skin problem and systemic disease. This chapter stresses the importance of using terms that patients and parents understand and of eliciting and relieving unwarranted anxieties they may have. Attention to detail is equally important in the physical examination, as illustrated in the selected case histories. Because most skin diseases are classified according to their general morphology, identification of the primary lesion enables you to assign a condition to a broad diagnostic group. After a time, you will find the variations on common dermatoses in each group to be easily recognizable. The system of clinical evaluation described here should help take the mystery and frustration out of the assessment of skin conditions in children.

SUGGESTED READINGS

Hurwitz S: Clinical Pediatric Dermatology, 2nd ed. Philadelphia, WB Saunders, 1993.
Meneghini EL, Bonifazi E: An Atlas of Pediatric Dermatology. Chicago, Year Book, 1998.
Schachner LA, Hanson RC: Pediatric Dermatology, 2nd ed. New York, Churchill Livingstone, 1995.

chapter 20

Caring for Children with Chronic Conditions and Their Families

RICHARD B. GOLDBLOOM

Providing the best possible care for a child with a chronic illness or disability calls for special skills if you are to be of maximum assistance to the child and family. While writing this chapter, I realized that those best equipped to speak with authority on this topic are the parents of children with chronic conditions and sometimes the youngsters themselves. Their years of firsthand experience, often dealing with multiple caregivers in and out of hospital, have left them with vivid memories of the clinical encounters that served them well and those that left them unhappy or dissatisfied. I have quoted the following people directly whenever it seemed appropriate:

Andrea Crowe: Andrea is an intelligent, articulate teenager who has spent much of her young life in the hospital with severe, disabling arthritis, chronic uveitis, and, more recently, a rare, poorly understood muscle disorder. Both Andrea and her mother, Ann, have strong views about the clinical skills that make for effective, sensitive care.

Carol and John Young: Years ago, Carol Young was a dedicated volunteer at a pediatric hospital. She began to care for Michael, an abandoned, desperately ill 3-month-old boy. Michael was blind from birth and had severe, chronic chloride-losing diarrhea. Carol and her husband, John, adopted Michael when the boy was 15 months old. Michael suffered from recurrent bouts of severe dehydration and was hospitalized repeatedly. Eventually his kidneys failed, and he received two successive renal transplants, both of which his body rejected. Michael was kept alive with hemodialysis and long-term peritoneal dialysis, the latter carried out mainly at home by Carol and John, for 3 years. Despite superb care from his parents, supported by several specialists, Michael died when he was 11 years old.

Donna and Ian Thompson: The Thompsons have raised two children, Robbie and Jane, both of whom were affected by cystic fibrosis. Robbie died as a young adult several years ago. As a family, the Thompsons have accumulated more than two decades of experience with health professionals and the health care system. They have also been outspoken, effective advocates, both nationally and internationally, for the improvement of care for children and adults with cystic fibrosis.

FIRST DISCLOSURE OF THE DIAGNOSIS TO PARENTS

The basic competencies required for initial disclosure of the diagnosis are the same, whether the child has cystic fibrosis, a congenital anomaly, cerebral palsy, Down syndrome, diabetes, or any other serious chronic condition. Physicians and students vary considerably in comfort level with the task of disclosing to parents the diagnosis and implications of their child's newly identified, chronic, possibly disabling condition. Some cannot wait to get the interview over with, talk far too fast, and without realizing it, may allow little time for interruptions or questions. Others may betray their personal discomfort by talking around the issues. From a parent's perspective, however, nothing makes the interview more unsatisfying and unhelpful than haste or circumlocution.

Carol Young: "Not every doctor has the comfort to sit down and talk to parents ... but honesty up front is the most important thing."

Donna Thompson (recalling how she and Ian first learned that their child had cystic fibrosis): "He [the doctor] had an intuitive sense of how much we could absorb at one time, so he had a paced way of delivering the information."

Several careful investigations have identified the specific factors that determine parents' level of satisfaction or dissatisfaction when they recall how their child's diagnosis was first disclosed to them. Their observations provide a very clear picture of "dos and don'ts." The key components that determined whether such parents remembered that conversation with appreciation or with rancor were (1) promptness, (2) honesty without abruptness, and (3) emphasizing the positive.

Promptness

Some parents have complained that "everyone knew the diagnosis before we did." Even when the news is bad, parents want to be told as soon as possible. When you cannot establish a definitive diagnosis immediately, parents usually accept the situation with understanding if you give them justifiable reasons for the delay. They simply want to know as soon as possible whether you have *any* concerns about their child, even if you are not yet sure of the exact nature of the condition.

Honesty Without Abruptness

Parents want the truth, but everyone needs time to absorb it and to come to terms with disturbing news. Parents who were dissatisfied with the manner in which their child's diagnosis was disclosed to them have often pinpointed the abruptness with which the information was delivered or the apparent lack of compassion on the part of the messenger.

Emphasizing the Positive

It is a lot easier for a parent to absorb and accept distressing news about a child when it is presented in a context that not only includes but emphasizes the child's positive attributes. The physician who opens the conversation "cold" with the bad news or focuses overwhelmingly on the negative or difficult aspects of the child's condition may inadvertently seem, in the eyes of the parents, to devalue the child. Such a message is guaranteed to induce anger, depression, or both.

Variations in individual styles of delivering bad news may reflect personality differences among caregivers. Each of us has personal endowments of optimism and pessimism, and the balance between the two may condition both the style of communicating bad news and the parents' reactions to hearing it. To illustrate this point, I sometimes ask medical students to indicate through role-play how they would deal (in actual language) with the following not-so-hypothetical situation:

"You have just carried out your initial examination of a newborn boy and discover that he has several major congenital anomalies. You consult an authoritative reference book on dysmorphic syndromes and learn that this particular condition carries a 5% risk of recurrence in subsequent children. What exactly do you say to the parents when they ask you about the recurrence risk?"

Some students reply that they would "tell them the truth," meaning that they would inform the parents that there was a 5% risk that the condition would reappear in a subsequent child. By contrast, others say they would begin by telling the parents that there was a 95% chance that any subsequent child would be completely normal, only *then* indicating the 5% recurrence risk. Mathematically, both approaches are equally accurate, but the impacts of the two styles of communication on the parents can be diametrically opposite.

By the same token, when starting an interview for the initial disclosure of a child's chronic condition, be it Down syndrome, a dysmorphic syndrome, or any other chronic condition, you can always open the conversation with comments that highlight the child's positive attributes. Also, you should *always but always* refer to the child by name, never as "he," "she," or "the baby." For example, you could start by saying, "I've examined Mary Ann. She is a lovely girl and her general health appears to be good. But she does have a problem I'm concerned about." At this point, as you reveal the specific reason for your concern, the conversation should immediately become a two-way interchange, during which you pause regularly to encourage the parents to ask questions. Never allow your disclosure to turn into a speech.

Conducting the First Interview

On the general principles outlined earlier, the essential ingredients that will make the first disclosure of a child's chronic condition least traumatic and as helpful as possible for the parents are as follows:

1. Both parents should be present. If only one parent can be present, a close relative or valued friend can provide important comfort and support. Other health care personnel

should be present *only* if they have a specific role to play in the child's care.

2. Everyone should be seated. Do not sit behind a desk if you can avoid it.

3. The infant should be present as well, unless she or he is too ill.

4. The setting should ensure comfort and privacy (turn off your beeper!).

5. Open the conversation with a positive statement about the baby, and balance the positive and negative elements of the baby's present and future condition throughout the discussion. (For goodness sake, *do not* ask the parents whether they've noticed anything odd about the baby!).

6. Avoid medical jargon. Encourage the parents to stop you if you use *any* words they do not understand. When parents nod assent, *do not* assume that they have understood you. Toward the end of the interview, always ask them to describe what they understand about the child's problem and the plan for investigating and managing it. Doing so gives you a clear picture of how well you have explained the issues and a chance to correct any misunderstandings.

7. Always take the initiative in encouraging and facilitating consultation with experts, either for confirmation of the diagnosis or for help with management. Parents appreciate this approach enormously.

8. Whenever possible, offer the parents correct and easily understood printed information or reliable Internet sources concerning the child's condition. It is often useful to put them in contact with other parents or support groups who are experienced in dealing effectively with children who have the same condition.

9. Try to sense, from both verbal and nonverbal cues, when the parents have had enough information for one session. All parents have limits of tolerance for how much bad news or complex information they can absorb at one sitting. Often, their full comprehension and acceptance may require several interviews.

10. Always conclude the interview by establishing a time and place for an early follow-up meeting with the parents—within 24 hours for a serious condition, but certainly within a few days. You could also take the initiative to telephone them later in the day to see whether they have further questions. Most parents do think of additional questions they want to ask; encourage them to keep a list of concerns to bring to your next meeting.

11. Finally, let them have some private time together at the conclusion of the interview.

Parental dissatisfaction with the initial disclosure interview is not inevitable. Nor is anger with the messenger who delivers the bad news. On the contrary, when you carry out the interview according to these principles, most parents remember the experience with appreciation despite its upsetting content. Above all, you must help them feel that they have a crucial role to play in ensuring their child the best possible future.

Not surprisingly, parents' initial reactions to disclosure of a child's diagnosis may sometimes recall parents' responses to bereavement, with mixtures of shock, disbelief, denial, and anger. Many parents search for causes or try to assign blame, often to themselves (see discussion of hidden agendas in Chapter 1). As with most clinical encounters, it is as important for you to understand the parents receiving the information as it is to be an authority on the child's condition.

SPECIAL SKILLS FOR CONTINUING CARE

Encouraging Shared Labor

Chapter 1 discussed the key role of labor sharing among family members as a determinant of emotional strength and resilience in families. Sharing the chores of everyday life is doubly important when the family includes a child with special needs. You can offer valuable guidance in ensuring that *both* parents, and often older siblings as well, share the responsibilities for the tasks of daily living and for the extra care the child requires.

Key Point

As often as possible, involve both parents when you discuss the child, and help them divide the responsibility for the tasks of daily care. Shared labor is a key contributor to every family's emotional strength and stability, but especially when the family includes a child with special needs.

Too often, health professionals unwittingly focus their attention on one parent only—more often the mother—thereby contributing to parental exhaustion and possibly increasing family tensions. Involving *both* parents as therapeutic partners serves both the child and family best.

John Young: "Often, doctors talk to mothers, rather than fathers. But both parents need to be partners with the doctor when there are decisions to be made."

It is important to assess parents' level of satisfaction with the quality of their child's care at regular intervals. The level of parents' satisfaction is often a reflection of the quality of the child's care.

Respecting Parents' Knowledge and Experience

Health professionals can learn a great deal about disease processes and principles of treatment from a combination of study and clinical experience. But no amount of either can confer the special, intimate knowledge that parents acquire about their own unique child. No one knows that child better than the parents.

> *Carol Young:* "Most parents of chronically ill children learn *so* much about how to care for their child, how to give medications and how to carry out complicated treatments, like home peritoneal dialysis and tracheostomy care, or how to help their child get through uncomfortable procedures. Sometimes they're better at it than the professionals."
>
> *Ian Thompson:* "You can't help but become pretty well informed—and you learn that there are times when the doctors are wrong and the parents are right."

Recognizing Emotional Overload, Exhaustion, and the Need for Respite

Parents rarely complain of "burnout" or ask for respite time, even when they have become totally exhausted by the daily demands of caring for a chronically ill or disabled child. Perhaps some believe that a confession of exhaustion would be interpreted as an admission of failure to fulfill their responsibilities. It is therefore essential that all health professionals involved in the child's care are sensitive to verbal and, especially, nonverbal signals that parents may be nearing "the end of the rope." Even the healthiest parents with the healthiest offspring need regular respite from each other and from their children. That need is magnified when the family includes a youngster who requires considerable additional care. Therefore, find out what parents do as a couple for regular diversion and recreation, and how often. Determining the family's external support systems (family members and close friends) is another key element in evaluating parent access to respite in practical terms.

> *Ian Thompson:* "Some parents simply won't leave their children. But all parents need periodic respite, right from Day 1. Those breaks are good for the children as well as the parents. On a day-to-day basis, parent respite includes simple things, like trying to avoid having to wake children during the night to give medications."

EVALUATING THE QUALITY OF LIFE IN CHILDREN WITH CHRONIC CONDITIONS

Because survival rates for many chronic conditions have improved dramatically over the last decades, many caregivers have turned their attention to evaluating and improving the quality of life (often abbreviated as QOL) in such children. In this context, *quality of life* refers to the area of the child's or adolescent's functioning directly affected by the disorder or by its treatment.

In developing the clinical skills necessary for assessing QOL in a child with a chronic disorder, you must consider four specific domains:

- The disease, its signs and symptoms.
- Functional status, which consists of cognitive function, self-help, mobility, physical activity, leisure activities, and academic performance.
- Psychosocial adjustment, including behavior problems, anxiety, and depression.
- Social adaptation, such as peer relationships and interactions with family members, teachers, and health professionals.

In addition, it may be important to evaluate the child's overall satisfaction with life and, for an adolescent, the level of satisfaction with personal appearance.

Key Point

Periodic, systematic assessment of the specific elements that determine the quality of a child's life can be a valuable way to determine overall adjustment and to identify the unmet needs of a youngster with a chronic, disabling condition.

Three generic parent rating scales have been widely used to develop an overall view of a child's general health and adjustment. They are as follows:

> *The Child Health Questionnaire (CHQ):* A 50-item questionnaire that assesses 14 health domains in children 5 years or older. It has established validity and reliability.
>
> *The Child Behavior Checklist (CBCL):* A parent rating scale that is valid and reliable for children aged 4 to 18 years. It includes a social competence scale and a behavior problem scale.
>
> *Children's Depression Inventory (CDI):* A well-validated instrument that has been widely used to assess depression in children with chronic illness.

Various questionnaire instruments have been developed to evaluate QOL in children or adolescents with specific chronic disease states, such as asthma, epilepsy, cystic fibrosis, diabetes, and malignant diseases. These instruments can provide clinically useful information, either as research tools to evaluate changes in management or as ways to follow the progress of individual children over time. Examples of such instruments are as follows:

- Pediatric Oncology Quality of Life Scales (POQOLS): Consists of separate scales for physical functioning, emotional distress, and treatment-related adjustment.
- Diabetic Quality of Life Instrument: Designed for adolescents.
- Cystic Fibrosis Problem Checklist
- Asthma Problem Behavior Checklist
- Child Epilepsy Questionnaire

Even if you do not use such instruments in the routine care of children with chronic conditions, you may find it valuable to become familiar with the questions they ask. Awareness of the principal domains you must evaluate to develop a clear picture of the quality of a child's life provides a knowledge base that will help you be of maximum benefit to the child and family. It is not enough to rely simply on common sense and intuition. The best form of intuition is the kind based on a thorough familiarity with existing knowledge.

PHYSICAL EXAMINATION OF A CHILD WITH A CHRONIC CONDITION

Andrea Crowe: "When a doctor who comes to examine me is someone I don't already know, I like him (or her) to come in, sit down, tell me his name and just talk to me, even if it's only for a minute or two. When he starts to examine me, I want him to respect my personal space. And when he's finished, he shouldn't just get up and leave. He should tell me what he's found and not simply write it down in the chart. Sometimes I wonder exactly what they're writing about me!"

Andrea also believes that the doctors who come to see her should read her chart beforehand. "Sometimes it's as if they haven't read it at all," she reports.

Remember that children have big ears and long antennae and that these receptors are especially well developed in youngsters who have spent significant time in the hospital. The unfortunate modern practice of conducting ward rounds largely in hospital corridors, poring over medical records and discussing patients in hushed tones, is a practice guaranteed to generate anxiety in the children and parents who observe but cannot hear those discussions.

Carol Young: "Chronically ill children grow up very quickly in some ways. They have big ears, and when they hear you talking, they don't always know if you're talking about them, or about someone else."

The detailed systematic physical examination of various systems is described in other chapters. One issue, however, deserves comment. In children with chronic conditions, it is often advisable to reorder the sequence of the examination so as to leave for last both the systems most affected by the child's condition and the procedures that may cause the child discomfort. Explain to older children what you are doing at every step. Tell them what you have found, and comment on normal findings and areas of improvement with approval. They usually appreciate this approach greatly.

TRANSITIONAL CARE

Too often, transferring responsibility for the care of an adolescent with a long-standing chronic condition from pediatric to adult specialists and facilities can cause the patient and the parents a lot of anxiety and discomfort. Such problems should be avoidable to a large extent. For many families, years of close association with and dependency on trusted pediatric health professionals and facilities have built a strong sense of confidence. Not surprisingly, many families feel anxious and destabilized by the prospect of change.

Many pediatric health centers have adopted a flexible policy about age limits for adolescents with chronic conditions. Ideally, the decision to transfer care to professionals who deal primarily with adult patients should be made jointly by the patient, the parents, and the caregivers. Once the decision is made, there should be as much overlap as possible between the two sets of caregivers, through mechanisms such as (1) having physicians and other professionals see the adolescent and family together and (2) "cross-over" visits between institutions to ensure that the transition will be as comfortable as possible for the adolescent or young adult and the family.

Some health professionals who deal exclusively with adults take an approach that suggests a belief that people who have reached the age of majority should stand on their own feet. Irrespective of the patient's age, however, chronic disabling illness makes all patients more dependent on others, most often on family members. Although self-sufficiency is a virtue that should be encouraged, the need for family-centered care does not disappear on a particular birthday. Effective transition from pediatric to adult care calls for special skills and sensitivity and for extremely close collaboration among all people concerned over a considerable time.

Donna Thompson: "It takes time to adapt to a new doctor. And when they have different views about treatment, it tends to shake your confidence."

Effective transitional care requires that the new caregivers maintain regular contact with the parents. The transition to adult care should be made as gradually as possible, rather than as a sudden break.

SUMMARY

Children with different chronic conditions and their families experience many common stresses, despite differences in disease process, degree of incapacity, and prognosis.

From the moment the diagnosis of a child's chronic, disabling condition is first disclosed to the parents, you need special clinical skills to help the family come to terms with the youngster's condition and to set the stage for optimum management and support. The specifics of what works best for sensitive, effective first disclosure of the child's diagnosis are well established. Caregivers must appreciate that many parents of children with chronic, disabling conditions need regular periods of respite, especially in situations that put heavy extra demands on them for the child's care. Acquiring the skills to evaluate the quality of the child's life can improve overall care and help you assess progress. All health professionals should cultivate a healthy respect for the knowledge, experience, and technical skills acquired by parents of chronically ill or disabled children. The physician's role can then

change, as it should, from that of the traditional, authoritarian prescriber of treatment to the far more valuable role of therapeutic partner.

REFERENCES

Achenbach TM: Manual for the Child Behavior Checklist/4–18 and 1991 profile. Burlington, VT, University of Vermont Department of Psychiatry.

Baird G, McConachie H, Scrutton D: Parents' perceptions of disclosure of the diagnosis of cerebral palsy. Arch Dis Child 83:475–480, 2000.

Buckstein DA: Evaluation of a short form for measuring health-related quality of life among pediatric asthma patients. J Allergy Clin Immunol 105:245–251, 2000.

Cottrell DJ, Summers K: Communicating an evolutionary diagnosis of disability to parents. Child Care Health Dev 16:211–218, 1990.

Cramer JA, Westbrook LE, Devinsky O, et al: Development of the Quality of Life in Epilepsy Inventory of Adolescents: The QOLIE-AD-48. Epilepsia 40:1114–1121, 1999.

Cunningham CC, Morgan PA, McGucken RB: Down syndrome: Is dissatisfaction with disclosure of diagnosis inevitable? Dev Med Child Neurol 26:33–39, 1984.

Ingersoll GM, Marrero DG: A modified quality-of-life measure for youths: Psychometric properties. Diabetes Educator 17:114–120, 1990.

Iveys HT, Perry JJ: Development and evaluation of a satisfaction scale for parents of children with special health care needs. Pediatrics 104:1182–1191, 1999.

Juniper EF, Guyatt GH, Feeny DH, et al: Measuring quality of life in children with asthma. Qual Life Res 5:35–46, 1996.

Landgraf JM, et al: Child Health Questionnaire (CHQ): A User's Guide. Boston, The Health Institute, New England Medical Center, 1996.

Quine L, Rutter DR: First diagnosis of severe mental and physical disability. J Child Psychol Psychiatr 35:1273–1287, 1994.

Skills for Assessing the Appropriate Role for Children in Health Decisions

NUALA P. KENNY and LINDA E. SKINNER

Medical decision-making in pediatric practice is ideally a collaborative process involving parents, the pediatrician, other members of the health care team, and, when appropriate, the children themselves. Pediatricians have a long tradition of helping parents make health decisions for their children. As these decisions become increasingly complex, practitioners require great skill in communicating medical prognosis as well as the risks and potential benefits of different interventions. The role of parents as primary decision-makers for infants and young children is clear. Caring and responsible parents are entrusted by society with the authority to give permission for health care decisions made in the "best interests" of their children.

Pediatricians owe ethical and legal duties to patients independent of parental authority. We recognize that medical decisions for children and adolescents must include the perspective and "voice" of the child.[1] Just as we have greater expectations for the ethical involvement of competent adults in health decisions, there are increasing expectations for the respectful involvement of children and adolescents. Pediatricians are expected to have the skills necessary to assess a child's capacities and to help parents determine the appropriate role for the child. This role is related not strictly to age but rather to the unique capacities of each child.

As children mature, their best interests increasingly include respectful involvement in decisions. Assessing the particular role of *this* child in *this* decision is important, because children are in a continuous process of decisional maturation.

THE DOCTOR-PATIENT RELATIONSHIP IN PEDIATRICS

The doctor-patient relationship in pediatrics has always been *both* with children and with their parents or care-givers. This focus on the child within the family is a particular strength of the specialty. Our focus on determining the appropriate involvement of the child does not mean setting up an adversarial relationship between parents and child. This determination is not about scoring points to determine who is the ultimate decision-maker. Rather, the aim is to recognize the balance between parents and maturing children. Decisional competence is a "necessary but not sufficient" condition on which to base respectful involvement.[2]

Competence is decision-specific. The context in which health decisions are made is extremely important in determining the appropriate role for a child. In primary care settings, the pediatrician's knowledge of the child and family is an invaluable resource in determining the best interests of the child and in helping parents determine the appropriate role of the child.

In hospital-based and specialty care, a number of other contextual features influence the involvement of the child. Acute illness and injury often require rapid decisions about diagnosis and treatment. There may not be sufficient time to assess the appropriate role for the child in such cases, so parental judgment is relied on. Children should, however, be involved as much as is reasonable. Children who experience chronic illness have knowledge and experience of health care decisions beyond their years. Their active involvement is essential for care. The clinician often has an established relationship with such a child and the family, enabling him or her to intimately understand both the child and the family and to identify potential or emerging conflicts in parent-child communications.

Life-threatening illness in children and adolescents poses particular challenges. Some parents refuse to have their children involved in any way in end-of-life decisions. Others explicitly forbid the pediatrician to speak honestly to their child or adolescent.

The ethical dilemmas created by such situations are beyond the scope of this chapter. Instead, we focus on the skills needed to continuously assess the child's capacities and to assist parents and children in their decisions.

THE ROLE OF PARENTS AND FAMILIES

Parents are primarily responsible for protecting and promoting their children's interests.[3] Children are raised in an increasingly complex set of parental or caregiver contexts, which may consist of a two-parent, single-parent, or blended family, foster care, or a homeless family. These familial and social factors shape the substance and context of decisions. Parents who are not neglectful, exploitive, or abusive of their children are generally granted wide discretion in making decisions for them. This discretion is granted for many reasons, some of which are (1) the child's incapacity, (2) parental knowledge of the child's best interests, (3) parental commitment to promoting those interests, (4) and parental burden of at least some of the consequences of decisions made on behalf of their children. Parents serve as *surrogate decision-makers* for their children as they take into account the unique characteristics of their child—age, illness, personality, and maturation. They may also need to balance their child's best interest with the family's best interest.[4]

Parents guide their children to decisional maturity in many and varied ways. The differences are related to the personality of the child and to the family's religious, ethnic, and cultural characteristics. Some parents are extremely protective of their children and limit all aspects of the child's involvement in decision-making, including disclosure of information. Others actively promote involvement of the child in decision-making from an early age.

A child's need to know medical information, especially about prognosis, can be a source of real conflict for parents, the pediatrician, and other members of the health care team. Even for a child who demonstrates decisional maturity, parents have good reasons to limit the child's present-day autonomy in favor of lifetime goals. Children's decisions are based on limited experience. Finally, family interests and goals are important too. Physicians provide only for a child's medical needs. The parents provide for all the child's needs and assume the consequences of medical decisions made for their children.

AUTONOMY, INFORMED CONSENT, AND CHILDREN

Respect for the autonomy of patients is a fundamental principle of contemporary ethical practice. Respect for children means respect for the developing autonomy even as they depend on parents and family.

Focusing the assessment on a child's capacity to make a competent decision helps make the decision regarding the appropriate involvement of the child an objective rather than intuitive process. The ethical requirements for decisional competence are as follows:

- Information (so that the decision is made knowingly)
- Capacity (for intelligent, competent decision-making)
- Freedom on voluntariness

Competence is content- and decision-specific. In general, the higher the levels of risk and harm, the greater the competence required. Decisional competence is a necessary but not a sufficient condition for determining the child's role in health care decisions. Even when children have not yet developed decisional maturity, their needs for information privacy, intimacy, confidentiality, truthfulness, and trust are essential. They still need support and care. The pediatrician's task is to balance respectful involvement of the child with parental authority and judgment. The real question is "What is the appropriate role for *this* child in *this* health care decision?"

The pediatrician must assess the following issues:

- What the child wants to know
- How much the child can understand
- The decisional capacity of the child's role in this decision
- What the child needs to know in order to participate appropriately

Professional guidelines have been developed to assist pediatricians with this assessment. The American Academy of Pediatrics (AAP) has identified the following three categories of children: (1) those lacking decisional capacity, (2) those with developing capacity, and (3) those older children and adolescents with capacity.[5] In attempting to provide this guidance, the AAP developed the concepts of assent and dissent; however, these concepts and the categories are confusing and contradictory in usage. The general categories have been further refined to identify the needs and capacities of children in four categories[6]:

1. Children with no communication (neonates and young children).
2. Children with some communication but no decisional maturity (younger school-aged children).
3. Children with some communication and developing decisional authority (older school-aged children).
4. Children with decisional maturity (i.e., equivalent to adult capacity for decisional maturity).

The role of parents for children in category 1 is clear. Parents are surrogate decisions-makers for their infants and young children. The pediatrician's role for such children is the traditional one of providing care for the child and information and support for the parental decision.

For children in categories 2 and 3, the role of a particular child in a given health decision must be determined. The pediatrician brings medical and developmental expertise to an assessment of such a child's capacity and need to participate. We outline here some specific assessment techniques that the pediatrician or other members of the health care team can use to identify more clearly the child's role. It is important to recognize the need for information and involvement even for the child who has not yet developed decisional maturity.

The role of adolescents (category 4) is complex. Some of the techniques identified for assessment of younger children are useful for young adolescents. We also address specific considerations regarding adolescents in a special section of this chapter.

ASSESSING THE APPROPRIATE ROLE FOR CHILDREN IN HEALTH DECISIONS

The pediatrician assesses the child's capacities for (1) communication, (2) reasoning, and (3) having a stable set of values—that is, a conception of "the good."

The Child's Capacity for Communication

ISSUES

Competence in decision-making requires a capacity for understanding and expressing language. Assessing the child's ability to understand basic concepts of health, illness, and treatment is essential for determining the proper role of the child in medical decisions. Although the development of verbal abilities is an early maturational task, everyone who listens to children knows that they can use language in ways that have different meanings from how adults understand the words.

Children's language and cognitive development must be sufficient to understand the medical information given to them. Understanding the meaning of certain concepts essential for decision-making, such as risk, pain, consequences, and death, requires certain life experience. Caregivers can have real concerns and conflicts about what the child truly understands about such concepts.

Conveying information to a child about medical interventions is a necessary step in determining the youngster's understanding. But how much information is enough? As in communications with parents, you

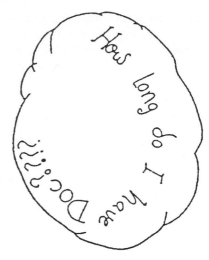

Figure 21–1 Child's drawing, "How long do I have Doc?" which the child used to ask a question that was too scary to ask with words.

must impart difficult or complex information gradually. If the child's threshold for understanding has been reached, more information might create anxiety and distress and should be withheld for the moment. Letting the child tell you how much he or she needs to know is an important strategy; it gives the child some sense of control of the situation. In Figure 21–1, reproduced from the work of Barbara Sourkes,[7] is the picture a 12-year-old drew and used to ask a question that was too scary to put into spoken words.

Listening is also important. Children can use specific language or direct questions to intellectualize their distress and thus appear to be more "comfortable" and to be coping better than they really are. This observation applies especially to the child with a chronic illness or disability.

Case History

Case 1

Rachel is an 8-year-old girl diagnosed with high-risk lymphocytic leukemia 4 months ago. She has experienced multiple complications, and the leukemia is not yet in remission. A systemic fungal infection is just being controlled. Rachel has been very ill since her diagnosis. Medical opinion is clear that chemotherapy must be continued. Her parents are extremely anxious that everything be done for this little girl. However, her primary care nurse and a Child Life Specialist, both of whom have become quite attached to her, have concerns. Rachel has stated repeatedly that she does not want the medicine. Over the past few weeks, she has begun to talk about wanting to be an "angel with God." She is markedly resistant to treatment and becomes angry about any medical intervention. The question now being raised is whether to honor her wishes about discontinuing therapy or "forcing" her to participate in it.

Rachel has experienced shock and loss as well as physical pain and distress since the diagnosis. To cope, she needs to understand what is happening to her. Her resistance to further treatment is a very common experience in such situations. Among other things, it may represent an opportunity for Rachel to exercise some control in a situation in which she feels totally out of control. However, the hoped-for medical benefit here is still cure. Familial beliefs and experiences color both her language and her understanding of the concepts involved. In this difficult situation, Rachel's parents alternate between finding solace in believing that Rachel is "comfortable with dying" and the fear that she has "given up" because she says she wants to be an angel.

In what ways are Rachel's language and understanding relevant to the medical decision? Is Rachel simply repeating words she has heard? Does she really equate "angel" with death? Much important communication from children of all ages is nonverbal. Children even younger than Rachel try to find some meaning in their illness. Spiritual understanding does call on religious understanding but goes beyond it.[8]

Strategies. At 8 years of age, Rachel is just developing reasoning abilities for probability and consequences. As well, she is able to use thought processes to assess events and has a concept of time and the relationship of events. However, she still demonstrates some elements of magical thinking. Many strategies are available that allow us to "listen" to children like Rachel to understand their fears and hopes.

Body Outline Doll. A soft, simple body-shaped doll (Fig. 21–2), the body outline doll is a useful tool for teaching the child about an illness or treatment and then assessing the child's understanding of the information he or she has been given. If a body outline doll is not available, the child's own doll or stuffed animal or a body outline drawing on cardboard can be used.

For Rachel, the body outline doll can represent the "angel" she wishes to be. Play and discussions involving the doll can help Rachel's parents and physician better understand how she pictures herself as an angel. Because children use concrete language, parents and caregivers may assume that they understand more than they do; however, children can and do express important issues if the communication tool is appropriate.

In their interactions with Rachel, her caregivers and parents use the body outline doll in play to represent an angel, and they ask her the following questions:

- Who lives with the angel?
- What does the angel do during the day?
- Where does the angel live?
- Who does the angel play with?

Rachel's answers make it clear to her family and her caregivers that her understanding of being an "angel" is very different from the adult perception. Rachel believes that as an "angel," she could stay with her family and play with her friends, and that for the most part, things could remain the way they have been.

Artwork. Children's artwork can contribute essential information about their awareness, understanding, and fears. Listening to children's interpretations of their own drawings is an important way for adults to assess their understanding of abstract situations. It is important for Rachel's physician and family to have a clear understanding of her beliefs. Rachel's explanation of her drawings of herself as an "angel" gives them another way of achieving this goal (Fig. 21–3). Asking her the same questions that were asked during play with the body outline doll will help the adults see the topic of angels through Rachel's eyes. If the child is unable or unwilling to draw the situation, action figures that represent specific individuals are a good substitute, as long as the person making the assessment is an active participant in the play and not an observer.

The use of dolls representing Rachel, her parents, caregivers, angels, and God helps her caregivers determine the meaning of these concepts for Rachel. Also, because young children's concepts of the causality of disease are often bound up with their sense of being "good" or "bad," the term "angels" may have an entirely different meaning for them. Rachel might have indicated that if she were good enough to be an angel, then she might get well again.

Comment. These strategies help Rachel's parents and caregivers understand that she is fearful but believes that if she refuses treatment, she can just go

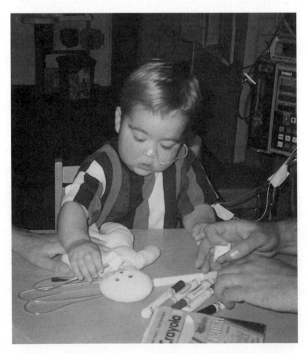

Figure 21–2 Child playing with a body outline doll.

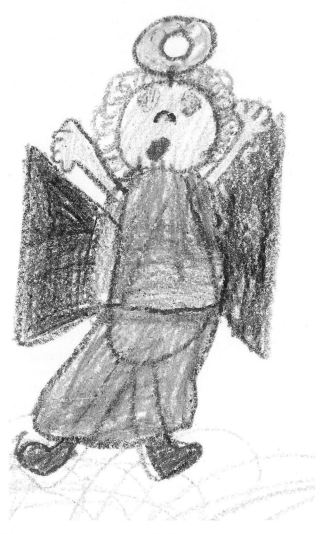

Figure 21–3 Child's drawing of self as an angel.

home. Death is not a meaningful concept for her. Rachel's parents can now see that she is not "ready for death" but is simply frightened and anxious. Rachel needs more participation in the medical decisions being made for her, not as primary decision-maker but as the central figure whose fears and expectations must be addressed if she is to participate in her care.

Key Point

It is important to listen to the child's explanation of artwork and stories and not to draw adult conclusions about them or read meaning into them that is not there.

Capacities for Reasoning

ISSUES

In addition to comprehension of concepts of health and disease, medical decision-making requires knowl-

edge of disease causation and the consequences of various choices. A young child's understanding of causation is often dominated by a belief that an illness was caused by something he or she failed to do. The child may therefore fantasize that being "good" may make him or her better or that having been "bad" justifies the illness.

Reasoning and deliberation require more than language skills. They call for an ability to deal with hypothetical reasoning—"if ... then" situations. Some ability to comprehend probability and risk is also essential. A child must have an awareness of the future and of consequences in order to make a valid choice. Research into children's development and capacities for consent has concluded that "we have practically no systematic information regarding children's understanding of the meaning of terms likely to arise in situations in which consent to treatment is sought."[9] Children who demonstrate capacities for reasoning and deliberation have developed sufficient linguistic skill to understand information if it is given in a sensitive, age-appropriate manner, so attention can focus on the child's ability to reason and take account of the consequences of choice.

A child's reasoning and deliberating capacity is more difficult to assess than his or her language. The child must have sufficient maturity to focus on the decision, reflect on the issues, deal with alternatives, understand risks and harms, and use both inductive and deductive reasoning. His or her experience of the illness itself, of medical interventions, of hospitalization, and of the family's response to the illness all affect this deliberation.

Children's ability to focus on decision-making depends largely on their sense of the locus of control. Children between 6 and 9 years of age do not generally see themselves as being decision-makers in any meaningful way. By 8 to 11 years of age, children are developing the role-playing skills necessary to weigh different options. By 12 to 14 years, these skills are quite well developed[10] and support a youngster's decision-making capacity. Regardless of age, seriously ill children feel overwhelmed and out of control, as evidenced by the touching drawing and poem shown in Figure 21–4. This lack of control can impair the child's ability to focus on the issues and decisions.

Deductive and inductive reasoning skills affect children's understanding of disease causation. Children 6 years and younger have magical views of disease causation. By 12 to 13 years of age, most children begin to understand that there are multiple causes of illness and that the body responds variably to both illness and treatments. Some children generate their own theories of disease to protect themselves against full awareness. Between 11 and 13 years of age, most children are developing sufficient capacity to understand medical choices and their consequences. By 14 years of age,

What am I?
A pincushion or a patient?
That's what I feel like.
What am I?
A helpless person
Or someone in need?
That's what I feel and know.

Angela Jean Ingersoll

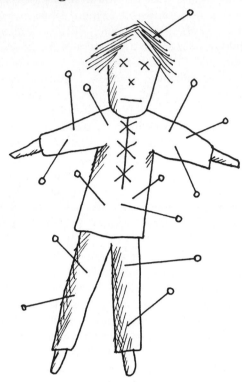

Figure 21–4 Drawing and poem by a child, expressing her feelings about being ill.

most adolescents have the cognitive skills necessary for complex decision-making; but other issues, such as emotional maturity, interdependence with families, and an enduring sense of the "good," should also be taken into account.

Case 2

Jason, now 11 years old, was diagnosed with renal failure at 3 years of age. SInce then, he has been dialysis-dependent. Currently, there are clear indications that he is rejecting his second kidney transplant despite optimum treatment. Once again, his name has been put on the transplant waiting list. Jason says clearly and consistently that he does not want another kidney transplant because it "won't work." His mother, a single parent caregiver, is distraught and confused. On the one hand, she desperately wants Jason to have another transplant; on the other, she hears him refusing to go through this again.

Strategies. Jason has been through a lot. At 11 years, he has spent most of his life with a chronic illness and multiple medical interventions. He has experienced the benefits and limitations of modern medicine firsthand. Certain strategies can help Jason express understandings, fears, and choices, including the use of "what if" games, role-playing, and story-telling.[11]

"What if." The "what if" activity can help Jason understand abstract situations in more concrete terms. Simple picture cards can be used to represent his choices of transplant list or no transplant list and the consequences of each choice (Fig. 21–5). This strategy is more successful if Jason identifies with the pictures. Therefore, photographs of him, his family, and their particular situations are best. Jason, at 11 years of age with 8 years of repeated medical interventions, may well show that he truly understands the consequence of refusing another transplant. His understanding of continued dialysis dependence can become clear. He may believe that the failure of the first two transplants is predictive of another failure. Alternatively, Jason may be depressed or may have lost faith in medicine because of his past experience. The "what if" cards may show logical and appropriate reasoning, magical thinking, or confusion.

Finish the Story/Drawing. The finish the story/drawing strategy could be useful in assessing Jason's understanding of the future implications of decision-making. He would be given a story and asked to finish it by depicting what he thought would happen if a specific course were followed. The key to this strategy is to use the story or drawing as a basis for discussing outcomes and the implications of choices.

It is important to clarify the child's understanding of both short- and long-term consequences. Causation and consequences are complex concepts that require considerable cognitive maturity for understanding. This case also illustrates the difficulty of assessing whether and how a young person understands the consequences of refusing an intervention.

Concept of the "Good"

ISSUES

Medical decisions involve balancing benefits hoped for from the interventions and the risks and harms resulting from no intervention or from the intervention itself. The concepts of benefits and harm are related to the "good." *Good* expresses the extent to which we judge that the benefits outweigh the harms. Values are endur-

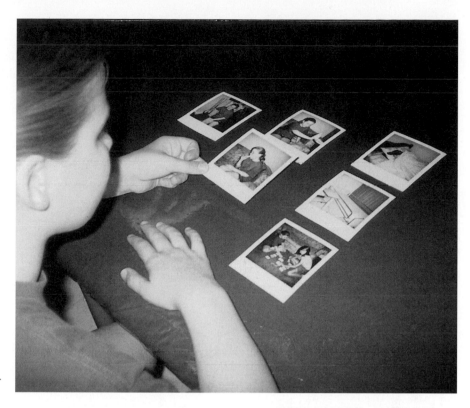

Figure 21–5 Cards for the "What if" activity.

ing, not unchanging but stable. How the values the child holds today relate to future interests is a key issue. Children 7 to 13 years of age still view the world in fairly concrete terms and seem to have great difficulty anticipating a real future. So what seems to be a here-and-now concrete good—no pain, no vomiting, going home—can overwhelm less tangible "goods" in a nebulous future.

Case 3

Adam, a 14-year-old with Duchenne muscular dystrophy, is demanding that he be connected to a ventilator if he experiences respiratory failure. His parents believe that he just does not know what this decision really means and that the burden of prolonging his suffering with ventilator dependency is wrong.

Children can fail to weigh future interests appropriately or may not appreciate how their future values may change. Determining the child's role in decision-making requires an assessment of a sufficient and enduring sense of the "goods" that are important for today and the future.

Everyone experiences a range of knowledge, motivation, and freedom of decision-making in the presence of risk. By 9 years of age, most children can make a reasonable decision; however, they may be less able to understand *all* the critical elements involved, especially the consequences of refusing an intervention and their freedom to refuse it. By 14 years of age, most children are comparable to adults in terms of the intellectual requirements for decision-making. However, children's life experience can be quite limited and may restrict their ability to consider future good effectively.

Strategies. Adam's demand presents an apparent adolescent-parent conflict. As a 14-year-old with muscular dystrophy, he has experienced health care interventions and their benefits and burdens. He should have the cognitive skills necessary to understand what this choice means. The particular issue seems to be Adam's sense of the "good" as he knows it and as he might experience it once he is started on continuous ventilation, contrasted with his parents' perception of the suffering such a step would entail.

Strategies for Adam include careful discussion with and listening to him. His experience of his illness and its limitations is relevant. He may be very clear and direct in his communication of the "good." However, because feelings and deeper issues of meaning are involved, other strategies may help clarify Adam's understanding and convey to his parents what "counts" for him.

Feelings Diary. The goal of the feelings diary is to give Adam the means to express his feelings by asking him to keep a daily record of his good and bad feelings and experiences. In a chart format (Fig. 21–6), Adam could record his feelings and experiences at different times of the day. A careful

Feelings Diary

Name: _____   Date: _____

	HAPPY	SAD	ANGRY	SCARED	LONELY	LUCKY	CHEERFUL	OTHER (name feeling)
MORNING 8:00								
9:00								
10:00								
11:00								
NOON 12:00								
1:00								
2:00								
3:00								
4:00								
5:00								
EVENING 6:00								
7:00								
8:00								
9:00								
10:00								
11:00								

Check the feeling next to the correct time of day and record what you were doing at the time of the feelings.

Figure 21-6   Patient form for a Feelings Diary.

review of Adam's diary would give him a visual inventory or "picture" of the mixture of feelings that he has and help him see that they are not all that bad. The next step is to offer counseling designed to build in more good experiences and fewer bad ones when possible. This procedure also gives Adam's parents and caregivers an idea of what makes him happy. His parents may begin to understand that listening to music and using his computer make Adam happy. Both activities are possible for a patient undergoing home ventilation.

The feelings diary can also elicit real conflicts. Adam may show feelings of anger toward his parents and the health care team. His statement that he wants to make a different choice for himself from that of his parents may be an attempt to "control" things, when, in fact, he feels very out of control and frightened. This strategy can expose deeper feelings that might adversely affect the freedom Adam needs for valid decision-making.

Finish the Story/Drawing. The choice of long-term ventilatory support is a major issue. The primary concern is Adam and his "best interest," but the decision has major consequences for his family as well.

Having Adam complete a story "When I need to go on the ventilator ..." can bring up new issues for discussion. Having him consider the story beginning "If I don't go on the ventilator ..." may open for discussion Adam's fear of dying.

Comment. In cases such as this, the apparent conflict between parental decisions and competent adolescent decisions evolves into a much more important discussion of the child's care during the terminal stages of illness. This case leads naturally to the next section, on special considerations for determining the appropriate involvement of adolescents in medical decisions.

Key Point

The concept of parental permission *and* child assent differs from the concept of parental consent alone. This approach to medical decision-making involves communication with both parents and child, recognizing the importance of supporting parental responsibility and of respecting children in decisions that affect them.

Special Considerations with Adolescents

ISSUES

The parents' role in decisions changes as children mature and become more independent. This changing role is most clearly demonstrated in decisions involving adolescents. Times have changed for adolescents, for their parents, and for the pediatricians who care for them. They are no longer merely the recipients of decisions made on their behalf. Numerous professional bodies in the United States and Canada have expanded the boundaries of adolescent decision-making. The result is a growing recognition that most developmentally normal adolescents older than 14 years have a capacity to make health care decisions equal to that of competent decision-makers.[12]

Although there is greater willingness on the part of parents and pediatricians to affirm this capacity, it requires careful determination and consideration of important contextual issues.[13] In addition, many workers in this field still doubt the capacity of adolescents to make truly important health decisions, especially those regarding life-threatening and terminal illnesses. In these circumstances, parents and pediatricians might feel comfortable acknowledging the agreement of an adolescent to the decisions made by parents and the health care team. Great difficulty arises, however, when the adolescent's choices are in conflict with those of the parents or pediatrician—such as when the adolescent refuses an intervention that others have decided should be undertaken or when the adolescent chooses an intervention that his or her parents disapprove.

Every day, adolescents cope with serious, chronic conditions and life-threatening illnesses. They think about their situations and choices. At least some of them want to give voice to their values, provide direction regarding their care, and ensure that their wishes and preferences are carried out.[14] Such situations reflect the uncertainty and complexity of medical care for adolescents. They raise some serious questions about the capacity of adolescents to make major health decisions. Do only *some* adolescents have that capacity? Do they have the capacity to agree but not to refuse?

Pediatricians play a critical role here. An expanding body of professional knowledge indicates that most adolescents are capable of making decisions and giving informed consent. Some characteristics of *young adolescents* (12 to 14 years) that must be taken into account, however, are that they (1) value peer recognition, (2) are making their first attempts at separation from family, and (3) can grasp abstract concepts in a limited way. Children in *middle adolescence* (15 to 17 years) are generally more mature but still not always realistic, especially about issues of risk and future consequences; further, they tend to feel intensely about

issues and, at times, their emotions can overmaster reasoned judgment. By *later adolescence* (16 to 18 years), most teenagers have the capacity to make competent decisions.

Adolescents may exhibit a greater tendency than adults to minimize their own vulnerability to harm. Some believe that risk perception is substantially different in the adolescent, making the parental duty to protect from harm an important consideration even when the adolescent has cognitive maturity. In fact, there is no strong empirical evidence that adolescents perceive risk of harm in medical decisions differently from most competent adults. Adolescents may have a tolerance for risk that is age-related and higher than that of adults. Adolescents may be less likely to have the stable lifelong goals necessary for truly authentic choice, but there is no strong empirical evidence that this is so.

Significant legal issues are involved in the actual participation of some adolescents in decisions about their treatment. The specific laws of the jurisdiction, province, or state must be taken into account. Many jurisdictions have moved from an age standard of competence to one of individual determination of capacity. Another change in the law involves exceptional categories for adolescents to make personal health decisions. Some young persons are "emancipated minors" and are treated as adults. Minors become "emancipated" by marriage, legal determination, consent of the parents, or failure by parents to meet legal responsibilities (adolescents rejected by their families). Adolescents who live apart from their families and are financially self-supporting are often judged "emancipated." Others are "mature minors" who are still dependent on families but have decision-making capacity for particular medical conditions. Over the past few years, the concept of "mature minors" has been expanded so that rather than age itself being the criterion for decisional authority, a determination of capacity is made for the individual adolescent. There are also "minor treatment statutes" specifying certain health problems for which legal minors can seek treatment without parental permission; these are the problems some adolescents would ignore if parental permission were required. Such statutes are typically limited to pregnancy, pregnancy prevention, sexually transmitted diseases, and alcohol or drug abuse.

The role of adolescent patients depends as much on the context of the intervention and the nature of the health care encounter as on the single issue of competence to consent. The role of parents in medical decision-making for adolescents is important but must be clarified in each situation. Generally, decisions regarding the treatment of adolescents without parental involvement are made in the office or clinic. The most common example is the prescription of contraceptives for sexually active adolescents. Chronic and life-threatening conditions necessitating aggressive interventions and hospitalization require family support even for an adolescent who fulfills the criteria for competent decision-making. The ability to assume the consequences of a decision is an important component of independent decision-making. The ideal is a balance of respect for the competence of adolescents with the need for family support.

Case Histories

Case 4

Karen, a 13-year-old girl who has been a patient in your practice for the past 8 years, arrives in the office asking to see you. She has been healthy and comes from a stable, supportive family environment. She says that she has come to see you because she wants to "go on the pill." She is quite anxious that you do not tell her parents that she has come to you. She says her mother would "just freak out" if she knew that Karen is sexually active and is requesting contraception. Karen herself tells you that she wants to be careful and responsible about her sexual activity, which is why she has come to you for help.

Strategies. Although adolescents can be presumed to have certain maturity in decision-making, their competence to consent in specific situations must be assessed. Because Karen is only 13, you must assess her competence carefully, particularly because her parents are not involved. The issue is complex and is not simply a question of Karen's intellectual understanding of the consequences of unprotected sexual activity.

Strategies for understanding the emotions involved in adolescent decision-making include activities for self-expression, such as keeping diaries, writing poetry, and art and music (Fig. 21–7). Karen needs to demonstrate some factual information

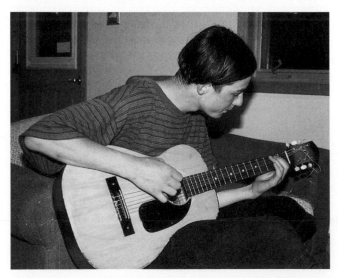

Figure 21–7 Adolescent engaging in an activity for self-expression.

about contraception. More importantly, however, you must determine why this 13-year-old girl is sexually active and plans to continue to be active. Why are her parents not involved in giving her information, guidance, and support?

In this case, you must balance your need to protect Karen from the consequences of unprotected sexual activity with the larger good of supporting a 13-year-old whose sexual activity may have psychological and moral consequences in the long term and who is, for reasons needing exploration, avoiding involving her parents in a major life decision.

Comment. In general, physicians need to make judgments about minimizing harms in situations such as that presented by Karen's request. Recognizing that notification of her parents in this situation is likely to create major difficulties in the patient-physician relationship and may even lead Karen to refuse further advice or treatment, most physicians would respond positively to Karen's request for contraception. Privacy and protection may determine the initial course of action, but there are larger issues of education and support for this teenager to which a caring physician must be committed over the "long haul."

Case 5

Thirteen-year-old Steven, who has Crohn disease, has been a patient in your practice for 5 years. During a recent flare-up, the consulting surgeon has recommended a resection to remove part of the diseased intestine. Steven believes that surgery is a drastic measure that he wants to avoid by continuing a combination of nutritional therapy and medication. Steven believes that he merely needs "to give my bowel a rest and eat really good food like my grandmother's." Steven's parents agree with the surgery, because they believe that Steven does not understand the impact of waiting to have the resection. They enlist your help to "persuade" Steven to agree to the surgery.

Strategies. Adolescents should be presumed to have decisional competence, Steven's capacity requires careful assessment. You must be clear about Steven's understanding of the implications of not having a resection, particularly because his views differ from his parents'. The issue is complex and is not simply a question of Steven's intellectual understanding of the consequences of not having the surgery. You must try to understand the emotional impact of Steven's chronic illness on his life, development, and coping, especially because he demonstrates some denial about the course of his illness and magical thinking about his grandmother's cooking. At 13, Steven is in the category of early adolescence, requiring careful assessment of cognitive, emotional, and familial issues in order to determine the appropriate roles for Steven and his parents in decisions made about his care.

SUMMARY

Parents and pediatricians share responsibility to act in the best interest of children requiring medical interventions. Although parents' roles in protection are crucial for all children, the appropriate role of children in medical decisions, especially as these decisions become more complex, more risky, and more intrusive, should be reconsidered, because of (1) new insights from child development, (2) changes in the laws regarding consent, and (3) ethical insights into the capacities necessary to make competent decisions. Communication strategies that both convey information to children and obtain information from children are essential components of clinical skills for physicians. Assessing the appropriate role for children in health decisions is an important function of caring and competent pediatric practice.

REFERENCES

1. Bartholme WG: A new understanding of consent in pediatric practice: Consent, parental permission, and child assent. Pediatr Ann 18:262–265, 1989.
2. Ross LF: Health care decision making by children: Is it in their best interest? Hastings Cent Rep 27:41–45, 1997.
3. Brock DW: Children's competence for health care decision making. In Kopelman LM, Myoscope JC (eds): Children and Health Care, Boston, Kluwer Academic, 1989, p 184.
4. Hardart G: Including the family's interests in medical decision making in pediatrics. J Clin Ethics 11:164–168, 2000.
5. American Academy of Pediatrics, Committee on Bio-ethics, Informed Consent: Parental permission and assent in pediatric practice. Pediatrics 95:314, 1995.
6. Baylis F, Downie J, Kenny N: Children and decision making in health research. IRB 21:5–10, 1999; reprinted in Health Law Review 8:3–9, 1999.
7. Sourkes B: Armfuls of Time. Pittsburgh, University of Pittsburgh Press, 1995.
8. Coles R: The Spiritual Life of Children. Boston, Houghton Mifflin, 1990.
9. Grisso T, Vierling L: Minor's consent to treatment: A developmental perspective. Prof Psychol 9:412, 1978.
10. Lewis CE: Decision-making related to health: When could/should children act responsibly? In Melton GB, Koocher GP, Saks MJ (eds): Children's Competence to Consent. New York, Plenum Press, 1983, p 75.
11. Gaynard L, Wolfer J, Goldberger J, et al: Psychosocial Care of Children in Hospitals: A Clinical Practice Manual from the ACCH Child Life Research Project. Bethesda, MD, Association for the Care of Children's Health.
12. Leikin L: Minors' assent or dissent to medical treatment. J Pediatr 102:169, 1983.
13. Weir RF, Peters C: Affirming the decisions adolescents make about life and death. Hastings Cent Rep 27:29–40, 1997.
14. Hyun I: When adolescents "mismanage" their chronic medical conditions. An ethical exploration. Kennedy Inst Ethics J10.147–163, 2000.

Index

Note: Page numbers followed by f indicate figures, and t indicates tables. Color plates are identified by the chapter and plate number, e.g., Plate 8–1.

A

Aarskog syndrome, 87, 88
Abdomen
  acute, 208
  assessment of, in trauma, 212–213
  auscultation of, 197, 209, 209f
  congenital anomalies of, 87, 213–215
  inspection of, 197, 208–209, 208f
  neonatal, 68–69, 213–214, 215
  palpation of, 68–69, 187, 197, 209
  percussion of, 209
  surgical assessment of, 207–222
  wall defects in, 214–215, 215f
Abdominal pain
  acute severe, 212
  approach to, 207–208
  assessment of, 194–197
  chronic, 212
  extra-abdominal causes for, 208
  from appendicitis, 210–211
  from intussusception, 195–196
  from trauma, 212–213
  functional, 196
  gynecologic, 211
  in biliary tract disease, 211
  in children and adolescents, 196–197
  in infants, 195–196
  in urinary tract disorders, 211–212
  nonspecific, 196
  origin of, 207–208
  parietal, 194–195
  physical examination for, 197, 208–210
  pyloric stenosis in, 221–222, 221f
  rectal examination in, 210
  recurrent, 196
  referred, 194
  rupture of hollow viscus in, 213
  visceral, 194, 195t
Abducens nerve (cranial nerve VI),
    232–233
Abduction of hip, 280, 280f
Abortion, cultural attitudes toward, 21
Abscess, peritonsillar, 123
Abstinence, 327
Acanthosis nigricans, 302–303, 303f, 307
Accidents, abdominal pain from, 212
Accommodation, ocular, 128
Acetaminophen, 266
Achalasia, 193
Achilles tendon, 263, 284
Achondroplasia, 29
Acne, 305
Acoustic nerve (cranial nerve VIII), 234
Acrocyanosis, 58
Acute abdomen, 208
Acute scrotum, 220–221
Addison disease, 303, 304f
Adenoma sebaceum, 239
ADHD (attention deficit hyperactivity
    disorder), 99–100
Adolescents
  abdominal pain in, 196–197

Adolescents (Continued)
  cardiovascular assessment of,
    188–189
  chest pain in, 153–154, 188
  communication with, 13–14
  confidentiality and, 13
  constipation in, 200–201
  contraception for, 327–329
  decisional competence in, 350–351,
    357–358
  depression in, 255
  diarrhea in, 203
  dysphagia in, 192–193
  eating disorders in, 254–255
  excel syndrome in, 188–189
  gastrointestinal bleeding in, 199
  gynecologic examination in, 321
  health decision making by, 357 358
  hyperbilirubinemia in, 204
  hyperventilation in, 154
  interviewing of, 13–15
    concluding visit in, 14–15
    hidden agendas in, 15
    "hot topics" and, 14
    nonverbal cues in, 13–14
    parental involvement in, 15
  physical examination of, 14
  pregnancy in, 327
  psychiatric assessment of, 249–250
  risk perception by, 357
  self-expression by, 358, 358f
  sexual behavior in, 322
  substance abuse by, 254
  suicidal behavior in, 256–257
Adrenal androgens, 297
Adrenal crisis, 303
Adrenal hyperplasia, congenital, 299–302
  hirsutism in, 302–303, 302f
  penile enlargement in, 301
  physical examination in, 301–302
  salt-losing, 69, 88, 300–301, 301f
  states of, 299t
  virilizing, 69, 299–301
Adrenal insufficiency
  causes of, 303
  congenital, 70
  physical examination in, 303
Adrenarche
  benign precocious, 299, 300f
  precocious, 302
  timing of, 47
Age of parents, congenital anomalies and,
    80
Agenda, hidden, 5–7, 15
Agglutination, labial, 319, 319f
AHC (anterior horn cell) disease, 226, 235
Airway obstruction, 164–165, 165f
Alae nasi, 157
Albinism, 85
Aldosterone, 297
Allergic rhinitis, 156
Allergic salute, 123, 156, 156f

Allergies, respiratory, 155–156
Allodynia, 266
Alopecia, assessment of, 339
Alopecia areata, 115, Plate 19–14
  diagnosis of, 339
  exclamation mark hairs in, 339f
Alström syndrome, 132
Alternative therapies, 23–24
Amblyopia
  definition of, 129
  in cataract, 130
  prevalence of, 129
  refractive, 132
Anal fissures, 198
Androgen excess, 298–303
Anemia, 49, 322
Aneuploidies, 80
Angel's kisses, 72
Anger, of parents, 16
Angina pectoris, 170, 188
Angioedema, 336
Angioma, facial, 225
Ankle, 284
Ankle reflex, 236
Ankylosing spondylitis, 266
Anorexia nervosa, 254–255
Anosmia, 230, 307
Antalgic gait, 271–272
Anterior horn cell (AHC) disease,
    226, 235
Anus
  imperforate, 200, 214
  neonatal, 69
  position of, 200
Anxiety
  assessment of, 255–256
  case history of, 256
  parental, 75
Aortic coarctation, 180
Aortic stenosis, 171, 180
Apgar score, 55–57, 56t
Aphasia, Wernicke, 229
Apnea
  case histories of, 167
  central, 159
  normal values of, 160
  obstructive, 160
  sleep, 159–160
Appendectomy, 211
Appendicitis
  acute, 210–211
  chronic, 211
  differential diagnosis of, 211
  pain from, 207–208
  palpation for, 209
  perforation in, 211
Appendix testis, 220–221
Apraxia, 230
Arachnodactyly, 88
Arciform lesions, of skin, 337
Arm span, 29, 40f
Arteriovenous malformations, 114

Arthritis. *See also* Rheumatoid arthritis, juvenile.
    definition of, 265
    monoarthritis, 267, 267t
    polyarthritis, 267–268
    psoriatic, 285
    septic, 263, 265
Artwork, communication through, 352–353, 353f
ASD (atrial septal defect), 180f, 181, 182
Ash leaf macules, Plate 19–15
Asphyxia
    Apgar score and, 55
    perinatal, 55, 57
Asthma
    common triggers of, 152, 152f
    developmental surveillance in, 91
    dyspnea in, 154
Asthma Problem Behavior Checklist, 347
Asymmetric tonic neck reflex (ATNR), 237, 238, 238f
Athletics, physical exam for. *See* Sports physical examination.
Atresia
    biliary, 204
    choanal, 66, 86
    duodenal, 213
    esophageal, 66–67, 192
    ileal, 213
Atrial septal defect (ASD), 180f, 181, 182
Atrioventricular (AV) conduction time, 178
Atrophic scar, 337
Atrophy of skin, 337
Attention deficit hyperactivity disorder (ADHD), 99–100
Auscultation
    abdominal, 197, 209, 209f
    cardiac, 174–175, 177–183
    of head, 114–115
    respiratory, 162–164, 164t
    sites for, 163f
    techniques for, 183–184
Autistic spectrum disorder, 99
Autonomy, 350–351
Autopsy, 21

B
Babinski sign, 236–237
Back
    congenital anomalies of, 87
    examination of, 71–72, 272–273, 273f
    pain in, 264–265
Bacterial cultures
    in gynecologic assessment, 320–321
    swabs for, 320, 321f
Bacterial infections, 265
Baker cyst, 282
Bardet-Biedl syndrome, 88
Barrel chest, 158, 158f
Basal ganglia disease, 226
Beckwith-Wiedemann syndrome, 86, 122
Behavior, in vision assessment, 134
Behavioral disorders
    assessment of, 99–100, 254–255, 346
    disruptive, 254
Bell's palsy, 225
Benign familial megalencephaly, 28
Benign hypermobility syndrome, 266, 266t
Benign precocious adrenarche, 299
Biceps reflex, 241
Bile, vomiting of, 194, 213, 214
Biliary atresia, 204
Biliary tract disease, 211
Bilirubin, 203, 204
Binocular vision, 128
Birth defects. *See* Congenital anomalies.

Birthmarks, 72
Blackheads, 336
Bladder abnormalities, 215
Blepharoconjunctivitis, 134, 135f
Blindness, 129–130
    hysterical, 231
    night blindness, 144
Blister, 332, 335
Blood pressure
    in adolescents, 14
    in infants, 175–177, 176f
    normal values for, 189f
Blount disease, 282
Body mass index, 36f–37f
Body outline doll, 352, 352f
Bone tumors, 265
Bowel movements, 8, 199
Bowel sounds, 209
Bowleg, 262, 262f, 282
Brachial pulses, 68, 184–185, 185f
Brachycephalic skull, 84
Brachydactyly, 88
Bradycardia, 186–187
Bragard test, 273
Breast
    cancer of, 48
    development of, 46–48
    gestational age and, 62
    neonatal hypertrophy of, 68
Breath smell, 121
Breath sounds
    adventitious, 164t
    auscultation and, 163–164, 164t
    diagnostic use of, 151
    neonatal, 68
    types of, 153
Breech presentation, 80
Brückner test, 136, 136f
Bruit, cranial, 114–115, 241
Buccal mucosa, 121
Buffalo hump, 298
Bulge sign, 282
Bulimia, 254–255
Bullae, 335
Burial, culture and, 21
Burnout, caregiver, 346
Burrows, in scabies, 336, 336f

C
Café au lait spots
    in neurofibromatosis, 73, 89, 239, 272
    in precocious puberty, 305, 305f
    in scoliosis, 272
    in tuberous sclerosis, 89
CAH (congenital adrenal hyperplasia). *See* Adrenal hyperplasia, congenital.
Camptodactyly, 88
Candida infections, 121, Plate 19–13
Capillary hemangioma, 131, Plate 8–3, Plate 19–4
Caput succedaneum, 63, 64f, 112
Carcinoma, thyroid, 295–296
Cardiac insufficiency, 179
Cardiorespiratory murmur, 183
Cardiovascular disorders
    assessment of, 169–190
    blood pressure and, 175–177, 176t
    clinical manifestations of, 172–175, 172f
    congestive heart failure onset and, 171
    crying and, 177
    heart murmurs in
        auscultation techniques for, 183–184
        continuous, 182–183
        diastolic, 181–182
        innocent, 180, 181, 187
        mechanisms of, 179, 180f

Cardiovascular disorders (*Continued*)
        systolic, 179–181
    heart sounds in
        gallop rhythm in, 178–179
        midsystolic click in, 179
        normal vs. abnormal, 177–178, 178f
    history-taking and, 171–174
    hyperkinetic circulation in, 187, 188f, 188t
    in adolescents, 188–189
    in infants, 169–177
    in preschool children, 177–187
    labor and delivery history in, 171–172
    physical examination for
        approach to, 172, 184
        auscultation in, 174–175, 183–184, 187
        liver size and position in, 173–174, 174f, 187
        observation in, 184
        of children, 184–187
        of infants, 172–177
        palpation in, 173, 173f, 187
        positioning for, 172
        pulses in, 175, 184–187
    respiratory distress in, 169–170
    signs and symptoms of, 169–171
    syncope in, 188
Caregivers, 345–346
Caries, nursing bottle, 121
Carotenemia, 203
Cataract, 130, 131
CBCL (Child Behavior Checklist), 346
CDI (Children's Depression Inventory), 346
Cellulitis, periorbital, 132
Central steady maintain fixation (CSMF) test, 137–138
Cephalhematoma (cephalohematoma), 63, 112
Cerebellar diseases, 228
Cerebral cortex, 229–230
Cerebral palsy
    differential diagnosis of, 244–245
    hemiparetic, 230
    labor complications and, 80
    toe-walking in, 263
Cerumen removal, 119–120
Cervical spine, 274, 276f
Cervix, 323–324, 324f
Chemosis, bulbar, 295
Chest
    circumference of, 61
    congenital anomalies of, 87
    expansion of, 160
    movement of, 158–159
    neonatal examination of, 68
    pain in, 153–154, 188
    palpation of, 187
    percussion of, 162
    wall shape and deformity in, 158, 158f, 159f
Chickenpox (varicella), 335, Plate 19–7
Child abuse
    abdominal pain in, 212
    assessment of, 257–258
    corporal punishment and, 21
Child Behavior Checklist (CBCL), 346
Child Epilepsy Questionnaire, 347
Child Health Questionnaire (CHQ), 346
Children's Depression Inventory (CDI), 346
Choanal atresia, 66, 86
Choking, from foreign bodies, 154
Chondromalacia patella, 264
Chorea, 226
Choreiform movement, 226
CHQ (Child Health Questionnaire), 346
Chronic conditions
    caregiver burnout in, 346
    caring for children with, 343–348

Chronic conditions (*Continued*)
  child decision-making about, 349
  cultural attitudes toward, 21, 23
  disclosure of diagnosis in, 343–345
  emphasizing positive in, 344
  encouraging shared labor in, 345–346
  honesty in communications about, 344
  interview in, 16, 344–345
  physical examination in, 347
  quality of life in, 346–347
  transitional care for, 347–348
Chvostek sign, 297
Cigarette paper wrinkling, 337
Clavicle fracture, 67–68
Cleft lip and palate, 86–87
  conditions associated with, 76
  examination of, 122
Clinodactyly, 77, 88, 88f
Clitoromegaly, 88
Clubbing of fingertips *See* Finger clubbing.
Clubfoot, 70
Cold sores, 121
Colds, 153
Colic
  diagnosis of, 195–196
  ureteral, 212
Colitis
  allergic, 198
  bleeding and, 199
  infectious, 202
Coloboma, 130, Plate 8–2
Color vision, 128
Colposcope, 326, 326f
Comedones, 336
Comitant strabismus, 133
Communication
  about chronic conditions, 343–345
  about death of child, 16–17
  about growth and development, 41–42, 42f
  body outline doll for, 352, 352f
  cross-cultural, 20–22, 24
  decisional competence and, 351–353, 351f
  forms of address in, 4
  in breaking difficult news, 17, 344
  in family interview, 1–2
  with adolescents, 13–14
  with angry parents, 16
Competence, decisional, 350–351
Condom, 328
Conduct disorders, 100
Confidentiality
  adolescents and, 13
  in neurological history-taking, 224
  in psychiatric interview, 250–252
Congenital adrenal hyperplasia (CAH). *See*
    Adrenal hyperplasia, congenital.
Congenital anomalies
  assessment of, 75–89
  constellations of, 77
  definitions of, 76–79
  diagnostic approach to, 75–76
  ethnicity in, 81
  four Cs of, 76
  growth and development in, 82
  history-taking for, 79–82
  in syndromes, 78–79
  isolated vs. multiple defects in, 76
  major malformations as, 76–77
  minor, 77
  of abdomen, 87
  of back, 87
  of ears, 85–86, 86f
  of eyes, 85, 85t
  of genitalia. *See* Genitalia, ambiguous.
  of head and scalp, 84–85

Congenital anomalies (*Continued*)
  of inguinal canal, 216–219, 216f–219f
  of intestinal tract, 214
  of limbs, 88–89
  of neck and chest, 87
  of nose and mouth, 86–87, 86f
  of skin, 89
  of testicular descent, 219–221
  parental age and, 80
  parental anxiety about, 75
  patterns in, 78–79
  physical examination in
    approaches to, 82–84
    normal variation in, 82
    specific assessments in, 84–89
  prevalence of, 75–76
  sequence in, 78
  subsequent pregnancies and, 76
Conjunctivitis, 134, 135f
Connective tissue disease, mixed, 266
Consanguinity
  in congenital anomalies, 81
  in congenital heart disease, 171
  questions about, 9
Constipation
  definition of, 199, 200–201
  functional, 196, 201, 201f
  in adolescents, 200–201
  in infants, 199–200
  in toddlers, 200, 200f
  normal elimination patterns and, 199
  rectal examination for, 201
Consultations, 15–16
Contact lenses, for infants, 130
Continuous heart murmurs, 182–183
Contraception
  for adolescents, 327–329, 328f, 357–358
  methods for, 327–329, 328f
  postcoital, 329
Contraceptive sponge, 327
Conversation, culturally effective, 21–22
Conversion disorder, 257
Cooing, 182
Coordination test, 226, 226f, 236, 240–241
Cornea
  cloudy, 134–135
  laceration of, 131
  light reflexes in, 135–136, 136f–137f, Plate 8–11
  size of, 134, 135f
  staining of, 142–143, 143f
Corneal reflex, 233, 233f
Corporal punishment, 21
Cortical thumb, 89
Cortisol, 297, 298
Cost-benefit analysis, 354–356
Costochondritis, 154
Cough
  case histories of, 167
  conditions associated with, 161t
  diagnostic use of, 160
  history of, 153
Counseling, genetic, 75
Cover test, 141–142, 141f
Cranial nerves. *See also specific nerves.*
  assessment of, 230–234
  lesions of, 225
  palsies of, 130f, 131–132
Craniofacial anomalies, 77
Craniosynostosis, 84, 112
Craniotabes, 114
Cremasteric fibers, 219
Cremation, 21
Crepitation, 283
Cri du chat syndrome, 58
Crigler-Najjar syndromes, 204

Crohn disease, 9, 211
Cross-eye (esotropia)
  corneal light reflexes in, 135f–136f
  definition of, 128, 130
Croup, 156
Crowing, 166
Cruciate ligaments, 284
Crusts (skin), 336, Plate 19–10
Crying
  asymmetric, 66, 67f
  cardiovascular disorders and, 177
  neonatal, 58
  normal, 195
Cryptorchidism, 70, 88, 219–220
CSMF (central steady maintain fixation) test, 137–138
Cultural competency, 20
Cultural factors
  alternative therapies and, 23–24
  chronic conditions and, 21, 23
  disciplinary practices and, 21
  family hierarchy and, 20
  hindsight and, 25
  in adolescent interviews, 14
  in breaking bad news, 24
  in developmental assessment, 22–23
  in family interview, 4
  in history-taking, 22–24
  in physical examination, 24–25
  in prescribing, 25
  in psychiatric assessment, 258
  informed consent and, 22
  interpreters and, 22
  language and, 20
  life and death issues and, 21
  looks and gestures in, 20–21
  naming systems and, 20
  pediatric practice and, 19–25
  recent immigrants and, 21
  stereotyping and, 19
Culture samples, collection of, 324–325
Cushing syndrome
  causes of, 298
  clinical features of, 298f
  diagnosis of, 51
  evaluation of, 298
Cutaneous diseases. *See* Skin, disorders of.
Cutis aplasia, 74
Cutis marmorata, 172
Cyanosis
  age of onset of, 171
  as diagnostic sign, 157, 172
  central, 170
  physical examination for, 24
  tetralogy of Fallot and, 171
Cystic fibrosis
  case histories of, 166–167
  diarrhea in, 202
  finger clubbing in, 160, 160f
  Pseudomonas infections in, 156
  symptoms of, 156
Cystic Fibrosis Problem Checklist, 347

D

Dactylitis, 284
Deafness, 105–106
Death
  cultural attitudes toward, 21
  fear of, 6–7
  informing parents of, 16–17
Decision-making, 20. *See also* Health
    decisions.
Defecation, 8, 199
Deformation, 76, 78
Delusions, 257
Dental development, 48, 48t, 121

Denver Development Screening Test II (DDST II), 92, 100
Depigmentation, 239, 239f
Depo-Provera (medroxyprogesterone acetate), 329
Depression
    ADHD and, 100
    assessment of, 255, 346
    maternal screening for, 3
Dermal compression test, 177
Dermatitis
    atopic, Plate 19–12
    definition of, 337
Dermatitis herpetiformis, 335
Dermatographism, 336, Plate 19–8
Dermatologic diseases. *See* Skin, disorders of.
Dermatomyositis, juvenile, 266
Dermatosis, 331
Desquamation, 336
Development
    abnormal
        case histories of, 105–108
        delayed growth in, 43
        head circumference and, 28
        parental guilt about, 6
        patterns of, 92
    assessment of, 91–109
        approach to, 100–103, 102f, 108–109
        behavior problems in, 99–100
        block tests for, 107f, 109f
        cultural factors in, 22–23
        equipment for, 100, 100f, 101f
        family history in, 92, 99
        gaining child's cooperation in, 101–103, 102f
        in hyperactive children, 103
        in inattentive children, 103
        in oppositional children, 102–103
        information sources for, 92
        intrusive parents and, 103
        shy and frightened children, 102, 102f
        social history in, 99
        surveillance in, 91–92, 99–100
    delayed, 82, 106–108
    milestones in, 91–92, 104–105
        infant and preschool child, 93t–96t
        school-aged child, 97t–98t
    physical examination of, 103–105
Diabetes insipidus, 288
Diabetes mellitus
    acanthosis nigricans in, 307
    checklist for, 309t
    clinical characteristics of, 307–308
    family history in, 307–308
    hirsutism in, 302–303
    ketoacidosis in, 308
    lipohypertrophy in, 310f
    skin conditions in, 310f
    symptoms of, 308
    type 1, 308
    type 2, 307–308
Diabetic Quality of Life Instrument, 347
Diaper rash, Plate 19–13
Diaphragm, 327
Diarrhea
    definitions of, 202
    in adolescents, 203
    in appendicitis, 210
    in infants, 202
    in toddlers, 202
    pathophysiology of, 202
Diastasis recti, 68, 216
Diastematomyelia, 72, 272, 273f
Diastolic murmurs, 181–182
DiGeorge syndrome, 297

Diplopia, 232
Disc space disease, 208
Discipline, 21
Discoid lesions, of skin, 337
Disruption (anomaly), 78
Disruptive behavior, 254
Diverticulosis, colonic, 199
Dolichocephaly, 29, 29f
Doll
    anatomically correct, 257
    body outline, 352, 352f
Doll's eye reflex, 232
Down syndrome
    appearance in, 225
    crying in, 58
    duodenal atresia in, 213
    minor anomalies in, 77
    palmar flexion crease in, 88f, 89
    skull in, 84
Dress, for family interview, 3
Droopy eyelid. *See* Ptosis.
Drugs, 25, 154
    reactions to, 333
Duchenne muscular dystrophy, 243–244
Duck-walk test, 271, 272f, 280
Duodenal atresia, 213
Dwarf, 29
Dysarthria, 225
Dyskinesia, oculotrigeminal, 145, 146f
Dyslexia, 231
Dysmorphology, 76, 85, 85t
Dyspepsia, 196
Dysphagia, 66, 156, 191–193
Dysphasia, 225
Dysplasia(s)
    ectodermal, 85, 115, 121
    frontonasal, 86
Dyspnea
    conditions associated with, 154
    definition of, 170
    in asthma, 154
    respiration and, 159
Dyspraxia, 241
Dystonic posturing, 226
Dysuria, 210

E
Eardrum, 118, 118f
Ears
    congenital anomalies of, 85–86, 86f
    examination of, 115–120, 157
        neonatal, 65
        otoscopy in, 116–118, 117f
        tympanic membrane in, 118, 118f
    gestational age and, 62, 62f
    low-set, 85
    shape and position of, 115–116
    wax removal from, 119–120
Eating disorders, 254–255
Ecchymoses, 58, 73
Echolalia, 99
Ectodermal dysplasias
    hair in, 85, 115
    teeth in, 121
Ectopia cordis, 215
Eczema
    crusts in, 336
    definition of, 337
    in respiratory disorders, 156
    subacute, Plate 19–12
Eczema herpeticum, 333
Edema
    idiopathic scrotal, 220–221
    peripheral, 170
Ejection click (heart), 177–178
Elbow, 278

Emancipated minors, 357
Emesis. *See* Vomiting.
Emotional disorders, 255–256, 258
Empathy, 1–2
Emphysema, subcutaneous, 162
Encephalopathy, bilirubin, 204
Encopresis, 100
Endocrine system
    adrenal disorders in, 297–303
    adrenarche and, 297, 299, 300f
    androgen excess in, 298–303
    calcium metabolism disorders in, 296–297, 296f
    clinical evaluation of, 287–310
    diabetes and. *See* Diabetes mellitus.
    growth hormone deficiency in, 287–290
    map of, 288f
    puberty and. *See* Puberty.
    signs and symptoms in, 297–298
    thyroid disorders in, 290–296
Enteritis, regional, 211
Enterocolitis, necrotizing, 194, 198, 214
Enthesitis, 283
Enuresis, 100
Environmental factors, respiratory, 155
Epicanthal fold
    corneal light reflexes and, 135–136, 136f, Plate 8–11
    definition of, 130
Epidermal necrolysis, toxic, Plate 19–6
Epidermolysis bullosa, 335
Epididymitis, 220–221
Epiglottis, 123
Epilepsy, assessment of, 347
Epiphora, 145–148
    diagnostic algorithm for, 147f
    differential diagnosis of, 147t
    lacrimal duct obstruction and, 147
    photophobia with, 145–146
Erosion (skin), 337
Erythema, 338, Plate 19–13
Erythema multiforme, 335, 337, Plate 19–11
Erythema toxicum, 73
Esodeviation, 130
Esophageal atresia, 66–67, 192
Esophageal obstruction, 66
Esophageal varices, 198
Esophagitis, reflux, 192–193
Esophoria, 130
Esotropia (cross-eye)
    corneal light reflexes in, 135f–136f
    definition of, 128, 130
Ethmoiditis, 132
Ethnicity
    congenital anomalies and, 81
    physical examination and, 24–25
    prescribing and, 25
Euthyroid states, 295
Ewing sarcoma, 265
Excel syndrome, 188–189
Excoriation, 337
Exophthalmos, 125, 295
Exotropia, 128, 135f
Exstrophy, of bladder, 215
Extraocular movements, assessment of, 138–139
    frame for, 139, 139f
    head twisting in, 139, 140f
    spinning in, 138–139, 139f
Extraocular muscles, innervation of, 131–132
Extrasystole, 68
Extremities
    neonatal, examination of, 70–71, 71f
    neurological assessment of, 235–241
Eye contact, cultural sensitivity in, 20–21

Eye(s)
  congenital anomalies of, 85
  lacerations of, 131
  movement of, in infants, 128
  neonatal, examination of, 64–65, 64f, 65f
Eyeball approximation, of measurement, 28

F

Face following, 127–128, 128f, 137
Facial asymmetry, 225
Facial nerve (cranial nerve VII), 233
Facial palsy, 66, 67f, 233
Failure to thrive, 52–53
False fluency, 22
Familial hypocalciuric hypercalcemia, 296
Family hierarchy, 20
Family history, 8–11
  congenital anomalies in, 80–81
  consanguinity in, 9
  diseases in, 9
  in chronic illness, 16, 344–345
  in developmental assessment, 92, 99
  obesity and, 50–51
  obtaining initial history in, 7–11
  occupational, of parents, 10
  psychosocial aspects of, 8–11
  respiratory disorders and, 155, 157
Family interview, 1–18. *See also* History-
      taking; Interviewing.
  communication and, 1–2
  cultural aspects of, 4, 24
  developmental surveillance and, 91–92,
      99–100
  disease vs. illness focus in, 1
  dressing for, 3
  encouraging second opinion in, 18
  establishing tone of, 4
  family dynamics in, 9–10
  fear of death and, 6–7
  ground rules for, 5
  hidden agendas in, 5–7
  household description in, 10–11
  interpreters and, 22
  occupying children during, 5
  parental guilt feelings in, 5–6
  parent-child relations in, 3
  parents' opening statement in, 5
  participation of both parents in, 5
  presenting vs. true complaint in, 5
  problem list and treatment plan in, 11–12,
      12t
  psychiatric, 253
  psychosocial aspects of, 10–11
  respecting time of others in, 4
  setting for, 4
  therapeutic nature of, 1, 2–3, 5–6, 12
  with adolescents, 13–15
FAS (fetal alcohol syndrome), 71, 86
Fatigue, 170
Febrile convulsions, 6–7
"Fecal fascination," 8
Feeding problems, 192
Feelings diary, 355–356, 356f
Feminization, testicular, 219, 301–302, 302f
Femoral epiphysis, slipped capital, 264
Femoral pulses, 68, 68f
Femoral torsion, internal, 261–262, 261f
Fencer position, 238, 238f
Fetal alcohol syndrome (FAS), 71, 86
Fetal growth, 79
Fetal hydantoin syndrome, 88
Fetal movements, 80
Fever, convulsions in, 6–7
Fibroma
  periungual, Plate 19–16
  sternocleidomastoid, 125–126

Fibromyalgia, 266
Finger clubbing
  assessment of, 160, 160f
  in cardiovascular assessment, 184,
      184f–185f
  in musculoskeletal assessment, 275
  in pulmonary disease, 151
Finish the story/drawing, 354, 356
Fissure, 337
Fisting, 240, 240f
Fixation, ocular, 137–138, 138f
Flat feet, 263, 284
Flexion contracture
  of hip, 280–281, 283f
  of knee, 281, 283f
FLK (funny-looking kid), 111
Floppy infant, 227, 235, 240, 240f
Flow murmurs
  diastolic, 182
  innocent, 181
  systolic, 181
Folk medicine, 23–24
Folliculitis, 335
Fontanels
  examination of, 113–114, 114f
  metopic, 113
  palpation of, 64, 114f
  persistent parietal foramina, 113
  tension in, 114
Foods, solid, 49
Foot
  congenital anomalies of, 70–71, 89
  examination of, 284
  flat, 263, 284
  pain in, 264
Footdrop, 227
Foramina, persistent parietal, 113
Forefoot adduction, 263, 263f
Formboard puzzles, 101f
Fragile X syndrome, 81, 106–108
Freckles, 334
Freiberg disease, 264
Frenulum, 122
Frog-leg position, 226
Frontal lobe lesions, 229
Frontonasal dysplasia, 86
Functional level, parent estimate of, 17
Funduscopy, 142, 231–232, 232f
Funnel chest, 158, 158f
Funny-looking kid (FLK), 111

G

Gag reflex, 121–122
Gait
  antalgic, 271–272
  in neurological diagnosis, 225
  observation of, 271–272
  tandem, 228
Gallop rhythm (heart), 178–179
Gastric distention, 213
Gastroenteritis, 202, 208
Gastroesophageal reflux (GER), 193, 194
Gastrointestinal bleeding, 197–199
  in infants, 197–198
  in older children and adolescents, 199
  in young children, 198–199
  types of, 197
  vomiting and, 198
Gastrointestinal disorder(s)/symptom(s)
  abdominal pain as, 194–197, 195t
  age factors in, 191
  constipation as, 199–201
  diarrhea as, 202–203
  dysphagia as, 191–193
  evaluation of, 191–206
  functional, 196

Gastrointestinal disorder(s)/symptom(s)
      (*Continued*)
  history-taking for, 191
  ischemic, 214
  jaundice as, 203–205
  vomiting as, 193–194
Gastroschisis, 78, 87, 215, 215f
Gelling phenomenon, 270
Genitalia
  abnormalities of, in older children, 88
  ambiguous, 70, 87–88, 219, 299–301, 300f,
      302f
  examination of, 69–70, 318–319
  female, 300f
  in precocious puberty, 306, 306f
  male, 46f
Genodermatoses, 331, 333
Genu valgum, 262, 262f
Genu varum, 262, 262f
Genu varus, 282
Geographic tongue, 122
GER (gastroesophageal reflux), 193, 194
Gestational age
  assessment of, 61–63
  correction for, 104
  ear and, 62, 62f
  genitalia and, 62, 63f
  scoring systems for, 63
  sole creases in, 61, 62f
Gestures, 20–21
Gilbert syndrome, 204
Gingiva, 121
Glaucoma, congenital
  definition of, 130
  epiphora in, 143–146
  ocular observations in, 134–135, 135f
Globus hystericus, 154
Glossopharyngeal nerve (cranial nerve IX),
      234
Glucocorticoids, 298, 299f
Goiter, 294, 295
Goldenhar syndrome, 115
Good, conception of, 354–356
Gower maneuver, 271, 272f
Gower sign, 235
Graphesthesia, 230
Grasp
  palmar, 59, 60f, 238
  pincer, 106f
  plantar, 59, 60f
  radial raking, 106f
Grasp reflex, neonatal, 57
Graves disease, 294–295
Growing pains, 154, 266
Growth. *See also* Growth charts.
  assessment of, 27–53
  communicating information about, 41–42
  constitutional deviations in, 27
  delayed, 43
  dental, 48, 48t
  failure to thrive and, 52–53
  in congenital anomalies, 82
  measurement of, 27–29, 40–41
    approximation in, 28
    arm span, 29, 40f
    ethnic factors in, 41
    head circumference, 28–29, 41
    height, 27–28, 28f
    height/weight graphs in, 41–42, 42f
    recording of, 29
    recumbent length, 27–28, 27f
    sequential, importance of, 40–41
    upper and lower segments, 40, 41f
    weight in, 28
  nutritional assessment in, 49–53
  proportion and disproportion in, 29, 40–41

Growth. (*Continued*)
  pubertal, stages of, 45–48
  short child, anxieties of, 43
  velocity in, 43–45, 44f, 45f
Growth charts
  for boys
    body mass index-for-age percentiles, 36f
    head circumference-for-age, 32f
    length-for-age, 30f
    stature-for-age and weight-for-age
      percentiles, 34f
    weight-for-age, 30f
    weight-for-length percentiles, 32f
    weight-for-stature percentiles, 38f
  for girls
    body mass index-for-age percentiles, 37f
    head circumference-for-age, 33f
    length-for-age, 31f
    stature-for-age and weight-for-age
      percentiles, 35f
    weight-for-age, 31f
    weight-for-length percentiles, 33f
    weight-for-stature percentiles, 39f
  neonatal, 61f
  sequential measurements and, 40–41
  use of, 29
Growth hormone deficiency
  case history of, 288
  characteristics of, 287–288
  hypoglycemia in, 287, 289f
  midline defects associated with, 287–288
  onset of, 288
  physical examination in, 288–290, 289f
  weight-to-height ratio in, 289f, 290
Growth plate injuries, 282
Guilt, parental, 5–6
Gynecologic assessment, 317–330
  adolescent contraception and, 325–327
  bacterial cultures in, 320–321, 321f
  for sexual abuse, 325–327
  history-taking in, 321–322
  of adolescent girls, 321
  pelvic examination in
    patient preparation for, 322
    procedure for, 323–325
  physical examination in, 317–321
    approach to, 317, 317f, 318f
    clitoral size in, 319
    of external genitalia, 318–319,
      318f–319f
    retroabdominal, 320–321
    vaginoscopy in, 319–320
  physician attitude toward, 317
  sexual activity and, 322
Gynecomastia, 306

H
Haemophilus influenzae, 132
Hair
  gestational age and, 62
  head examination and, 115
  in Cushing syndrome, 298
  in skin disorders, 339
  in Waardenburg syndrome, 85
Halitosis, 121
Hallucinations, 257
Hamstring muscles, 273, 283, 284
Hand
  congenital anomalies of, 88–89
  examination of, 275–276
  joint palpation in, 276
  swelling of, 275, 278f
  weakness of, 225
Harlequin color change, 58
Hashimoto disease, 291, 292
Hay fever, 156

Head
  congenital anomalies of, 84
  craniotabes in, 114
  examination of, 111–124
    auscultation in, 114–115
    ears in, 115–120
    general observations in, 111
    hair in, 115
    mouth in, 120–123
    neonatal, 63–67
    nose in, 123–124
  fontanels in, 64, 113–114
  shape of, 112
  skull growth in, 112
  support of, in newborns, 67, 67f
  sutures in, 63
  transillumination of, 64
Head circumference
  developmental delay and, 28
  growth charts for, 32f, 33f
  measurement of, 28–29, 41, 60–61, 60f,
    112–113, 113f
  of parents, 28, 113
Head position, in vision assessment, 134
Head tilt, 130, 130f, 132
Head turn, 130–131, 130f, 132
Headache, 9, 241–243, 242t
Health care, culture and, 20
Health decisions. *See also* Informed consent.
  assessing adolescent role in, 357–358
  assessing child's role in, 349–359
    communication capacity in, 351–353,
      351f
    conception of "good" in, 354–356
    emotional expression in, 354f
    feelings diary in, 355–356, 356f
    finish the story/drawing in, 354, 356
    reasoning capacity in, 353–354
    "what if" activities in, 354, 355f
    with artwork, 352–353, 353f
    with body outline doll, 352, 352f
  competence of children for, 350–351
  parent and family role in, 350
  patient autonomy in, 350–351
Hearing, assessment of, 115
Heart defects, congenital, 171, 172
Heart diseases. *See also* Cardiovascular
    disorders.
  classification of, 169
  consanguinity in, 171
Heart failure, congestive
  case history of, 175
  clinical manifestations of, 172–175, 172f
  in infants, 170, 171
  liver enlargement in, 174
Heart murmurs, 179–183
  auscultation for, 183–184
  cardiorespiratory, 183
  continuous, 182–183
  diastolic, 181–182
  in mitral valve prolapse, 183
  in patent ductus arteriosus, 182–183
  innocent, 180, 181, 187
  mechanisms of, 179, 180f
  presystolic, 181
  systolic, 179–181
    flow, 181
    obstructive, 180
    regurgitant, 179–180
    vibratory, 180
  venous hum, 182, 182f
Heart rate, 68, 186, 186t
Heart sounds
  evaluation of, 177–179
  in infants, 174–175
  normal vs. abnormal, 177–178, 178f

Heart sounds (*Continued*)
  numbering of, 177
  triple rhythm in, 178–179
Heartburn, 192
Heel walking, 227
Height
  adult, prediction of, 43
  growth charts for, 34f, 35f
  growth velocity and, 43–45, 44f, 45f
  measurement of, 27–28, 28f
Hemangioma
  capillary, 131, Plate 8–3, Plate 19–4
  definition of, 131
  neonatal, 58, 72
  orbital, 131
  skin changes and, 89
  strawberry, 73
Hematemesis
  color of, 197
  esophageal varices and, 198
  in older children and adolescents, 199
  in peptic ulcer, 199
Hematochezia
  causes of, 199
  definition of, 197
  juvenile polyps in, 198
  Meckel diverticulum in, 198
Hemiparesis, 225, 239
Hemivertebra, 268
Hemolytic-uremic syndrome (HUS), 199
Hemorrhage, life-threatening, 212
Hemorrhagic disease of newborn, 198
Hemorrhoids, 199
Henoch-Schönlein purpura (HSP), 196
Hepatitis, 204
Hepatosplenomegaly, 205
Herbal remedies, 23–24
Hernia
  diastasis recti, 216
  epigastric, 216
  incarcerated, 218
  inguinal. *See* Inguinal hernia.
  neonatal, 70
  umbilical, 87, 215–216, 215f
Herpes simplex, 121, 335
Heterochromia iridis, 82
Hidden agenda, 5–7, 15
Hip
  abduction in, 280f
  congenital dislocation of, 70, 71f, 87
  examination of, 70, 71f, 280–281
  flexion contracture in, 280–281, 283f
  leg length in, 280, 281f
  pain in, 263–264
  rotation in, 281f
Hirschsprung disease, 213, 214
Hirsutism, 302–303, 302f
History-taking, 1–18. *See also* Family
    interview; Interviewing
  adolescents and, 13–15
  alternative therapies in, 23–24
  antenatal, 55, 56t
  bowel movements in, 8
  chief complaints in, 7
  confidentiality in, 224
  cross-cultural, 22–24
  differential diagnosis in, 12
  family and psychosocial history in, 8–11
  feeding problems in, 7–8
  format for, 7–8
  growth and development in, 8
  immunizations in, 8
  labor and delivery in, 7
  neonatal period in, 7
  prenatal history and, 7
  present illness in, 7

History-taking (*Continued*)
  previous illnesses in, 8
  problem list and treatment plan
      development from, 11–12, 12t
  review of systems in, 8, 9t
Hives, 335–336
HLA-B27 marker, 270
Hoffman reflex, 241
Holoprosencephaly, 85, 86
Honesty, 344
Hospital rounds, 15
HOTV vision test, 138, 138f
Household, 10–11
HSP (Henoch-Schönlein purpura), 196
Human Genome Project, 79
Hurler syndrome, 137
HUS (hemolytic-uremic syndrome), 199
Hydrocele, 217f
  assessment of, 217–219
  communicating vs. noncommunicating, 217
  definition of, 77
  inguinal hernia and, 217–219, 218f–219f
  neonatal, 70
Hydrocephalus, 64, 112
11–Hydroxylase deficiency, 301
21–Hydroxylase deficiency, 299
3β-Hydroxysteroid dehydrogenase
      deficiency, 301
Hymen, 318–319, 318f, 319f
Hyperactivity disorder, 99–100
Hyperbilirubinemia
  classification of, 203
  direct-reacting, 204–205
  idiopathic unconjugated, 204
  indirect-reacting, 203–204
Hypercalcemia, 296, 296f
Hypercalciuria, 212
Hyperextensibility, of fingers, 88
Hyperinsulinism, 302
Hyperkinetic circulation, 187, 188f, 188t
Hyperphoria, 131
Hyperpigmentation, 338
Hyperplasia
  adrenal. *See* Adrenal hyperplasia,
      congenital.
  Leydig cell, 305f
Hyperpnea, 159
Hypersensitivity, oral, 192
Hypertelorism, 83f, 85
Hypertension
  persistent pulmonary, in infants, 171–172
  pheochromocytoma in, 297
  portal, 198, 205
Hyperthyroidism, 290
Hypertrophic scar, 337
Hypertropia, 131, 135f
Hyperventilation, 154
Hyphemia, 131, Plate 8–4
Hypocalcemia, 296–297
Hypochondriasis, 257
Hypoglossal nerve (cranial nerve XII), 234
Hypoglycemia, 287, 289f
Hypogonadism, hypothalamic, 307
Hypoparathyroidism, 296, 297
Hypophoria, 131
Hypophosphatemic rickets, 297
Hypopigmentation, 49, 89, 338
Hypopnea, 159
Hyposmia, 307
Hypospadias, 69, 70, 88, 301
Hypotelorism, 85
Hypothalamic hypogonadism, 307
Hypothalamic-pituitary disease, 291
Hypothyroidism
  acquired, 292

Hypothyroidism (*Continued*)
  appearance in, 291f
  causes of, 291–292
  congenital, 58, 291–292, 292f, 295
  evaluation of, 290–291, 290t
  hair in, 115
  reflexes in, 236
  tongue size in, 122
  treatment of, 294
Hypotonia, 235
Hypotropia, 131
Hypoxia, 170
Hysterical blindness, 231

I
Ichthyosis, congenital, 72
Idiopathic scrotal edema, 220–221
Ileal atresia, 213
Ileus, meconium, 213
Illiterate E vision chart, 138
Immunizations
  cultural factors in, 22
  in history-taking, 8
  respiratory disorders and, 155
Imperforate anus, 200, 213
Impetigo, 335, Plate 19–10
Incarceration, of hernia, 218
Incomitance, 136
Infantile spasm, 246
Infants. *See also specific conditions, in infants.*
  abdominal pain in, 195–196
  cardiovascular assessment of, 169–177
  color vision in, 128
  developmental milestones in, 93t–96t
  diarrhea in, 202
  hyperbilirubinemia in, 203–204
  reflex assessment in, 237–238
  visual development in, 127–128
  vomiting in, 194
Infarct, vasculitic, 275, 277f
Infection, 265, 331. *See also specific type,
      e.g., Candida infection.*
Informed consent. *See also* Health decisions.
  by adolescents, 357–358
  by children, 350–351
  cultural sensitivity and, 22
Inguinal canal
  abnormalities of, 216–219
  development of, 216, 216f
Inguinal hernia, 216–219, 217f–219f
  diagnosis of, 218, 218f–219f
  direct vs. indirect, 216
  embryology of, 216
  in cryptorchidism, 220
  in girls, 219
  intermittent nature of, 217
  manual reduction of, 218
  palpation of, 218
  patent processus vaginalis in, 217–219,
      218f–219f
  physical examination for, 217–218
Intercostal muscles, 154
Internal strabismus, patellar, 261–262, 261f
Interphalangeal joints, 276, 278f
Interpreters, 22
Interviewing. *See also* History-taking.
  culture and, 4, 14
  dress and, 3
  explaining purpose of, 13
  interpreters and, 22
  introductory conversation in, 4
  nonverbal cues in, 13–14
  note-taking in, 2
  of adolescents, 13–15
  of family. *See* Family interview.
  question styles in, 2–3

Interviewing (*Continued*)
  skills for, 2–7
In-toeing, 261–262, 261f
Intracranial pressure, 114
Intrauterine device (IUD), 328
Intussusception, 195–196
Iris lesions, of skin, 337
Iritis, 286
Iron deficiency, 49
Irritable bowel syndrome
  constipation in, 201
  definition of, 196–197
  diagnostic criteria for, 197t
Itching, 332
IUD (intrauterine device), 328

J
Jargon, 1
Jaundice, 203–205
  definition of, 203
  examination of liver and spleen in, 205
  in hepatitis, 204
  in infants, 203–204
  in older children and adolescents, 204–205
Jaw jerk reflex, 233
Jaw-winking phenomenon, 145, 146f
Jittery eyes. *See* Nystagmus.
Joints. *See also specific joints, e.g.,* Hip.
  hypermobility of, 266, 266t
Juvenile rheumatoid arthritis. *See*
      Rheumatoid arthritis, juvenile.

K
Kawasaki disease, 122
Kayser-Fleischer rings, 204
Keloid, 337
Kernicterus, 204
Ketoacidosis, diabetic, 308
Khamis-Roche height prediction method, 43
Kidney calculi, 212
Kinky hair syndrome, 85, 115
Klinefelter syndrome, 307
Knee
  angulation in, 282
  examination of, 281–284
  flexion of, 283
  flexion contracture of, 281, 283f
  pain in, 264
  palpation of, 282–283
Knee reflex, 236
Knock knee, 262, 262f, 282
Köhler disease, 264
Koplik spots, 338
Korotkoff sounds, 176
Kyphoscoliosis, 159, 159f
Kyphosis, 264–265, 272

L
Labia
  agglutination in, 319, 319f
  examination of, 317, 317f–318f
  gestational age and, 62, 63f
  neonatal, 69
Labor and delivery
  congenital anomalies and, 80
  in cardiovascular disorders, 171–172
  ophthalmic injuries in, 127
Lacerations, ocular, 131
Lacrimal duct
  drainage of, 142, 143f, 147
  examination of, 142, 143f
  obstruction of, 131
Language, 20, 22
Laryngomalacia, 166, 166f
Larynx, infantile, 166
Lasègue test, 273

Laurence-Moon-Biedl syndrome, 51, 51f, 132
Learning disorders, 100, 108
Legal blindness, 129
Legg-Calvé-Perthes disease, 263–264, 271
Leg(s)
    length discrepancy in, 272, 273f
    measurement of, 280, 281f
    proximal weakness of, 225
    scissoring of, 236, 236f
Length, recumbent
    growth charts for, 30f–33f
    measurement of, 27–28, 28f, 61, 61f
Leprechaunism, 83f
Leukemia, 265
Leukocoria, Plate 8–5
    definition of, 130, 131
    diagnostic algorithm for, 149f
    differential diagnosis in, 149t
    evaluation of, 148
    in PHPV, 132
Leukodystrophy, 223
Levonorgestrel (Norplant), 329
Leydig cell hyperplasia, 305f
Lichen planus
    buccal mucosa plaques in, 338
    itching in, 332
    papules in, 334
Lichenification, 337
Lid ptosis. See Ptosis.
Life events, 11
Limp, 267, 267t
Lingual thyroid, 294, 294f
Lip abnormalities, 86–87
Lip pits, 86, 86f
Lip-licker's rash, 121
Lipohypertrophy, 310f
Lipomeningocele, 72
Liver, 205, 205f
Liver diseases, 204–205
Log roll test, 280
Lordosis, 272, 274
Lower extremities
    muscle tone in, 235–236
    neonatal, examination of, 70–71, 71f
    neurological assessment of, 235–239
    power in, 235
Lupus erythematosus, systemic, 266, 333
Lyme disease, 265, 270
Lymph nodes, 125, 125f
Lymphadenitis, mesenteric, 211
Lymphangioma, 131, 131f

M
Macular umbo, 127, Plate 8–1
Macule, 334
Maculopapular patches, 334
Malformation, 76, 77–78
Mallory-Weiss syndrome, 199
Malnutrition, 43t. See also Nutritional
    assessment.
Marble skin, 58, 58f, 172
Marcus Gunn oculotrigeminal dyskinesia,
    145, 146f
Marfan syndrome, 171, 188
Marital stability, 11
Masseter muscles, 233
Maze puzzle, 226, 226f
McCune-Albright syndrome, 305, 305f, 306
McMurray test, 283
Meckel diverticulum, 198–199, 211
Meconium, 213
Mediastinal crunch, 183
Medications, 25, 154
    reactions to, 333
Medroxyprogesterone acetate (Depo-
    Provera), 329

Medullary carcinoma, 296
Megalencephaly, benign familial, 28, 60–61
Melanoma, 333
Melena, 197, 199
Memory, tests for, 229, 229f
Menarche, 321
Meningitis, 124, 132
Menkes syndrome, 85, 115
Menorrhagia, 322
Menstruation, 321, 322
Mental disorders. See Psychiatric disorders.
Mental retardation, 81, 258
Mesenteric lymphadenitis, 211
Metacarpal sign, 51, 52f
Metacarpophalangeal joints, 276
Metatarsophalangeal joints, 284, 285f
Metatarsus varus, 263, 263f
Micrognathia, 274, 277f
Micropenis, 88
Midget, 29
Midgut malrotation, 214
Midsystolic click, 179
Migraine, 9
Milia, 72
Minors, decision-making by, 357
Mitochondrial diseases, 145
Mitral regurgitation, 179, 182
Mitral valve prolapse, 179, 183
Mitral valve stenosis, 181
Mixed connective tissue disease, 266
Molluscum contagiosum, 334, Plate 19–1
Mongolian spots, 24, 73, 338
Monoarthritis, 267, 267t
Morning stiffness, 270
Moro reflex, 59, 59f, 115, 237–238
Motor aphasia, 229
Motor neuron lesions
    assessment of, 229
    signs of, 223, 224f
    upper vs. lower, 223, 224f
Mouth
    congenital anomalies of, 86–87, 86f
    examination of, 120–123
        breath in, 121
        buccal mucosa in, 121, 338
        epiglottis in, 123
        gingiva in, 121
        lips in, 121
        neonatal, 66–67, 66f
        palate in, 122
        pharyngeal wall in, 123
        position for, 120, 120f
        teeth in, 121
        tongue in, 121–122
        tonsils in, 122–123
    tongue tie in, 66, 66f
Moving, of household, 10
Mucocolpos, 318f
Mucopolysaccharidoses, 85, 134
Multiculturalism, 19
Munchausen syndrome by proxy, 202
Murmurs. See Heart murmurs.
Muscle strength
    assessment of, 284–285
    observation of, 225
    of lower extremities, 235, 235t
    of pelvic girdle, 271, 271f
    of upper extremities, 239–240, 240f
    proximal, 227–228
    scales for, 285t
    tests for, 271, 271f
Muscle tone
    in lower extremities, 235–236
    in newborn infant, 58–59
    in upper extremities, 240, 240f
    observation of, 225–226

Muscular dystrophy, 225, 235
Musculoskeletal disorders, 261–286
    age range for, 269t
    history-taking in, 268–271
    limp in, 267, 267t
    medical examination in, 285
    monoarthritis in, 267, 267t
    multiple swollen joints in, 267–268
    muscle assessment in, 284–285
    normal variants vs., 261–263
    observation in, 271–272, 271f
    ocular manifestations of, 285–286
    pain in
        aggravating and relieving factors in,
            269–270
        diffuse idiopathic, 266
        generalized causes of, 265–267
        infections and, 270
        local causes of, 263–265
        localized idiopathic, 266–267
        locating sites of, 268–269
        stress in, 268
        symptoms and signs of, 270–271
        timing of symptoms in, 268
        trauma and, 270
    physical examination for, 271–285
        ankle and foot in, 284
        back in, 272–273, 273f
        cervical spine in, 274, 276f
        elbow in, 278
        forearm supination and pronation in, 278
        hand in, 275–276
        hip in, 280–281, 280f–283f
        knee in, 281–284, 283f
        peripheral joints in, 275
        shoulder in, 278–279, 279f
        temporomandibular joint in, 274–275
        wrist in, 276–278
    sex factors in, 269t
    single swollen joint in, 267, 267t
    skeletal deformities in, 268
    sports physical and, 311–316, 312f–315f,
        312t
    stress in, 268
Myasthenia gravis, 145, 233
Myelinated nerve fiber layer, 131, Plate 8–6
Myocardial infarction, 9
Myoclonus, 226, 246
Myotonia, 226
Myotonic dystrophy, 225–226

N
Nabothian cysts, 323, 324f
Nails
    examination of, 275, 277f, 338–339
    hypoplasia of, 88
Names, cultural differences in, 20
Nasal discharge, 123
Nasal flaring, 157
Nasal speculum, 123
Nasogastric intubation, 66–67
Nasolacrimal duct blockage, 127
Nebulizers, 154
Neck
    anomalies of, 87, 125–126
    examination of
        approach to, 124
        lymph nodes in, 125, 125f
        neonatal, 67–68
        observation in, 111
        trachea in, 125
    stiffness of, 124
    webbing of, 125
Necrobiosis lipoidica diabeticorum, 310f
Necrolysis, toxic epidermal, Plate 19–6
Neonates. See Newborn infant.

Neural tube defects, 72
Neuroblastoma, 265
Neurocutaneous syndromes, 239
Neurofibroma, plexiform, 132, 133f
Neurofibromatosis
   café au lait spots in, 73, 89, 239, 272
   congenital, 73
   diagnosis of, 239
   in precocious puberty, 305
   scoliosis and, 268
   skin anomalies in, 89
Neurological examination, 223–247
   abnormal movements in, 226
   approach to, 223
   case histories in, 241–246
   coordination in, 226, 226f, 236, 240–241
   differential diagnosis in, 241–246
   equipment for, 246f
   history-taking in, 223–225
   motor neuron lesion signs in, 223, 224f
   muscle strength in, 225, 239–240
   muscle tone in, 225–226, 240
   neonatal, 58
   observation in, 225–227, 227f
   physical examination in, 227–241
      of cortical function, 229–230
      of cranial nerves, 230–234
      of lower extremities, 235–239
      of preschool-aged child, 228–229
      of school-aged child, 227–228
      of upper extremities, 239–241
   reflexes in, 236–238, 241
   sensation in, 238–239, 241
Nevus
   compound, Plate 19–18
   congenital, Plate 19–17
   giant congenital, Plate 19–19
Newborn infant
   acrocyanosis in, 58
   anomalies of. See Congenital anomalies.
   antenatal history of, 55, 56t
   Apgar score of, 55–57, 56t
   assessment of, 55–74
      abdominal, 68–69, 213–214
      back, 71–72
      chest, 68
      clinical observations in, 57–58
      extremities, 70–71, 71f
      first examination in, 55–57
      genitalia, 69–70
      gestational age, 61–63
      head, 63–67
      hips, 70
      neck, 67–68
      neurological, 58
      parent participation in, 57, 57f
      second examination in, 57
      skin, 72–74
      third examination in, 57
   crying in, 58
   cutis marmorata in, 58, 58f
   hernia in, 70, 87, 215–216, 215f
   history-taking for, 7, 55–57
   hydroceles in, 70
   muscle tone in, 58–59
   rash in, 73
   reflexes in, 57, 59–60, 59f, 60f
   sex determination of. See Sex assignment.
   skin changes in, 72
   umbilical discharge in, 215
   weighing and measuring of, 60–61
Night blindness, 144
Nikolsky sign, 335, Plate 19–6
Nodules
   definition of, 335
   vascular, Plate 19–4

Noisy breathing, 153, 160, 161t
Nonverbal cues, 13–14
Noonan syndrome, 85, 125
Normal variation, 82
Norplant (levonorgestrel), 329
Nose
   congenital anomalies of, 86
   discharge from, 123
   examination of, 65–66, 123–124, 157
   inferior turbinate vs. polyp in, 123–124
Note-taking, 2
Nuchal rigidity, 124
Nummular lesions, of skin, 337
Nursing bottle caries, 121
Nutrition disorders, 43t
Nutritional assessment
   energy intake and requirements in, 52–53, 53t
   failure to thrive and, 52–53
   iron deficiency in, 49
   obesity in, 49–52
   solid food intake in, 49
Nyctalopia, 144
Nystagmus
   causes of, 135
   definition of, 131
   diagnosis of, 143–144, 144t
   optokinetic (opticokinetic), 137, 137f, 231
   with night blindness, 144

O

Obesity
   Cushing syndrome and, 298
   evaluation of, 49–52
   genetic factors in, 50
   history-taking in, 50–51
   in diabetes, 307–308
   physical examination in, 51
   physician attitude toward, 50
   self-esteem in, 50–51
   syndromes related to, 51
Obsessive-compulsive disorder, 256
Obstructive apnea, 160
Obstructive murmurs, 180, 181
Occipital lobe lesions, 230
Occult blood, gastrointestinal, 197, 199
Occupational history, 10
Oculomotor nerve (cranial nerve III), 232–233
Oculotrigeminal dyskinesia, 145, 146f
Odynophagia, 192
Olfactory nerve (cranial nerve I), 230
Omphalocele, 87, 214, 215f
Onycholysis, 338
Onychomycosis, 338
Opening snap (heart), 177–178
Ophthalmia neonatorum, 131
Ophthalmology. See Visual system.
Ophthalmoscopy, 65
Oppenheim reflex, 236
Oppositional-defiant disorder, 100
Optic nerve (cranial nerve II)
   hypoplasia of, 130, 131, Plate 8–7
   testing of, 230–232
Optokinetic (opticokinetic) nystagmus (OKN), 137, 137f, 231
Oral candidiasis, 121
Oral contraceptives, 328–329
Orbital hemangioma, 131
Orchidometer, 306f
Orchidopexy, 220
Organ transplantation, cultural factors in, 21
Orthopnea, 159, 170–171
Ortolani test, 281
Osgood-Schlatter disease, 264, 281, 283
Osler-Weber-Rendu disease, 199
Osteochondritis dissecans, 264, 271, 283

Osteoid osteoma, 265
Osteomyelitis, 265
Osteoporosis, 298, 299f
Osteosarcoma, 265
Otitis media, 156
Otoscopy
   handling of otoscope in, 116–118, 117f
   landmarks in, 118
   pneumatic, 118–119, 119f
   positioning child for, 116, 117f
Ottawa Ankle Rules, 284
Overanxious parents, 7

P

Pain
   abdominal. See Abdominal pain.
   musculoskeletal. See Musculoskeletal disorders, pain in.
   referred, 194, 207, 208
   somatic, 207
   visceral, 194, 195t, 207, 207f
   vomiting and, 193–194
Palate, 122
Pale child, 49
Palmar flexion creases, 88f, 89
Palmar grasp, 59, 60f, 238
Palpation
   abdominal, 68–69, 187, 197, 209
   for cardiovascular disorders, 173, 173f
   in pelvic examination, 325
   in respiratory diagnosis, 160, 162, 162f
   of chest, 187
   of finger joints, 276
   of inguinal hernia, 218
   of knee, 282–283
   of liver, 173–174, 174f, 205
   of pulses, 175, 184–187, 185f
   of spine, 273
   of spleen, 205
   of suprasternal notch, 173, 173f
   of thyroid gland, 292, 293f–294f
Pancreatitis, 211
Papanicolaou (Pap) smear, 324–325, 324f
Papule, 334
Papulosquamous eruptions, 335, Plate 19–2, Plate 19–3
Paranasal sinuses, 124
Parents
   as surrogate decision-makers, 350–351
   disclosure of diagnosis to, 343–345
   face following and bonding with, 127–128, 128f
   hostility in, 16
   intrusive, 103
   knowledge and experience of, 346
   psychiatric interview with, 252
   screening questions for, 3
Parents' Evaluation of Developmental Status (PEDS), 91
Paresthesia, 296–297
Parietal lobe lesions, 230
Parietal pain, 194–196
Parotid gland, 124
Patches (skin), 334
Patella
   dislocation of, 264
   internal strabismus of, 261–262, 261f
Patellar tab, 282
Patellofemoral malalignment, 264
Patent ductus arteriosus, 171, 182–183
Patient compliance, medications and, 154
PCOS (polycystic ovary syndrome), 302
Pectus carinatum, 158, 159f
Pectus excavatum, 158, 158f
Pediatric Oncology Quality of Life Scales (POQOLS), 347

Pedigree, 80–81, 81f
Pelvic examination, 323–325
 cervical examination in, 323–324, 324f
 culture samples in, 324–325, 324f
 palpation in, 325
 Pap smear in, 324–325, 324f
 patient preparation for, 322
 rectoabdominal, 323
 rectovaginal, 325
 tailoring of, 323
 vaginal instrumentation in, 323–324
 vaginal specula for, 323, 323f
Pelvic inflammatory disease, 328
Pemphigoid, bullous, 335
Pemphigus, 335
Pena-Shokeir syndrome, 89
Penis, 69, 88
Peptic ulcer, 199
Percussion, 162, 209
Pericardial friction, 183
Perineal hypospadias, 301
Periodontal disease, 121
Periorbital cellulitis, 132, Plate 8–8
Peripheral neuropathies, 227
Peritoneal fluid, 217
Peritonsillar abscess, 123
Periungual fibroma, Plate 19–16
Persistent hyperplastic primary vitreous
  (PHPV), 132, 132f
Persistent parietal foramina, 113
Perspiration, 170
Pes cavus, 235, 235f
Petechiae
 cultural factors in, 24
 neonatal, 73
 on palate, 122
Pets, 155
Peutz-Jeghers syndrome, 199
Phakomatosis, 89
Pharynx, 123
Pheochromocytoma, 297, 298
Phoria, 130
Photophobia, 134, 145–146
Physical examination. *See also specific*
  systems and conditions.
 cross-cultural skills in, 24–25
 for sports participation, 311–316
 gynecologic, 317–321
 in chronic conditions, 347
 in psychiatric disorders, 258
 neurological, 227–241
 of adolescents, 14
 of congenital anomalies, 82–84
 of development, 103–105, 104f
 seating during, 103–104, 104f
Physical growth. *See* Growth.
Physician-patient relations
 antenatal, 55
 chronic illness and, 16, 343–345
 communication and, 1, 343–345
 consultants and, 15–16
 death of child and, 16–17
 difficult news and, 17, 24, 344
 empathy in, 1–2
 in neurological assessment, 223–224
 in pediatric care, 349–350
 irate parents and, 16
 time and, 1
Pica, 49
Pierre Robin syndrome, 86–87
Pigeon breast, 158, 159f
Pigmentation abnormalities, 338
Pilonidal dimple, 72, 72f
Pink eye, 134, 135f
Pirouette test, 228
Pityriasis rosea, 339–340, Plate 19–3

Placing reflex, 60
Plaque, 334–335
Plexiform neurofibroma, 132, 133f
Pneumomediastinum, 162
Pneumonia, 208
Pneumothorax, 162
Poison ivy dermatitis, 332, 335, Plate 19–5
Poland syndrome, 87
Polyarthritis, 267–268
Polycyclic lesions, of skin, 337
Polycystic ovary syndrome (PCOS), 302
Polycythemia, 203
Polydactyly, 71, 88
Polyp, nasal, 123–124
Popliteal cyst, 282
POQOLS (Pediatric Oncology Quality of Life
  Scales), 347
Port-wine stains, 72, 334
Portal hypertension, 198, 205
POSSUM, 82
Prader-Willi syndrome, 51, 88
Precocious puberty. *See* Puberty,
  precocious.
Precocious thelarche, 305–306, 306f
Pregnancy
 history of, 7, 24, 79–80
 in adolescents, 325
Premature infant
 gestational age assessment in, 61–63
 head shape in, 112
Premature synostosis, 28–29, 29f
Preparticipation physical, for sports. *See*
  Sports physical examination.
Preschool children
 cardiovascular assessment of, 177–187
 developmental screening of, 92, 93t–96t
 neurological examination of, 224–225,
  228–229
 pulse-taking in, 184–187
Privacy, in psychiatric interview, 250
Problem list, 11–12, 12t
Processus vaginalis
 obliteration of, 216, 216f
 persistent patency of, 217–219, 217f–219f,
  220
Projectile vomiting, 221
Prolactinoma, 307
Promptness, in disclosure of diagnosis, 344
Pronator sign, 228, 228f
Proprioception, 228, 238, 238f
Proptosis, 135, 295
Propulsive reflex, 60
Protruding eyes, 135, 295
Proximal strength, 227–228
Prune belly, 215
Pruritus, 332
Pseudoanemia, 49
Pseudohypertrophy, 235
Pseudohypoparathyroidism, 51, 52f, 297,
  307f
Pseudomonas infections, 156
Pseudostrabismus
 corneal light reflexes in, 135–136, Plate
  8–11
 definition of, 130
Psoriasis, Plate 19–2
 nail pitting in, 275, 277f, 338
Psoriatic arthritis, 285
Psychiatric disorders
 assessment of, 249–259
 behavioral, 254–255
 classification of, 253
 clinical interview for, 249–250
  child interview in, 252–253
  confidentiality in, 250–252
  cultural considerations in, 258

Psychiatric disorders (*Continued*)
 clinical interview for
  family interview in, 253
  format for, 249–251
  history-taking in, 251–252
  in mentally retarded patients, 258
  length of, 250
  multiple informants in, 251, 253
  parent interview in, 252
  setting for, 250
 eliciting information about, 253
 emotional, 255–257
 physical examination in, 258
 prevalence of, 249
 psychosocial history and, 11
 standardized interviews and
   questionnaires for, 258–259
Psychogenic pain, abdominal, 196
Psychosis, 257
Psychosocial history
 cross-cultural factors in, 22
 household description in, 10–11
 in developmental assessment, 99
 omission of, 8
 parent occupations in, 10
 screening issues in, 10
Psychosomatic disorders, 154, 196
Ptosis
 cranial nerve lesions in, 233
 diagnostic algorithm for, 145f
 in differential diagnosis, 144–145, 146t
 in mitochondrial diseases, 145
 in myasthenia gravis, 145, 233
Puberty
 definitions in, 304
 delayed, 306–307, 307t
 genitalia development in, 46f
 hirsutism and, 302
 history-taking for, 304–305
 onset of, 47
 precocious, 304–306
  breast development in, 305–306, 306f
  café au lait spots in, 305, 305f
  causes of, 304t
  genitalia in, 306, 306f
  Leydig cell hyperplasia in, 305f
  physical examination in, 305–306,
   305f–306f
  testicular examination in, 306, 306f
 pubic hair development in, 46f, 47f
 staging of, 45–48
Pubic hair, 46f, 47f
Pulmonary hypertension, persistent, 171–172
Pulses
 brachial, 68, 184–185, 185f
 collapsing, 185, 185f
 femoral, 68, 68f
 in cardiovascular disorders, 173, 175
 normal rate for, 186, 186t
 radiofemoral delay in, 186f
 taking of, 184–187
 variations in, 184–187
Pulsus alternans, 186
Pulsus bisferiens, 186
Pulsus paradoxus, 160, 162, 185–186
Pupil(s)
 dilation of, 142
 movements of, 128
 red reflex in, 136–137, 136f, 297, Plate
  8–11, Plate 8–12
 response of, 232
Purpura, 338
Pustules, 335
Pyloric stenosis, 221–222, 221f
Pyloromyotomy, 222
Pyrosis, 192

Q

Quality of life, 346–347
Questions, 2–3

R

Rachitic rosary, 297
Radiation, thyroid tumors and, 295
Radiofemoral pulse delay, 177
Range of motion
    in cervical spine, 274
    in shoulder, 279, 279f
Ranula, 122
RAP (recurrent abdominal pain), 196
Rash
    disease processes in, 331
    itching and, 332
    neonatal, 73
    questions regarding, 332
Reading, 99
Reasoning, 353–354
Recall, tests for, 229–230, 229f
Recreational activities, 11
Rectal examination
    for constipation, 201
    in abdominal pain, 210
    neonatal, 214
Rectovaginal examination, 325
Recurrent abdominal pain (RAP), 196
Red eye, 134, 135f
Red reflex, 136–137, 136f, 297, Plate 8–12
Referred pain
    abdominal, 207
    evaluation of, 194
    mechanisms for, 208
Reflex(es)
    ankle, 236, 237f
    assessment of, 236–238, 241
    asymmetric tonic neck, 237, 238, 238f
    biceps, 241
    corneal, 233, 233f
    doll's eye, 232
    gag, 121–122
    Hoffman, 241
    in infants, 237–238
    knee, 236, 237f
    Moro, 59, 59f, 237–238
    Oppenheim, 236
    palmar grasp, 59, 60f
    placing and propulsive, 60
    plantar grasp, 60, 60f
    primitive, 59–60, 103, 104f
    red, 136–137, 136f, 297, Plate 8–12
    rooting, 66, 66f
    sucking, 66
    testing of, 236–238
    tonic neck response, asymmetric, 59
    triceps, 241
    vestibular, 65, 65f
Regurgitant murmurs
    diastolic, 181
    in mitral valve prolapse, 183
    systolic, 179–180
Regurgitation, 193, 194
Reiter syndrome, 285
Repetitive stress injuries, 270
Respiration
    accessory muscles in, 157
    evaluation of, 159–160
    neonatal, 68
    normal values for, 157t
    retractions in, 157–158
    rhythm of, 159–160
Respiratory disorders, 151–168
    abdominal pain in, 208
    airway obstruction and, 164–165, 165f
    allergies and, 155–156

Respiratory disorders (*Continued*)
    cardiovascular implications of, 169–177
    case histories of, 166–167
    cough in, 160
    exercise-related, 155
    finger clubbing in, 160, 160f
    history-taking for, 151–157
        associated conditions in, 155–157
        chief complaints in, 152–154
        family history and, 155, 157
        medications and, 154
        previous hospitalization in, 154
        unusual infections in, 156
    in infants, 169–170
    parental tolerance of, 153
    physical examination for
        approach to, 157
        auscultation in, 162–164, 163f, 164f
        chest-abdominal movement in, 158–159
        chest wall in, 158, 158f, 159f
        general signs in, 157–158
        palpation in, 160, 162, 162f
        percussion in, 162
        positioning for, 157f
        respiration and, 159–160
        respiratory noises in, 160, 161t
    recurring, 153
    school absenteeism and, 155
Retention cyst, 122
Retina, myelinated nerve fibers in, 131,
        Plate 8–6
Retinal hemorrhage, congenital, 127
Retinitis pigmentosa, 132, 144, Plate 8–9
Retinoblastoma, 131, 132, Plate 8–10
Retinopathy of prematurity (ROP), 133
Rhabdomyosarcoma, 133
Rheumatic diseases, 266
Rheumatic fever, 265
Rheumatoid arthritis, juvenile
    cervical spine extension in, 274, 276f
    definitions of, 265
    hand in, 276–278, 278f
    knee deformities in, 281, 283f
    medical examination for, 285
    rheumatoid nodules in, 285
    temporomandibular joint in, 274–275, 277f
    uveitis in, 133
    wrist swelling in, 276–278, 278f
Rhinitis, allergic, 156
Rickets, 282, 297
Rieger syndrome, 87
Rinne test, 234
Risk perception, 357
Robinow syndrome, 87
Romberg test, 228, 238, 239
Rooting reflex, 66, 66f
ROP (retinopathy of prematurity), 133
Rotation, of hip, 280, 281f
Rourke Baby Record, 91
RWT height prediction method, 43

S

Saccades, 137
Salivary glands, 124
Sandifer syndrome, 268
Scabies
    burrows in, 336, 336f
    chronic, 336, Plate 19–9
    differential diagnosis of, 340–341
    nodular, Plate 19–9
Scalded skin syndrome, staphylococcal, 341
Scaling (skin), 336
Scalp, 84–85, 339
Scaphocephalic head, 112
Scar, 337
Scarf test, 240

Scheuermann disease, 264, 272–273
Schmorl nodes, 265
School absenteeism, 155
School performance, 224
Scissoring of legs, 236, 236f
Scleral hemorrhage, 64, 64f
Sclerodactyly, 275, 277f
Scleroderma, 266
Scoliosis
    back examination for, 272, 274f
    café au lait spots in, 272
    definition of, 268
Scratching, 332
Scrotum
    acute, 220–221
    gestational age and, 62, 63f
    idiopathic edema of, 220–221
    neonatal, 69
Second opinion, 18
Self-esteem, 100
Sensory perception, 230, 241
Septic arthritis, 263, 265
Sex assignment
    delay in, 299
    explaining problems to parents in, 87–88
    factors in, 70
    physical examination and, 301–302
    testicular feminization in, 219
Sexual abuse
    assessment of, 257, 325–327
        equipment for, 326, 326f
        history-taking in, 325–326
        physical examination in, 326–327
        sexually transmitted disease in, 326, 327
    musculoskeletal pain and, 268
Sexual activity, 322
Sexually transmitted diseases, 325, 326, 327
Shagreen plaque, 340
Shaking hands, 20–21
Shoes, 225–226, 262–263
Short child, 43, 287
Shortness of breath, 154
Shoulder, 278–279, 279f
SIDS (sudden infant death syndrome), 21
Sinus arrhythmia, 186
Sinus disorders, 156
Skin
    clinical assessment of, 331–342
        buccal mucosa in, 338
        case histories in, 339–341
        color changes in, 338
        eczema and dermatitis in, 337
        history-taking in, 332–333
        nails in, 338–339
        physical examination in, 333–338
        scalp and hair in, 339
        special patterns in, 337
        surface examination in, 334
    congenital anomalies of, 89
    disorders of
        drug reactions in, 333
        familial factors in, 333
        infectious diseases and, 331
        morphologic classification of, 331t
        prevalence of, 331
        primary lesions in, 334–336
        secondary lesions in, 336–337
        terminology for, 332t
    neonatal, examination of, 72–74
        angiomatous lesions of, 72
        erythema toxicum in, 73
        milia in, 72
        petechiae in, 73
        pigmented and depigmented lesions in,
            73–74, 74f
        postmaturity changes in, 72

Skin tag, 51, 51f, 71, 88
Skull, 112
Sleep, REM, 158–159
Sleep apnea, 159–160, 167
Slipped capital femoral epiphysis, 264
Smell, disorders of, 307
Smith-Lemli-Opitz syndrome, 70, 89
Smoking, 155
Snoring, 156
Somatic pain, 207
Somatoform disorders, 257
Spasticity
    assessment of, 227–228, 235
    in neurological diagnosis, 225–226
Spatial perception, 229, 229f
Spermicides, 327–328
Sphygmomanometry, 14
Spina bifida occulta, 72
Spinal accessory nerve (cranial nerve XI), 234
Spinal dimples, 272, 273f
Spine
    disorders of, 208
    flexation tests for, 273, 275f
    palpation of, 273
    rotation tests for, 273, 275f
Spinning, 138–139, 139f
Spleen, 205
Spondylitis, ankylosing, 266
Spondyloarthropathies, 266
Spondylolisthesis, 273
Spondylolysis, 264
Sports physical examination, 311–316
    orthopedic, 311–312, 312f–315f, 312t
    re-injury prevention and, 311
    timing of, 311
    value of, 311
Squatting, 170
Staphylococcal scalded skin syndrome, 341
Stein-Leventhal syndrome, 302
Stereotyping, 19
Sternocleidomastoid fibroma, 125–126
Sternocleidomastoid muscle, 274
Sternomastoid tumor, fibrous, 67
Stork bite, 72
Strabismus
    assessment of, 136
    comitant, 133, 139f
    cover test for, 141–142, 141f
    definition of, 133
    diagnostic algorithm for, 148f
    evaluation of, 147–148, 148t
    incomitant, 136, 139
    internal femoral, 261–262, 261f
Strawberry hemangioma, 73
Strawberry tongue, 122
Strength, proximal, 227–228, 235
Streptococcal infections, 122
Stress, psychological, 268
Stretch marks, 51, 298
Striae, 51, 298
Stridor
    in airway obstruction, 164–165, 165f
    in diagnosis, 151
    in laryngomalacia, 166
    in tracheomalacia, 165
Sturge-Weber syndrome, 225, 239
Subcostal indrawing, 170, 173
Submandibular gland, 124
Substance abuse
    ADHD and, 100
    assessment of, 254
    in psychosocial history, 11
Sucking reflex, 66
Sudden infant death syndrome (SIDS), 21
Suicidal behavior, 256–257
Sun damage, 333

Support systems, 11
Suprasternal notch, 173, 173f
Surveillance, developmental, 91–92, 99–100
Swallowing difficulties. See Dysphagia.
Sweating, 170
Swinging flashlight test, 232
Symptoms, duration of, 152
Syncope, cardiac, 188
Syndactyly, 70, 71f, 77, 88
Synostosis, premature, 28–29, 29f
Synovial plicae, 264
Synovitis
    abdominal pain in, 208
    muscle wasting in, 284
    transient, 263
Systemic lupus erythematosus, 266, 333
Systolic murmurs, 179–181

T

Tachypnea, 170
Tandem gait, 228
Target lesions, 337, Plate 19–11
Tarsal coalition, 264
Tay-Sachs disease, 81
Tearing. See Epiphora.
Teenagers. See Adolescents.
Teeth, examination of, 121
Teething, 48, 48t, 121
Telangiectasia, hereditary hemorrhagic, 199
Telecanthus, 82, 83f, 85
Telogen effluvium, 339
Telogen hairs, 339
Temporal lobe lesions, 229
Temporomandibular joint, 274–275, 277f
Tendonitis, 284
Tenosynovitis, 276, 277
Terminal care, 349–350
Testicular feminization, 219, 301–302, 302f
Testis(es)
    abdominal pain and, 208
    acute scrotum and, 220–221
    appendix, 220
    cremasteric fibers in, 219
    descent of, 219–221
    ectopic, 220
    gestational age and, 62, 63f
    in precocious puberty, 306, 306f
    neonatal, 69
    puberty and, 47
    retractile, 220
    torsion of, 220
Tetralogy of Fallot, 170, 171
Thalassemia, 81
Thelarche, 47, 47f
    precocious, 305–306, 306f
Therapeutic contract, 12, 15
Thomas test, 281, 283f
Throat, 157
Thrush, 121
Thyroglossal duct cyst, 125, 294, 294f
Thyroid, lingual, 294, 294f
Thyroid bruits, 295
Thyroid disorder, 290–296
    characteristics of, 290–292
    euthyroid states in, 295
    eye examination in, 295
    hyperthyroidism as, 290
    hypothyroidism as. See Hypothyroidism.
    physical examination for, 292–296
        observation in, 292, 293f
        of children and adolescents, 292, 294–295
        of infants, 292, 294f
        palpation in, 292, 293f, 294f
    radiation exposure in, 296
    signs and symptoms of, 290
    tumors in, 295–296

Thyroid gland, 292, 293f, 294f
Thyroiditis
    autoimmune, 291, 292
    lymphocytic, 291
    silent, 295
    subacute, 294
L-Thyroxine, 294
Tibial torsion, internal, 262
Tic disorders, 100
Tics, definition of, 226
Tietze syndrome, 154
Time, respecting value of, 4
Tinea capitis, 339
Tinea versicolor, 334
Toe deformities, 284
Toeing-out, 262–263
Toe-walking, 263
Tongue, 121–122
Tongue depressor
    fear of, 111, 120
    use of, 120, 121–122
Tongue-tie, 66, 66f, 122, 192
Tonic neck response, asymmetric, 59
Tonsillitis, 123, 208
Tonsils, 122–123
TORCH lesions, ocular, 133
Torsion, testicular, 220
Torsional phenomenon(a), 261–263
    bowleg as, 262, 262f
    femoral, 261–262, 261f
    flat feet as, 263
    knock knees as, 262, 262f
    metatarsus varus as, 263, 263f
    tibial, 262
    toe-walking as, 263
    toeing-out as, 262–263
Torticollis
    characteristics of, 268
    congenital anomalies and, 87
    examination for, 274, 276f
Touch, cultural sensitivity in, 20–21
Tourette syndrome, 226
Toxic epidermal necrolysis, Plate 19–6
Toxic nodular goiter, 295
Toxocara canis, 133
Trachea, 160, 162f
Tracheoesophageal fistula, 67
Tracheomalacia, 165–166, 166f
Transient synovitis, 263
Transillumination
    of hydrocele, 217
    of neonatal head, 64
Transitional care, 347–348
Trauma. See Wounds and injuries.
Treatment plan, 11–12, 12t
Tremor, 226
Trendelenburg test, 225, 225f, 272, 281, 283f
Triceps reflex, 241
Trichotillomania, 115, 339
Tricuspid regurgitation, 179–180, 182
Tricuspid valve stenosis, 181
Trigeminal nerve (cranial nerve V), 233
Triggering, in tenosynovitis, 276
Triple rhythm (heart), 178–179
Trisomy 13, 74, 89
Trisomy 18, 84, 89
Trochlear nerve (cranial nerve IV), 232–233
Tropia, 130
Trousseau sign, 297
Tuberous sclerosis
    café au lait spots in, 89
    depigmentation in, 73, 73f, 239, 239f
    differential diagnosis of, 245–246
    skin anomalies in, 89, 239, 340, Plate 19–15, Plate 19–16
Tuck sign, 278, 278f

Tumor(s)
  of bone, 265
  of breast, 48
  sternomastoid, 67
  thyroid, 295–296
Tunica vaginalis, 216, 220
Tuning fork, 238, 239
Turner syndrome
  delayed puberty in, 307
  diagnosis of, 307, 307f
  fisting in, 297
  gastrointestinal bleeding in, 199
  hairline in, 85
  metacarpal sign in, 52f, 89
  neck webbing in, 125
Tympanic membrane, 118, 118f

U

Ulcer, 337
Umbilical cord
  discharge from, 215
  evaluation of, 69
  single artery in, 87
Umbilical hernia, 87, 215–216, 215f
Upper extremities, 239–241
  neonatal, examination of, 71
Ureteral colic, 212
Urinary calculi, 212
Urinary tract anomalies, 88
Urinary tract infection (UTI), 208, 211–212
Urticaria, 335–336
Uveitis, 133, 133f
Uvula, bifid, 87

V

Vaginal culture techniques, 320, 321f
Vaginoscopy, 319–320, 320f
Vagus nerve (cranial nerve X), 234
Van der Woude syndrome, 86–87
Varicella, 335, Plate 19–7
Vasculitis, systemic, 266
Venous hum, 182, 182f
Ventral suspension maneuver, 104f
Ventricular septal defect (VSD), 172f
  familial factors in, 171
  heart murmurs in, 179, 180, 180f, 182
Vernix caseosa, 72
Vesicle, 335
Vesiculobullous eruptions, 335, 336

Vestibular reflex, 65, 65f
Vestibulocochlear nerve (cranial nerve VIII), 234
Vibratory murmurs, 180
Virilization, antenatal, 299–301, 300f
Visceral pain, 194, 195t, 207, 207f
Visual-motor skills, 101f
Visual system
  binocular vision in, 128
  birth-related injuries to, 127
  case histories of, 143–148
  cover test for, 141–142, 141f
  examination of, 127–150, 230–232
    behavior in, 134
    corneal light reflexes in, 135–136, 135f–136f, Plate 8–11
    corneal staining in, 142–143, 143f
    equipment for, 129t, 130f
    extraocular movements in, 138–139, 139f, 140f
    eye appearance in, 134–135
    facial features in, 134
    fixation behavior in, 137–138, 138f
    funduscopy in, 142, 231–232, 232f
    general observation in, 134
    head position in, 134
    lacrimal sac in, 142, 143f
    ocular observations in, 134–137
    red reflexes in, 136–137, 136f, 297, Plate 8–11, Plate 8–12
    sequential logical assessment in, 143–148
    techniques for, 137–143, 144t
  face following and, 127–128, 128f, 137
  history-taking for, 133
  macular umbo in, 127, Plate 8–1
  normal development of, 127–128
  terminology of, 129–133, 129t
  visual acuity in
    single vs. dual eye testing for, 138
    tests for, 137–138, 231, 231f
  visual fields in, 139, 141, 141f, 230–231, 230f
  volumetric relationship in, 127
Vitamin A, 296
Vitamin D, 296
Vitamin D deficiency, 297
Vitamin K deficiency, 198
Vitiligo, 338

Vitreous, persistent hyperplastic primary (PHPV), 132, 132f
Vocabulary cards, 101f
Vocal fremitus, 160
Volvulus, midgut, 198, 214
Vomiting
  age factors in, 194
  assessment of, 193–194
  bilious, 194, 213, 214
  cyclic, 194
  gastrointestinal bleeding and, 198
  pain and, 193–194
  projectile, 221
  regurgitation vs., 193
VSD. *See* Ventricular septal defect (VSD).
Vulnerable child syndrome, 7

W

Waardenburg syndrome, 82, 85, 115
Weber's lateralizing test, 234
Weight
  as percentage of ideal, 42–43
  growth charts for, 30f–35f, 38f–39f
  measurement of, 28
  neonatal, 61
Werdnig-Hoffmann disease, 226
Wernicke aphasia, 229
Wharton jelly, 69
Wheal, 335
Wheelbarrow test, 239, 240f
Wheeze
  diagnostic use of, 151
  in airway obstruction, 164–165, 165f
  in tracheomalacia, 165
White coats, interview and, 3
Whiteheads, 336
Whoop, 183
Williams syndrome, 71, 296, 296f
Wilson disease, 204–205
Witches' milk, 68
Wood lamp, 338, 339
Wounds and injuries
  abdominal assessment in, 212–213
  gastric distention in, 213
  musculoskeletal pain in, 265
  rupture of hollow viscus in, 213
Wrist, 276–278
Wryneck, 125–126, 268